CURRENT CLINICAL UROLOGY

ERIC A. KLEIN, MD, SERIES EDITOR
PROFESSOR OF SURGERY
CLEVELAND CLINIC LERNER COLLEGE OF MEDICINE HEAD,
SECTION OF UROLOGIC ONCOLOGY
GLICKMAN UROLOGICAL AND KIDNEY INSTITUTE
CLEVELAND, OH

For further volumes:
http://www.springer.com/series/7635

Steven C. Campbell · Brian I. Rini
Editors

Renal Cell Carcinoma

Clinical Management

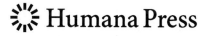 Humana Press

Editors

Steven C. Campbell, MD, PhD
Center for Urologic Oncology
Glickman Urological and Kidney Institute
Cleveland Clinic
Cleveland, OH, USA

Brian I. Rini, MD, FACP
Cleveland Clinic Lerner College
  of Medicine
Case Western Reserve University;
Cleveland Clinic Taussig Cancer Institute
Department of Solid Tumor Oncology
Cleveland, OH, USA

ISBN 978-1-62703-061-8   ISBN 978-1-62703-062-5 (eBook)
DOI 10.1007/978-1-62703-062-5
Springer New York Heidelberg Dordrecht London

Library of Congress Control Number: 2012945009

Printed on acid-free paper

Humana Press is a brand of Springer
Springer is part of Springer Science+Business Media (www.springer.com)

Preface

Kidney cancer, more than any other malignancy, has undergone a fundamental transformation over the past decade, with seminal discoveries related to tumor biology and prognostication, molecular genetics, and pathologic classification. The evaluation and management of this disease has likewise been revolutionized by the introduction of novel targeted agents and innovative surgical approaches. This textbook provides a timely update on these advances with a strong emphasis on clinical management.

A greater appreciation of the importance of renal function and competing risks have complicated management for patients with localized disease, and there are now a wide spectrum of options ranging from active surveillance to surgical excision, much of which can now be accomplished through minimally invasive techniques. Partial nephrectomy is now established as the reference standard, but overtreatment remains a major concern. The role of biopsy is still debated, and efforts to provide truly rational care for this sizeable group of patients remain a work in progress.

Locally advanced kidney cancer has always been primarily a surgical domain, yet increased response rates with targeted agents, particularly in the primary tumor, have stimulated efforts to reassess treatment paradigms, with neoadjuvant protocols followed by consolidative surgery being investigated more intensively. The optimal approaches to integrate surgery and targeted therapies remain controversial, although there is a strong consensus that there are great opportunities to improve management for this challenging patient population.

Advanced kidney cancer has seen perhaps the greatest transformation with extended survival and better quality of life now a reasonable expectation for many patients with metastatic disease. A fundamental comprehension of the VEGF, mTOR, and related pathways is a key to understanding where we are now and how we will move into the future. Again, integration of surgery has been revisited with new perspectives. While targeted molecular agents have moved to the forefront, immunotherapy, both conventional and investigational, still holds promise for many patients. All of these advances are reviewed with an emphasis on routine clinical management along with the many unique challenges that are often encountered in this field.

We are grateful to all of our authors for their outstanding contributions and trust that you will find this textbook up-to-date and informative. We have been fortunate to have international leaders in each branch of the field participate and provide their expertise for this textbook, which should serve as a resource for educating physicians about kidney cancer and ultimately should advance the care of patients with this malignancy.

Cleveland, OH, USA   Steven C. Campbell, MD, PhD
                                                              Brian I. Rini, MD, FACP

Contents

Contributors

Kamran Ahrar Department of Diagnostic Radiology and Section of Interventional Radiology, The University of Texas MD Anderson Cancer Center, Houston, TX, USA

Leonard J. Appleman Division of Hematology/Oncology, UPMC Cancer Pavilion, University of Pittsburgh Physicians, Pittsburgh, PA, USA

Alexandra Arreola Departments of Medicine and Genetics, Lineberger Comprehensive Cancer Center, University of North Carolina, Chapel Hill, NC, USA

Frédéric D. Birkhäuser Department of Urology, David Geffen School of Medicine, University of California, Los Angeles, Los Angeles, CA, USA

Steven C. Campbell Center for Urologic Oncology, Glickman Urological and Kidney Institute, Cleveland Clinic, Cleveland, OH, USA

Daniel Canter Division of Urologic Oncology, Department of Surgical Oncology, Fox Chase Cancer Center, Philadelphia, PA, USA

Michel Choueri Division of Genitourinary Medical Oncology, University of Texas MD Anderson Cancer Center, Houston, TX, USA

Stephen H. Culp Department of Urology, University of Virginia Health System, Charlottesville, VA, USA

Mellar Davis Taussig Cancer Institute, Cleveland Clinic, Cleveland Clinic Lerner School of Medicine, Case Western Reserve University, Cleveland, OH, USA

Ithaar H. Derweesh Division of Urology, Department of Surgery, Moores UCSD Cancer Center, University of California San Diego Medical Center, La Jolla, CA, USA

Khaled S. Hafez Division of Urologic Oncology, Department of Urology, University of Michigan, Ann Arbor, MI, USA

Huiying He Department of Pathology, Health Science Center, Peking University, Beijing, China

Daniel Y.C. Heng Department of Oncology, Tom Baker Cancer Centre, University of Calgary, Calgary, AB, Canada

Brian R. Herts Section of Abdominal Imaging, Imaging & Glickman Urological and Kidney Institute, Cleveland Clinic, Cleveland, OH, USA

Eric Jonasch Department of Genitourinary Medical Oncology, The University of Texas MD Anderson Cancer Center, Houston, TX, USA

Simon P. Kim Department of Urology, Mayo Clinic, Rochester, MN, USA

Nils Kroeger Department of Urology, David Geffen School of Medicine, University of California, Los Angeles, Los Angeles, CA, USA

Alexander Kutikov Division of Urologic Oncology, Department of Surgical Oncology, Fox Chase Cancer Center, Philadelphia, PA, USA

Brian R. Lane Michigan State University College of Human Medicine, Van Andel Research Institute, Minimally Invasive Surgery Program, Spectrum Health, Department of Urologic Oncology, Spectrum Health Cancer Program, Urology Division, Spectrum Health Medical Group, Grand Rapids, MI, USA

Bradley C. Leibovich Department of Urology, Mayo Clinic, Rochester, MN, USA

Surena F. Matin Departments of Urology and Minimally Invasive New Technology in Oncologic Surgery (MINTOS), The University of Texas MD Anderson Cancer Center, Houston, TX, USA

Jeffery S. Montgomery Division of Urologic Oncology, Department of Urology, University of Michigan, Ann Arbor, MI, USA

Allan J. Pantuck Department of Urology, Institute of Urology Oncology, David Geffen School of Medicine, University of California, Los Angeles, Los Angeles, CA, USA

Armida Parala-Metz The Harry R. Horvitz Center for Palliative Medicine and Supportive Oncology, Taussig Cancer Institute, Cleveland Clinic Health Systems, Cleveland, OH, USA

Thom Powles Department of Medical Oncology, Barts Cancer Institute, St Bartholomew's Hospital, Queen Mary University of London, London, UK

Andrei S. Purysko Section of Abdominal Imaging, Imaging Institute, Cleveland Clinic, Cleveland, OH, USA

W. Kimryn Rathmell Departments of Medicine and Genetics, Lineberger Comprehensive Cancer Center, University of North Carolina, Chapel Hill, NC, USA

Erick M. Remer Section of Abdominal Imaging, Imaging Institute, Cleveland Clinic, Cleveland, OH, USA

Brian I. Rini Department of Solid Tumor Oncology, Cleveland Clinic Taussig Cancer Institute, Case Western Reserve University, Cleveland Clinic Lerner College of Medicine, Cleveland, OH, USA

Paul Russo Department of Surgery, Urology Service, Memorial Sloan Kettering Cancer Center, Weill Medical College, Cornell University, New York, NY, USA

Matthew N. Simmons Center for Urologic Oncology, Glickman Urological and Kidney Institute, Cleveland Clinic, Cleveland, OH, USA

Marc C. Smaldone Division of Urologic Oncology, Department of Surgical Oncology, Fox Chase Cancer Center, Philadelphia, PA, USA

Cora N. Sternberg Department Medical Oncology, San Camillo-Forlanini Hospital, Rome, Italy

Sean P. Stroup Division of Urology, Department of Surgery, Moores UCSD Cancer Center, University of California San Diego Medical Center, La Jolla, CA, USA

Robert G. Uzzo Division of Urologic Oncology, Department of Surgery, Fox Chase Cancer Center, Philadelphia, PA, USA

Michael M. Vickers Department of Oncology, Tom Baker Cancer Center, University of Calgary, Calgary, AB, Canada

Alon Z. Weizer Division of Urologic Oncology, Department of Urology, University of Michigan, Ann Arbor, MI, USA

Christopher G. Wood Department of Urology, The University of Texas MD Anderson Cancer Center, Houston, TX, USA

Ming Zhou Department of Pathology, New York University Tisch Hospital, New York, NY, USA

Part I

Localized Disease

Etiology of Renal Cell Carcinoma: Incidence, Demographics, and Environmental Factors

Frédéric D. Birkhäuser, Nils Kroeger, and Allan J. Pantuck

Incidence

Kidney cancer was estimated to be the 14th most common malignancy worldwide in 2008 [1], although this cancer is much more common in certain countries or regions of the world. More than 85% of kidney cancers arise in the renal parenchyma, with the overwhelming majority representing renal cell carcinomas (RCCs), while the remainder arise in the renal pelvis, of which the vast majority are urothelial carcinomas [2, 3]. RCC is considered to be the most lethal of all the common urologic cancers. Worldwide incidence rates vary considerably by geographical region, age, and ethnicity. The highest incidences are observed in Northern America, Europe, and Australia/New Zealand, while substantially lower incidence rates are found in Africa, the Pacific and Asia (Figs. 1.1 and 1.2) [1]. The World Health Organization (WHO) has estimated the worldwide incidence of kidney cancers to be 273,500 cases (169,000 in men, 104,500 in women) for the year 2008, representing 2.2% of all adult cancer cases [1]. Worldwide, the incidence of kidney cancer rose 2.4% per year from 1975 to 1990 and 1.3% per year from 1990 to 2001 [3] and is still reported to be rising. Particularly in the Western world, kidney cancer has been among the tumors with the highest upward trend in incidence, both for men and for women (Fig. 1.3) [1, 4–6].

United States of America

In the United States of America (USA), the American Cancer Society estimated that 58,240 cases of kidney cancer (35,370 in men, 22,870 in women) were diagnosed in 2010 [7]. From 1988 to 2006, the overall age-standardized incidence rate for kidney cancer was 9.4 per 100,000 person-years. Temporal trends showed that incidence rates rose from 7.6 per 100,000 person-years in 1988 to 11.7 per 100,000 person-years in 2006 (Fig. 1.4) [8]. For localized stages, the rate was 5.7 per 100,000 person-years, while for regional and distant stages, the rates were 1.8 and 2.0 per 100,000 person-years, respectively. Also stage-specific incidence rates have revealed changes over time, with the greatest increase being noted for localized tumors. In localized stages, the incidence rate rose from 3.8 in 1988 to 8.2 per 100,000 person-years in 2006. Among distant stages, the rate slightly decreased from 2.1 in 1988 to 1.8 per 100,000 person-years in 2006. However, during the same time period, the incidence rate of regional stages remained stable with 1.6 per 100,000 person-years from 1988 to 2006 [8].

F.D. Birkhäuser, MD • N. Kroeger, MD
• A. J. Pantuck, MD, MS, FACS (✉)
Department of Urology, David Geffen School of Medicine, Institute of Urologic Oncology, University of California-Los Angeles, 924 Westwood Boulevard, Suite 1050, Los Angeles, CA 90095-7207, USA
e-mail: apantuck@mednet.ucla.edu

S.C. Campbell and B.I. Rini (eds.), *Renal Cell Carcinoma: Clinical Management*, Current Clinical Urology, 3
DOI 10.1007/978-1-62703-062-5_1, © Springer Science+Business Media New York 2013

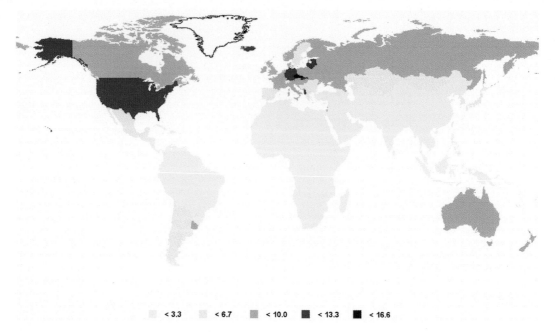

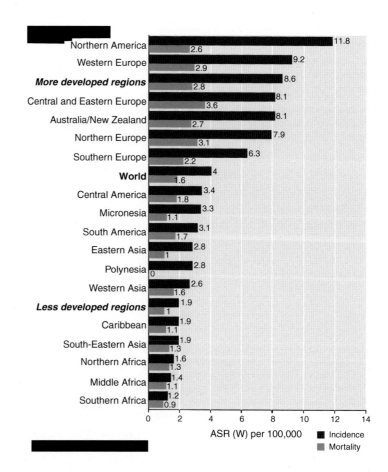

| < 3.3 | < 6.7 | < 10.0 | < 13.3 | < 16.6 |

Fig. 1.1 Map of estimated age-standardized incidence rates of kidney cancer per 100,000 person-years worldwide, by countries, including both sexes and all ages (from Ferlay J, Shin HR, Bray F, Forman D, Mathers C and Parkin DM. GLOBOCAN 2008, Cancer Incidence and Mortality Worldwide: IARC CancerBase No. 10 [Internet]. Lyon, France: International Agency for Research on Cancer; 2010)

Fig. 1.2 Estimated age-standardized incidence and mortality rates per 100,000 person-years of kidney cancer worldwide, by regions, including both sexes and all ages (from Ferlay J, Shin HR, Bray F, Forman D, Mathers C and Parkin DM. GLOBOCAN 2008, Cancer Incidence and Mortality Worldwide: IARC CancerBase No. 10 [Internet]. Lyon, France: International Agency for Research on Cancer; 2010)

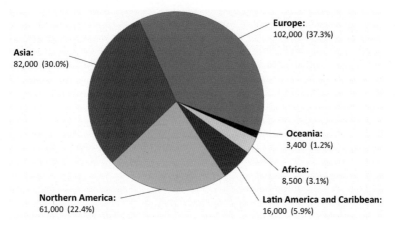

Fig. 1.3 Estimated worldwide incidence of kidney cancer, including both sexes and all ages (adapted with permission from Ferlay J, Shin HR, Bray F, Forman D, Mathers C and Parkin DM. GLOBOCAN 2008, Cancer Incidence and Mortality Worldwide: IARC CancerBase No. 10 [Internet]. Lyon, France: International Agency for Research on Cancer; 2010)

SEER Observed Incidence, SEER Delay Adjusted Incidence and US Death Rates[a]
Cancer of the Kidney and Renal Pelvis, by Race and Sex

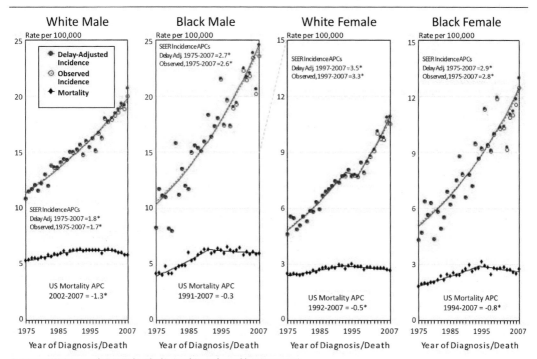

[a] Source: SEER 9 areas and US Mortality Files (National Center for Health Statistics, CDC).
Rates are age-adjusted to the 2000 US Std Population (19 age groups – Census P25-1103).
Regression lines and APCs are calculated using the Joinpoint Regression Program Version 3.4.3, April 2010, National Cancer Institute.
The APC is the Annual Percent Change for the regression line segments. The APC shown on the graph is for the most recent trend.
* The APC is significantly different from zero (p < 0.05).

Fig. 1.4 Age-standardized incidence and mortality rates per 100,000 person-years of kidney cancer in the United States, by race and sex (Altekruse SF, Kosary CL, Krapcho M, et al. SEER Cancer Statistics Review, 1975–2007, National Cancer Institute. Bethesda, MD, http://seer.cancer.gov/csr/1975_2007/, based on November 2009 SEER data submission, posted to the SEER web site, 2010)

Overall, the lifetime risk of developing cancer of the kidney for men and women born in the USA today, based on rates from 2005 to 2007, is 1 in 67, or 1.49% [9].

Europe

In Europe, the incidence of malignant tumors of the kidney was estimated to be 102,000 cases (62,800 in men, 39,200 in women) for the year 2008 [1]. This corresponds to an age-standardized incidence rate of 8.1 per 100,000 person-years for both sexes (11.3 in men, 5.5 in women). For the European Union (EU-27), 73,200 new diagnosed cases (46,200 men, 27,000 women) and an age-standardized rate of 8.0 per 100,000 person-years for both sexes (11.2 in men, 5.2 in women) has been estimated for the same year 2008 [1]. However, in Europe kidney cancer incidence and mortality rates show substantial

regional differences and trends between regions and countries over time. Countries of Central and Eastern Europe have the highest rates, with the Czech Republic having the highest incidence and mortality rates for many years. In contrast, countries from Western and Southern Europe report substantially lower rates (Fig. 1.5) [1]. Interestingly, if one considers only the last 10 years, a shift towards stabilization or even to a decrease in incidence could be observed in some countries in both sexes. Moreover, as an outlier to the general European trends, Sweden showed a decreasing incidence rate for both sexes for the last 30 years (Fig. 1.6) [1].

Future Worldwide RCC Incidence

The World Health Organization predicts a rising incidence of RCC for the entire world until at least 2030, with a faster rise in the incidence for

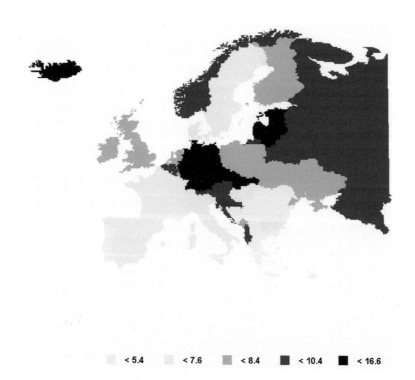

< 5.4   < 7.6   < 8.4   < 10.4   < 16.6

Fig. 1.5 Map of estimated age-standardized incidence rates per 100,000 person-years of kidney cancer in Europe, by countries, including both sexes and all ages (from Ferlay J, Shin HR, Bray F, Forman D, Mathers C and Parkin DM. GLOBOCAN 2008, Cancer Incidence and Mortality Worldwide: IARC CancerBase No. 10 [Internet]. Lyon, France: International Agency for Research on Cancer; 2010)

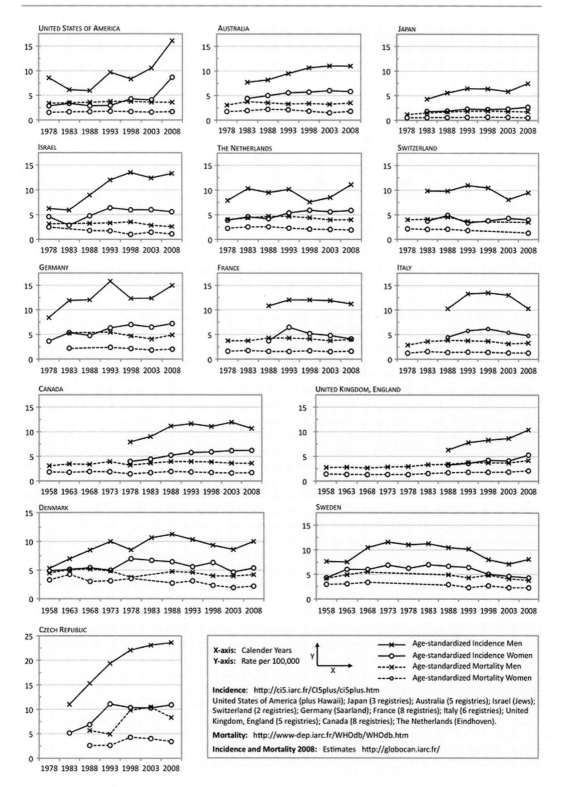

Fig. 1.6 Trends of age-standardized incidence and mortality rates per 100,000 person-years of kidney cancer in 14 different countries around the world

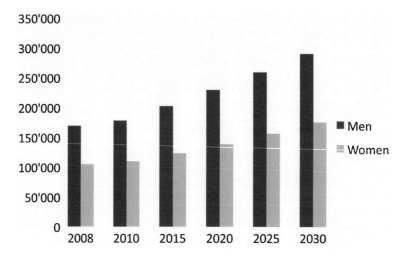

Fig. 1.7 Prediction of future worldwide incidence of kidney cancer until 2030

men compared to women. In 2030, a total incidence of 466,000 cases is expected to occur, representing 290,500 new cases for men and 175,500 new cases in women (Fig. 1.7). The steepest rise in incidence is predicted to occur in the Americas and the Western Pacific region, whereas in the European region the incidence will rise more slowly but will remain near the top regarding absolute incidence numbers [1].

Incidence Rate, Tumor Size, and Stage

As noted above, the most pronounced increase in the incidence of new RCC cases was for localized and small tumors <2.0 cm. According to recent data from the surveillance, epidemiology, and end results (SEER) program, the percentage of kidney cancer diagnosed in the localized stage ranges between 59% and 73%, depending on race and sex. This trend for small, low-stage tumors has been proposed to be a reflection of earlier diagnosis primarily as a result of the widespread and increasing use of noninvasive abdominal imaging modalities such as ultrasound (US), computerized tomography (CT), and magnetic resonance imaging (MRI) [10]. This trend becomes even more obvious when considering that, in just the USA alone, the total number of CT examinations performed annually has risen from approximately three million in 1980 to nearly 70 million in

2007 [11, 12], and that approximately 13–27% of abdominal imaging studies will incidentally identify some type of kidney lesion [13, 14], though the majority of these lesions will be small simple cysts that will not require treatment.

However, increased abdominal imaging and enhanced detection does not explain the continued increase of larger and more advanced tumors, or the increase in tumor size-specific mortality noted among kidney cancer patients [5, 6]. In the SEER data, nearly one-third of new cases will still present with advanced disease at the time of first diagnosis [15]. Thus, the increased incidence rate likely reflects both a real increase and increased detection, which, however, varies considerably among demographic groups. The failure to detect a true stage migration with both increased small tumors and with fewer advanced tumors may be due to other reasons, such as the concomitant rise in the presence of environmental or other RCC risk factors like obesity [16] and hypertension [17].

Prevalence

Included in disease prevalence calculations are the numbers of all patients alive who had previously been diagnosed with kidney cancer, including both patients with active disease and those who had already been cured of their disease. At the beginning of 2007, there were approximately

281,000 patients (165,000 men, 116,000 women) alive in the USA having a history of kidney cancer [9]. In the USA, paralleling the incidence of new cases, prevalence rates have increased over the last decades. However, the stage-specific prevalence has varied significantly. From 1988 to 2006, the prevalence for localized RCCs rose from 51.2% to 70.8%. Conversely, reflecting the enhanced detection of low-stage RCC with a greater propensity to be cured and for patients to live longer, the prevalence of regional stages declined from 20.9% to 13.6%, and for distant stages from 27.9% to 15.6%, for the same time points [8]. Looking to the next several years, at least in the more developed countries, RCC prevalence is likely to further increase, reflecting increased incidence, longer survival rates, as well as aging of the population, which will lead in the future to even more kidney cancer diagnoses.

Mortality

Worldwide, the number of deaths due to malignant tumors of the kidney was estimated to be 116,500 (72,000 in men, 44,500 in women) in 2008 [1]. Mortality rates show important variations when countries around the world are analyzed (Fig. 1.6).

United States of America

The American Cancer Society estimated that in 2010 there would be 13,040 deaths due to malignant tumors of the kidney (8,210 in men, 4,830 in women) [7], making RCC the tenth leading cause of cancer deaths in men. Over the past 30 years, the death rate for kidney cancer increased slightly from 3.6 per 100,000 person-years in 1975 to 4.3 per 100,000 person-years in 2001 [3]. Based on patients who died in 2003–2007 in the USA, the age-standardized death rate for cancer of the kidney and renal pelvis was 4.1 per 100,000 men and women per year [9]. However, in the last decade this trend seems to have stabilized or even to have slightly decreased [18]. Mortality rates vary considerably according to different geographic states, as shown in (Fig. 1.8). The 5-year overall survival of kidney cancer has nearly doubled from 34% in 1954 to 67% in 1996–2004 [18]. Current data from the USA indicate a median age at death for cancer of the kidney and renal pelvis of 71 years. Approximately 0.5% died under the age of 20; 0.5% between 20 and 34; 2.2% between 35 and 44; 10.0% between 45 and 54; 20.2% between 55 and 64; 25.0% between 65 and 74; 28.0% between 75 and 84; and 13.6% at 85 years of age or above [9].

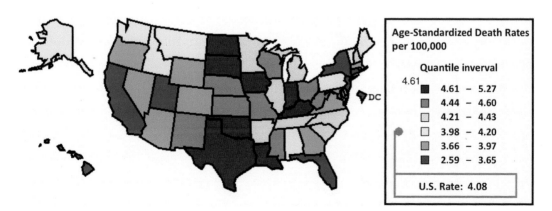

Fig. 1.8 Age-standardized death rates per 100,000 person-years of kidney cancer in the USA, by States, including both sexes (Altekruse SF, Kosary CL, Krapcho M, et al. SEER Cancer Statistics Review, 1975-2007, National Cancer Institute. Bethesda, MD, http://seer.cancer.gov/csr/1975_2007/, based on November 2009 SEER data submission, posted to the SEER web site, 2010)

Europe

In Europe, it was estimated that there were 45,100 deaths due to kidney cancer in 2008, including 28,300 deaths occurring in men and 16,800 in women [1]. For the European Union (EU-27), 31,300 deaths (19,600 in men, 11,700 in women) were estimated for the same time period. Mortality from kidney cancer increased throughout the European Union until the late 1980s or early 1990s. Thereafter, it tended to stabilize or even decline. In men, age-standardized mortality rates from kidney cancer peaked at 4.8 per 100,000 person-years in 1990–1994, and then declined to 4.1 (−13%) in 2000–2004. In women, the corresponding values were 2.1 in 1990–1994, and 1.8 (−17%) in 2000–2004 [19]. The greatest decreases took place in Scandinavian and other Western European countries. In most countries of Central and Eastern Europe, kidney cancer mortality rates tended to stabilize, even if values remained exceedingly high, e.g., in the Czech Republic, Hungary, Poland, and the Baltic countries (Fig. 1.6) [20].

Demographics

Age

Incidence rates worldwide, and especially in the USA and Europe, increase consistently with age [1]. The steepest increase has been noted in young men and women between 25 and 50 years of age. With age up to 70–75 years, the velocity of increase slows, which may be a result of less frequent and rigorous diagnostic testing in elderly people (Fig. 1.9). The vast majority of kidney cancers are diagnosed at age over 65 [3]. As the population ages in several regions worldwide, further increases of incidence are expected (Fig. 1.7). From 2003 to 2007 in the USA, the median age at diagnosis for cancer of the kidney and renal pelvis was 64 years of age. For men, the median age was 64 years, and for women it was 66 years [9]. Approximately 1.3% of kidney cancers were diagnosed under age 20; 1.6% between 20 and 34; 6.1% between 35 and 44; 16.4% between 45 and 54; 24.9% between

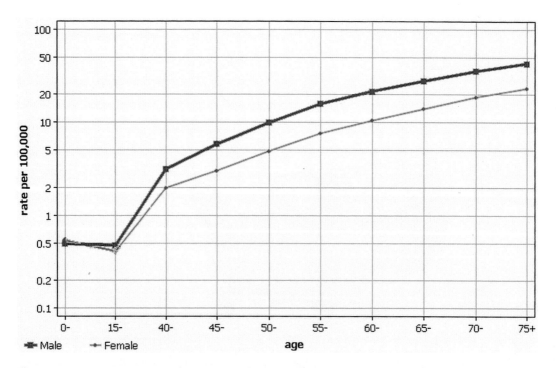

Fig. 1.9 Estimated world-incidence rates per 100,000 person-years of kidney cancer, by age (from Ferlay J, Shin HR, Bray F, Forman D, Mathers C and Parkin DM. GLOBOCAN 2008, Cancer Incidence and Mortality Worldwide: IARC CancerBase No. 10 [Internet]. Lyon, France: International Agency for Research on Cancer; 2010)

55 and 64; 24.2% between 65 and 74; 19.8% between 75 and 84; and 5.8% at years of age 85 and above [9].

Sex

Both age-standardized incidence and mortality rates of kidney cancer, in particular from the more developed regions of the world, have consistently been reported to be higher among men than women. This pattern is likewise observed throughout the rest of the world, with the exception of some Western and Central Africa countries, where reported incidence rates appear to be equal or even

higher among women (Figs. 1.6 and 1.10) [1]. In various regions worldwide, a trend to steeper rising incidence rates in women compared to men has been observed. In the USA between 1975 and 1995, the incidence rate of kidney cancer increased annually by 2.3% among white men, 3.1% among white women, 3.9% among black men, and 4.3% among black women (Fig. 1.4) [10]. In the USA in 2009, kidney cancer was expected to be the seventh leading cause of cancer in men and the eighth leading cause of cancer in women, corresponding to about 5% of all cancers in men and 3% of all cancers in women [18]. Over the last 20 years, 62% of all cases of kidney cancer were in men and 38% were in women [8].

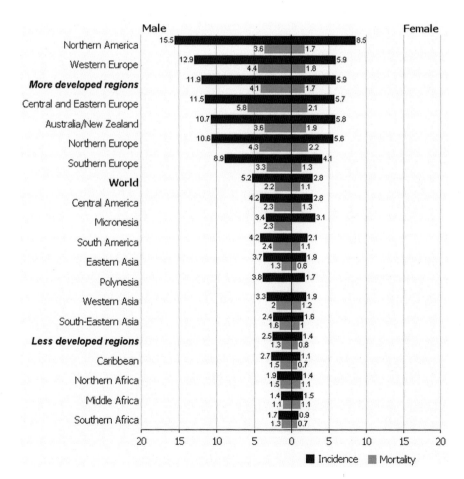

Fig. 1.10 Estimated age-standardized incidence rates per 100,000 person-years of kidney cancer by World regions, by men and women (from Ferlay J, Shin HR, Bray F, Forman D, Mathers C and Parkin DM. GLOBOCAN 2008, Cancer Incidence and Mortality Worldwide: IARC CancerBase No. 10 [Internet]. Lyon, France: International Agency for Research on Cancer; 2010)

Ethnicity

Wide differences in incidence and mortality rates in many countries and regions around the world have been well documented. However, these data, usually collected in national or regional cancer registries, may be difficult to compare strictly in regards to differences in ethnicity due to various concomitant biasing factors, including access to and quality of health care, lifestyle-associated or environmental risk factors, and to differences in socioeconomic status. Another general limitation to most large cancer data sets is that they often indicate overall but not disease specific survival. Thus, ethnical disparities in comorbidities may bias survival data. Fortunately, the SEER database in the USA compares different demographic groups in a single country, which potentially may reduce biasing factors. Considering the therein-recorded demographic groups, the incidence rates of kidney cancer have clearly been rising for all demographic groups during the last decades. However, both incidence rate and velocity of rise have differed significantly between different ethnic groups. American Indians and Alaska Natives had the highest incidence rate, but the slowest rise. On the other hand, Asian and Pacific Islanders had the lowest incidence rate. Between the extremes of those two ethnical groups, African Americans, Caucasians, and Hispanics showed similar incidence rates and trends. When age and race are considered together, African American men under 60 had the most rapid rise in incidence of kidney cancer (Fig. 1.4) [21].

When looking at the mortality rate, a significant increase in RCC-related deaths in both African Americans and Caucasians was observed until the 1990s, with African Americans having the steepest increase in mortality rate over the last years (Fig. 1.11) [3, 9]. Since that time, the trend appears to have stabilized for all ethnicities reflected in the SEER database [3]. Compared to Caucasians, however, African Americans have experienced worse survival; from 1975 to 1990, the survival for African Americans under 60 years of age presenting with localized tumors was 190 months, while for Caucasians having the same age and stage, it was 259 months. Also for age above 60 years, survival for African Americans was worse [3]. The reasons underlying this observation are not well understood, but may be due to either different biological behavior of the disease between ethnicities, to underlying somatic genetic differences in various ethnic populations, or to different comorbid conditions occurring in various ethnic groups [21].

When migrating to nonnative geographic regions, ethnic populations may eventually either change or preserve their native incidence rates. An unchanged and low incidence rate has been observed in Asians, both in the majority of Asian countries and in the USA [1, 4, 5]. In contrast, incidence rates are highest among African Americans in the USA [5, 9], whereas they have been reported to be much lower in the same groups living in many African countries [1, 4]. These observations provide indirect evidence that the risk of developing kidney cancer may not only vary between ethnicities, but may also involve gene–environment interactions, as well as differences in access to health care, frequency of diagnostic imaging, and to the prevalence of lifestyle-associated or environmental risk factors.

Environmental Risk Factors for RCC

Smoking

Smoking and RCC: Biological Background
Cigarette smoke contains more than 4,500 chemical compounds of which more than 60 are well-established carcinogens [22], including various chemical classes such as polycyclic aromatic hydrocarbons (PAHs), *N*-nitrosamines, aromatic amines, aldehydes, volatile organic hydrocarbons, and metals. Many other, less well investigated carcinogens are also components of cigarette smoke [23]. Chemical components of tobacco smoke are generally metabolized by phase I and phase II enzymes through the liver, and cleared through the urinary tract. Carcinogenic components are therefore concentrated in the kidneys. Because of this excretory pathway, the urinary tract is exposed to much higher concentrations of the carcinogenic substances present in

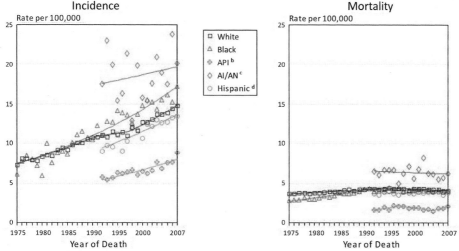

SEER Incidence and US Death Rates[a]
Cancer of the Kidney and Renal Pelvis, Both Sexes
Joinpoint Analyses for Whites and Blacks from 1975-2007
and for Asian/Pacific Islanders, American Indians/Alaska Natives and Hispanics from 1992-2007

Source: Incidence data for whites and blacks are from the SEER 9 areas (San Francisco, Connecticut, Detroit, Hawaii, Iowa, New Mexico, Seattle, Utah, Atlanta). Incidence data for Asian/Pacific Islanders, American Indians/Alaska Natives and Hispanics are from SEER 13 Areas (SEER 9 Areas, San Jose-Monterey, Los Angeles, Alaska Native Registry and Rural Georgia). Mortality data are from US Mortality Files, National Center for Health Statistics, CDC.

[a] Rates are age-adjusted to the 2000 US Std Population (19 age groups – Census P25-1103).
   Regression lines are calculated using the Joinpoint Regression Program Version 3.4.3, April 2010, National Cancer Institute. Joinpoint analyses for Whites and Blacks during the 1975-2007 period allow a maximum of 4 joinpoints. Analyses for other ethnic groups during the period 1992-2007 allow a maximum of 2 joinpoints.
[b] API = Asian/Pacific Islander.
[c] AI/AN = American Indian/Alaska Native. Rates for American Indian/Alaska Native are based on the CHSDA (Contract Health Service Delivery Area) counties.
[d] Hispanic is not mutually exclusive from whites, blacks, Asian/Pacific Islanders, and American Indians/Alaska Natives. Incidence data for Hispanics are based on NHIA and exclude cases from the Alaska Native Registry. Mortality data for Hispanics exclude cases from Connecticut, the District of Columbia, Maine, Maryland, Minnesota, New Hampshire, New York, North Dakota, Oklahoma, and Vermont.

Fig. 1.11 Age-standardized incidence and mortality rates of kidney cancer in the USA for various ethnic groups, including both sexes. Joint analyses for Whites and Blacks from 1975 to 2007 and for Asian/Pacific Islanders, American Indians/Alaska Natives and Hispanics from 1992 to 2007 (Altekruse SF, Kosary CL, Krapcho M, et al. SEER Cancer Statistics Review, 1975–2007, National Cancer Institute. Bethesda, MD, http://seer.cancer.gov/csr/1975_2007/, based on November 2009 SEER data submission, posted to the SEER web site, 2010)

tobacco smoke than many other organ systems in humans (even, surprisingly, the respiratory system). The major established pathway of cancer causation by smoking is described by a report of the US Surgeons General as follows [23]: (1) the exposure to carcinogens from tobacco smoke leads to (2) formation of covalent bonds between the carcinogens and DNA (DNA adduct formation), and (3) the resulting accumulation of permanent somatic mutations in critical genes leading to conversion of the affected cells to cancerous cells (Fig. 1.12). These pathological changes are followed by clonal outgrowth, additional mutations, and genetic instability that ultimately leads to the development of cancer [23].

One example of a carcinogenic component found in tobacco smoke is benzo[α]-pyrene diol epoxide (BPDE). From four known enantiomers, one (BPDE-N^2-deoxyguanosine) has been reported to be strongly carcinogenic [24]. Two critical targets of the BPDE adducts are known: mutational spots in the p53 tumor-suppressor gene and the KRAS oncogene [23]. Zhu et al. recently reported a higher frequency of BPDE-associated 3p deletions in the lymphocytes of RCC patients. 3p deletions are known as the most commonly chromosomal aberrations in RCC. The authors concluded that chromosome 3p may be a specific target of cigarette carcinogens like BPDE [25]. Other authors have shown an N-nitrosdimethylamine (NMDA) dosage-dependent induction of kidney tumors in rats [26, 27]. Furthermore, 4-(methylnitrosamino)-1-(3-pyridiyl)-1-butanone (NNK)-induced DNA damage is associated with a

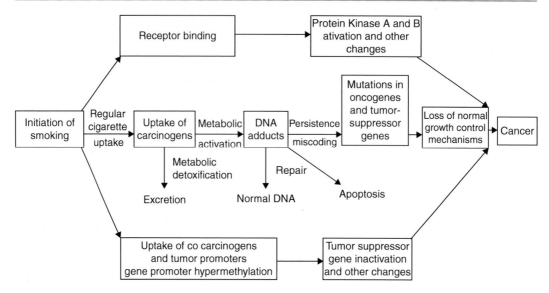

Fig. 1.12 Relationship between cancer and smoking (from How Tobacco Smoke Causes Disease: The Biology and Behaviroal Basis for Smoking Attributable Disease: A Report of the Surgeon General. Rockville, MD: Department of Health and Human Services; 2010: 221–350)

higher risk for kidney cancer [28]. In general, because tobacco smoke contains such a high number and variety of carcinogens, it is difficult to fully tease out the RCC-causative effect of any one single component of cigarette smoke. Together, however, epidemiological and biological data strongly support the conclusion that kidney cancer is a smoking-related disease.

Smoking and RCC: Cancer Development

Tobacco smoking has been declared a causal risk factor for the development of RCC by both the International Agency for Research on Cancer [29] and the US Surgeon General [30]. Numerous studies have investigated the relationship between smoking and the development of RCC. Despite having differing study designs (cohort studies, hospital- and population-based case–control studies, etc.), the majority of these studies have shown consistent results in both sexes: tobacco exposure is linked to a higher risk for developing RCC [29, 31].

In a meta-analysis of 24 studies, Hunt et al. found that the relative risk (RR) for smokers was 1.38 (95% CI: 1.27–1.50) that of lifetime non-smokers [31]. Their findings of gender-specific differences are notable: whereas women smokers had an RR of 1.22 (95% CI: 1.09–1.36), men who had smoked had a greater RR of 1.54 (95% CI: 1.42–1.68). Furthermore, the authors demonstrated a dose-dependent effect of smoking on the development of kidney cancer, showing a 1.60 (95% CI: 1.21–2.12), 1.83 (95% CI: 1.30–2.57), and 2.03 (95% CI: 1.51–2.74) higher risk in men who smoked, 1–9, 10–20, and 21 or more cigarettes/day, respectively. The impact of the same dosage exposure is different for women than for men; women who smoked the same dosage of 1–9, 10–20, and 21 or more cigarettes/day had no higher risk (RR 0.98, 95% CI: 0.71–1.35), 38% higher risk, (RR 1.38; 95% CI: 0.90–2.11), and 58% (RR 1.58%; 95% CI: 1.14–2.20) higher risk, respectively, than nonsmoking women for developing kidney cancer. Smoking cessation is reported to be associated with a reduction in the RR for developing kidney cancers, but the risk does not seem to diminish until a long latency period of over 10 years [31].

It has been estimated that 1.3 billion people in the world are currently smokers. If the trends of smoking and population growth continue, the number of smokers is expected to reach two billion worldwide in 2030. The prevalence of tobacco consumption, however, has shifted from developed countries to the developing world: the highest prevalence of smoking currently is found in Eastern Europe, the former Soviet Union, China, and Indonesia. About 50% of the men and 9% of women in developing countries, compared to 35% of the men and 22% of women in developed countries, are currently smokers. On average, the consumption of tobacco will continue to fall in developed countries, but rise in low- and medium-resource countries [32]. These developments raise concern that the number of RCC cases in developing countries will increase in the future.

Smoking and RCC: Cancer-Specific Survival Outcome

While most of the studies which have investigated the relationship between smoking and kidney cancer have focused on the development of kidney cancer, few studies have investigated the relationship between smoking and the outcome of kidney cancer patients. Sweeny et al. reported in a case–control study of 555 patients that current smokers experienced a worse overall and cancer-specific survival than nonsmokers (HR 1.7, 95% CI: 1.2–2.5). However, when smoking was considered in this study as part of a multivariate Cox hazard proportional model, it was not retained as an independent factor of survival outcome. The authors explained the survival differences with reference to the higher pT stages of the patients [33]. In another study, Parker et al. also reported a worse cancer-specific survival outcome of current smokers compared to nonsmokers (HR 1.31; 95% CI: 1.09–1.58). However, again, after adjustment for TNM stage group and tumor grade, this difference was no longer significant [34]. Many studies of smoking and RCC outcomes have been limited by small cohort size, limited follow-up, and inability to substratify patients according to RCC histological subtype and according to tobacco exposure dosage. Furthermore, since many studies have been epidemiologically based, they have generally been unable to further investigate the genetic and molecular mechanisms that might underlie the worse survival outcome seen in smokers.

Obesity

Obesity and RCC: Biological Background

The mechanisms that are associated with kidney cancer development potentially related to obesity are poorly understood. To date, however, both in vitro and in vivo studies have provided evidence that key pathways for cancer development and progression are altered through host factors associated with obesity and the "metabolic syndrome." These host factors include leptin, adiponectin, steroid hormones, reactive oxygen species (ROC), insulin, and insulin-like growth factor [35]. Furthermore, obesity is associated with a state of chronic, low-grade systemic inflammation, and inflammation is in turn associated with both cancer and cancer progression. The levels of several cytokines, such as tumor necrosis factor (TNF)-α, soluble TNF receptor, IL-1β, IL-6, IL-1 receptor antagonist, and C-reactive protein, have been found to be two- to threefold increase in obese people compared to nonobese people [36]. Metabolic stress and the special cytokine environment associated with inflammatory changes provoke oxidative stress, resulting in higher levels of ROS. ROS are highly reactive radicals, which lead to damage of lipids, proteins, and nucleic acids. Interestingly, the P13K/akt pathway, an important activator of the mTOR pathway whose function has implications for both the pathogenesis and the treatment of RCC [37–39], can be activated through ROS [35].

Insulin resistance and hyperinsulinemia are conditions typically found in obese patients. Both have been shown to increase the risk for tumor progression in different cancer types [40, 41]. The effects of insulin and IGF-1 occur through their binding to cell surface receptors on tumors or precancerous cells, and represent another mechanism for the subsequent activation of the P13/Akt pathway [40, 42]. Furthermore, IGF-1 has been shown to interact with the p53 tumor suppressor [43]. The (mal)-function of the p53 tumor suppressor has been implicated in the development of RCC, as it has been in many other cancers [44, 45].

The metabolic function of the liver is a crucial factor in the inactivation of environmental and dietary carcinogens. Epidemiologic studies have suggested that 1–3% of the western population has nonalcohol-related liver disease, and that a considerable percentage of these patients suffer eventual progression towards liver inflammation, fibrosis, and cirrhosis. These processes result in a restriction of the metabolic and detoxification functions of the liver [46]. Many toxic substances, whether in original form or as metabolic byproducts of phase I and phase II metabolism, are cleared through the urinary tract. Impaired liver function may in some situations result in higher concentrations of toxic substances that are in turn delivered to the kidney [27]. Many hormones, including steroid hormones (estrogens, progesterone, and adrenal steroids), leptin, and adiponectin have been shown to be associated with carcinogenesis and tumor progression [47]. Consistent with studies showing the association of estrogens and carcinogenesis with tumor progression, Nicodemus et al. found that women who reported estrogen use in the past had a 62 higher risk for the development of RCC. Elevated estrogen levels have also been reported to be associated with obesity [48].

Obesity and RCC: Cancer Development

Obesity is a complex disease, which is influenced by underlying genetic factors, as well as lifestyle factors such as high caloric intake and low physical activity. It is difficult to distinguish the impact and individual influence of each of these intertwined factors on the risk of kidney cancer development. The evaluation of obesity, therefore, necessarily includes consideration of all of its associated risk factors. Nevertheless, diet alone is considered an important risk factor for the development of cancer in general [47, 49]. The following paragraphs investigate the role of obesity, and the factors which are involved in the development of obesity and which therefore may indirectly affect the development of RCC.

Obesity has been rising in prevalence through the last few decades in the USA and many others countries [50]. Several studies worldwide have demonstrated the influence of body weight on the risk of kidney cancer development [51, 52]. Renehan et al. demonstrated in a meta-analysis of prospective observational studies that 40% of the RCC cases in the USA and 30% in Europe are associated with excessive bodyweight [53]. The risk for the development of kidney cancer has been reported to be directly correlated with increased weight. Comparisons between obese and nonobese patients have shown a 48% higher risk for RCC in obese patients, with each unit increase in body mass index (BMI) leading to a 4% increased risk of developing RCC (HR 1.04, 95% CI: 1.02–1.06, $p = 0.001$) [54]. Interestingly, clear cell RCC is the histological subtype that appears to be the most obesity associated [54]. The role of fat distribution in RCC development was investigated in one study. Among women, an increased risk of RCC was observed with respect to elevated body weight (highest vs. lowest quintile, RR 2.13, 95% CI: 1.16–3.90, $p = 0.003$), BMI, (2.25, 1.14–4.44, $p = 0.009$), wider waists (1.67, 0.94–2.98, $p = 0.003$), and wider hip circumference (2.30, 1.22–4.34, $p = 0.01$), but waist and hip circumference was not longer significant after controlling for body weight [52].

Individual macro and micronutrient variation in the diet may further modify the risk associated with excessive caloric intake alone. For example, a high fruit and vegetable intake has been reported to be associated with a decreased risk of RCC in a pooled analysis of 13 prospective studies [55]. The authors were able to show a reduction or RCC risk with the consumption of six or more servings of fruits and vegetables a day. Lindblad et al. observed a 50–60% reduction in risk of RCC (highest vs. lowest quartile of intake) with respect to consumption of total fruit, apple, and citrus fruits [56]. However, data from the European Prospective Investigation into cancer and nutrition, the largest prospective population-based study of diet and disease, has found no consistent correlation between fruit and vegetable intake and RCC risk [57].

Fat and protein intake of animal origin is a risk factor for a number of cancer types, especially colon cancer. However, in a pooled study as well as in a large prospective cohort study, neither fat nor protein was found to be associated with a higher risk of RCC [58, 59]. Allen et al. concluded that there is no association between these macronutrients and the risk of RCC. However, Mellemgaard et al. reported in a smaller study of 351 RCC cases and 340 controls, that both high caloric and fat intakes are associated with a higher risk of RCC in both men and women [60].

For a long time, it was hoped that a high intake of antioxidant vitamins such as vitamins A, C, and E could be associated with a reduction in cancer risk. However, data from studies focusing on the influence of antioxidant nutrients has delivered inconsistent results. Lee et al., for example, were able to demonstrate that vitamin A, C, and carotenoid intake correlated with a decreased risk of RCC, though vitamin E did not appear to influence the risk of RCC development [61]. On the other hand, other studies have demonstrated a positive relationship between vitamin C and E intake and RCC risk [48, 62, 63].

The consumption of fatty fish (such as salmon and tuna) has been considered to be an important protective factor in cardiovascular diseases. A study on 61,433 Swedish women reported a 44% decrease in the risk of RCC for a consumption of one or more servings of fatty fish per week. Moreover, women who reported consistent consumption of at least 1–3 servings of fatty fish per month, over at least 10 years, had a 74% lower risk of developing RCC [64]. However, another study did not find a protective effect of fatty fish consumption with respect to RCC development [60].

Another confounding lifestyle and dietary factor to consider is alcohol consumption. Moderate consumption of alcohol has been reported to decrease the risk of RCC. In a pooled analysis of 12 studies, Lee et al. reported a decreased risk of 28% (95% CI: 0.60–0.86) for moderate alcohol consumption of ≥15 g/day, equivalent to slightly more than one alcoholic drink per day [65]. The alpha-tocopherol, beta carotene (ATBC) cancer prevention study suggested that these findings were particularly true for the highest quartile of alcohol intake (RR 0.53, 95% CI: 0.34–0.83). Another study showed that these findings in men are in agreement with the data for women (RR 0.50, 95% CI: 0.2–0.9).

Lower physical activity has been reported to be associated with an increased risk of RCC for women [66]. In a prospective study of 482,386

participants and 1,238 cases, Moore et al. found a reduction of RCC incidence of 23% [95% CI: 0.64, 0.92; p(trend) = 0.10] for women currently exercising, 16% [95% CI: 0.57, 1.22; p(trend) = 0.03] for routine physical activity, and 18% [95% CI: 0.68, 1.00; p(trend) = 0.05] for activity during adolescence [67]. However, other studies did not find evidence of a protective effect for physical activity and the risk of RCC. A prospective cohort study of 17,241 Swedish twins having a follow-up of 30 years identified 102 cases of RCC. In that study, neither occupational nor leisure physical activity was associated with a decreased risk for RCC [68]. Data from the Netherlands Cohort Study on Diet and Cancer showed a slight risk reduction of RCC for occupational physical activity in men, for work comparable to 8–12 kJ/min (RR 0.98; 95% CI: 0.64–1.49) and >12 kJ/min (RR 0.86; 95% CI: 0.50–1.46). For nonoccupational physical activity, risk reduction was demonstrated for 30–60 min/day (RR 0.46; 95% CI: 0.28–0.77), 60–90 min/day (RR 0.67; 95% CI; 0.38–1.17) and >90 min/day (RR 0.66; 95% CI: 0.41–1.07), respectively. For women, a risk reduction at 30–60, 60–90 and >90 min/day of nonoccupational physical activity of RR 0.95 (95% CI: 0.54, 1.68), RR1.07 (95% CI: 0.59, 1.94) and RR 0.85 (95% CI; 0.44, 1.63) was found. For both men and women, these results were considered significant by p trend [68].

In conclusion, the influence of obesity, irrespective of the fat distribution, on the development of RCC has moderate support in the epidemiological literature. Dietary factors such as high energy intake, low physical activity, and low consumption of fatty fish, vegetables, and fruit that are more common in patients with obesity are associated with an increased risk for development of RCC. Moderate alcohol consumption may decrease the risk. The field of nutrition, diet and lifestyle modification warrants further prospective interventional study.

Obesity and RCC: Cancer-Specific Survival Outcome

The overweight, obesity, and mortality from cancer study, a prospective study of US adults, found higher mortality rates from all types of cancer (52% higher for men and 62% higher for women) for the heaviest members of the study cohort (BMI > 40) compared to men and women of normal weight. Compared to the group of normal weight women (BMI 18.5–24.9), the RRs of female patients with a BMI of 25.0–29.9, 30.0–34.9, 35.0–39.9, and ≥40 were, 1.33 (95% CI: 1.08–1.63), 1.66 (95% CI: 1.23–2.24), 1.70 (95% CI: 0.94–3.05), and 4.75 (95% CI: 2.50–9.04), respectively. For men in the same BMI groups, the RRs were 1.18 (95% CI: 1.02–1.37), 1.36 (95% CI: 1.06–1.74), and 1.70 (95% CI: 0.99–2.92).

Several studies, conversely, have demonstrated a favorable overall and cancer-specific survival outcome in patients who presented with obesity [69–71]. In contrast to the overweight, obesity, and mortality from cancer study, however, these studies were all case–control studies. The biggest of these studies, with 1,338 clear cell RCC patients, retained obesity as an independent predictor for cancer-specific survival in localized RCC; in metastatic patients, obesity was not retained as an independent factor predicting survival in multivariate analysis. This study, however, had several limitations. The authors did not control their study population for important confounders, such as smoking and ECOG performance status [69]. Parker et al. reported that obesity retained only borderline significance in their analysis (HR 0.77, 95% CI: 0.57–1.05, $p = 0.096$), after adjustment for TNM stage group, nuclear grade, and necrosis [71]. In particular, the results of Parker et al. suggest that the role of obesity is of at most minor importance for the survival outcome of RCC patients.

Hypertension

Hypertension and RCC: Biological Background

The biological mechanisms that mediate the epidemiological association between hypertension and RCC risk are poorly understood. Hypertension is associated with cell proliferation and lipid peroxidation in the renal tubule. These processes can lead to inflammation, angiogenesis, and oxidative damage which are risk factors for the development of kidney cancer [72]. One of the hallmarks of hypertension is rarefaction of microvessels and increased expression of angiogenic growth factors such as VEGF, and this may predispose to malignancy in the kidney [73]. In addition, rarefaction of microvessels induces tissue hypoxia, and in this setting, hypoxia inducible factor (HIF) is not degraded and is instead expressed constitutively [73]. Of interest, both angiogenic growth factors and HIF are key players in the development of RCC; however, further investigation into the potential biological effects of hypertension that may predispose to RCC is necessary.

Hypertension and RCC: Cancer Development, Use of Antihypertensive Medication and Cancer-Specific Outcome

Prospective cohort studies have shown an association between hypertension and risk for RCC [74–76]. One of the largest prospective cohort studies, involving 363,992 Swedish men, investigated RCC risk in relation to hypertension. Over a follow-up period of 25 years, workers underwent physical examination with blood pressure measurement every 2–5 years. Overall, 759 men developed RCC. The authors found that those with diastolic blood pressure of 90 mm Hg or more had twice the risk for RCC compared to patients with a diastolic blood pressure of 70 mm Hg or less. Further, compared to patients with a median systolic blood pressure of 120 mm Hg, patients with a median systolic blood pressure of 150 mm Hg or more were at 60–70% higher risk of RCC. Even after controlling for other risk factors, the authors were able to demonstrate a correlation between hypertension and the development of RCC. Furthermore, this investigation also showed a "dose–response" relationship between hypertension and the risk of RCC [74]. Vatten et al. showed similar results for women in a study of 36,688 women from Norway. Women with a systolic blood pressure of 130–149 mm Hg had an RR of 1.7 (95% CI: 0.9–3.5); with levels of 150–169 mm Hg, the RR was 2.0 (95% CI: 0.9–4.2), and with levels ≥170 mm Hg, it reached 2.0 (95% CI: 0.9–4.6). Interestingly, women who had never used antihypertensive medication and had a systolic blood pressure of ≥170 mm Hg had an RR of 3.4 (95% CI: 0.8–2.2) compared to those with a blood pressure of <130 mm Hg. This result raises the possibility for using effective blood pressure management as a strategy for the reduction of RCC risk [77].

The investigation of an independent influence of hypertension on RCC risk is complicated by the inevitable use of antihypertensive medication in patients with hypertension [78]. Moreover, the use of particular types of antihypertensive medication itself has also been implicated in increasing the risk of RCC. Numerous studies have investigated the relationship between diuretics and the risk of RCC. While Flaherty et al. did not find an increased RCC risk associated with the use of thiazide diuretics [75]; other studies have shown a positive association between diuretic use and RCC. A pooled meta-analysis of 18 studies has shown an increased risk of RCC for diuretic (RR 1.43; 95% CI: 1.12–1.83) and nondiuretic hypertensive medications (RR 1.51; 95% CI: 1.21–1.87). However, further analysis suggested that the effect of diuretics was significant only in women but not in men [79]. Other large studies have suggested, on the other hand, that hypertension alone rather than the use of antihypertensive medication, increases RCC risk [76, 80, 81]. For example, Shapiro et al. reported a higher risk of RCC for women on antihypertensive medications (OR = 1.8; 95% CI: 1.0–3.1), but only in univariate analysis.

The role of hypertension in the outcome of RCC patients was investigated in a cohort study of 576,562 Korean men. An increased risk for cancer-specific mortality was found only for current smokers who were also hypertensive (RR 2.80; 95% CI: 1.64–4.79). For nonsmokers and former smokers, on the other hand, hypertension was not found to be an independent risk factor for cancer-specific mortality [82]. This study is, to our knowledge, the only one which found a significant effect of hypertension on the survival of RCC patients. The result of this study, however, is questionable because other studies have reported worse cancer-specific survival for current smokers alone [33, 34], and the ability to differentiate between the effects of smoking and hypertension on the survival of RCC patients is fraught with difficulty. It is possible, therefore, that the observed effect was more likely an effect of smoking than an effect of hypertension.

In summary, the data to date has shown uncertain results in terms of demonstrating an independent relationship between the use of antihypertensive medication and an increased risk of RCC. Experimental studies and better controls for other risk factors in epidemiological studies are necessary to determine whether there indeed is a relationship. Nevertheless, the results from epidemiological cohort studies appear to be sufficient to support a relationship between hypertension and the risk of RCC.

Summary

The worldwide incidence of kidney cancer has been increasing and is expected to continue to rise for the next several decades. The increased incidence of RCC likely reflects numerous factors, including increased utilization of abdominal imaging leading to the increased incidental diagnosis of small renal tumors, as well as the aging of the population and the increased prevalence of environmental and lifestyle risk factors for RCC such as obesity, hypertension, and smoking. The number of new cases presenting at advanced stages, however, has remained at a stable but relatively high level, comprising approximately one-third of all newly diagnosed cases. Regardless of this trend, both 5-year survival and mortality rates for RCC have improved. A wide variability in geographic, gender, and ethnic differences has been observed relative to RCC around the world. The majorities of these gene/environment interactions remain poorly understood and are still a matter of ongoing research. Tobacco use, obesity, and hypertension have emerged as the primary environmental factors that predispose to RCC. However, since many of these risk factors are modifiable, future investment in research directed at the biological mechanisms that underlie the pathogenesis of RCC and the development of evidence-based screening and prevention programs are warranted.

References

1. World Health Organization (WHO). Globocan 2008. Cancer incidence and mortality worldwide; 2008. http://globocan.iarc.fr/. Accessed Nov 2010.
2. Devesa SS, Silverman DT, McLaughlin JK, Brown CC, Connelly RR, Fraumeni Jr JF. Comparison of the descriptive epidemiology of urinary tract cancers. Cancer Causes Control. 1990;1(2):133–41.
3. Surveillance, Epidemiology, and End Results (SEER) Program Public-Use Data (1973–2002), National Cancer Institute, Division of Cancer Control and Population Sciences, Surveillance Research Program, Cancer Statistics Branch, released April 2005, based on the November 2004 submission; 2005.
4. Mathew A, Devesa SS, Fraumeni Jr JF, Chow WH. Global increases in kidney cancer incidence, 1973–1992. Eur J Cancer Prev. 2002;11(2):171–8.
5. Hollingsworth JM, Miller DC, Daignault S, Hollenbeck BK. Rising incidence of small renal masses: a need to reassess treatment effect. J Natl Cancer Inst. 2006;98(18):1331–4.
6. Chow WH, Linehan WM, Devesa SS. Re: rising incidence of small renal masses: a need to reassess treatment effect. J Natl Cancer Inst. 2007;99(7):569–70 [author reply 570–1].
7. American Cancer Society. Cancer facts & figures 2010. Atlanta: American Cancer Society; 2010.
8. Sun M, Thuret R, Abdollah F, et al. Age-adjusted incidence, mortality, and survival rates of stage-specific renal cell carcinoma in North America: a trend analysis. Eur Urol. 2011;59(1):135–41.
9. Altekruse SF, Kosary CL, Krapcho M, et al. SEER Cancer statistics review, 1975–2007. Bethesda: National Cancer Institute. http://seer.cancer.gov/csr/1975_2007/. Accessed Nov 2010.
10. Chow WH, Devesa SS, Warren JL, Fraumeni Jr JF. Rising incidence of renal cell cancer in the United States. JAMA. 1999;281(17):1628–31.
11. IMV Medical Information Division. CT census database and market summary report. Greenbelt; MD IMV2008.
12. Amis Jr ES, Butler PF, Applegate KE, et al. American College of Radiology white paper on radiation dose in medicine. J Am Coll Radiol. 2007;4(5):272–84.
13. Tada S, Yamagishi J, Kobayashi H, Hata Y, Kobari T. The incidence of simple renal cyst by computed tomography. Clin Radiol. 1983;34(4):437–9.
14. Hara AK, Johnson CD, MacCarty RL, Welch TJ. Incidental extracolonic findings at CT colonography. Radiology. 2000;215(2):353–7.
15. Chow WH, Devesa SS. Contemporary epidemiology of renal cell cancer. Cancer J. 2008;14(5):288–301.
16. World Health Organization (WHO). Fact sheet N311. Obesity and overweight; 2011. http://www.who.int/mediacentre/factsheets/fs311/en/index.html.
17. Kearney PM, Whelton M, Reynolds K, Muntner P, Whelton PK, He J. Global burden of hypertension: analysis of worldwide data. Lancet. 2005;365(9455):217–23.
18. Jemal A, Siegel R, Ward E, Hao Y, Xu J, Thun MJ. Cancer statistics, 2009. CA Cancer J Clin. 2009;59(4):225–49.
19. Levi F, Ferlay J, Galeone C, et al. The changing pattern of kidney cancer incidence and mortality in Europe. BJU Int. 2008;101(8):949–58.
20. Levi F, Lucchini F, Negri E, La Vecchia C. Declining mortality from kidney cancer in Europe. Ann Oncol. 2004;15(7):1130–5.
21. Vaishampayan UN, Do H, Hussain M, Schwartz K. Racial disparity in incidence patterns and outcome of kidney cancer. Urology. 2003;62(6):1012–7.
22. Sopori M. Effects of cigarette smoke on the immune system. Nat Rev Immunol. 2002;2(5):372–7.
23. Centers for Disease Control and Prevention (US); National Center for Chronic Disease Prevention and Health Promotion (US); Office on Smoking and Health (US). How tobacco smoke causes disease: the biology and behavioral basis for smoking-attributable disease: A report of the surgeon general. Atlanta (GA): Centers for Disease Control and Prevention (US); 2010. Available from: http://0-www.ncbi.nlm.nih.gov.elis.tmu.edu.tw/books/NBK53017/.
24. Thakker DR, Yagi H, Levin W, Wood AW, Conney AH, Jerina DM. Polycyclic aromatic hydrocarbons: metabolic activation to ultimate carcinogens. In: Anders MW, editor. Bioactivation of foreign compounds. New York: Academic; 1985. p. 177–242.
25. Zhu Y, Horikawa Y, Yang H, Wood CG, Habuchi T, Wu X. BPDE induced lymphocytic chromosome 3p deletions may predict renal cell carcinoma risk. J Urol. 2008;179(6):2416–21.
26. Shiao YH, Rice JM, Anderson LM, Diwan BA, Hard GC. von Hippel-Lindau gene mutations in N-nitrosodimethylamine-induced rat renal epithelial tumors. J Natl Cancer Inst. 1998;90(22):1720–3.
27. Swann PF, Kaufman DG, Magee PN, Mace R. Induction of kidney tumours by a single dose of dimethylnitrosamine: dose response and influence of diet and benzo(a)pyrene pretreatment. Br J Cancer. 1980;41(2):285–94.
28. Clague J, Shao L, Lin J, et al. Sensitivity to NNKOAc is associated with renal cancer risk. Carcinogenesis. 2009;30(4):706–10.
29. IARC monographs on the evaluation of carcinogenic risks to humans tobacco smoke and involuntary smoking, vol 83. Lyon: World Health Organization International Agency for Research on Cancer; 2004. p. 339–70. Available from: http://apps.who.int/bookorders/anglais/detart1.jsp?sesslan=1&codlan=1&codcol=72&codcch=83.
30. US Department of Health and Human Services. The health consequence of smoking: a report of the surgeon general. Atlanta: Centers for Disease Control and Prevention, National Center for Chronic Disease Prevention and Health Promotion, Office on Smoking and Health; 2004.
31. Hunt JD, van der Hel OL, McMillan GP, Boffetta P, Brennan P. Renal cell carcinoma in relation to cigarette

smoking: meta-analysis of 24 studies. Int J Cancer. 2005;114(1):101–8.

32. Thun MJ, DeLancey JO, Center MM, Jemal A, Ward EM. The global burden of cancer: priorities for prevention. Carcinogenesis. 2010;31(1):100–10.

33. Sweeney C, Farrow DC. Differential survival related to smoking among patients with renal cell carcinoma. Epidemiology. 2000;11(3):344–6.

34. Parker A, Lohse C, Cheville J, Leibovich B, Igel T, Blute M. Evaluation of the association of current cigarette smoking and outcome for patients with clear cell renal cell carcinoma. Int J Urol. 2008;15(4):304–8.

35. Hursting SD, Berger NA. Energy balance, host-related factors, and cancer progression. J Clin Oncol. 2010;28(26):4058–65.

36. Ceciliani F, Giordano A, Spagnolo V. The systemic reaction during inflammation: the acute-phase proteins. Protein Pept Lett. 2002;9(3):211–23.

37. Pantuck AJ, Seligson DB, Klatte T, et al. Prognostic relevance of the mTOR pathway in renal cell carcinoma: implications for molecular patient selection for targeted therapy. Cancer. 2007;109(11):2257–67.

38. Hudes G, Carducci M, Tomczak P, et al. Temsirolimus, interferon alfa, or both for advanced renal-cell carcinoma. N Engl J Med. 2007;356(22):2271–81.

39. Motzer RJ, Escudier B, Oudard S, et al. Phase 3 trial of everolimus for metastatic renal cell carcinoma: final results and analysis of prognostic factors. Cancer. 2010;116(18):4256–65.

40. Masur K, Vetter C, Hinz A, et al. Diabetogenic glucose and insulin concentrations modulate transcriptom and protein levels involved in tumour cell migration, adhesion and proliferation. Br J Cancer. 2011;104(2):345–52.

41. Mussig K, Haring HU. Insulin signal transduction in normal cells and its role in carcinogenesis. Exp Clin Endocrinol Diabetes. 2010;118(6):356–9.

42. Pollak M. Insulin and insulin-like growth factor signalling in neoplasia. Nat Rev Cancer. 2008;8(12): 915–28.

43. Takahashi K, Suzuki K. Association of insulin-like growth-factor-I-induced DNA synthesis with phosphorylation and nuclear exclusion of p53 in human breast cancer MCF-7 cells. Int J Cancer. 1993;55(3):453–8.

44. Klatte T, Said JW, de Martino M, et al. Presence of tumor necrosis is not a significant predictor of survival in clear cell renal cell carcinoma: higher prognostic accuracy of extent based rather than presence/absence classification. J Urol. 2009;181(4):1558–64 [discussion 1563–4].

45. Noon AP, Vlatkovic N, Polanski R, et al. p53 and MDM2 in renal cell carcinoma: biomarkers for disease progression and future therapeutic targets? Cancer. 2010;116(4):780–90.

46. Tilg H, Moschen AR. Evolution of inflammation in nonalcoholic fatty liver disease: the multiple parallel hits hypothesis. Hepatology. 2010;52(5):1836–46.

47. Hursting SD, Smith SM, Lashinger LM, Harvey AE, Perkins SN. Calories and carcinogenesis: lessons learned from 30 years of calorie restriction research. Carcinogenesis. 2010;31(1):83–9.

48. Nicodemus KK, Sweeney C, Folsom AR. Evaluation of dietary, medical and lifestyle risk factors for incident kidney cancer in postmenopausal women. Int J Cancer. 2004;108(1):115–21.

49. Gonzalez CA, Riboli E. Diet and cancer prevention: contributions from the european prospective investigation into cancer and nutrition (EPIC) study. Eur J Cancer. 2010;46(14):2555–62.

50. James PT, Leach R, Kalamara E, Shayeghi M. The worldwide obesity epidemic. Obes Res. 2001;9 Suppl 4:228S–33.

51. Sawada N, Inoue M, Sasazuki S, et al. Body mass index and subsequent risk of kidney cancer: a prospective cohort study in Japan. Ann Epidemiol. 2010;20(6):466–72.

52. Pischon T, Lahmann PH, Boeing H, et al. Body size and risk of renal cell carcinoma in the European prospective investigation into cancer and nutrition (EPIC). Int J Cancer. 2006;118(3):728–38.

53. Calle EE, Kaaks R. Overweight, obesity and cancer: epidemiological evidence and proposed mechanisms. Nat Rev Cancer. 2004;4(8):579–91.

54. Lowrance WT, Thompson RH, Yee DS, Kaag M, Donat SM, Russo P. Obesity is associated with a higher risk of clear-cell renal cell carcinoma than with other histologies. BJU Int. 2010;105(1):16–20.

55. Lee JE, Mannisto S, Spiegelman D, et al. Intakes of fruit, vegetables, and carotenoids and renal cell cancer risk: a pooled analysis of 13 prospective studies. Cancer Epidemiol Biomarkers Prev. 2009;18(6): 1730–9.

56. Lindblad P, Wolk A, Bergstrom R, Adami HO. Diet and risk of renal cell cancer: a population-based case-control study. Cancer Epidemiol Biomarkers Prev. 1997;6(4):215–23.

57. Weikert S, Boeing H, Pischon T, et al. Fruits and vegetables and renal cell carcinoma: findings from the European prospective investigation into cancer and nutrition (EPIC). Int J Cancer. 2006;118(12): 3133–9.

58. Allen NE, Roddam AW, Sieri S, et al. A prospective analysis of the association between macronutrient intake and renal cell carcinoma in the European prospective investigation into cancer and nutrition. Int J Cancer. 2009;125(4):982–7.

59. Lee JE, Spiegelman D, Hunter DJ, et al. Fat, protein, and meat consumption and renal cell cancer risk: a pooled analysis of 13 prospective studies. J Natl Cancer Inst. 2008;100(23):1695–706.

60. Mellemgaard A, McLaughlin JK, Overvad K, Olsen JH. Dietary risk factors for renal cell carcinoma in Denmark. Eur J Cancer. 1996;32A(4):673–82.

61. Lee JE, Giovannucci E, Smith-Warner SA, Spiegelman D, Willett WC, Curhan GC. Intakes of fruits, vegetables, vitamins A, C, and E, and carotenoids and risk of renal cell cancer. Cancer Epidemiol Biomarkers Prev. 2006;15(12):2445–52.

62. Hu J, Mao Y, White K. Diet and vitamin or mineral supplements and risk of renal cell carcinoma in Canada. Cancer Causes Control. 2003;14(8):705–14.

63. Wolk A, Gridley G, Niwa S, et al. International renal cell cancer study. VII. Role of diet. Int J Cancer. 1996;65(1):67–73.

64. Wolk A, Larsson SC, Johansson JE, Ekman P. Long-term fatty fish consumption and renal cell carcinoma incidence in women. JAMA. 2006;296(11):1371–6.

65. Lee JE, Hunter DJ, Spiegelman D, et al. Alcohol intake and renal cell cancer in a pooled analysis of 12 prospective studies. J Natl Cancer Inst. 2007;99(10): 801–10.

66. Chiu BC, Gapstur SM, Chow WH, Kirby KA, Lynch CF, Cantor KP. Body mass index, physical activity, and risk of renal cell carcinoma. Int J Obes (Lond). 2006;30(6):940–7.

67. Moore SC, Chow WH, Schatzkin A, et al. Physical activity during adulthood and adolescence in relation to renal cell cancer. Am J Epidemiol. 2008;168(2):149–57.

68. Bergstrom A, Terry P, Lindblad P, et al. Physical activity and risk of renal cell cancer. Int J Cancer. 2001;92(1):155–7.

69. Waalkes S, Merseburger AS, Kramer MW, et al. Obesity is associated with improved survival in patients with organ-confined clear-cell kidney cancer. Cancer Causes Control. 2010;21(11):1905–10.

70. Haferkamp A, Pritsch M, Bedke J, et al. The influence of body mass index on the long-term survival of patients with renal cell carcinoma after tumour nephrectomy. BJU Int. 2008;101(10):1243–6.

71. Parker AS, Lohse CM, Cheville JC, Thiel DD, Leibovich BC, Blute ML. Greater body mass index is associated with better pathologic features and improved outcome among patients treated surgically for clear cell renal cell carcinoma. Urology. 2006;68(4):741–6.

72. Andreotti G, Boffetta P, Rosenberg PS, et al. Variants in blood pressure genes and the risk of renal cell carcinoma. Carcinogenesis. 2010;31(4):614–20.

73. Sane DC, Anton L, Brosnihan KB. Angiogenic growth factors and hypertension. Angiogenesis. 2004;7(3): 193–201.

74. Chow WH, Gridley G, Fraumeni Jr JF, Jarvholm B. Obesity, hypertension, and the risk of kidney cancer in men. N Engl J Med. 2000;343(18):1305–11.

75. Flaherty KT, Fuchs CS, Colditz GA, et al. A prospective study of body mass index, hypertension, and smoking and the risk of renal cell carcinoma (United States). Cancer Causes Control. 2005;16(9): 1099–106.

76. Weikert S, Boeing H, Pischon T, et al. Blood pressure and risk of renal cell carcinoma in the European prospective investigation into cancer and nutrition. Am J Epidemiol. 2008;167(4):438–46.

77. Vatten LJ, Trichopoulos D, Holmen J, Nilsen TI. Blood pressure and renal cancer risk: the HUNT Study in Norway. Br J Cancer. 2007;97(1):112–4.

78. Weikert S, Ljungberg B. Contemporary epidemiology of renal cell carcinoma: perspectives of primary prevention. World J Urol. 2010;28(3):247–52.

79. Corrao G, Scotti L, Bagnardi V, Sega R. Hypertension, antihypertensive therapy and renal-cell cancer: a meta-analysis. Curr Drug Saf. 2007;2(2):125–33.

80. Shapiro JA, Williams MA, Weiss NS, Stergachis A, LaCroix AZ, Barlow WE. Hypertension, antihypertensive medication use, and risk of renal cell carcinoma. Am J Epidemiol. 1999;149(6):521–30.

81. McLaughlin JK, Chow WH, Mandel JS, et al. International renal-cell cancer study. VIII. Role of diuretics, other anti-hypertensive medications and hypertension. Int J Cancer. 1995;63(2):216–21.

82. Choi MY, Jee SH, Sull JW, Nam CM. The effect of hypertension on the risk for kidney cancer in Korean men. Kidney Int. 2005;67(2):647–52.

Pathology of Renal Cell Carcinoma

2

Ming Zhou and Huiying He

Arising from the renal tubular epithelial cells, renal cell carcinoma (RCC) accounts for more than 90% of primary kidney tumors in adults. It encompasses a group of heterogeneous tumors with diverse clinical, pathological, and molecular characteristics as well as distinct prognosis and therapeutic responses. It is therefore of paramount importance to accurately classify renal tumors. In this chapter, we review the pathological and molecular characteristics of major histological subtypes of RCC that are recognized by the 2004 World Health Organization (WHO) classification of renal tumors [1]. We also discuss several newly described subtypes of RCC and RCC associated with inherited cancer syndromes. The prognostic significance of various histological parameters will also be highlighted [2–4].

Pathological Classification of RCC

In addition to rendering an accurate diagnosis, pathological classification of RCC also provides relevant prognostic information and guidance to therapy. The current classification of renal tumors was introduced by WHO in 2004 (Table 2.1) [1]. It is based primarily on morphology but has also incorporated characteristic genetic and molecular features of renal tumors. These ten tumors represent the most common RCC subtypes encountered clinically. However, many other less common subtypes of RCC have been described with distinct clinical, pathological, and genetic features, and it is likely that additional ones will be identified in the future. As the molecular mechanisms of renal tumors have been increasingly elucidated, molecular classification will eventually replace morphological classification [2–4].

Pathologic and Molecular Characteristics of RCC Histologic Subtypes

Renal Cell Carcinoma, Clear Cell (CCRCC) Type

Clinical Features

CCRCC type is the most common histological subtype and accounts for 60–70% of all RCCs. Although it may occur in all age groups, it most commonly affects patients in their sixth to seventh decades of life and the majority are males with a ratio of approximately 2:1 [5]. Most CCRCC arises sporadically, with only 2–4% of the cases presenting as part of an inherited cancer syndrome, including von Hippel–Lindau (VHL) syndrome, Birt–Hogg–Dube (BHD) syndrome,

M. Zhou, MD, PhD (✉)
Department of Pathology, New York University Langone Medical Center, 560 First Avenue, TCH-461, New York, NY 10016-6497, USA
e-mail: Ming.Zhou@nyumc.org

H. He, MD, PhD
Department of Pathology, Health Science Center, Peking University, Beijing, China

Table 2.1 2004 World Health Organization classification of renal cell carcinoma

Renal cell carcinoma
Clear cell renal cell carcinoma
Multilocular clear cell renal cell carcinoma
Papillary renal cell carcinoma
Chromophobe renal cell carcinoma
Carcinoma of the collecting ducts of Bellini
Renal medullary carcinoma
Xp11 translocation carcinomas
Carcinoma associated with neuroblastoma
Mucinous tubular and spindle cell carcinoma
Renal cell carcinoma, unclassified

and constitutional chromosomal 3 translocation syndrome [6, 7]. As a general rule, familial CCRCC presents at a younger age and is much more likely to be multifocal and bilateral.

Pathology

Grossly, CCRCC usually presents as a unilateral and unicentric, round and well-demarcated mass with a fibrous capsule. The cut surface often has characteristic golden yellow color with variable degree of hemorrhage, necrosis, cystic degeneration, and calcification (Fig. 2.1a). Bilaterality and/or multicentricity occur in <5% of sporadic CCRCC cases but are more common in inherited cancer syndromes.

Microscopically the tumor cells are arranged in compact nests, sheets, alveolar, or acinar structures separated by thin-walled blood vessels. Tumor cells have clear cytoplasm (Fig. 2.1b) due to loss of cytoplasmic lipid and glycogen during tissue processing and slide preparation. In high-grade and poorly differentiated tumors, cells lose their cytoplasmic clearing and acquire granular eosinophilic cytoplasm (Fig. 2.1c).

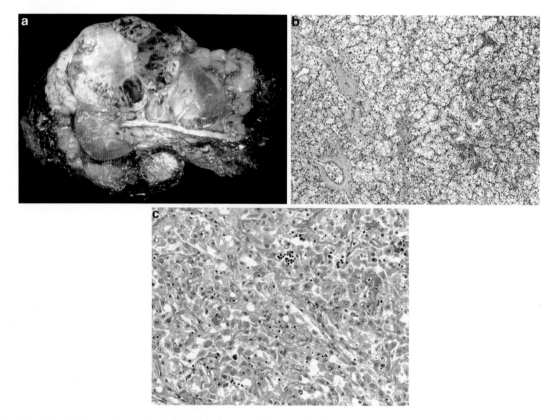

Fig. 2.1 (**a**) Large clear cell renal cell carcinoma with characteristic *bright golden yellow color* extends into perinephric and sinus fat. Adrenal metastasis is also seen on the *bottom of the image* (**a**). Clear cell RCC is com- posed of compact nests of tumor cells with clear cytoplasm separated by delicate arborizing vasculature (**b**). High-grade clear cell RCC can show eosinophilic and granular cytoplasm (**c**)

Molecular Genetics

Seventy to ninety percent of CCRCCs harbor chromosome 3p alterations which comprise deletion, mutation, or methylation of several important genes, including *von Hippel–Lindau* (*VHL*) gene on chromosome 3p25-26, *RASSF1A* on 3p21 and *FHIT* on 3p14.2. Duplication of 5q22 is the second most common cytogenetic finding and may be associated with better prognosis. Other cytogenetic alterations involve loss of chromosomes 6q, 8p12, 9p21, 9q22, 10q, 17p, and 14q [3, 8, 9].

Somatic mutations in *VHL* gene have been found in 18–82% of sporadic CCRCC cases. Loss of heterozygosity at the *VHL* locus has been reported in up to 98% of cases [10–12]. Hypermethylation of the *VHL* gene promoter resulting in gene inactivation has been detected in 5–20% of patients without gene alteration. The

vast majority of CCRCC showing somatic *VHL* mutations also exhibit allelic loss or LOH at the *VHL* locus, consistent with Knudson's two-hit model of tumorigenesis.

VHL protein plays a critical role in the cellular response to hypoxia (Fig. 2.2). Hypoxia-inducible factor (HIF) is a transcriptional factor whose cellular level is regulated by VHL. Under normoxic condition, HIF is hydroxylated, and the wild-type VHL protein binds and targets this form of HIF for degradation in proteosomes. Consequently, HIF levels are kept low within normal cells under normoxic conditions through the action of functional VHL. Under hypoxic condition, however, HIF is not hydroxylated and cannot be recognized by VHL, and therefore begins to accumulate. This in turn activates many downstream hypoxia-driven genes, including genes that promote angiogenesis [vascular endothelial growth

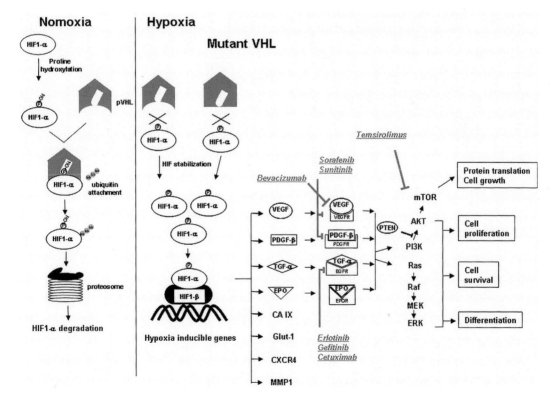

Fig. 2.2 Molecular pathways involving the *VHL* gene. Under normoxic condition, VHL directs HIF for proteolytic degradation. Under hypoxic condition or when VHL gene expression is inactivated by mutation or promoter hypermethylation, HIF accumulates and activates multiple target genes and signal transduction pathways to control cell proliferation, survival, growth, and differentiation. Several small molecule inhibitors can block various critical steps in these pathways and are currently used to treat advanced stage disease

factor (*VEGF*) and platelet-derived growth factor β (*PDGF-β*)], cell growth or survival [transforming growth factor α (*TGF-α*)], anaerobic metabolism (*Glut-1*), acid base balance (*CA IX*), and red cell production (*erythropoietin*). Along the way numerous intracellular signal transduction pathways are activated, including PI3 kinase-Akt-mTOR pathway and Ras-raf-erk-mek pathway, which are involved in various cellular processes, including cell proliferation, survival, and differentiation [12, 13]. These signal transduction pathways serve a beneficial role by stimulating angiogenesis and compensatory metabolic changes in normal cells coping with hypoxia. When *VHL* gene is inactivated by mutation or promoter hypermethylation, no functional VHL is produced. The end result is activation of the aforementioned cellular processes which are no longer controlled by normal physiological mechanisms and therefore contribute to the tumorigenesis and many of the clinical manifestations of CCRCC. Recent clinical trials have targeted the critical components of these pathways in patients with advanced stage CCRCC, including VEGF using neutralizing antibody bevacizumab; VEGFR and PDGFR using small molecule inhibitors of tyrosine kinase, such as sorafenib and sunitinib; EGFR using erlotinib, and mTOR using temsirolimus [14, 15] (Fig. 2.2).

Renal Cell Carcinoma, Papillary Type (Papillary RCC)

Clinical Features

Papillary RCC (PRCC) is the second most common type of RCC and accounts for 10–15% of RCCs. The gender and age distribution are similar to those of CCRCC. However, PRCC has a better prognosis with a 5-year survival approaching 90% [5]. The vast majority of tumors occur sporadically, but some develop in members of families with hereditary PRCC (HPRCC) [16] or rarely in hereditary leiomyomatosis and renal cell cancer (HLRCC) [17].

Pathology

Grossly, PRCC typically presents as a well-circumscribed mass enclosed within a pseudocapsule. Some tumors appear entirely necrotic and friable (Fig. 2.3a). PRCC is more likely to be bilateral and multifocal than the other types of RCC.

Microscopically, PRCC is composed of varying proportions of papillae, tubulopapillae, and tubules. Occasionally it has tightly packed tubules or papillae and imparts a solid appearance. The papillae characteristically contain delicate fibrovascular cores infiltrated by foamy histiocytes (Fig. 2.3b). Necrosis, hemorrhage, acute and chronic inflammation, hemosiderin deposition, and psammoma bodies are common.

Two subtypes of PRCC are recognized based on the histology [18]. Accounting for about two-thirds of PRCC, type I tumor contains papillae that are delicate and short, lined with single layer of tumor cells with scant cytoplasm and low-grade nuclei (Fig. 2.3b). In contrast, papillae in type II PRCC are large and lined with cells having abundant eosinophilic cytoplasm and large pseudostratified nuclei with prominent nucleoli (Fig. 2.3c). Patients with type I PRCC have a better prognosis than those with type II tumor.

Molecular Genetics

Trisomy or tetrasomy 7, trisomy 17, and loss of Y chromosome (in men) are the most common cytogenetic changes in PRCC [19]. Types I and II PRCC have distinct genetic features, for example, gain of 7p and 17p is more common in type I tumors [20]. Deletion of 9p is present in approximately 20% of PRCC and loss of heterozygosity at 9p13, limited to type II tumors in recent studies, has been linked to shorter survival [21].

Renal Cell Carcinoma, Chromophobe Type (Chromophobe RCC)

Clinical Features

Chromophobe RCC (ChRCC) accounts for approximately 5% of RCCs and is believed to arise from the intercalated cells of the collecting ducts [22]. ChRCC can occur in patients of wide age range. Males and females are affected almost equally. The prognosis is significantly better than that of CCRCC, with disease recurrence in <5%

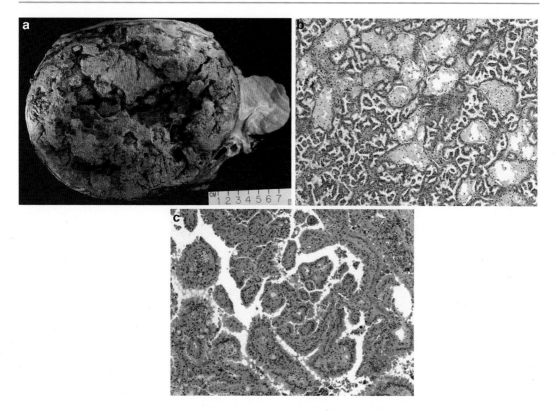

Fig. 2.3 Papillary renal cell carcinoma has a thick tumor capsule and extensive necrosis (**a**). Type I tumors are composed of papillae covered by a single layer of tumor cells with scant cytoplasm and low-grade nuclei. The fibrovascular cores are expanded with foamy histiocytes (**b**). Type II tumor cells have abundant eosinophilic cytoplasm and large pseudostratified nuclei with prominent nucleoli (**c**)

of patients [5]. Most cases arise sporadically, while some familial cases are associated with BHD syndrome [23, 24].

Pathology

ChRCC is typically a solitary, well-circumscribed and nonencapsulated mass with homogenous light brown solid cut surface (Fig. 2.4a). Hemorrhage and/or necrosis are uncommon. A central stellate scar can be seen in large tumors.

Microscopically, the tumor cells are usually arranged in solid sheets with some cases demonstrating areas of tubulocystic architecture. The classic ChRCC tumor consists of large and polygonal cells with finely reticulated cytoplasm due to numerous cytoplasmic microvesicles, and prominent "plant cell like" cell membrane. The nuclei are typically irregular, hyperchromatic and

wrinkled with perinuclear haloes (Fig. 2.4b). Not infrequently the tumor consists predominantly of cells with intensely eosinophilic cytoplasm, termed eosinophilic variant [25]. However, there is no substantial difference in the clinical characteristics between the two variants.

Molecular Genetics

ChRCC harbors extensive chromosomal loss, most commonly involving chromosomes Y, 1, 2, 6, 10, 13, 17, and 21 [26]. Occasionally, ChRCC occurs in BHD syndrome, characterized by mutations in Birt–Hogg–Dube gene (*BHD*) on 17p11.2, which encodes the protein folliculin [27]. However, *BHD* mutations are rarely found in sporadic ChRCC. It has been proposed that ChRCC may evolve from oncocytoma after acquiring additional cytogenetic abnormality [28].

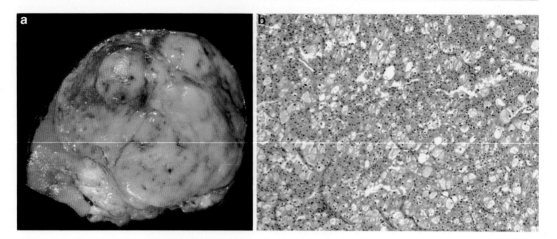

Fig. 2.4 Chromophobe renal cell carcinoma forms a circumscribed, nonencapsulated mass with a homogenous *light brown* cut surface (**a**). The large and polygonal tumor cells have finely reticulated cytoplasm, prominent cell border, and irregular nuclei with perinuclear clearing (**b**)

Other Uncommon Subtypes of Renal Cell Carcinoma

Other subtypes of RCC are uncommon and collectively account for <5% of RCC cases in the kidney. However, they have clinical, pathological, and genetic characteristics distinct from the more common types discussed previously. The clinical, pathological, and genetic features of these uncommon RCC subtypes are summarized in Table 2.2 (Figs. 2.5–2.9).

Renal Cell Carcinoma, Unclassified Type

RCC, unclassified type, is a term for the designation of RCC that does not fit into any of the accepted categories. It is important to understand that this is a diagnostic category rather than a true biological entity. These tumors represent a heterogeneous group of malignancies with poorly defined clinical, morphological, or genetic features and therefore cannot be classified using the current criteria. Most unclassified tumors are poorly differentiated and are associated with a poor prognosis. As our understanding of RCC improves, this category is destined to diminish and perhaps eventually disappear. There are several other entities that were identified very

recently and were not included in the 2004 WHO classification. Several of these entities are reviewed in Table 2.3 (Fig. 2.10).

Renal Cell Carcinomas in Inherited Cancer Syndromes

Less than 5% of RCC occur in the setting of inherited cancer syndromes, including von Hippel–Lindau disease (VHLD), HPRCC, hereditary leiomyomatosis and renal cell cancer (HLRCC), and BHD syndrome [6]. Each inherited cancer syndrome predisposes patients to distinct subtypes of RCC which often occur at a young age and have a higher incidence of bilaterality and multifocality [56].

von Hippel–Lindau Disease

VHLD is an autosomal-dominant hereditary condition with stigmata including CCRCCs, central nervous system hemangioblastomas, pheochromocytomas, pancreatic cysts and endolymphatic sac tumors of the inner ear [13]. It is caused by germline mutations in *VHL* gene. VHLD patients are born with a germline defect in one of the alleles. Inactivation of the second allele results in

Table 2.2 Clinical, pathological, and genetic features of uncommon RCC subtypes included in the 2004 WHO classification of RCC

RCC subtype	Clinical features	Pathology		Genetics	Prognosis	Reference
		Grossly	Microscopically			
Multilocular cystic RCC (Fig. 2.5)	Variant of CCRCC (5% of CCRCC) Mean age 51 years (range 20–76) Male:female = 2–3:1	Well-circumscribed, entirely cystic mass; no grossly visible nodules expanding the septa; necrosis is absent	Variably sized cysts lined with one or several layers of flat or plump cellular cells; no expansile cellular nodules; low grade nuclei (Fuhrman nuclear grade 1 or 2)	3p deletion as observed in CCRCC	Favorable No local or distant metastasis after complete surgical removal	[29, 30]
Carcinoma of the collecting ducts of Bellini (Fig. 2.6)	<1% of all renal tumors; arising in the collecting ducts of Bellini Often seen in 4th to 7th decade with mean age 55 years Male:female = 2:1	Poorly circumscribed; usually centrally located; cut surface usually gray, white and firm	High-grade tumor cells form complex tubulocystic structures; prominent desmoplastic stroma	Variable results LOH on chromosomes 1q, 6p, 8p.9p, 13q, 19q32 and 21q; c-erB2 amplification associated with unfavorable outcome	Poor; 1/3 presenting with metastasis 2/3 patients dead of disease within 2 years of diagnosis	[31–34]
Medullary carcinoma (Fig. 2.7)	Exceedingly rare; almost exclusively in patients with sickle cell hemoglobinopathies or traits; majority are African-Americans Mean age 19 years (5–69) Male:female = 2:1	More common in right kidney; poorly circumscribed, centrally located; tan to gray, with varying degrees of hemorrhage and necrosis	High-grade tumor cells with reticular, microcystic or solid pattern; Desmoplastic stroma; may have abundant neutrophils	Not well defined	Highly aggressive 95% presenting with metastasis; often dead of disease within 6 months of diagnosis	[35, 36]
Xp11.2 translocation carcinoma (Fig. 2.8)	Predominantly affecting children and young adults; accounts for 40% of RCCs in this age group; occurs post-chemotherapy in some cases male = female also affects adult patients with a striking female predominance	Usually circumscribed; may resemble PRCC	Most distinctive features: papillary structures lined with clear cells (Fig. 2.8a) Confirmatory test: positive nuclear immunostain for TFE3 protein (Fig. 2.8b)	Chromosomal translocation involving TFE3 gene on Xp11.2 resulting in overexpression of the TFE3 protein; has several Translocation partner genes	Present at advanced stage, but with indolent clinical course in children; Adult patients may pursue more aggressive course	[37–43]
Mucinous tubular spindle cell carcinoma (Fig. 2.9)	Mean age 53 years (range 13–82) Affects predominantly female patients (male:female = 1:4) incidental finding in most cases	Sharply circumscribed; gray–white with myxoid appearance; many have minimal hemorrhage and/or necrosis	Elongated compressed tubules and bland spindle cells embedded in a lightly basophilic myxoid stroma Low-grade nuclei	Not well defined Losses involving chromosomes 1, 4, 6, 8, 9, 11, 13, 14, 15, 18, 22 reported; 3p alterations and gain of chromosome 7, and 17 not present	Favorable; majority of patients remain disease free after surgical resection	[44–47]
Post-neuroblastoma renal cell carcinoma	In long-term survivors of neuroblastoma; male = female; neuroblastoma diagnosis in the first 2 years of life; mean age of RCC diagnosis 13.5 years (range 2–35)	Same as CCRCC	Limited data: many tumors are typical CCRCC; some tumors have cells with abundant granular cytoplasm and arranged in solid, nests or in papillae	Not well defined Loss of multiple chromosomal loci observed	Similar to other common RCC subtypes	[48, 49]

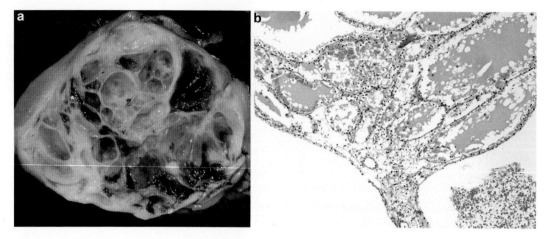

Fig. 2.5 Multilocular cystic renal cell carcinoma is a well-circumscribed entirely cystic mass (**a**). The cystic septa are delicate without solid tumor nodules. The cysts are lined with one or several layers of tumor cells with clear cytoplasm and uniformly small, dense and low grade nuclei (**b**)

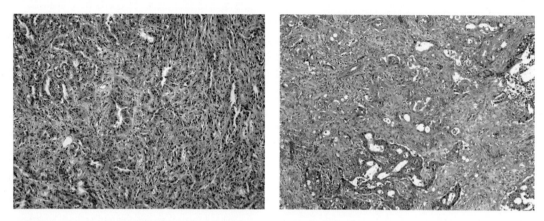

Fig. 2.6 Collecting duct carcinoma consists of high-grade tumor cells forming complex tubules or tubulopapillary structures embedded in a remarkably desmoplastic stroma

Fig. 2.7 Renal medullary carcinoma comprises high-grade tumor cells arranged in irregular nests with microcystic formation. The stroma is desmoplastic

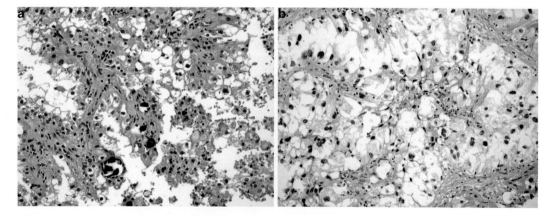

Fig. 2.8 ASPL-TFE3 renal cell carcinoma with *t*(X;17) (p11.2;q25) chromosomal translocation shows nests or pseudopapillary structures lined by cells with abundant clear, sometimes eosinophilic cytoplasm and vesicular nuclei with prominent nucleoli. Psammomatous calcification is also present (**a**). The tumor cells are positive for nuclear TFE3 protein by immunostaining (**b**)

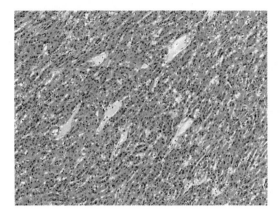

Fig. 2.9 Mucinous tubular and spindle cell carcinoma is composed of elongated cords and collapsed tubules with slit-like spaces embedded in a lightly basophilic myxoid background. The tumor cells have low-grade nuclear features

uncontrolled cell growth and tumor formation. Renal lesions in VHLD are always CCRCC and tend to be bilateral and multifocal. Dozens or even hundreds of microscopic tumor foci can be identified in resected kidney specimens. VHLD-related RCC develops early with a mean age of onset of 37 years as compared to 61 years for sporadic CCRCC. Although metastasis typically only occurs when tumors are greater than 3 cm, RCC is nevertheless the leading cause of death in this syndrome. However, VHLD patients with renal involvement have better 10-year survival than their sporadic counterparts [6].

Hereditary Papillary Renal Cell Carcinoma

HPRCC is an inherited renal cancer characterized by a predisposition to develop multiple bilateral papillary renal tumors of type I histology. To date, kidney is the only organ to be affected in these patients [16]. HPRCC is associated with a germline mutation in the tyrosine kinase domain of the *c-met* proto-oncogene on chromosome 7q31. *c-met* gene encodes a cell surface receptor protein for hepatocyte growth factor (HGF) and has tyrosine kinase activity [57]. Gain-of-function mutations result in activated cellular processes that contribute to carcinogenesis, including angiogen-

esis, cell motility, proliferation, and morphogenic differentiation. The tyrosine kinase domain of MET is a promising therapeutic target [58].

Hereditary Leiomyomatosis and Renal Cell Cancer

HLRCC is an autosomal-dominant disease and predisposes patients to cutaneous leiomyomas, uterine leiomyomas in women, and PRCC of type II histology. The renal tumors are often solitary, unilateral, and more likely to be aggressive and lethal. Only 20–35% of patients develop RCC. Germline mutations are identified in the fumarate hydratase (*FH*) gene on chromosome 1 (1q42.3–43) [59], which is an essential regulator of the Krebs cycle. Inactivation of *FH* impairs the Krebs cycle, thereby activating anaerobic metabolism and upregulation of HIF and hypoxia-inducible genes.

Birt–Hogg–Dube Syndrome

RCC is also part of the BHD syndrome, an autosomal-dominant disorder characterized by benign skin tumors (fibrofolliculomas, trichodiscomas of hair follicles, and skin tag), renal epithelial neoplasms, lung cysts, and spontaneous pneumothorax [24]. Renal neoplasms are often multifocal and bilateral, the most common being hybrid oncocytic tumors (50%) with features of both ChRCC and oncocytoma [60]. Renal tumors can also include ChRCC (33%), oncocytomas (5%), and occasionally CCRCC or PRCC. *BHD*, the gene implicated in the syndrome, is a potential tumor suppressor gene on 17p11.2 and encodes the protein folliculin.

Common Benign Renal Tumors

Papillary Adenoma

By WHO definition, papillary adenoma constitutes epithelial neoplasms with papillary and/or tubular architecture, <5 mm in size and low-grade nuclei.

Table 2.3 Uncommon subtypes of renal cell carcinoma not included in 2004 WHO classification [4]

RCC subtype	Clinical features	Pathology		Genetics	Prognosis	Reference
		Grossly	Microscopically			
Tubulocystic carcinoma	Occurs in 5th and 6th decades (range 30–94 years); male:female = 7:1	Usually solitary; circumscribed and unencapsulated; spongy cut surface resembling "bubble wrap"	Circumscribed collection of tubules and cysts of varied sizes; separated by fibrous stroma; no desmoplastic reaction; the lining cells usually exhibit high-grade nuclei and eosinophilic cytoplasm	Gain in chromosome 7 and 17 in some cases; may be related to PRCC	Not fully established; majority cases are have indolent clinical course; recurrence or metastasis in a few cases	[50–52]
Clear cell tubulopapillary carcinoma	Mean age 60 years; male=female	Small tumor with mean size of 2.4 cm; the majority are cystic and have prominent fibrous capsule and stroma	Branching tubules, acini and/or clear cell ribbons with low-grade nuclei; positive for CK7 and negative for CD10	Limited data; do not exhibit the genetic changes characteristic of CCRCC and PRCC	Low-grade and low-stage tumor; mostly biological indolent tumors	[53]
Thyroid-like follicular carcinoma	Very rare; mean age 45 years	Wide size range; tan colored	Prominent pseudocapsule; micro- and macrofollicles lined with low-grade cells; colloid-like material present in >50% of follicles; negative for TTF-1 and thyroglobulin	Limited data	Not well defined; available cases are free of disease after surgical resection	[54]
Acquired cystic kidney disease (ACKD)-associated RCC (Fig. 2.10)	2–7% incidence in ACKD patients; occur in relatively young patients; male predominance	Frequently multicentric and bilateral; generally well circumscribed	About 40% are classic CCRCC, PRCC or ChRCC; various architectures; 80% of tumor cells show abundant intratumoral calcium oxalate crystals	Limited data; gains in chromosomes 1, 2, 6, and 10	Less aggressive than sporadic RCC	[55]

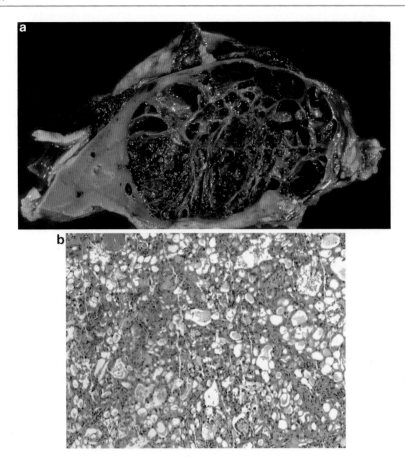

Fig. 2.10 Acquired cystic disease-associated renal cell carcinoma forms a well-circumscribed mass with cysts and solid nodules (**a**). The non-neoplastic kidney is atrophic with several cysts. The tumor exhibits tubulocystic architectures and contains calcium oxalate crystals (**b**)

Clinical Features

Adenoma is the most common renal cell neoplasm, frequently presenting as incidental findings after nephrectomy or at autopsy. In one autopsy study, papillary adenomas were found in up to 40% of patients older than 70 years of age. Its incidence increases with age and also in patients on long-term dialysis.

Pathology

Papillary adenomas appear as small (<5 mm), well circumscribed, yellow or white nodules in the renal cortex. They have papillary, tubular, or tubulopapillary architecture, similar to PRCC [61]. The tumor cells have uniform small nuclei and inconspicuous nucleoli equivalent to Fuhrman grade 1 or 2 nuclei (Fig. 2.11).

Molecular Genetics

Papillary adenomas share many genetic alterations with PRCC; both have combined gains of chromosomes 7 and 17 and loss of the Y chromosome in men. PRCCs acquire additional genetic alterations, including trisomy 12, 16, or 20. The cytogenetic findings support the hypothesis that papillary adenoma is a precursor of PRCC [62].

Renal Oncocytoma

Clinical Features

Renal oncocytoma accounts for 5% of surgically resected nonurothelial renal neoplasms. Patients vary greatly in age with a peak incidence in the seventh decade of life. The male-to-female ratio

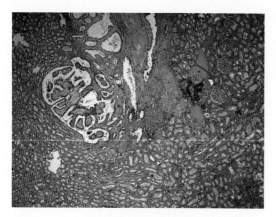

Fig. 2.11 Papillary adenoma comprises collection of papillae that are lined with cells with uniform small nuclei and inconspicuous nucleoli. The tumor size is less than 5 mm

is 1.7:1. Most cases are sporadic, although familial cases have been reported in association with BHD syndrome and familial renal oncocytoma syndrome.

Pathology

Oncocytoma is typically solitary, well circumscribed and has varying degrees of encapsulation (Fig. 2.12a). The cut surface exhibits a characteristic homogeneous mahogany-brown color. A central stellate scar can be seen in one-third of the cases, more commonly in larger tumors. More

than 10% of cases have multifocal or bilateral lesions.

Microscopically, oncocytoma is characterized by bright eosinophilic cells, termed oncocytes, arranged in nested, acinar or microcystic pattern associated with a loose hypocellular and hyalinized stroma (Fig. 2.12b). Extension of oncocytoma into the perinephric fat, or rarely into vascular space, can be found sometimes and does not adversely affect the benign prognosis of the lesion.

Molecular Genetics

Most oncocytomas are composed of a mixed population of cells with normal and abnormal karyotypes [63]. Combined loss of chromosomes 1 and X/Y is the most frequent chromosome abnormality. Translocations involving chromosome 11, with a breakpoint at 11q12-13, have also been reported. Other rare chromosome rearrangements have been reported, such as t(1;12) (p36;q13), loss of chromosome 14 and gain of chromosome 12 [64]. Oncocytoma can be a manifestation of BHD syndrome.

Whether oncocytoma and ChRCC are related is still controversial. They not only have overlapping morphological features but also share some cytogenetic changes, such as the loss of heterozygosity at chromosome 1 [65]. However, monosomy of chromosomes 2, 10, 13, 17, and 21 occurred exclusively in ChRCC [66].

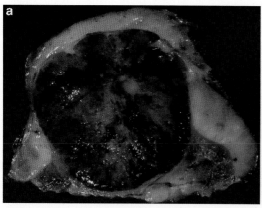
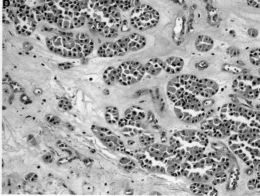

Fig. 2.12 Renal oncocytoma forms a solitary, well-circumscribed, nonencapsulated mass with homogeneous *dark-brown* cut surface (**a**). It consists of bright eosinophilic cells nested in a loose stroma. The tumor cells are uniform, round to polygonal with granular eosinophilic cytoplasm and regular round nuclei (**b**)

Pathological Prognosis Parameters for Renal Cell Carcinoma

Fuhrman Nuclear Grading

Currently, the four-tiered Fuhrman grading scheme, first described in 1982, remains the most commonly used grading system for RCC [67]. Fuhrman grade, based on the nuclear size and shape, chromatin and nucleolar prominence, is categorized into G1–4 (Table 2.4) (Fig. 2.13). Most studies have confirmed that Fuhrman nuclear grade is an independent prognostic predictor for CCRCC [68]. Simplified two-tiered (G1–2 vs. G3–4) or three-tiered (G1–2 vs. G3 vs. G4) Fuhrman systems have been proposed to improve interobserver agreement and still preserve its prognostic significance [69]. Grade 1 and grade 2 may be grouped together as low grade since the two are not prognostically different in multivariate analysis. However, studies have shown that grade 3 and grade 4 tumors should not be grouped together as grade 3 tumors have better 5-year cancer-specific survival than grade 4 tumors (45–65% in grade 3 cancers vs. 25–40% in grade 4 cancers). A recent study showed that the three-tiered Fuhrman grading system is an appropriate option for the prognostication of CCRCC in both univariate analysis and multivariate model setting [70]. The use of a simplified Fuhrman nuclear grading system in clinical practice requires further clarification and preferably a consensus between pathologists and urologists.

The prognostic value of Fuhrman grading for nonclear cell RCC, however, remains controversial. For PRCC, it is significantly associated with survival in univariate analysis but this significance is lost in multivariate models. One recent study demonstrated that only nucleolar prominence is significantly associated with survival in both univariate and multivariate analyses [71]. Another study showed that Fuhrman grade, not the nucleolar grade, is an independent prognostic factor and should be used as the standard grading system for PRCC [72]. Only a few studies addressed the prognostic significance of Fuhrman grading system for ChRCC using univariate analysis. A recent study found that Fuhrman grading does not correlate with survival, therefore is not appropriate for ChRCC [73]. A new grading system was recently proposed for ChRCC based on the assessment of geographic nuclear crowding and anaplasia. This grading scheme was shown to be an independent predictor of clinical outcomes for ChRCC [74].

Sarcomatoid and Rhabdoid Differentiation

Sarcomatoid differentiation is present in about 5% of RCCs and can be observed in any RCC subtype [75]. Therefore, sarcomatoid RCC is not considered a distinct subtype of RCC by 2004 WHO classification; rather, it is thought to represent a high-grade and poorly differentiated component.

RCC with sarcomatoid differentiation typically has other adverse pathological features, including large tumor size, extension into perinephric fat and vessels, and presence of hemorrhage and necrosis. It is also significantly associated with an increased likelihood of distant metastasis and cancer-specific death. It is an adverse independent prognostic indicator in both univariate and multivariate analyses [76]. Any

Table 2.4 Fuhrman nuclear grading system [67]

Grade	Nuclear size	Nuclear shape	Chromatin	Nucleoli
1	<10 μm	Round	Dense	Inconspicuous
2	15 μm	Round	Finely granular	Small, not visible at 10× magnification
3	20 μm	Round/oval	Coarsely granular	Prominent, visible at 10× magnification
4	>20 μm	Pleomorphic, multilobated	Open, hyperchromatic	Macronucleoli

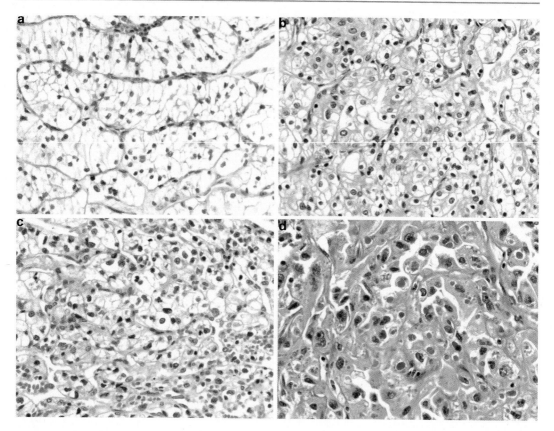

Fig. 2.13 Fuhrman grading system is based on the nuclear size, irregularity of the nuclear membrane and nucleolar prominence. Grade I RCC has uniformly small and dense nuclei (**a**). Grade 2 nuclei have smooth open chromatin but inconspicuous nucleoli (**b**). In grade 3 RCC, nuclei have open chromatin and prominent nucleoli visible at low magnification (**c**). Grade 4 nuclei are markedly pleomorphic, hyperchromatic with single or multiple macronucleoli (**d**)

RCC with sarcomatoid differentiation is assigned a Fuhrman grade 4.

Sarcomatoid components usually appear as bulging, lobulated areas with white to gray, firm and fibrous cut surface within a tumor (Fig. 2.14). Histologically, the sarcomatoid component ranges from malignant spindle cells to those resembling leiomyosarcoma, fibrosarcoma, angiosarcoma, rhabdomyosarcoma, and other sarcomas. The coexisting RCC component, including clear cell, papillary, chromophobe RCC and sometimes collecting duct RCC, can often to be identified and is used to subtype the RCC with sarcomatoid differentiation. However, such subtyping may not be possible if the sarcomatoid component overruns RCC epithelial components, a rare occurrence.

Rhabdoid differentiation can be identified in approximately 5% of RCCs with tumor cells having large eccentric nuclei, macronucleoli and prominent acidophilic globular cytoplasm (Fig. 2.15). The presence of rhabdoid component is also associated with high grade and high stage with frequent extrarenal extension. The rhabdoid foci may account for 5–90% of the tumor area. It is a marker of high risk for metastasis and poor prognosis even when the rhabdoid component is limited [77].

Tumor Necrosis

For CCRCC, tumor necrosis, identified either macroscopically or microscopically, is an adverse

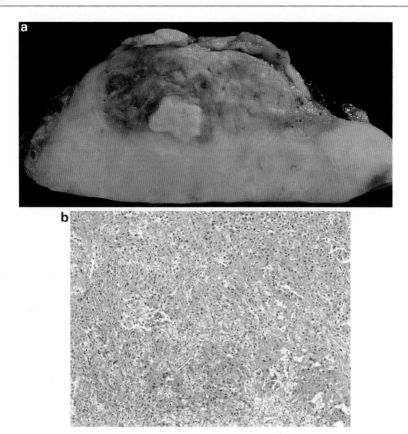

Fig. 2.14 Renal cell carcinoma with sarcomatoid differentiation. The *upper portion* of this renal tumor is *golden yellow*, characteristic of clear cell RCC. The *lower portion* has a fleshy appearance, suggestive of sarcomatoid differentiation (**a**). Microscopically the sarcomatoid component shows the malignant spindle cells (**b**)

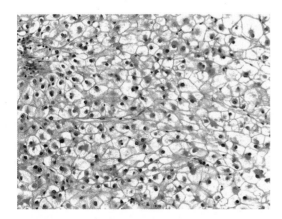

Fig. 2.15 Renal cell carcinoma with so-called "rhabdoid" morphology contains large eccentric nuclei, macronucleoli and prominent acidophilic globular cytoplasm

pathological factor and is associated with worse clinical outcomes in both uni- and multivariate analyses. Studies from Mayo Clinic clearly showed that histological necrosis is associated with twice the cancer-specific death rate compared to those without necrosis [5]. The presence and extent of histological necrosis in CCRCC are independent predictors of survival in localized but not metastatic cases, although one recent study showed limited prognostic value [78]. Two outcome prediction models, SSIGN from Mayo Clinic, and the postoperative outcome nomogram from MSKCC, both incorporate tumor necrosis in their models [79, 80]. A few recent studies also reported that the proportional extent of necrosis correlated with a worse cancer-specific death [81, 82]. The data on the prognostic role of tumor necrosis in nonclear cell RCC is limited.

Microvascular Invasion

Microvascular invasion (MVI), defined as neoplastic cells invading the vessel wall or neoplastic emboli in the intratumoral vessel detected microscopically, is present in 13.6–44.6% of RCC. It is more common in RCC of high stage and grade, and large size. An important prognostic factor in various malignancies including liver, testis, bladder and upper tract urothelial carcinoma, its prognostic role in RCC is controversial. Several studies have demonstrated that MVI may have an independent predictive role for either disease recurrence or cancer-specific mortality after adjusting for other clinical and pathologic covariates [83, 84]. Further studies are needed to better define its prognostic significance.

Summary

RCC encompasses a group of heterogeneous tumors with diverse clinical, pathological, and molecular characteristics as well as distinct prognosis and therapeutic responses. The current classification is based primarily on morphology but genetic features of renal tumors have been increasingly incorporated into the classification scheme. Many histological parameters obtained from routine pathological examination of renal tumor provide invaluable prognostic values. The clinical, pathological, and genetic features in combination will eventually enable urologists to predict individual tumor behavior and stratify patients into more sophisticated risk groups, ultimately rendering individualized management and treatment options.

References

1. Eble JN, Sauter G, Epstein JI, Sesterhenn IA. Pathology and genetics, tumors of the urinary system and male genital organs, vols 9–88. Lyon: IAPC Press; 2004.

2. Murphy WM, Grignon DG, Perlman EJ. Tumors of the kidney, bladder, and related urinary structures. Washington: American Registry of Pathology; 2004.

3. Cheng L, Zhang S, MacLennan GT, Lopez-Beltran A, Montironi R. Molecular and cytogenetic insights into the pathogenesis, classification, differential diagnosis, and prognosis of renal epithelial neoplasms. Hum Pathol. 2009;40:10–29.

4. Srigley JR, Delahunt B. Uncommon and recently described renal carcinomas. Mod Pathol. 2009;22 Suppl 2:S2–23.

5. Cheville JC, Lohse CM, Zincke H, Weaver AL, Blute ML. Comparisons of outcome and prognostic features among histologic subtypes of renal cell carcinoma. Am J Surg Pathol. 2003;27:612–24.

6. Cohen D, Zhou M. Molecular genetics of familial renal cell carcinoma syndromes. Clin Lab Med. 2005;25:259–77.

7. Rosner I, Bratslavsky G, Pinto PA, Linehan WM. The clinical implications of the genetics of renal cell carcinoma. Urol Oncol. 2009;27:131–6.

8. Strefford JC, Stasevich I, Lane TM, Lu YJ, Oliver T, Young BD. A combination of molecular cytogenetic analyses reveals complex genetic alterations in conventional renal cell carcinoma. Cancer Genet Cytogenet. 2005;159:1–9.

9. Hoglund M, Gisselsson D, Soller M, Hansen GB, Elfving P, Mitelman F. Dissecting karyotypic patterns in renal cell carcinoma: an analysis of the accumulated cytogenetic data. Cancer Genet Cytogenet. 2004;153:1–9.

10. Banks RE, Tirukonda P, Taylor C, et al. Genetic and epigenetic analysis of von Hippel–Lindau (VHL) gene alterations and relationship with clinical variables in sporadic renal cancer. Cancer Res. 2006;66:2000–11.

11. Gimenez-Bachs JM, Salinas-Sanchez AS, Sanchez-Sanchez F, et al. Determination of vhl gene mutations in sporadic renal cell carcinoma. Eur Urol. 2006;49:1051–7.

12. Gossage L, Eisen T. Alterations in VHL as potential biomarkers in renal-cell carcinoma. Nat Rev Clin Oncol. 2010;7:277–88.

13. Kaelin Jr WG. The von Hippel–Lindau tumor suppressor protein and clear cell renal carcinoma. Clin Cancer Res. 2007;13:680s–4.

14. Lane BR, Rini BI, Novick AC, Campbell SC. Targeted molecular therapy for renal cell carcinoma. Urology. 2007;69:3–10.

15. Linehan WM, Bratslavsky G, Pinto PA, et al. Molecular diagnosis and therapy of kidney cancer. Annu Rev Med. 2010;61:329–43.

16. Zbar B, Tory K, Merino M, et al. Hereditary papillary renal cell carcinoma. J Urol. 1994;151:561–6.

17. Launonen V, Vierimaa O, Kiuru M, et al. Inherited susceptibility to uterine leiomyomas and renal cell cancer. Proc Natl Acad Sci U S A. 2001;98:3387–92.

18. Delahunt B, Eble JN, McCredie MR, Bethwaite PB, Stewart JH, Bilous AM. Morphologic typing of papillary renal cell carcinoma: comparison of growth

kinetics and patient survival in 66 cases. Hum Pathol. 2001;32:590–5.

19. Brunelli M, Eble JN, Zhang S, Martignoni G, Cheng L. Gains of chromosomes 7, 17, 12, 16, and 20 and loss of Y occur early in the evolution of papillary renal cell neoplasia: a fluorescent in situ hybridization study. Mod Pathol. 2003;16:1053–9.

20. Jiang F, Richter J, Schraml P, et al. Chromosomal imbalances in papillary renal cell carcinoma: genetic differences between histological subtypes. Am J Pathol. 1998;153:1467–73.

21. Schraml P, Muller D, Bednar R, et al. Allelic loss at the D9S171 locus on chromosome 9p13 is associated with progression of papillary renal cell carcinoma. J Pathol. 2000;190:457–61.

22. Storkel S, Steart PV, Drenckhahn D, Thoenes W. The human chromophobe cell renal carcinoma: its probable relation to intercalated cells of the collecting duct. Virchows Arch B Cell Pathol Incl Mol Pathol. 1989;56:237–45.

23. Zbar B, Alvord WG, Glenn G, et al. Risk of renal and colonic neoplasms and spontaneous pneumothorax in the Birt–Hogg–Dube syndrome. Cancer Epidemiol Biomarkers Prev. 2002;11:393–400.

24. Adley BP, Smith ND, Nayar R, Yang XJ. Birt–Hogg–Dube syndrome: clinicopathologic findings and genetic alterations. Arch Pathol Lab Med. 2006;130:1865–70.

25. Thoenes W, Storkel S, Rumpelt HJ, Moll R, Baum HP, Werner S. Chromophobe cell renal carcinoma and its variants – a report on 32 cases. J Pathol. 1988;155:277–87.

26. Brunelli M, Eble JN, Zhang S, Martignoni G, Delahunt B, Cheng L. Eosinophilic and classic chromophobe renal cell carcinomas have similar frequent losses of multiple chromosomes from among chromosomes 1, 2, 6, 10, and 17, and this pattern of genetic abnormality is not present in renal oncocytoma. Mod Pathol. 2005;18:161–9.

27. Vira M, Linehan WM. Expanding the morphological and molecular genetic phenotype of kidney cancer. J Urol. 2007;177:10–1.

28. Al-Saleem T, Cairns P, Dulaimi EA, Feder M, Testa JR, Uzzo RG. The genetics of renal oncocytosis: a possible model for neoplastic progression. Cancer Genet Cytogenet. 2004;152:23–8.

29. Suzigan S, Lopez-Beltran A, Montironi R, et al. Multilocular cystic renal cell carcinoma: a report of 45 cases of a kidney tumor of low malignant potential. Am J Clin Pathol. 2006;125:217–22.

30. Halat S, Eble JN, Grignon DJ, et al. Multilocular cystic renal cell carcinoma is a subtype of clear cell renal cell carcinoma. Mod Pathol. 2010;23:931–6.

31. Antonelli A, Portesi E, Cozzoli A, et al. The collecting duct carcinoma of the kidney: a cytogenetical study. Eur Urol. 2003;43:680–5.

32. Karakiewicz PI, Trinh QD, Rioux-Leclercq N, et al. Collecting duct renal cell carcinoma: a matched analysis of 41 cases. Eur Urol. 2007;52:1140–5.

33. Tokuda N, Naito S, Matsuzaki O, et al. Collecting duct (bellini duct) renal cell carcinoma: a nationwide survey in Japan. J Urol. 2006;176:40–3 [discussion 43].

34. Selli C, Amorosi A, Vona G, et al. Retrospective evaluation of c-erbB-2 oncogene amplification using competitive PCR in collecting duct carcinoma of the kidney. J Urol. 1997;158:245–7.

35. Leitao VA, da Silva Jr W, Ferreira U, Denardi F, Billis A, Rodrigues Netto Jr N. Renal medullary carcinoma. case report and review of the literature. Urol Int. 2006;77:184–6.

36. Watanabe IC, Billis A, Guimaraes MS, et al. Renal medullary carcinoma: report of seven cases from brazil. Mod Pathol. 2007;20:914–20.

37. Argani P, Ladanyi M. Renal carcinomas associated with Xp11.2 translocations/TFE3 gene fusions. In: Eble J, Sauter G, Epstein J, et al., editors. World Health Organization classification of tumours: pathology and genetics of tumors of the urinary system & male genital organs. Lyon: IARC; 2004. p. 37–8.

38. Argani P, Olgac S, Tickoo SK, et al. Xp11 translocation renal cell carcinoma in adults: expanded clinical, pathologic, and genetic spectrum. Am J Surg Pathol. 2007;31:1149–60.

39. Armah HB, Parwani AV. Xp11.2 translocation renal cell carcinoma. Arch Pathol Lab Med. 2010;134:124–9.

40. Argani P, Lal P, Hutchinson B, Lui MY, Reuter VE, Ladanyi M. Aberrant nuclear immunoreactivity for TFE3 in neoplasms with TFE3 gene fusions: a sensitive and specific immunohistochemical assay. Am J Surg Pathol. 2003;27:750–61.

41. Ross H, Argani P. Xp11 translocation renal cell carcinoma. Pathology. 2010;42:369–73.

42. Argani P, Antonescu CR, Illei PB, et al. Primary renal neoplasms with the ASPL-TFE3 gene fusion of alveolar soft part sarcoma: a distinctive tumor entity previously included among renal cell carcinomas of children and adolescents. Am J Pathol. 2001;159:179–92.

43. Argani P, Antonescu CR, Couturier J, et al. PRCC-TFE3 renal carcinomas: morphologic, immunohistochemical, ultrastructural, and molecular analysis of an entity associated with the t(X;1)(p11.2;q21). Am J Surg Pathol. 2002;26:1553–66.

44. Fine SW, Argani P, DeMarzo AM, et al. Expanding the histologic spectrum of mucinous tubular and spindle cell carcinoma of the kidney. Am J Surg Pathol. 2006;30:1554–60.

45. Yang G, Breyer BN, Weiss DA, MacLennan GT. Mucinous tubular and spindle cell carcinoma of the kidney. J Urol. 2010;183:738–9.

46. Cossu-Rocca P, Eble JN, Delahunt B, et al. Renal mucinous tubular and spindle carcinoma lacks the gains of chromosomes 7 and 17 and losses of chromosome Y that are prevalent in papillary renal cell carcinoma. Mod Pathol. 2006;19:488–93.

47. Brandal P, Lie AK, Bassarova A, et al. Genomic aberrations in mucinous tubular and spindle cell renal cell carcinomas. Mod Pathol. 2006;19:186–94.

48. Eble JN. Mucinous tubular and spindle cell carcinoma and post-neuroblastoma carcinoma: newly recognised entities in the renal cell carcinoma family. Pathology. 2003;35:499–504.

49. Argani P. The evolving story of renal translocation carcinomas. Am J Clin Pathol. 2006;126:332–4.

50. Zhou M, Yang XJ, Lopez JI, et al. Renal tubulocystic carcinoma is closely related to papillary renal cell carcinoma: implications for pathologic classification. Am J Surg Pathol. 2009;33:1840–9.

51. Amin MB, MacLennan GT, Gupta R, et al. Tubulocystic carcinoma of the kidney: clinicopathologic analysis of 31 cases of a distinctive rare subtype of renal cell carcinoma. Am J Surg Pathol. 2009;33:384–92.

52. Osunkoya AO, Young AN, Wang W, Netto GJ, Epstein JI. Comparison of gene expression profiles in tubulocystic carcinoma and collecting duct carcinoma of the kidney. Am J Surg Pathol. 2009;33:1103–6.

53. Aydin H, Chen L, Cheng L, et al. Clear cell tubulopapillary renal cell carcinoma: a study of 36 distinctive low-grade epithelial tumors of the kidney. Am J Surg Pathol. 2010;34:1608–21.

54. Amin MB, Gupta R, Ondrej H, et al. Primary thyroid-like follicular carcinoma of the kidney: report of 6 cases of a histologically distinctive adult renal epithelial neoplasm. Am J Surg Pathol. 2009;33:393–400.

55. Pan CC, Chen YJ, Chang LC, Chang YH, Ho DM. Immunohistochemical and molecular genetic profiling of acquired cystic disease-associated renal cell carcinoma. Histopathology. 2009;55:145–53.

56. Coleman JA, Russo P. Hereditary and familial kidney cancer. Curr Opin Urol. 2009;19:478–85.

57. Lubensky IA, Schmidt L, Zhuang Z, et al. Hereditary and sporadic papillary renal carcinomas with c-met mutations share a distinct morphological phenotype. Am J Pathol. 1999;155:517–26.

58. Giubellino A, Linehan WM, Bottaro DP. Targeting the met signaling pathway in renal cancer. Expert Rev Anticancer Ther. 2009;9:785–93.

59. Sudarshan S, Pinto PA, Neckers L, Linehan WM. Mechanisms of disease: hereditary leiomyomatosis and renal cell cancer – a distinct form of hereditary kidney cancer. Nat Clin Pract Urol. 2007;4:104–10.

60. Murakami T, Sano F, Huang Y, et al. Identification and characterization of Birt–Hogg–Dube associated renal carcinoma. J Pathol. 2007;211:524–31.

61. Grignon DJ, Eble JN. Papillary and metanephric adenomas of the kidney. Semin Diagn Pathol. 1998;15:41–53.

62. Wang KL, Weinrach DM, Luan C, et al. Renal papillary adenoma – a putative precursor of papillary renal cell carcinoma. Hum Pathol. 2007;38:239–46.

63. Brown JA, Takahashi S, Alcaraz A, et al. Fluorescence in situ hybridization analysis of renal oncocytoma reveals frequent loss of chromosomes Y and 1. J Urol. 1996;156:31–5.

64. Yusenko MV. Molecular pathology of renal oncocytoma: a review. Int J Urol. 2010;17:602–12.

65. Cochand-Priollet B, Molinie V, Bougaran J, et al. Renal chromophobe cell carcinoma and oncocytoma. A comparative morphologic, histochemical, and immunohistochemical study of 124 cases. Arch Pathol Lab Med. 1997;121:1081–6.

66. Yusenko MV, Kuiper RP, Boethe T, Ljungberg B, van Kessel AG, Kovacs G. High-resolution DNA copy number and gene expression analyses distinguish chromophobe renal cell carcinomas and renal oncocytomas. BMC Cancer. 2009;9:152.

67. Fuhrman SA, Lasky LC, Limas C. Prognostic significance of morphologic parameters in renal cell carcinoma. Am J Surg Pathol. 1982;6:655–63.

68. Novara G, Martignoni G, Artibani W, Ficarra V. Grading systems in renal cell carcinoma. J Urol. 2007;177:430–6.

69. Rioux-Leclercq N, Karakiewicz PI, Trinh QD, et al. Prognostic ability of simplified nuclear grading of renal cell carcinoma. Cancer. 2007;109:868–74.

70. Hong SK, Jeong CW, Park JH, et al. Application of simplified Fuhrman grading system in clear-cell renal cell carcinoma. BJU Int. 2010;107:409–15.

71. Sika-Paotonu D, Bethwaite PB, McCredie MR, William Jordan T, Delahunt B. Nucleolar grade but not Fuhrman grade is applicable to papillary renal cell carcinoma. Am J Surg Pathol. 2006;30:1091–6.

72. Klatte T, Anterasian C, Said JW, et al. Fuhrman grade provides higher prognostic accuracy than nucleolar grade for papillary renal cell carcinoma. J Urol. 2010;183:2143–7.

73. Delahunt B, Sika-Paotonu D, Bethwaite PB, et al. Fuhrman grading is not appropriate for chromophobe renal cell carcinoma. Am J Surg Pathol. 2007;31:957–60.

74. Paner GP, Amin MB, Alvarado-Cabrero I, et al. A novel tumor grading scheme for chromophobe renal cell carcinoma: prognostic utility and comparison with fuhrman nuclear grade. Am J Surg Pathol. 2010;34:1233–40.

75. de Peralta-Venturina M, Moch H, Amin M, et al. Sarcomatoid differentiation in renal cell carcinoma: a study of 101 cases. Am J Surg Pathol. 2001;25:275–84.

76. Cheville JC, Lohse CM, Zincke H, et al. Sarcomatoid renal cell carcinoma: an examination of underlying histologic subtype and an analysis of associations with patient outcome. Am J Surg Pathol. 2004;28:435–41.

77. Gokden N, Nappi O, Swanson PE, et al. Renal cell carcinoma with rhabdoid features. Am J Surg Pathol. 2000;24:1329–38.

78. Isbarn H, Patard JJ, Lughezzani G, et al. Limited prognostic value of tumor necrosis in patients with renal cell carcinoma. Urology. 2010;75:1378–84.

79. Frank I, Blute ML, Cheville JC, Lohse CM, Weaver AL, Zincke H. An outcome prediction model for patients with clear cell renal cell carcinoma treated with radical nephrectomy based on tumor stage, size, grade and necrosis: the SSIGN score. J Urol. 2002;168:2395–400.

80. Sorbellini M, Kattan MW, Snyder ME, et al. A postoperative prognostic nomogram predicting recurrence for patients with conventional clear cell renal cell carcinoma. J Urol. 2005;173:48–51.

81. Klatte T, Said JW, de Martino M, et al. Presence of tumor necrosis is not a significant predictor of survival in clear cell renal cell carcinoma: higher prognostic

accuracy of extent based rather than presence/absence classification. J Urol. 2009;181:1558–64 [discussion 1563–4].

82. Katz MD, Serrano MF, Grubb 3rd RL, et al. Percent microscopic tumor necrosis and survival after curative surgery for renal cell carcinoma. J Urol. 2010;183: 909–14.

83. Antunes AA, Srougi M, Dall'Oglio MF, et al. Microvascular invasion is an independent prognostic factor in patients with prostate cancer treated with radical prostatectomy. Int Braz J Urol. 2006;32:668–75 [discussion 675–7].

84. Madbouly K, Al-Qahtani SM, Ghazwani Y, Al-Shaibani S, Mansi MK. Microvascular tumor invasion: prognostic significance in low-stage renal cell carcinoma. Urology. 2007;69:670–4.

Familial Renal Cell Carcinoma

3

Simon P. Kim and Bradley C. Leibovich

Introduction

Recently our understanding of the biologic mechanisms underlying the development of renal cell carcinoma (RCC) has undergone a remarkable evolution. Extensive research on familial kidney cancer has served as the basis for better understanding of the pathology and molecular genetics of this malignancy. This has in turn facilitated the introduction of novel targeted therapeutic agents that continue to change and refine the clinical management for both familial and sporadic forms of this malignancy.

RCC represents the prototypical example of a malignancy in which discoveries related to the familial syndromic forms of this malignancy have transformed treatment paradigms. It is therefore paramount to have a critical understanding of the genetic mechanisms in hereditary kidney cancer given the high prevalence of these genetic abnormalities that have been identified in sporadic cases. To date, four forms of familial kidney cancer have been well characterized: (1) von Hippel–Lindau (VHL); (2) hereditary papillary renal cell carcinoma (HPRCC); (3) Birt–Hogg–Dubè (BHD); and (4) hereditary leiomyomatosis renal cell carcinoma (HLRCC). Each of these heredi-

tary familial cancer syndromes has distinct clinical manifestations and treatment challenges. Herewith, we will provide an overview of the genetics, clinical syndromes, and management of hereditary kidney cancer syndromes.

Overview

In 2010, approximately 58,240 patients were diagnosed with RCC, which remains one of the most lethal of the common urologic malignancies [1]. Although most patients diagnosed with RCC present with sporadic unilateral tumors, approximately 3–4% of incident cases are due to familial kidney cancer syndromes [2]. At present, four hereditary RCC syndromes have been well characterized with each having a clearly identified genetic abnormality responsible for the specific histologic subtype of RCC and unique clinical manifestations (Table 3.1).

von Hippel–Lindau Disease

VHL is an autosomal dominant hereditary RCC syndrome in which affected individuals develop clear cell RCC. Though the prevalence of VHL has been estimated to affect approximately 1 in every 36,000 individuals, it is the most common form of familial RCC [3]. The molecular genetics of VHL has important implications in both the familial and sporadic forms of clear cell RCC [4, 5]. VHL gene mutation has clinically relevant

S.P. Kim, MD, MPH • B.C. Leibovich, MD (✉)
Department of Urology, Mayo Clinic, 200 First Street
SW, Rochester, MN 55905, USA
e-mail: Leibovich.Bradley@mayo.edu

Table 3.1 Hereditary familial RCC syndromes

Syndrome	Genetic element (location)	Gene product	Patterns of inheritance	Type of RCC and manifestation
von Hippel–Lindau	VHL gene (3p25-26)	pVHL	Autosomal dominant	Clear cell RCC Solid and/or cystic Multiple and bilateral
Hereditary papillary RCC	c-MET proto-oncogene (7q31)	MET	Autosomal dominant	Type I papillary RCC Multiple and bilateral renal tumors
Birt–Hogg–Dubè	BHD gene (17p12q11)	Folliculin	Autosomal dominant	Hybrid oncocytyic RCC Chromophobe RCC Oncocytoma Clear cell RCC
Familial leiomyatosis RCC	FLCN (1.q42.3-q43)	Fumarate hydratase	Autosomal dominant	Type II papillary RCC Solitary and aggressive

implications in sporadic cases, as mutation has been associated with improved survival compared to cases without the VHL mutation [6–9]. It is also noteworthy that the VHL mutation is specific to clear cell RCC and has not been identified in the remaining histologic subtypes [10–14].

Through molecular genetic linkage analysis of affected families, the gene mutation responsible for the familial form of clear cell RCC has been identified as the VHL tumor suppressor gene (Fig. 3.1). The VHL gene, which has been located at chromosome 3p.25-26, has been fully sequenced and encodes a 213 amino acid protein. The VHL gene produces a protein that binds elongins B and C and Cul2, forming a protein complex that facilitates ubiquitin-mediated degradation of hypoxia-inducible factors (HIF-1α and HIF-2α) [15–17]. HIFs function as critically important intracellular proteins in regulating the cellular response to hypoxia and stress. Under conditions of hypoxia, there is an accumulation of HIF proteins causing an upregulation in the transcription of epidermal growth factor receptor (EGFR), glucose transporter (GLUT-1), platelet-derived growth factor (PDGF), and vascular endothelial growth factors (VEGFs). All of these downstream mediators play an adaptive role under hypoxic conditions. Under normoxic conditions and a normal functioning VHL gene, HIF-1α and HIF-2α are hydroxylated through an oxygen-mediated process by HIF prolyl hydroxlase (HPH). Hydroxylated HIFs are readily recognized and bound by the VHL protein complex and targeted for degradation. However,

inactivation of the VHL gene leads to accumulation of HIF-α, resulting in increased production of downstream products, such as EGFR, GLUT-1, PDGF, and VEGF [18–20]. It is the dysregulation of this process that results in the angiogenesis and tumorigenesis responsible for the development of clear cell RCC.

The clinical criteria for the diagnosis of VHL syndrome are based on the presence of one or more major manifestations and/or a family history of VHL disease (Table 3.2). The major manifestations of VHL include clear cell RCC, pheochromocytoma, retinal angiomas, and central nervous system hemangioblastomas (brainstem, cerebellum, or spinal cord). Evaluation of affected families has demonstrated that two types of the VHL syndrome exist and each has varying degrees of tumor risk in the CNS and visceral organs [21]. Molecular differences in the type of mutation in the VHL gene contribute to the heterogeneity of clinical findings and the varying degrees of expression in the two types of VHL (Table 3.3) [22–26].

In type 1 VHL, individuals carrying the gene mutation have increased risks of clear cell RCC, CNS hemangioblastomas, and pancreatic endocrine tumors or cysts, but a low risk in the development of pheochromocytoma. Type 1 is also the most common form of VHL, accounting for 75% of familial cases. Mutations for type 1 VHL are due to partial or complete deletion and nonsense, missense, and frame shift mutations, thereby altering the ability of the VHL to bind to elongin C and preventing HIF degradation [27].

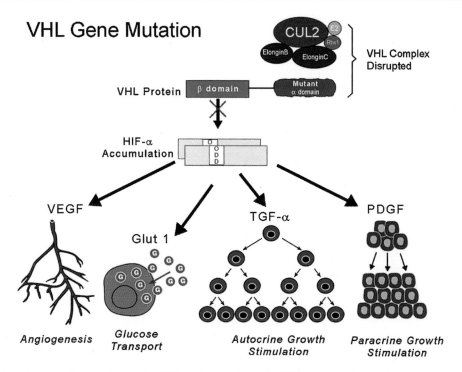

Fig. 3.1 Molecular pathway and targeting VHL pathway in clear cell renal carcinoma. A mutation in the VHL gene prevents binding to elongin B and C causing an intracellular accumulation of hypoxia-inducible factors (HIF). Under hypoxia, HIF-1α accumulates and promotes downstream production of vascular endothelial growth factors (VEGFs), glucose transporters (GLUT-1), transforming growth factor (TGF-α), and platelet-derived growth factor (PDGF) [2]

Table 3.2 Clinical criteria for a diagnosis of familial VHL disease

Patients with a family history of VHL and
One major manifestation
Central nervous system hemangioblastoma
Retinal angiomas
Pheochromocytoma
Clear cell RCC
Patients without a family history and
Two major manifestations
Two or more central nervous system hemangioblastoma
One hemangioblastoma and pheochromocytoma or clear cell RCC

Type 2 VHL has been further subdivided into three distinct phenotypic subtypes (2A, 2B, and 2C) based on the different clinical manifestations and types of mutation resulting in HIF accumulation. All three subgroups in type 2 VHL are caused by missense mutations in the VHL gene and carry a high predisposition of pheochromocytoma. VHL types 2A and 2B also share a high risk for CNS hemangioblastomas, but differ in that VHL type 2B carries a high risk of clear cell RCC while type 2A does not. Type 2B is associated with a high risk pancreatic endocrine tumors and cysts. Type 2C is unique in that the only visceral organ at risk is the adrenal gland (pheochromocytoma).

Hereditary Papillary Renal Cell Carcinoma

In 1994, HPRCC was described as another hereditary renal cancer syndrome, in which affected families were reported to have an increased risk of bilateral multifocal tumors with type I papillary renal carcinoma histologic subtype [28]. HPRCC is a rare autosomal dominant familial kidney cancer with the only phenotypic manifestation occurring in the kidney [23, 28]. The causal genetic mechanism of HPRCC has been identified

Table 3.3 Major manifestations by genotype–phenotype correlations for VHL disease

VHL type	Genotype	Phenotype
Type I	Deletion, truncation	High risk of clear cell RCC Low risk of pheochromocytoma High risk of CNS hemangioblastoma Pancreatic endocrine tumor or cyst
Type 2		
2A	Missense	High risk of pheochromocytoma Low risk of clear cell RCC High risk of CNS hemangioblastoma
2B	Missense	High risk of pheochromocytoma High risk of clear cell RCC Pancreatic endocrine tumor and cyst
2C	Missense	High risk of pheochromocytoma

as a proto-oncogene, the MET gene, located on the chromosome 7q31.3 [29–31].

The function of the protein encoded by the MET gene has been defined as a transmembrane tyrosine kinase receptor with hepatocyte growth factor, also located on chromosome 7, identified as the ligand for activation [32]. Activation of the tyrosine kinase receptor by a gain-of-function mutation in the MET gene leads to unregulated proliferation and growth. It is this molecular mechanism that results in familial HPRC and a small subset (approximately 10%) of sporadic type 1 papillary RCC. Mutations in the MET gene also lead to upregulation of HIFα, although HIF-α promotion in this instance is due to a VHL independent pathway.

In the clinical manifestations for HPRCC, the MET gene mutation causes a high propensity for bilateral, multifocal type I papillary renal carcinoma in young adulthood [33]. Of all the hereditary kidney cancer syndromes, HPRCC has the highest degree of penetration, such that 90% of affected individuals develop multiple tumors with type I papillary RCC histology over the course of a lifetime [30]. It has been shown that HPRCC patients will go onto develop an average of 3,400 microscopic papillary tumors per kidney [34].

Birt–Hogg–Dubè Syndrome

BHD is a rare autosomal dominant inherited familial RCC syndrome with an estimated preva-lence of 1 in every 200,000 individuals. Although BHD was first described based on the classic dermatologic presentation of fibrofolliculomas in 1977, it was later documented that these individuals were also at increased risk for developing multiple renal tumors and pulmonary cysts, which manifest as a spontaneous pneumothorax [35–38]. The risk of renal tumors varies among families with BHD. Investigators have documented that 25–35% of affected individuals will ultimately develop renal tumors [36, 38–40]. The pathologic features of renal tumors in individuals with BHD have been shown to have several different types of histologic features. Pavlovich and colleagues documented that a majority of renal tumors in BHD consist of an oncocytic-hybrid, which was initially described as a chromophobe-oncocytoma renal carcinoma (50%), followed by chromophobe renal carcinoma (34%), clear cell carcinoma (9%), oncocytoma (5%), and papillary renal carcinoma (2%).

The folliculin (FLCN) gene on the short arm of chromosome 17p11.2 is now established as the germline mutation responsible for BHD [41, 42]. The FLCN gene contains 14 exons and encodes the folliculin protein that has been hypothesized to function as a tumor suppressor gene. However, its function in the pathogenesis of BHD has yet to be fully elucidated. Baba and colleagues identified folliculin-interacting protein1 (FNIP1) that facilitates phosphorylation of folliculin and interacts with 5′ AMP-activated protein kinase (AMPK). This pathway serves to functions as a negative regulator of the mTOR pathway [43]. mTOR appears to modulate folliculin since blockade of AMPK or MTOR will inhibit folliculin phosphorylation by FNIP1. These findings suggest that mTOR inhibitors may have efficacy in the treatment of renal carcinoma in patients with BHD.

Given the various organ systems affected and differing degrees of phenotypic expression within each organ system, a validated and accepted diagnostic criteria system for BHD would facilitate ease of diagnosis and a uniform measure of disease severity. While a formal clinical criteria for identifying individuals considered to be likely carriers of BHD has yet to be established or validated, Menko and colleagues recently proposed a clinical classification to further facilitate recognition and diagnosis of this uncommon hereditary kidney cancer syndrome (Table 3.4) [39]. The diagnostic criteria have two components—major and minor criteria. In the major criteria, an individual will have at least five fibrofolliculomas

Table 3.4 Major and minor diagnostic criteria for BHD

Major criteria
Five or more fibrofolliculomas
Pathogenic FCLN germline mutation
Minor criteria
Multiple bilateral lung cysts located at the base
Renal cell carcinoma with early age onset (<50 years)
First-degree relative with BHD syndrome

(Fig. 3.2), one of which is histologically confirmed; or a pathogenic *FCLN* mutation. The minor criteria may be one or more of the following: multiple lung cysts that are located at the base of each lung bilaterally; early multifocal or bilateral renal carcinoma of early age onset or renal carcinoma with a histology consistent of mixed chromophobe renal carcinoma and oncocytoma; or a first-degree relative with BHD.

Pulmonary cysts will present with spontaneous pneumothorax and are the most commonly observed clinical feature in BHD. Approximately 80% of BHD individuals will have pulmonary cysts on CT of the chest. While spontaneous pneumothorax has been traditionally described in apical pulmonary cysts, BHD individuals have a 50 times higher rate of pneumothorax due to large basal pulmonary cysts [36]. Toro and colleagues have estimated that the prevalence of pneumothorax in BHD is 24% with a median age of presentation of 38 years [39, 45]. The clinical appearance of the pulmonary cysts has been characterized histologically as emphysematous changes [46, 47].

Individuals suspected to have BHD, even those who have unclear clinical presentations, should undergo genetic testing for the FCLN (folliculin mutation) or referral to a medical geneticist. Detection of an FCLN mutation is pathognomonic and confirmatory in the diagnosis of BHD. Moreover, genetic testing is essential

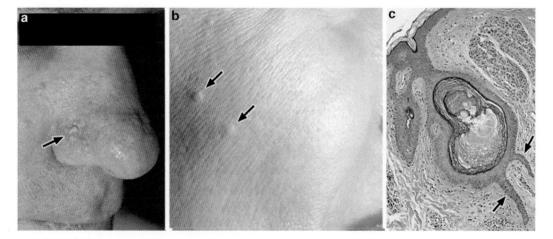

Fig. 3.2 Cutaneous lesions and histology of fibrofolliculomas in Birt–Hogg–Dubè syndrome [44]

given the clinical variability of BHD and the need to test family members due to the autosomal dominant transmission.

Hereditary Leiomyomatosis Renal Cell Carcinoma

HLRCC is a familial kidney cancer syndrome distinctly different from others in that the associated renal tumors typically behave aggressively, with a propensity for early metastasis from small solitary renal tumors. In this syndrome, affected individuals have an increased risk of developing cutaneous and uterine leiomyomas and type II papillary renal carcinoma. HLRCC was initially described as multiple cutaneous and uterine syndrome, or reed syndrome in 1972 [48]. In the original description, the clinical findings of uterine and cutaneous leiomyomas were the only manifestations initially reported. In 2001, however, Launonen and colleagues demonstrated that Reed Syndrome was also associated with type II papillary renal carcinoma and further localized the genetic mutation as a loss of chromosome 1q through genetic linkage

analysis among 11 affected family members [49]. It was later determined that the genetic aberration in HPRCC resulted in loss of function of the fumarate hydratase (FH) gene, located on the chromosome 1q42. -q43 [50].

FH is a Krebs cycle enzyme and is typical for genetic mutations in RCC in that it affects metabolic pathways. Mutation of FH leads to a VHL independent accumulation of HIF-α and its associated downstream products. FH mutations have been established as the major molecular pathway responsible for HPRCC, since this mutation has been identified in more than 90% of clinically affected individuals. Under normal conditions, HIF-α is degraded by HPH and fumarate is converted to malate by FH. However, fumarate and HIF-α directly compete for the same binding site of HPH, and a mutation in FH causes fumarate to accumulate and bind to HPH, thereby preventing hydroxylation and subsequent degradation of HIF (Fig. 3.3). As a result, mutations in FH create a pseudohypoxic environment, where accumulation of intracellular HIF leads to the same downstream products from VHL, although through an independent pathway [52].

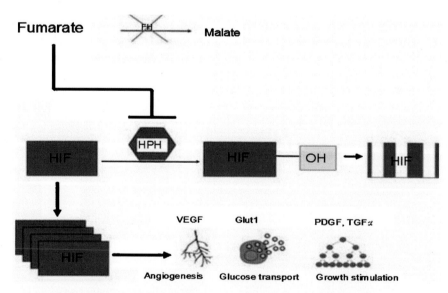

Fig. 3.3 Molecular pathway in HLRCC. Mutations in fumarate hydratase (FH), a critical enzyme in the Kreb cycle, cause an accumulation of fumarate and compete with HIF for HIF prolyl hydroxlase (HPH), thereby creating a pseudohypoxic state. This causes an increase in intracellular HIF and downstream transcription of vascular endothelial growth factor (VEGF), glucose transporter (GLUT-1), platelet-derived growth factor (PDGF), and transforming growth factor (TGF-α) [51]

In HPRCC, the phenotypic expression involves cutaneous and uterine leiomyomas and type II papillary renal carcinoma. Historically, the classic presentation is that of young female who may undergo hysterectomy for multiple large leiomyomas. It is also noteworthy that uterine leiomyomas due to HPRCC have low malignant potential for leiomyosarcoma [49, 53, 54]. Leiomyomas also present as a dermatologic manifestation. Cutaneous leiomyomas are often painful and located on the torso or extremities in a grouped, segmental, or disseminated and segmental pattern, affecting 80% of individuals with HPRCC [55]. While HPRCC has been shown to have a high prevalence in the phenotypic expression of uterine and cutaneous leiomyomas, the degree of penetration of renal tumors with type II papillary renal carcinoma is lower. It has been estimated that approximately 15% of affected individuals will develop type II papillary renal carcinoma in HLRCC [49, 53–55].

Management of renal masses in HLRCC is unique from the other familial renal cancer syndromes due to the highly aggressive nature of the solitary small renal tumors with type II papillary RCC histology and predilection for early metastasis [56]. As a result, immediate aggressive surgical intervention is recommended for renal tumors in patients with HLRCC.

Management

Surgical Treatment

Current recommendations in the management of renal masses in familial kidney cancer syndromes (with the exception of HLRCC) are based on the observation that these tumors have little metastatic potential when under 3 cm in size [57]. Consequently, patients should be observed with serial imaging until one or more tumors approach a size threshold of 3 cm to initiate surgical intervention, or rapid increases in renal tumor size are noted on interval imaging. Delaying intervention until renal tumors reach the size threshold minimizes the frequency of surgery and treatment related morbidity.

Nephron-sparing surgery remains the mainstay in the urologic management of patients with renal cancer syndromes for multiple reasons. Patients with inherited syndromes resulting in renal tumors tend to present early in life and most will have multiple renal tumors over their lifetime. For example, patients with VHL are at risk for developing over 1,000 cysts and 600 tumors per kidney, while patients with HPRCC may have up to 3,000 renal tumors per kidney [34, 58, 59]. While patients undergoing kidney surgery for renal carcinoma have other competing risks of cancer and chronic renal insufficiency from surgical extirpation, there is increasing evidence to suggest that nephron-sparing surgery may reduce the risk of chronic renal insufficiency and mortality [60–65]. Although existing studies in the surgical management of familial kidney cancer are limited to single institution, retrospective series, Herring and colleagues reported that a large proportion of patients with VHL, HPRCC, or BHD avoided stage V chronic kidney disease and dialysis by undergoing multiple parenchymal-sparing surgeries [57, 66, 67].

With patients likely to require multiple surgeries over a lifetime, minimally invasive treatment with ablation also has been evaluated in individuals with hereditary renal cancer syndromes in order to reduce morbidity and complications associated with open surgery. Though a large prospective study evaluating the effectiveness of ablation of renal tumors among individuals with familial kidney cancer syndromes has yet to be undertaken, several smaller cohort studies suggest that percutaneous radio frequency ablation can be performed safely and offers some efficacy following short-term and intermediate follow-up with limited complications [68, 69]. Further studies with longer follow-up are needed to determine the long-term effectiveness of ablation in patients with hereditary forms of RCC (with exception to HLRCC).

Although delaying surgical intervention until the size threshold of 3 cm and nephron-sparing surgery is the current recommended treatment for most familial kidney cancer syndromes, the surgical treatment for HLRCC differs given the highly aggressive nature of the associated renal tumors and early risk of metastasis [56]. These patients should have early and aggressive surgical resection. Although the clinical benefit of a lymph node dissection is debatable for patients diagnosed with HLRCC, most of these patients should undergo a radical nephrectomy at a minimum given the highly aggressive nature of these associated renal tumors.

Conclusion

Although familial kidney cancer syndromes occur infrequently, our understanding of the molecular mechanism responsible for the clinical manifestations has led to advances in novel targeted agents and altered the management of metastatic disease for all patients. It is also important to understand the unique clinical challenges and differences in the surgical management of renal masses among individuals with familial kidney cancer. Since there remains a significant risk of recurrent multifocal renal tumors, expectant management with serial imaging until the renal mass reaches ≥3 cm in size and nephron-sparing surgery are the key features in the surgical management for most familial kidney cancer syndromes with exception to HLRCC-associated tumors. Given the highly aggressive nature of renal tumors associated with HLRCC, early surgical intervention with a radical nephrectomy and lymph node dissection is recommended. In the future, targeted agents may also play an important role in reducing renal recurrences for individuals affected by familial kidney cancer syndromes. Though clinical guidelines for hereditary RCC syndromes have yet be developed, the ideal clinical management should be undertaken at institutions with a high volume of clinical experience using a multidisciplinary approach with urologists, medical oncologists, and medical geneticists.

References

1. Jemal A, Siegel R, Xu J, Ward E. Cancer statistics, 2010. CA Cancer J Clin. 2010;60(5):277–300.
2. Pfaffenroth EC, Linehan WM. Genetic basis for kidney cancer: opportunity for disease-specific approaches to therapy. Expert Opin Biol Ther. 2008;8(6):779–90.
3. Maher ER, Iselius L, Yates JR, et al. Von Hippel–Lindau disease: a genetic study. J Med Genet. 1991;28(7):443–7.
4. Latif F, Tory K, Gnarra J, et al. Identification of the von Hippel–Lindau disease tumor suppressor gene. Science. 1993;260(5112):1317–20.
5. Stolle C, Glenn G, Zbar B, et al. Improved detection of germline mutations in the von Hippel–Lindau disease tumor suppressor gene. Hum Mutat. 1998;12(6):417–23.
6. Yao M, Yoshida M, Kishida T, et al. VHL tumor suppressor gene alterations associated with good prognosis in sporadic clear-cell renal carcinoma. J Natl Cancer Inst. 2002;94(20):1569–75.
7. Kim HL, Seligson D, Liu X, et al. Using tumor markers to predict the survival of patients with metastatic renal cell carcinoma. J Urol. 2005;173(5):1496–501.
8. Patard JJ, Rioux-Leclercq N, Masson D, et al. Absence of VHL gene alteration and high VEGF expression are associated with tumour aggressiveness and poor survival of renal-cell carcinoma. Br J Cancer. 2009;101(8):1417–24.
9. Patard JJ, Fergelot P, Karakiewicz PI, et al. Low CAIX expression and absence of VHL gene mutation are associated with tumor aggressiveness and poor survival of clear cell renal cell carcinoma. Int J Cancer. 2008;123(2):395–400.
10. Maher ER, Yates JR. Familial renal cell carcinoma: clinical and molecular genetic aspects. Br J Cancer. 1991;63(2):176–9.
11. Gnarra JR, Tory K, Weng Y, et al. Mutations of the VHL tumour suppressor gene in renal carcinoma. Nat Genet. 1994;7(1):85–90.
12. Shuin T, Kondo K, Torigoe S, et al. Frequent somatic mutations and loss of heterozygosity of the von Hippel–Lindau tumor suppressor gene in primary human renal cell carcinomas. Cancer Res. 1994;54(11):2852–5.
13. Neumann HP, Bender BU, Berger DP, et al. Prevalence, morphology and biology of renal cell carcinoma in von Hippel–Lindau disease compared to sporadic renal cell carcinoma. J Urol. 1998;160(4):1248–54.
14. Nickerson ML, Jaeger E, Shi Y, et al. Improved identification of von Hippel–Lindau gene alterations in clear cell renal tumors. Clin Cancer Res. 2008;14(15):4726–34.
15. Duan DR, Pause A, Burgess WH, et al. Inhibition of transcription elongation by the VHL tumor suppressor protein. Science. 1995;269(5229):1402–6.
16. Kibel A, Iliopoulos O, DeCaprio JA, Kaelin Jr WG. Binding of the von Hippel–Lindau tumor suppressor protein to Elongin B and C. Science. 1995;269(5229):1444–6.
17. Pause A, Lee S, Worrell RA, et al. The von Hippel–Lindau tumor-suppressor gene product forms a stable complex with human CUL-2, a member of the Cdc53 family of proteins. Proc Natl Acad Sci USA. 1997;94(6):2156–61.
18. Maxwell PH, Wiesener MS, Chang GW, et al. The tumour suppressor protein VHL targets hypoxia-inducible factors for oxygen-dependent proteolysis. Nature. 1999;399(6733):271–5.

19. Ohh M, Park CW, Ivan M, et al. Ubiquitination of hypoxia-inducible factor requires direct binding to the beta-domain of the von Hippel–Lindau protein. Nat Cell Biol. 2000;2(7):423–7.

20. Stebbins CE, Kaelin Jr WG, Pavletich NP. Structure of the VHL-ElonginC–ElonginB complex: implications for VHL tumor suppressor function. Science. 1999;284(5413):455–61.

21. Zbar B. Von Hippel–Lindau disease and sporadic renal cell carcinoma. Cancer Surv. 1995;25:219–32.

22. Neumann HP, Bender BU. Genotype-phenotype correlations in von Hippel–Lindau disease. J Intern Med. 1998;243(6):541–5.

23. Zbar B, Klausner R, Linehan WM. Studying cancer families to identify kidney cancer genes. Annu Rev Med. 2003;54:217–33.

24. Chen F, Kishida T, Yao M, et al. Germline mutations in the von Hippel–Lindau disease tumor suppressor gene: correlations with phenotype. Hum Mutat. 1995;5(1):66–75.

25. Friedrich CA. Genotype–phenotype correlation in von Hippel–Lindau syndrome. Hum Mol Genet. 2001;10(7):763–7.

26. Verine J, Pluvinage A, Bousquet G, et al. Hereditary renal cancer syndromes: an update of a systematic review. Eur Urol. 2010;58(5):701–10.

27. Clifford SC, Maher ER. Von Hippel–Lindau disease: clinical and molecular perspectives. Adv Cancer Res. 2001;82:85–105.

28. Zbar B, Glenn G, Lubensky I, et al. Hereditary papillary renal cell carcinoma: clinical studies in 10 families. J Urol. 1995;153(3 Pt 2):907–12.

29. Schmidt L, Duh FM, Chen F, et al. Germline and somatic mutations in the tyrosine kinase domain of the MET proto-oncogene in papillary renal carcinomas. Nat Genet. 1997;16(1):68–73.

30. Schmidt L, Junker K, Weirich G, et al. Two North American families with hereditary papillary renal carcinoma and identical novel mutations in the MET proto-oncogene. Cancer Res. 1998;58(8):1719–22.

31. Schmidt L, Junker K, Nakaigawa N, et al. Novel mutations of the MET proto-oncogene in papillary renal carcinomas. Oncogene. 1999;18(14):2343–50.

32. Kovacs G. Molecular cytogenetics of renal cell tumors. Adv Cancer Res. 1993;62:89–124.

33. Zbar B, Tory K, Merino M, et al. Hereditary papillary renal cell carcinoma. J Urol. 1994;151(3):561–6.

34. Ornstein DK, Lubensky IA, Venzon D, Zbar B, Linehan WM, Walther MM. Prevalence of microscopic tumors in normal appearing renal parenchyma of patients with hereditary papillary renal cancer. J Urol. 2000;163(2):431–3.

35. Birt AR, Hogg GR, Dube WJ. Hereditary multiple fibrofolliculomas with trichodiscomas and acrochordons. Arch Dermatol. 1977;113(12):1674–7.

36. Zbar B, Alvord WG, Glenn G, et al. Risk of renal and colonic neoplasms and spontaneous pneumothorax in the Birt–Hogg–Dube syndrome. Cancer Epidemiol Biomarkers Prev. 2002;11(4):393–400.

37. Roth JS, Rabinowitz AD, Benson M, Grossman ME. Bilateral renal cell carcinoma in the Birt–Hogg–Dube syndrome. J Am Acad Dermatol. 1993;29(6):1055–6.

38. Toro JR, Glenn G, Duray P, et al. Birt–Hogg–Dube syndrome: a novel marker of kidney neoplasia. Arch Dermatol. 1999;135(10):1195–202.

39. Menko FH, van Steensel MA, Giraud S, et al. Birt–Hogg–Dube syndrome: diagnosis and management. Lancet Oncol. 2009;10(12):1199–206.

40. Pavlovich CP, Walther MM, Eyler RA, et al. Renal tumors in the Birt–Hogg–Dube syndrome. Am J Surg Pathol. 2002;26(12):1542–52.

41. Schmidt LS, Nickerson ML, Angeloni D, et al. Early onset hereditary papillary renal carcinoma: germline missense mutations in the tyrosine kinase domain of the met proto-oncogene. J Urol. 2004;172(4 Pt 1):1256–61.

42. Khoo SK, Bradley M, Wong FK, Hedblad MA, Nordenskjold M, Teh BT. Birt–Hogg–Dube syndrome: mapping of a novel hereditary neoplasia gene to chromosome 17p12–q11.2. Oncogene. 2001;20(37):5239–42.

43. Baba M, Hong SB, Sharma N, et al. Folliculin encoded by the BHD gene interacts with a binding protein, FNIP1, and AMPK, and is involved in AMPK and mTOR signaling. Proc Natl Acad Sci USA. 2006;103(42):15552–7.

44. Pavlovich CP, Grubb RL, Hurley K, et al. Evaluation and management of renal tumors in the Birt–Hogg–Dube' syndrome. J Urol. 2005;173(5):1482–6.

45. Toro JR, Wei MH, Glenn GM, et al. BHD mutations, clinical and molecular genetic investigations of Birt–Hogg–Dube syndrome: a new series of 50 families and a review of published reports. J Med Genet. 2008;45(6):321–31.

46. Butnor KJ, Guinee Jr DG. Pleuropulmonary pathology of Birt–Hogg–Dube syndrome. Am J Surg Pathol. 2006;30(3):395–9.

47. Ayo DS, Aughenbaugh GL, Yi ES, Hand JL, Ryu JH. Cystic lung disease in Birt–Hogg–Dube syndrome. Chest. 2007;132(2):679–84.

48. Reed WB, Walker R, Horowitz R. Cutaneous leiomyomata with uterine leiomyomata. Acta Derm Venereol. 1973;53(5):409–16.

49. Launonen V, Vierimaa O, Kiuru M, et al. Inherited susceptibility to uterine leiomyomas and renal cell cancer. Proc Natl Acad Sci USA. 2001;98(6):3387–92.

50. Tomlinson IP, Alam NA, Rowan AJ, et al. Germline mutations in FH predispose to dominantly inherited uterine fibroids, skin leiomyomata and papillary renal cell cancer. Nat Genet. 2002;30(4):406–10.

51. Sudarshan S, Linehan M, Neckers L. HIF and fumarate hydratase in renal cancer. Br J Cancer. 2007;96(3):403–7.

52. Isaacs JS, Jung YJ, Mole DR, et al. HIF overexpression correlates with biallelic loss of fumarate hydratase in renal cancer: novel role of fumarate in regulation of HIF stability. Cancer Cell. 2005;8(2):143–53.

53. Toro JR, Nickerson ML, Wei MH, et al. Mutations in the fumarate hydratase gene cause hereditary leiomyomatosis and renal cell cancer in families in North America. Am J Hum Genet. 2003;73(1):95–106.

54. Alam NA, Olpin S, Leigh IM. Fumarate hydratase mutations and predisposition to cutaneous leiomyomas, uterine leiomyomas and renal cancer. Br J Dermatol. 2005;153(1):11–7.

55. Wei MH, Toure O, Glenn GM, et al. Novel mutations in FH and expansion of the spectrum of phenotypes expressed in families with hereditary leiomyomatosis and renal cell cancer. J Med Genet. 2006;43(1):18–27.

56. Grubb 3rd RL, Franks ME, Toro J, et al. Hereditary leiomyomatosis and renal cell cancer: a syndrome associated with an aggressive form of inherited renal cancer. J Urol. 2007;177(6):2074–9. discussion 2079–80.

57. Walther MM, Choyke PL, Glenn G, et al. Renal cancer in families with hereditary renal cancer: prospective analysis of a tumor size threshold for renal parenchymal sparing surgery. J Urol. 1999;161(5):1475–9.

58. Walther MM, Lubensky IA, Venzon D, Zbar B, Linehan WM. Prevalence of microscopic lesions in grossly normal renal parenchyma from patients with von Hippel–Lindau disease, sporadic renal cell carcinoma and no renal disease: clinical implications. J Urol. 1995;154(6):2010–4. discussion 2014–5.

59. Poston CD, Jaffe GS, Lubensky IA, et al. Characterization of the renal pathology of a familial form of renal cell carcinoma associated with von Hippel–Lindau disease: clinical and molecular genetic implications. J Urol. 1995;153(1):22–6.

60. Huang WC, Elkin EB, Levey AS, Jang TL, Russo P. Partial nephrectomy versus radical nephrectomy in patients with small renal tumors–is there a difference in mortality and cardiovascular outcomes? J Urol. 2009;181(1):55–61. discussion 61–52.

61. Miller DC, Schonlau M, Litwin MS, Lai J, Saigal CS. Renal and cardiovascular morbidity after partial or radical nephrectomy. Cancer. 2008;112(3):511–20.

62. Thompson RH, Boorjian SA, Lohse CM, et al. Radical nephrectomy for pT1a renal masses may be associated with decreased overall survival compared with partial nephrectomy. J Urol. 2008;179(2):468–71. discussion 472–463.

63. Thompson RH, Siddiqui S, Lohse CM, Leibovich BC, Russo P, Blute ML. Partial versus radical nephrectomy for 4 to 7 cm renal cortical tumors. J Urol. 2009;182(6):2601–6.

64. Weight CJ, Larson BT, Gao T, et al. Elective partial nephrectomy in patients with clinical T1b renal tumors is associated with improved overall survival. Urology. 2010;76(3):631–7.

65. Weight CJ, Lieser G, Larson BT, et al. Partial nephrectomy is associated with improved overall survival compared to radical nephrectomy in patients with unanticipated benign renal tumours. Eur Urol. 2010;58(2):293–8.

66. Herring JC, Enquist EG, Chernoff A, Linehan WM, Choyke PL, Walther MM. Parenchymal sparing surgery in patients with hereditary renal cell carcinoma: 10-year experience. J Urol. 2001;165(3):777–81.

67. Walther MM, Choyke PL, Weiss G, et al. Parenchymal sparing surgery in patients with hereditary renal cell carcinoma. J Urol. 1995;153(3 Pt 2):913–6.

68. Pavlovich CP, Walther MM, Choyke PL, et al. Percutaneous radio frequency ablation of small renal tumors: initial results. J Urol. 2002;167(1):10–5.

69. Hwang JJ, Walther MM, Pautler SE, et al. Radio frequency ablation of small renal tumors intermediate results. J Urol. 2004;171(5):1814–8.

Imaging of Renal Cell Carcinoma

4

Andrei S. Purysko, Erick M. Remer, and Brian R. Herts

Introduction

With the expanded use of imaging in recent decades, there has been an increase in the detection of asymptomatic, incidental renal cell tumors [1–7]. While most incidentally detected lesions are benign cysts, solid renal tumors are predominantly renal cell carcinomas (RCCs). Occasionally, though, solid masses are other benign renal neoplasms [8, 9]. When malignant, these incidentally discovered tumors are more frequently lower stage and lower grade tumors, with a better prognosis than tumors in patients who present with hematuria or flank pain [10–13].

The introduction of thin slice, multidetector computed tomography (MDCT) and advanced magnetic resonance (MR) imaging hardware and software have helped radiologists confidently characterize masses as enhancing and, therefore, solid tumors rather than cysts [14]. While imaging technology has advanced, there has been a contemporaneous development of a number of surgical and ablative therapies to treat renal tumors. These include partial nephrectomy, laparoscopic total or partial nephrectomy, and percutaneous ablative procedures. These newer techniques are typically used for patients with smaller size, lower stage tumors. The radiological imperatives for these patients include not only accurate staging, but also a more sophisticated anatomical analysis than was needed when radical nephrectomy was the standard of care.

This chapter will discuss imaging of RCC as it relates to the detection of RCC and its characterization and the differential diagnoses of renal masses. We will briefly summarize the current status of ultrasound (US), CT, and MR for detection and staging of RCC, including presurgical planning, and will also compare their strengths and weaknesses. The imaging features of different histologies of RCC and other solid renal masses will then be discussed. Finally, we will review postprocedural imaging, including imaging after partial nephrectomy, tumor ablation, and targeted antiangiogenic therapy.

Imaging Methods for the Detection of Renal Cell Carcinoma

Detection of renal lesions on US is dependent upon either a contour abnormality or a difference in echogenicity between the lesion and normal parenchyma. Detection of renal lesions on CT and MR is possible because of a difference in

A.S. Purysko, MD
Section of Abdominal Imaging, Imaging Institute, Cleveland Clinic, 9500 Euclid Avenue-A21, Cleveland, OH 44195, USA

E.M. Remer, MD (✉) • B. R. Herts, MD
Section of Abdominal Imaging, Imaging Institute, Cleveland Clinic, 9500 Euclid Avenue-A21, Cleveland, OH 44195, USA

Glickman Urological and Kidney Institute, Cleveland Clinic, Cleveland, OH 44195, USA
e-mail: remere1@ccf.org

S.C. Campbell and B.I. Rini (eds.), *Renal Cell Carcinoma: Clinical Management*, Current Clinical Urology, DOI 10.1007/978-1-62703-062-5_4, © Springer Science+Business Media New York 2013 density or signal intensity from the normal renal parenchyma. This occurs not only because the kidneys filter contrast, but also because contrast is concentrated within the collecting tubules as water is reabsorbed. Normal renal parenchyma becomes denser on CT and has higher signal intensity on T1-weighted MR as contrast is concentrated. The degree of contrast concentration is dependent upon the relative function of nephrons and the volume and concentration of contrast given [15]. Neither cysts nor renal tumors will concentrate contrast. Therefore, the kidneys should be imaged at peak concentration of contrast with the highest contrast load to maximize detection of renal lesions. Unfortunately, for patients with impaired renal function the risk of contrast-induced nephropathy is increased while detection and characterization of renal masses is diminished.

Ultrasound

Ultrasound is ideal for distinguishing between cystic and solid renal masses [16]. Ultrasound is not considered the best test for the detection and characterization of renal tumors because small renal tumors are often similar in echogenicity to normal parenchyma, making the lesions difficult to detect. Also, the ability to detect fat within a lesion and, therefore, identify an angiomyolipoma (AML) is less robust with US than other cross-sectional imaging methods. Renal tumors that are large, contour-deforming, or partially cystic, however, can be detected sonographically (Fig. 4.1). On ultrasound, RCC can be less echogenic, equally echogenic or more echogenic than normal renal parenchyma. Advantages of renal ultrasound include its noninvasive nature, no need for potentially nephrotoxic iodinated contrast agents, and lack of radiation exposure.

Ultrasound is performed with a 3–6 MHz transducer and images are obtained through each kidney in both the axial and longitudinal planes. Tissue harmonic imaging can be used to increase the sensitivity of US for renal masses. Cysts appear as round or oval, anechoic structures with thin or imperceptible walls and increased through transmission. The sensitivity of US for the detection of RCC is dependent upon the size and location of the lesion. In general, smaller isoechoic intraparenchymal lesions are more difficult to detect, and some exophytic lesions can be obscured by bowel gas [17]. Ultrasound has also been investigated for screening for RCC in select patient populations, although the cost is problematic and generalized screening is not recommended in the USA [18, 19].

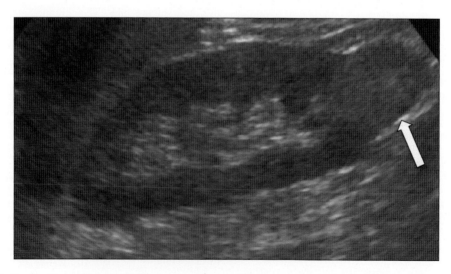

Fig. 4.1 Renal cell carcinoma on ultrasound. Partially exophytic lower renal pole solid mass (*arrow*), with slightly increased and heterogeneous echogenicity

The use of Doppler ultrasound has been accessed to improve the detection of renal masses. Kitamura et al. compared color flow Doppler (CFD) US to contrast-enhanced CT for the detection of renal tumors [17]. In this study, approximately 90% of clear cell carcinomas seen on CT were identifiable as hypervascular lesions on CFD US; however, there was no additional benefit gained by using CFD US.

Microbubble ultrasound contrast agents are able to depict renal vessels and show enhancement without the use of iodinated intravenous contrast material. These agents, therefore, may be especially useful in the problematic situation of a patient who has both a suspected renal mass and renal insufficiency. The sensitivity of US for the detection of renal tumors appears to be improved with the use of intravenous microbubble contrast agents; in one study the sensitivity was 97% compared to 70% for gray scale US alone [20]. The accuracy of ultrasound intravenous microbubble contrast to predict benign vs. malignant histology of renal masses is currently under investigation (http://clinicaltrials.gov/ct2/show/NCT00671411). Another use of ultrasound contrast agents is to improve characterization of complex renal cysts. Strong enhancement of the vascularity in septations and mural nodules improves lesion classification [21]. Finally, by depicting similar blood flow to normal renal parenchyma, ultrasound contrast can be used to exclude tumors in renal pseudotumors [21]. Ultrasound contrast agents are available for use with Doppler US systems but are not in general usage and are not FDA approved for this indication in the USA. The use of contrast eliminates ultrasound's main advantage by making it minimally invasive instead of noninvasive [22–24].

Computed Tomography

Computed tomography is the gold standard for the detection and characterization of renal masses, with a sensitivity for the detection of RCC ranging from 88% to 100%. Dedicated renal CTs should routinely include pre- and post-contrast imaging if possible, because renal tumors are generally isoat-tenuating to normal parenchyma on unenhanced scans and lesion enhancement is key to the diagnosis. The optimal time to image the kidney is during the nephrographic or parenchymal phase of enhancement when there is peak contrast concentration. This occurs 90–150 s after the initiation of a bolus of 100–150 mL of iodinated contrast. Early imaging in the corticomedullary phase (CMP) is less sensitive for focal renal masses [25] and some may even be obscured [26].

After a standard dose of IV contrast, most RCC enhance more than 120 HU on CT [27]; some tumors, such as papillary and chromophobe carcinomas, are much less vascular and enhance less avidly [28]. In the era of conventional CT, a change of 10 Hounsfield units (HU) between unenhanced and enhanced scans was deemed evidence of enhancement. The introduction of helical CT scanning has led to increasing image noise leading some authors to suggest 15–20 HU as an appropriate threshold to determine enhancement, while others consider a 10–20 HU change as indeterminate and suggest other imaging such as MRI [29]. One caveat is that with the detection of smaller lesions there is more variability in the HU density. This occurs because the thickness of small lesions may be similar to the thickness of the CT slice, and therefore, pixels from outside the lesion may be included in attenuation measurements (so-called partial volume averaging).

Multiphasic CT Technique

A three-phase CT scan is considered the optimal technique for detecting and characterizing renal masses, as well as staging RCC. This includes an unenhanced scan, a vascular or CMP scan and a parenchymal or nephrographic phase (NP) scan (Fig. 4.2). Several studies have shown that the NP is the most sensitive for the detection of renal tumors, although in one study more lesions were seen when a combination of unenhanced, CMP and NP scans were used [29–34].

The CMP is useful for assessing the renal vasculature, and enhancement seen in this phase can also be useful for characterizing lesions [35–37]. When used alone, however, the CMP can result in missed lesions and false positive diagnoses of medullary lesions [38, 39].

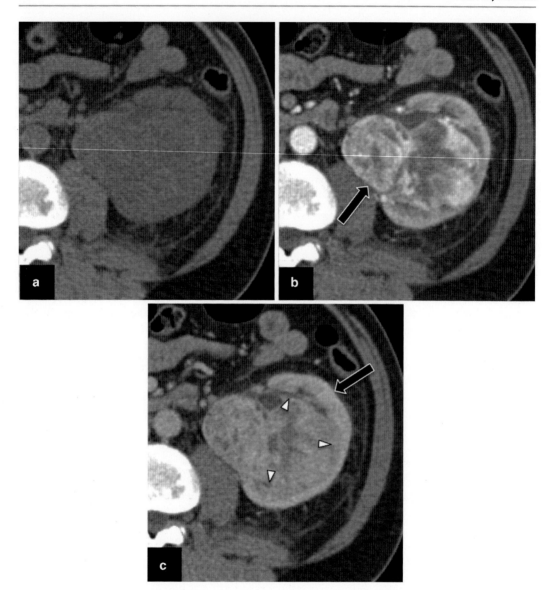

Fig. 4.2 Renal cell carcinoma (clear cell type) on multiphasic computed tomography. (**a**) Pre-contrast; (**b**) corticomedullary phase; (**c**) nephrographic phase. Large central renal mass extending into the renal sinus (*arrow* on **b**), with intense and heterogeneous contrast enhancement in the corticomedullary phase. The renal parenchyma concentrates the contrast more homogenously and becomes hyperdense compared to the mass in nephrographic phase (*arrow* on **c**), improving the tumor outlining (*arrowheads* on **c**)

Pseudoenhancement

Pseudoenhancement refers to an artificial attenuation change in a lesion between unenhanced and enhanced scans. It is thought to be due to the image reconstruction algorithm used in helical CT scanners. In one study, more than 95% of cysts demonstrated a change in attenuation value less than 10 HU, most less than 8 HU [40]. However, some simple cysts can have a measurable increase of more than 10 HU after contrast administration. Pseudoenhancement occurs most often when the cyst is surrounded by enhancing renal parenchyma. Many are small (<2 cm) and are completely intrarenal [29]. Therefore, one needs to take the lesion size and location into consideration when using change in attenuation value to characterize renal lesions [41, 42].

Surgical Planning

With the introduction of multidetector high-speed CT scanners, high-resolution MR imaging and three-dimensional (3D) postprocessing imaging software, surgical planning can now be performed using CT and MRI [43–48]. While 2D multiplanar reformations can depict pertinent surgical anatomy, real-time volume rendered 3D representations provide spatial cues that help plan a surgical approach, resection margins, and vascular control. 3D images from the corticomedullary or vascular phase scans provide a detailed depiction of the number, size and locations of all renal arteries and veins, major segmental arterial branches, the left adrenal vein, the gonadal veins, and any prominent lumbar veins (Fig. 4.3). The renal parenchymal phase (NP) is used to render the renal position, renal tumor location, depth of extension and relationship of the tumor to the pelvocalyceal system, and position of the adrenal gland (Fig. 4.4).

Magnetic Resonance Imaging

MR imaging can also be used to characterize and stage RCC and is the test of choice in patients with contrast allergies and mild renal insufficiency. At clinical doses, gadolinium-based MR contrast agents do not appear to have substantial nephrotoxic effects [49]. Recently an association between gadolinium-based MR contrast agents and nephrogenic systemic fibrosis (NSF) [34, 38, 50], a potentially crippling, life-threatening skin disorder, has been described in patients with compromised renal function. Further studies are necessary to determine what the exact relationships are between gadolinium-containing contrast agents, patient renal function and NSF. Currently, the development of NSF is thought be linked to the administration of relatively high doses (e.g., >0.2 mM/kg) and to agents in which the gadolinium is least strongly chelated. The Federal Drug Administration recommends that until further information is available, gadolinium contrast agents should not be administered to patients with either acute or significant chronic kidney disease

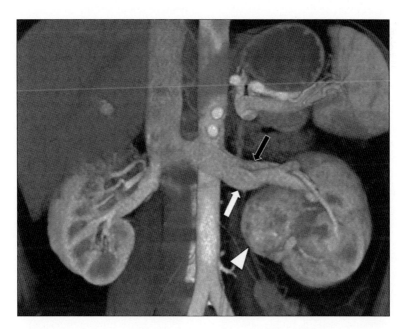

Fig. 4.3 Contrast-enhanced computed tomography (corticomedullary or vascular phase) using 3D volume rendering reconstruction technique for anatomical evaluation of patient with left lower pole renal mass (*arrowhead*), being considered for partial nephrectomy. Single left renal artery (*black arrow*) and single left renal vein (*white arrow*) with typical course anterior to the aorta are demonstrated

Fig. 4.4 Computed tomography (excretory phase) using 3D volume rendering reconstruction technique, demonstrating relation of exophytic renal lesion (*arrow*) with contrast-filled renal pelvis (*asterisk*)

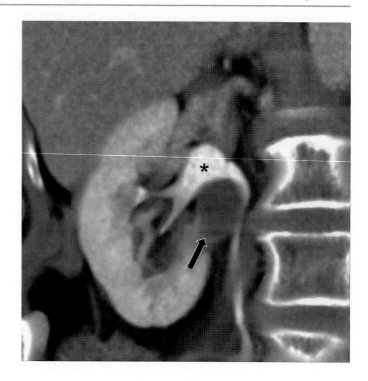

(estimated GFR <30 mL/min/1.73 m), recent liver or kidney transplant or hepatorenal syndrome, unless a risk-benefit assessment suggests that the benefit of administration in the particular patient clearly outweighs the potential risk(s) [38]. Since the implementation of these guidelines, the incidence of NSF has abated considerably [51].

In addition to characterizing and staging renal masses, MR imaging is used to attempt characterization of lesions that are indeterminate on CT. MRI is more contrast-sensitive than CT, i.e., MRI is better at detecting enhancement. Similar to CT, MR imaging must be performed before and after contrast. T1-weighted images (T1WI), usually with a fat-suppressed breath-hold sequence, are obtained before contrast and after contrast during several phases, in both axial and coronal planes [36, 52]. Before contrast, T2-weighted imaging (T2WI) is performed to characterize cysts. Other techniques (in- and out-of-phase imaging and chemical selective fat suppression) are used to detect fat within lesions. MR is highly sensitive for renal tumors, approaching 100%, and has some advantages over CT for the characterization of subcentimeter cysts. There is no universally

agreed upon method to quantify enhancement on MRI. Signal intensity in MR images is based on a relative scale, not on absolute density, as is the Hounsfield unit scale [37]. Therefore, most authors recommend a subtraction between pre- and post-contrast MR sequences to eliminate the subjectivity of determining enhancement after contrast on MR. A threshold of 15% increase in signal intensity has also been advocated to identify enhancement in renal tumors [53, 54]. Identification of calcium in renal masses on MRI is limited because calcium appears as a signal void.

The sensitivity for the detection of RCC is reported to be as high as 88–100% for CT and 78–100% for MR [39, 55–57]. In direct comparison studies, the sensitivity for detecting renal tumors is similar between MR and CT, and both are more sensitive than ultrasound [58, 59].

Renal Mass Detection

Currently, more than 60% of RCCs are detected incidentally at imaging [10, 11]. In the era when most renal masses were found due to patient symptoms, it was dogma that any solid renal mass was an RCC until proven otherwise. Even today, excluding infections and AMLs, most solid renal masses in adults are RCC [13]. However, with the detection of an increasing number of renal lesions, recent pathological series have found a higher than previously known proportion of small, solid renal masses to be benign [7, 8, 13, 60]. One series of 2,770 renal tumor resections [60] found a benign rate of 12.8%. It is noteworthy that the likelihood of the solid renal mass being malignant was generally proportional to its size: 25% for masses smaller than 3 cm, 30% for masses smaller than 2 cm, and 44% for masses smaller than 1 cm.

Solid Masses

The typical appearance of RCC is a heterogeneous, enhancing solid mass following contrast administration (Fig. 4.2) [61]. While the majority of RCC are solid, rounded, or ovoid mass lesions, some RCC are infiltrating or complex cystic mass lesions. Clear cell, papillary, and chromophobe RCC subtypes are usually solid on CT, US, and MRI. Unfortunately, both benign (e.g., oncocytoma, angiomyolipoma) and other malignant (e.g., some transitional cell carcinoma and metastatic disease) lesions are also solid, mass lesions.

There are only a few imaging features of solid lesions that have been found to suggest a benign diagnosis. Solid masses that contain regions of macroscopic fat on imaging are benign AMLs. AML is a type of perivascular epitheloid cell tumor and is composed of a variable amount of vessels, muscle, and adipose tissue. The fat content is seen as low attenuation on CT (Fig. 4.5) and can be identified with fat suppression sequences on MRI (Fig. 4.6). Approximately 5% of AML have small amounts of fat that are not detectable on imaging studies, and therefore mimic RCCs [62]. Identifying small regions of fat with CT pixel analysis can help identify these AMLs, but is a relatively insensitive technique [63]. Masses that are high attenuation before contrast and enhance homogeneously may prove to be AMLs with minimal histological lipid content [19, 64]. Oncocytoma is a benign solid neoplasm that has a classic imaging features of a central, stellate scar (Fig. 4.7). This feature, unfortunately, is neither sensitive nor specific for the diagnosis [65]. Therefore, in general, imaging cannot be used to differentiate benign from malignant solid masses. Short of resection of these masses, diagnostic options are limited to observation and percutaneous biopsy. With the increasing realization that small, hyperattenuating, homogeneously enhancing renal masses are more frequently benign than other solid renal masses, there is currently an emerging role of percutaneous biopsy at some institutions [13].

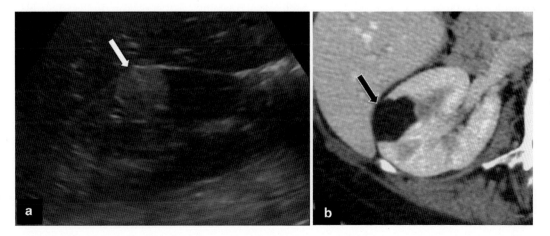

Fig. 4.5 Angiomyolipoma. (**a**) Hyperechoic rounded renal lesion on ultrasound (*arrow*). (**b**) Same lesion on contrast-enhanced CT demonstrating predominantly fat attenuation

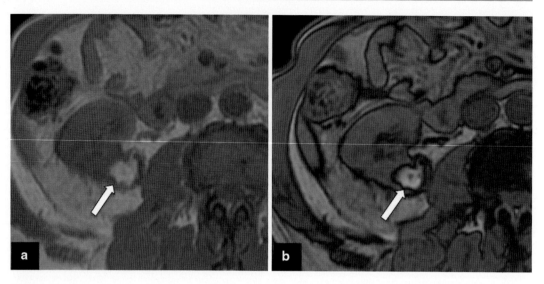

Fig. 4.6 Angiomyolipoma on MRI. T1-weighted image "in-phase" showing partially exophytic renal lesion (*arrow* on **a**) with fat content that is characterized by a low signal intensity rim (India ink artifact) surrounding the lesion on T1-weighted imaging "out-of-phase" indicating a fat-soft tissue interface (*arrow* on **b**)

Cysts and Complex Cystic Renal Masses

RCC can have a cystic growth pattern that can be unilocular, multilocular, or necrotic, and RCC can develop within the wall of an otherwise benign cyst [66]. Renal epithelial cysts are common and contain simple serous fluid. Other benign cysts can contain fluid with a high protein content, hemorrhage, or infection, making the differentiation between a benign cyst and cystic RCC difficult [67, 68]. Different imaging-based classification methods have been proposed to help predict the likelihood of a cystic lesion being malignant; one used by both radiologists and urologists was originally described in 1986 by Bosniak and has since been modified. Bosniak originally proposed four categories, each predicting an increasing likelihood of malignancy. This classification system has been modified more recently to include a fifth category [69–72].

Category I cysts are simple unilocular cysts, either round or oval, with a thin, noncalcified walls (Fig. 4.8a). These cysts contain simple serous fluid measuring less than 10–20 HU at CT and have MR signal characteristics of simple fluid (low signal intensity on T1- and high signal intensity on T2-weighted sequences). There is no solid, soft tissue density in the lesion or enhancement after intravenous contrast.

Category II cysts are minimally complicated cysts either with high-density fluid due to a increased protein content or hemorrhage within the cysts (higher than 20 HU density, a "hyperdense" cyst), or are multilocular with a few septa (Fig. 4.8b) or thin peripheral calcifications. Category II cysts do not demonstrate enhancement after intravenous contrast and are almost always benign [73, 74]. Contrast is needed to distinguish between a hyperdense cyst and a homogeneous solid renal neoplasm. Both lesions may appear similar on pre- or post-contrast scans, but the hyperdense cyst will not enhance after contrast, whereas the homogeneous solid renal neoplasm will enhance. Hyperdense cysts tend to be higher in attenuation and more homogeneous than RCCs on unenhanced CT [75]. On nephrographic phase contrast-enhanced CT scans, attenuation greater than 70 HU or moderate or marked internal heterogeneity favor a diagnosis of RCC over a diagnosis of high-attenuation renal cyst [58]. Category II cysts have a less than 15% change of malignancy and, therefore, may be followed to document stability over time.

Category IIF cysts are complex lesions that have multiple septa or calcifications that have a relatively

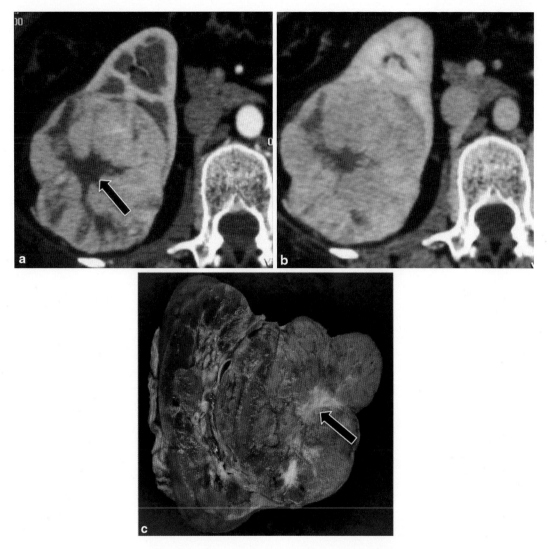

Fig. 4.7 Oncocytoma. Large right renal mass on contrast-enhanced CT corticomedullary (**a**) and nephrographic (**b**) phases, showing central stellate-shaped low attenuation area (*black arrow* on **a**) which corresponds to white fibrous tissue in pathological specimen (*black arrow* on **c**). While this pattern is typical for oncocytoma, it is not specific and can be seen in renal cell carcinomas

benign appearance (Fig. 4.8c). Calcifications, once felt to be a potential sign of malignancy, are now considered less important [26]. Category IIF cysts are thought to be benign, but need interval follow-up to confirm their stability [59].

Category III cysts are complicated cystic lesions that have some features suggesting malignancy—multiple septa, thick or irregular rims—or heterogeneity suggesting necrosis (Fig. 4.8d). Category III cysts have an approximately 50–60% chance of being a cystic RCC according to published studies

[28, 76]. Typically, these lesions are surgically explored. While biopsy has been studied in these patients [33, 77], finding a "definitive" diagnosis in 61–88% of lesions, these studies suffer from the fact that negative results were supported by interval follow-up rather than histopathology [13].

Category IV cysts contain solid, soft tissue enhancing elements seen either within the cyst or as part of a complex cystic mass (Fig. 4.8e). These lesions are almost always cystic RCC and should be treated as such.

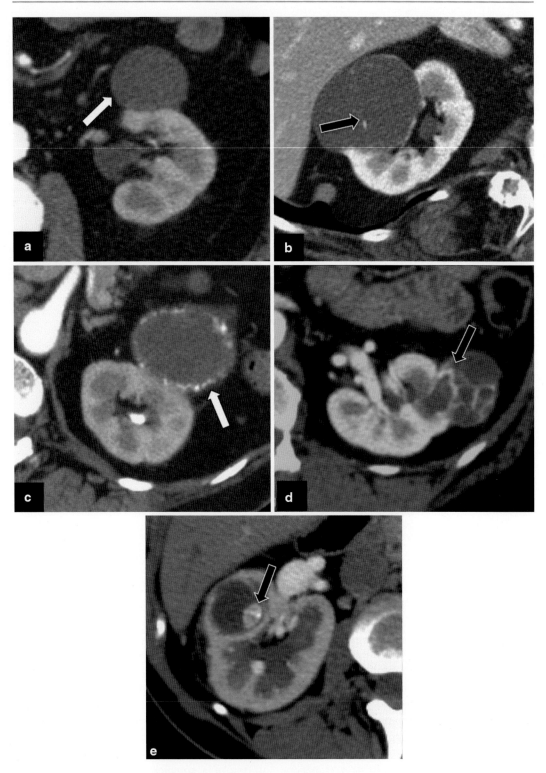

Fig. 4.8 Spectrum of cystic renal lesions. (**a**) Thin-walled simple cyst (*arrow*) with homogenous low attenuation content—Bosniak I; (**b**) cystic lesion with thin (<~1 mm) partially calcified internal septum (*arrow*)—Bosniak II; (**c**) slightly thicker wall cystic lesion with peripheral calcifications (*arrow*)—Bosniak IIF; (**d**) exophytic cystic renal lesion with multiple thick (>1 mm) enhancing septa (*arrow*)—Bosniak III; (**e**) cystic renal lesion with solid enhancing mural nodule (*arrow*)—Bosniak IV

While one typically expects Bosniak III or IV lesions to represent cystic clear cell carcinomas, there are a number of benign cystic neoplasms that mimic this diagnosis. These include cystic nephroma (CN) (Fig. 4.9) and mixed epithelial and stromal tumor (MEST) of the kidney (Fig. 4.10). In one series, 70% of 22 CN were characterized as Bosniak III lesions and 70% of 10 MEST had enhancing solid elements [78]. These tumors are much more commonly seen in women or men receiving exogenous hormones and are frequently symptomatic [58].

Management guidelines for complex renal cysts are based on this classification scheme. In general, category I lesions do not need further evaluation; category II lesions, if larger than 3 cm or irregular, and category IIF lesions should be followed for interval growth or change, which suggest malignancy; category III lesions should be explored or resected; and category IV lesions appropriately treated as presumed RCC. Biopsy of indeterminate cystic renal masses can also be considered, although concerns about tumor spillage and false negative results persist. It is important to note that the Bosniak criteria are guidelines for describing and managing cystic renal masses. Other factors, including risk factors for RCC, a genetic disorder that predisposes the individual to cystic renal tumors, age, and comorbid conditions should influence any management decision.

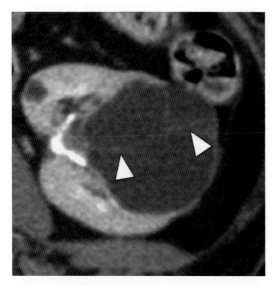

Fig. 4.9 Cystic nephroma. Large cystic renal mass with multiple enhancing septa (*arrowheads*) insinuating into the renal sinus, consistent with a Bosniak III lesion

Infiltrative Renal Masses

While most renal tumors exhibit radial growth patterns with a space-occupying mass and may occasionally have a cystic growth pattern, RCC can also infiltrate within the renal parenchyma along the interstitium [79]. In these instances, the renal contour is maintained but the involved portion of the kidney is typically enlarged. Infiltrating tumors encase rather than displace the vasculature and renal collecting structures. On CT, infiltrating lesions are poorly marginated areas of relatively decreased enhancement reflecting the disruption of the normal tubular concentration of contrast (Fig. 4.11). On ultrasound, these are often similar in echogenicity to normal parenchyma, making their detection and definition by sonography difficult. Only occasionally are infiltrating renal lesions slightly hypoechoic or hyperechoic compared to normal renal parenchyma.

Several tumors other than RCC demonstrate an infiltrating pattern on imaging [40]. Transitional cell carcinoma (TCC) comprises 90% of urothelial

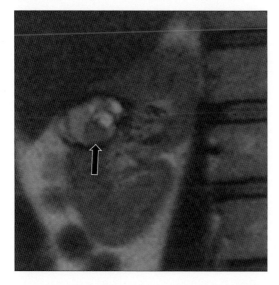

Fig. 4.10 Mixed epithelia and stromal tumor (MEST). Coronal T2-weighted image showing complex cystic lesion with peripheral solid nodular component (*arrow*)

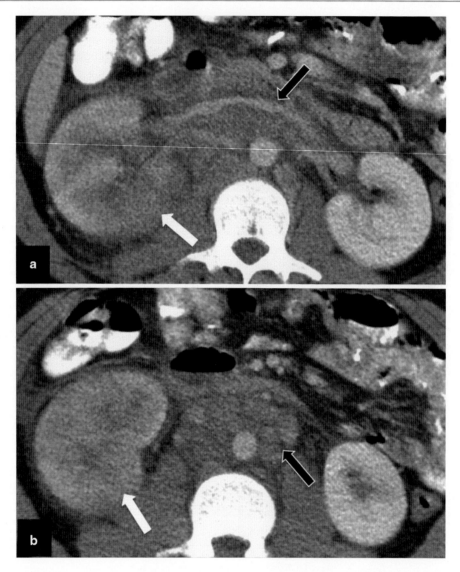

Fig. 4.11 Infiltrative renal cell carcinoma (medullary type). Contrast-enhanced CT shows ill-defined infiltrative hypoenhancing right renal mass (*white arrow* on **a** and **b**), associated with confluent retroperitoneal lymphadenopathy encasing the renal veins (*black arrow* on **a**) and aorta (*black arrow* on **b**)

tumors and when it involves renal parenchyma is characteristically infiltrative in its growth pattern. While typically a slow-growing papillary tumor, TCC of the kidney is occasionally high grade and infiltrating. A key to the imaging diagnosis is its central location in the kidney or in the renal sinus and lack of visualization or displacement of renal collecting structures.

Primary renal non-Hodgkin's lymphoma (NHL) can arise in the renal parenchyma or renal hilar lymph nodes. Extranodal lymphoma is more common with Hodgkin's disease than with NHL. Perinephric confluent tissue is more suggestive of NHL than RCC (Fig. 4.12a). In general, however, renal involvement in lymphoma is associated with systemic disease. On CT and MR, renal lymphoma is typically hypovascular with multiple solid or infiltrating masses (Fig. 4.12b) [80].

Leukemia is always infiltrating in its growth pattern, typically causing renal enlargement [81].

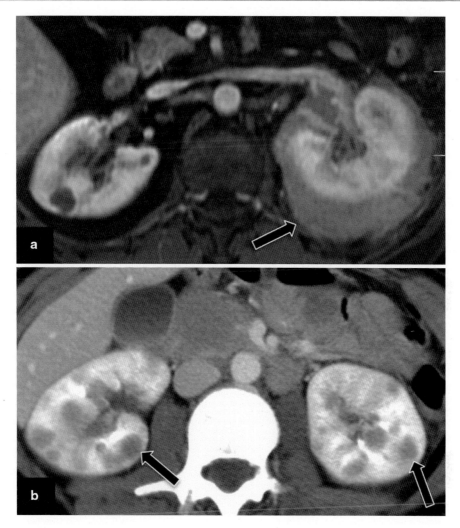

Fig. 4.12 Lymphoma. (**a**) Enhancing tissue rind surrounding the left kidney on contrast-enhanced T1-weighted MR image (*arrow*). (**b**) Multiple bilateral low attenuation renal nodules (*black arrows*) on contrast-enhanced CT

Metastatic disease to the kidneys is seen as multiple, bilateral, poorly marginated solid lesions that can occasionally demonstrate an infiltrative pattern [82, 83].

Some nonmalignant conditions can demonstrate an infiltrating pattern on imaging, and it is vitally important to recognize these entities. Acute pyelonephritis is seen as wedge-shaped areas of decreased enhancement that extend from the papilla to the cortex. Differential enhancement of infected and uninfected parenchyma occurs from tubular obstruction from inflammatory debris, interstitial edema, and vasospasm. This appearance should be distinguished from tumor infiltration, especially with a history of fever, flank pain, and pyuria.

Imaging Features of Renal Carcinoma Subtypes

Renal cell neoplasms can be classified as clear cell, chromophobe, papillary, collecting duct, medullary, mixed cell types or as adenocarcinoma not specified; or as small cell carcinoma, juxtaglomerular tumor or carcinoid [84–86].

Since prognosis differs among the different types of RCC, it is worth reviewing the more common features of each on imaging studies.

Clear Cell Renal Cell Carcinoma

Clear cell carcinoma, the most common type of RCC, originates from the proximal convoluted tubule and accounts for 70–80% of all RCC. Clear cell carcinomas are typically hypervascular after contrast administration on CT, with more avid enhancement than that displayed by other RCC subtypes (Fig. 4.2) [51, 87, 88]. A hypervascular pattern is present in nearly 50% of clear cell carcinomas, compared to approximately 15% of papillary and 4% of chromophobe RCCs. The degree of enhancement is significantly different among the clear cell, papillary and chromophobe subtypes in the corticomedullary and excretory phases as well [82]. The chromophobe subtype shows homogeneous enhancement in 75% of cases in comparison with 45% and 65% of clear cell and papillary subtypes. Clear cell carcinoma also has heterogeneous peripheral enhancement more frequently than papillary and chromophobe RCC [81].

On MRI, clear cell RCC is typically isointense on T1-weighted images and isointense to hyperintense on T2-weighted images compared to normal renal parenchyma (Fig. 4.13) [89]. Clear cell carcinomas are commonly more aggressive tumors than other cell types and they may directly involve and invade the renal collecting system [90].

Cystic degeneration is also more common (15%) in the clear cell subtype than in the other subtypes irrespective of tumor size. Tumor necrosis can also cause a cystic appearance on imaging, but this feature confers a worse prognosis than a true cystic clear cell carcinoma [91]. Calcification occurs in 21–25% of each of the clear cell, papillary and chromophobe subtypes.

Overall, enhancement is the most valuable parameter used to differentiate the subtypes of RCC. The degree of enhancement, presence or absence of cystic degeneration, vascularity and enhancement patterns can serve a supplemental role in differentiating RCC subtypes.

Papillary Renal Cell Carcinoma

Papillary renal cell carcinoma (PRCC) comprises 10–15% of RCC [92, 93]. Most studies suggest that it has a greater tendency to lower stage and better prognosis than clear cell RCC. On CT, papillary RCC is typically a hypovascular, homogeneous solid mass [52, 94]. A tumor that enhances less than 25% of the attenuation value (Hounsfield units) of normal parenchyma in the CMP and NP is significantly more likely to be a PRCC. Conversely, tumors that enhance more than 25% of the enhancement of the normal renal parenchyma are rarely papillary RCC [52]. Papillary RCC rarely invades the collecting system, and locally invasive behavior is less common [84]. On MR, PRCC can be hemorrhagic, leading to heterogeneous signal intensity on T1-weighted images and a decreased signal intensity on T2-weighted images compared to normal renal parenchyma (Fig. 4.14) [83]. Enhancement is lower and delayed in papillary RCC compared to clear cell RCC [95].

An important feature of papillary RCC is that is more commonly bilateral and multifocal than other RCC subtypes [96]. Papillary RCC is often smaller in size than clear cell carcinoma [97]. There are histologic descriptions of two different types of papillary RCC: those with small basophilic cells (Type 1) and those with eosinophilic cells (Type 2) [98]. Survival is worse for type 2 and one small series that found that type 2 tumors have less distinct margins, are more heterogeneous, generally present at more advanced stages, and frequently grow centripetally [99].

PRCC that are more than 3 cm in diameter may have heterogeneous attenuation and areas of necrosis and hemorrhage. PRCC may occasionally show cystic growth that can be from necrosis, but such changes are much less common than in clear cell RCC.

Chromophobe Renal Cell Carcinoma

The chromophobe subtype accounts for only a small percentage of RCC [100]. Chromophobe RCC is typically hypovascular at CT, similar to papillary RCC [81]. In one study of 11 patients

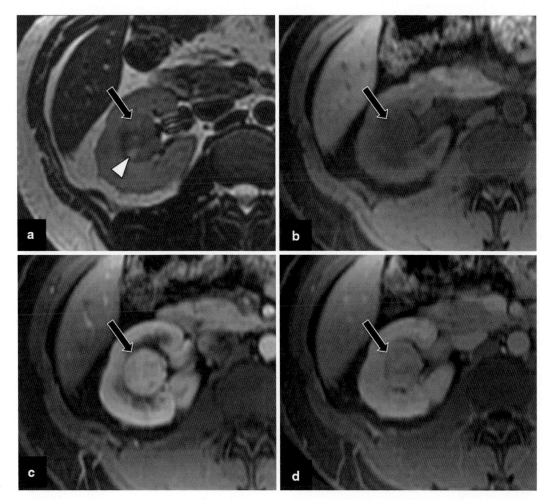

Fig. 4.13 Renal cell carcinoma (clear cell type). (**a**) Central right renal mass with slightly heterogeneous signal on T2-weighted image, and small focus of hyperintense signal (*arrow*), consistent with areas of cystic degeneration. (**b**) On T1-weighted image the lesion is slightly hypointense compared to the surrounding renal parenchyma (*arrow*). (**c, d**) The lesion demonstrates intense contrast enhancement in the corticomedullary phase (*arrow* on **c**), and becomes slightly hypointense in the nephrographic phase (*arrow* on **d**)

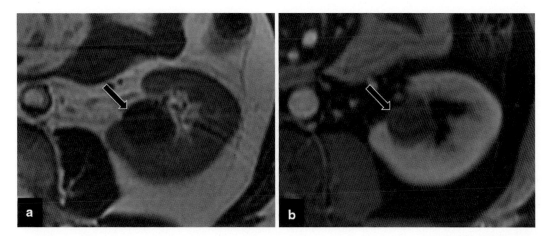

Fig. 4.14 Papillary renal cell carcinoma. Left interpolar renal mass with low T2-weighted signal intensity (*arrow* on **a**), demonstrating poor enhancement on T1-weighted post-contrast image (*arrow* on **b**), typical features of papillary RCC

with the chromophobe cell type, there was a spoke-like enhancement pattern with a central stellate form [101]. This can be seen with chromophobe RCC and oncocytoma and is, therefore, not specific for either tumor. Hale's colloidal iron stain has been used to differentiate between the two pathologically.

Collecting/Bellini Duct Carcinoma

Collecting duct (Bellini duct) carcinomas are uncommon, comprising 1–2% of all RCC. Histologically, these tumors are characterized by a tubular or tubulopapillary infiltrative growth pattern, which is reflected in the CT appearance. Collecting duct RCC (CDRCC) are medullary and infiltrating in the central sinus and only rarely reported in the renal cortex [102–105]. Metastases are more common at presentation than other types of RCC, occurring in 35–40% of patients [94, 97]. When bone metastases occur, they are frequently osteoblastic, unlike metastases from clear cell RCC, which are osteolytic [94]. On CT and angiography, CDRCC are hypovascular tumors [97].

In one study reporting 11 cases of CDRCC, the vast majority of CDRCC were hyperechoic on ultrasound and hyperintense on T2WI on MRI. The differential diagnosis of CDRCC includes sarcomatoid variants of RCC, high grade infiltrating TCC or squamous cell carcinoma of the renal pelvis, and NHL [106].

Sarcomatoid Renal Cell Carcinoma

Sarcomatoid RCC is a highly aggressive variant of other histological subtypes and typically has an infiltrating appearance on imaging. The vast majority are symptomatic at presentation [107]. Renal sarcoma and sarcomatoid RCC should be considered when there is an extensively infiltrating tumor with spread into the perinephric space and adjacent organs. The differential diagnosis of sarcomatoid RCC includes other infiltrating tumors such as TCC, NHL, fibrosarcoma, and leiomyosarcoma [108].

Medullary Carcinoma

Medullary carcinoma is often considered a distinct entity, but may be an aggressive form of CDRCC that occurs in children and young adults. Medullary renal carcinoma has been associated with sickle cell trait, but not sickle cell disease. As with CDRCC, medullary RCC is typically infiltrating and aggressive with centrally located tumors. Large size, venous and lymphatic invasion and regional lymph node metastases are usually present at presentation (Fig. 4.11). Medullary carcinoma can demonstrate necrosis and hemorrhage [40, 98].

Other Primary and Secondary Renal Neoplasms

Oncocytoma

Stellate central scars (Fig. 4.7) on CT and MR and spoke-wheel enhancement on angiography have both been described as imaging features suggestive of renal oncocytoma. Oncocytoma is hypervascular, similar to clear cell carcinoma, and homogeneous in attenuation [65]. Although these imaging features can be used to raise suspicion for oncocytoma, none is sufficiently diagnostic and a tissue diagnosis is needed [109]. The histopathologic features of oncocytoma allowing differentiation from RCC on biopsy have only recently been described [110, 111].

Cystic Nephroma/Mixed Epithelial and Stromal Tumor

CN or multilocular CN is a tumor characterized by varying sized cysts, thin septa, and no solid elements. MEST is a biphasic tumor with complex stromal and epithelial elements. They share pathological similarities and are grouped together as mixed mesenchymal and epithelial tumor in the 2004 World Health Organization of renal neoplasms [112]. CN have a complex cystic appearance with multiple septa without soft tissue components (Fig. 4.9). They characteristically project or herniate into the renal sinus and may extend into the renal pelvis. Patients have a bimodal distribution, with CN often occurring in younger males or middle-aged females. MEST have similar features to CN on imaging, but also have solid, enhancing elements (Fig. 4.10) [78]. Their imaging features have been described in small series to date [78, 113].

Metastatic Disease

Metastatic disease to the kidneys is particularly common with lung and breast carcinoma, melanoma, and lymphoma [44, 114]. Lesions are usually multiple and bilateral. When there is a history of a nonrenal primary tumor, as many as 50–85% of solitary renal masses are metastatic disease [43, 115]. Conversely, nearly 90% of patients with pathologically proven metastatic disease to the kidney have a history of a primary malignancy [44].

Renal Lymphoma

Renal lymphoma can be primary, involving the renal or perirenal lymphatics, or secondary with associated lymphadenopathy. On CT and MRI, lymphoma can be seen as either a focal mass or have an infiltrative appearance (Fig. 4.12) [41, 116]. Lymphoma is typically homogeneous and enhances less than normal renal parenchyma. Renal lymphoma should be considered when there is splenomegaly, bulky retroperitoneal or mesenteric lymphadenopathy, and organ involvement, such as bowel, that is not typical of RCC. Biopsy should be considered to differentiate renal lymphoma from RCC when there are other imaging findings suggesting lymphoma or the patient has a history of lymphoma.

Angiomyolipoma and Other Fat-Containing Renal Tumors

AML is a benign renal hamartoma containing lipomatous, smooth muscle, and vascular elements. Most AML have macroscopic fat associated with the lipomatous elements and can, therefore, be diagnosed on imaging (Figs. 4.5 and 4.6). About 5% of AML, however, have small amounts of fat that cannot be identified preoperatively at CT. AML with minimal fat is radiographically similar to RCC on CT. It may be higher in attenuation than normal renal parenchyma on unenhanced CT [117], a finding that is atypical for RCC. Kim et al. described prolonged enhancement and homogeneous enhancement in AML with minimal fat as opposed to heterogeneous, transient enhancement in clear cell RCC. Both findings together have a 91% positive predictive value (PPV) for AML [118]. When calcification is seen in a lesion with no or minimal fat, it is most likely an RCC and not an AML [119, 120]. On ultrasound, AML are generally smaller and are frequently hyperechoic; shadowing from a renal lesion is also more suggestive of an AML than an RCC. On MRI, the diagnosis of AML can be made when macroscopic fat can be discerned with fat suppression techniques. Minimal fat AMLs tend to have low signal intensity on T2WI, a finding also seen in PRCC, but not clear cell carcinoma. More avid enhancement after contrast is typical of AML, unlike papillary RCC which tends to enhance only minimally.

An exophytic AML can usually be differentiated from a retroperitoneal or renal capsular liposarcoma by the presence of a renal parenchyma defect, large blood vessels feeding the mass, and aneurysms or varices [121, 122].

Staging of Renal Cell Carcinoma by CT and MRI

Accuracy of Imaging for Staging

The TNM system is now primarily used for staging RCC [123–128]. Overall, the accuracy for CT and MR for staging RCC appears to be similar [129–134]. The accuracy of contrast-enhanced CT for RCC staging ranges from 72% to 91% [133, 135] and the accuracy of MRI ranges from 78% to 98% [59, 76, 136]. In one study, there was no difference between overall CT and MR accuracy [76], but in another MRI showed higher accuracy than CT [59]. MRI was better than CT for stage 2 disease and worse than CT for stage 4 disease [137].

The major limitation of imaging for staging is identifying tumors that have spread beyond the renal capsule which increases the tumor stage from T1 or T2 to T3a by the TNM system. Criteria such as a discrete nodule or thickening of a septum, either greater than 3 mm, in the perinephric space are neither sensitive nor specific for spread beyond the renal capsule. Most studies demonstrate understaging by CT [138]. This understaging by CT, however, does not appear to affect patient's overall prognosis. A study that compared patients with clinical stage T1 disease and pathologic stage T1 disease to patients with clinical stage T1 disease and pathologic stage T3 disease found no statistically significant difference in 5-year survival between the groups [139]. The lack of perinephric fat infiltration on MRI has been shown to have a high negative predictive value for extracapsular tumor invasion [140].

Ultrasound is not generally recommended for RCC staging. Ultrasound is inferior to CT and MR in large part because of poor lymph node visibility [128]. Ultrasound may be accurate for assessing renal vein involvement and can be used as an adjunct to CT or MR if equivocal or limited in any way.

Renal Central Sinus Invasion and Urothelial Invasion

Invasion of the central sinus fat may have significant prognostic implications in patients with RCC, similar to extension outside the renal capsule [141]. Now staged as T3a in the 2010 TNM staging system, sinus invasion can be difficult to accurately detect on CT [142]. It is considered the most common site for extrarenal extension of RCC. Some authors have suggested that urothelial invasion should be an added criterion for staging because it was associated with a worse prognosis in one series [84]. In this study patients with pathologically determined T2 tumors with urothelial invasion did worse than patients with T2 tumors without urothelial invasion.

Tumor Size

Final pathological tumor size is an important prognostic staging criterion in the current TNM staging system. Several studies have compared CT tumor size with pathologic size [132–134]. In general, there has been excellent correlation between CT size and pathological size with correlation coefficients ranging from 0.90 to 0.95 [143, 144]. The size of smaller tumors tends to be overestimated by CT [132]. Clear cell tumors have also been shown to be overestimated by CT. In one study of 30 tumors larger than 4 cm, 22 clear cell RCC were overestimated by more than 1 cm [145]. This discrepancy may be explained by shrinkage of the pathological specimen in comparison with in vivo imaging due to lack of vascular perfusion. This also may account for the larger discrepancy that has been found between CT size and pathological size for the more vascular clear cell RCC compared to hypovascular RCC. Another factor that might create a difference between measured CT and pathologic sizes is that the tumors may have been measured only in the axial plane when some tumors had the longest dimension in another plane.

Pelvic and Chest CT

Pelvic CT may not be needed for the initial staging evaluation of RCC. Most studies have shown that there are few significant findings on pelvic CT for most patients with renal tumors [146, 147]. For expected low-stage disease with small primary tumors, a normal chest X-ray will likely suffice for pulmonary staging [148]; for larger tumors and patients with extensive regional disease or pulmonary symptoms, chest CT is indicated.

Lymphadenopathy

Both CT and MR are highly sensitive for metastatic lymphadenopathy using a criterion of 1 cm short-axis diameter. Computed tomography sensitivity for lymph node involvement is 89–100% [59, 122]. The imaging features of lymph node metastases often mimic that of the primary tumor. For example, lymph node metastases from clear cell RCC are frequently hypervascular.

Adrenal Metastases

Adrenal gland involvement by RCC is uncommon, particularly so in the modern era with earlier detection, smaller and lower grade tumors, and asymptomatic, incidental presentation [149]. In one series, adrenal gland involvement ranged from less than 1% in early, low-stage disease to 8% in advanced disease [150]. Computed tomography has a reported 94–100% negative predictive value for adrenal involvement [138, 151, 152]. Therefore, when the CT demonstrates a normal ipsilateral adrenal gland, the gland is almost certainly not involved. Moreover, when the adrenal is not seen or the renal tumor obscures visualization of the adrenal, the adrenal is still only involved in a small percentage of cases [141]. PPV of standard enhanced CT for adrenal metastasis is low, only 11–26%. This is likely due to the high prevalence of benign adrenal adenomas. When an adrenal nodule coexists with a renal tumor, unenhanced CT or MR with in- and out-of-phase imaging can be used to distinguish between lipid-rich adenomas and metastatic disease; performing a bolus and delayed phase scan at 10–15 min and calculating washout can further increase the sensitivity for adrenal adenomas by identifying lipid-poor adenomas [153, 154].

Renal Vein and Inferior Vena Cava Tumor

The identification of renal vein or inferior vena cava (IVC) tumor thrombus and its precise localization are critical for proper staging [144]. Level I tumor thrombus extends only within the renal vein (Fig. 4.15), or into the renal vein and IVC within 2 cm of the renal vein ostia; level II extends within the IVC more than 2 cm from the renal vein ostia but not into the intrahepatic IVC; level III extends into the intrahepatic IVC but not above the hepatic veins; and level IV extends above the hepatic veins including into the right atrium. The presence of renal vein invasion not only increases the stage of what may otherwise have been a stage I or II tumor to stage III, but it also directly affects surgical management [155–157]. The level of extension of tumor thrombus within the IVC can be evaluated by transesophageal echo, ultrasound, MR, and CT. MR has excellent sensitivity and specificity for renal vein

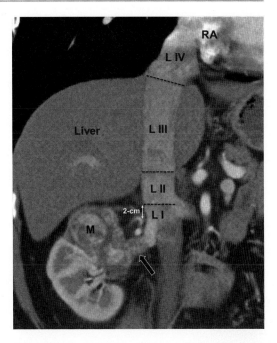

Fig. 4.15 Contrast-enhanced computed tomography showing large left upper pole renal mass (M), with enhancing tumor-thrombus invading the left renal vein (*arrow*). *Dashed lines* demarcate different levels of invasion (see text for full description). *L* level, *RA* right atrium

involvement: 90–100% [158–162]. Earlier reports noted that CT was not as sensitive as MR [59, 122, 147, 150]; however, with the use of state-of-the-art MDCT with multiphase and multiplanar imaging, CT at 87% is essentially equivalent to MR sensitivity [123, 149].

Ultrasound can also be used to assess renal vein and IVC involvement, but is frequently technically inadequate [149]. Ultrasound with CFD in experienced hands nearly matches the sensitivity of CT, but is not recommended for staging for the reasons described earlier.

Metastatic Disease

Up to 30% of patients with a new diagnosis of RCC can have metastasis at presentation [163]. RCC can metastasize to almost any organ (Fig. 4.16), but lung, brain, and bone are the most common sites. The appearance of the metastasis, whether hypervascular, hypovascular, or cystic, typically resembles the primary lesion. Lung metastases appear at chest X-ray or CT as multiple round pulmonary nodules of varying size and

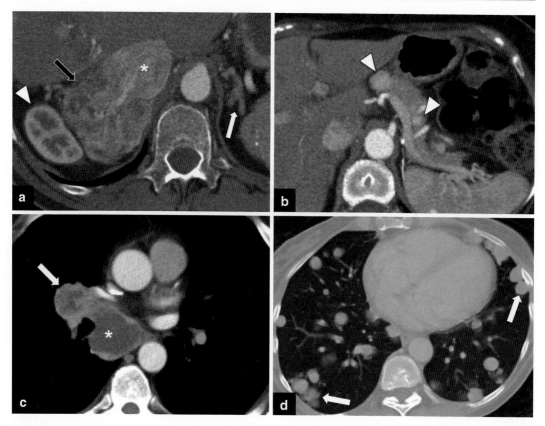

Fig. 4.16 Renal cell carcinoma metastases. (**a**) Large hypervascular right adrenal metastasis (*black arrow*) invading the inferior vena cava (*asterisk*). Normal left adrenal gland (*white arrow*); (**b**) hyperenhancing pancre- atic metastases (*arrowheads*); (**c**) hypervascular mediasti- nal and right hilar metastatic adenopathy (*arrow*), with areas of central necrosis (*asterisk*); (**d**) numerous pulmo- nary metastases (*arrows*)

are from hematogenous spread [137]. Mediastinal lymphadenopathy is more common with more extensive pulmonary metastatic disease.

Bone metastases tend to be expansile and osteolytic. Patients with metastatic RCC may have spread to the liver, adrenal glands, and soft tissue. Pancreas metastases are more commonly recognized due to improvements in scanning techniques [164, 165].

Postoperative Imaging

Patients who have had partial nephrectomy undergo routine initial follow-up at 4–6 weeks with serum creatinine and an excretory urogram to evaluate the reconstructed kidney (Fig. 4.17)

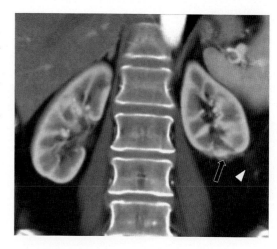

Fig. 4.17 Partial nephrectomy. Contrast-enhanced CT showing typical appearance after partial nephrectomy of the left lower renal pole (*black arrow*) with expected mild adjacent retroperitoneal fat stranding (*white arrowhead*)

[166]. Earlier imaging is performed in patients who have clinical findings such as fever or elevated white blood cell count, decreasing hematocrit, or increased output from surgical drains. These patients are imaged to assess for abscess, hematoma, or urinary leak [167, 168]. Generally, CT scan with intravenous contrast is utilized, although if a urine leak is the main consideration, then excretory urography is an appropriate alternative. Urine leaks appear as contrast-filled collections that may extend outside the renal contour or be confined to it. Hematomas are heterogeneous, soft tissue attenuation collections. Abscesses may have an enhancing wall or contain internal gas foci. Patients who present with hematuria may have an uncommon but significant complication: a pseudoaneursym (Fig. 4.18). Pseudoaneurysms are seen after <1% of open partial nephrectomies [169] and <2% of laparoscopic partial nephrectomies [170].

Strategies to assess for recurrent tumor and metastases depend on metastatic or recurrent disease risk. Because tumors that are treated with nephron-sparing surgery tend to be smaller and lower stage than those that are treated by radical nephrectomy, conventional postsurgical imaging algorithms are not used. A number of surveillance protocols have been reported. Some rely predominantly on pathologic tumor stage [171, 172] and others are more complex, integrating other factors such as tumor size, tumor grade, and degree of tumor necrosis.

One study evaluated 327 patients with sporadic RCC who underwent open nephron-sparing surgery [171]. The incidences of local recurrence and metastatic disease based on initial pathological staging were: 0 and 4.4% for stage T1, 2.0 and 5.3% for stage T2, 8.2 and 11.5% for stage T3a, and 10.6 and 14.9% for stage T3b. Including all the patients in the study, local recurrence in the remaining renal remnant occurred in 4% of patients with a peak time interval of 6–24 months. One or more metastatic lesions were seen without local recurrence in 7.6% of patients, with a peak time interval of longer than 48 months. Another study showed that patients who had pathological T1 tumors that recur had symptoms and/or thoracic metastases 81% of the time suggesting that clinical follow-up and chest radiographs are the most important components in the surveillance process [172].

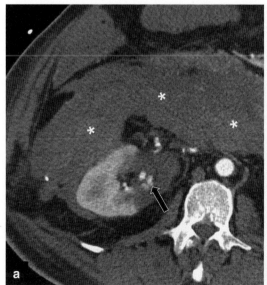
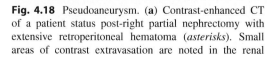
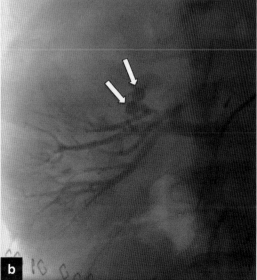

Fig. 4.18 Pseudoaneurysm. (**a**) Contrast-enhanced CT of a patient status post-right partial nephrectomy with extensive retroperitoneal hematoma (*asterisks*). Small areas of contrast extravasation are noted in the renal parenchyma (*black arrow*). (**b**) Renal arteriography confirms the presence of small rounded areas of contrast opacification (*arrows*), diagnostic of pseudoaneurysms

Taken together, this data suggests that postoperative surveillance for recurrent disease can be tailored based upon the initial pathological stage of the tumor and the clinical status of the patient [166]. All patients should be evaluated annually with a history and physical examination and blood tests including serum calcium, alkaline phosphatase, liver function tests, BUN, serum creatinine, and electrolytes. Patients with T_1 tumors based on the 1997 TNM classification ($pT_1 < 2.5$ cm and organ confined) do not require postoperative imaging due to very low risk of recurrent malignancy. A yearly chest radiograph is recommended for T_2 or T_3 tumors because the lung is the most common site of metastasis. Patients with T_2 tumors should also have abdominal and pelvic CT every 2 years. Patients with T_3 tumors have a higher risk of developing local recurrence, shorter time to recurrence, and more commonly recur within the abdomen; they should have a CT every 6 months for 2 years then at 2-year intervals.

The strategy discussed above is only one example of a post-therapy algorithm. Many others have been published, some including more variables. Frank et al. showed that metastases in the abdomen, lung, bone, and brain can be predicted by independent variables such as TNM stage, tumor size, tumor grade, and degree of tumor necrosis [173]. Similarly, the group from the University of California, Los Angeles, proposed a surveillance protocol based on prognostic categories that combine TNM stage, Fuhrman grade and ECOG performance status [174].

Postprocedural imaging is less standardized after renal tumor ablation. Typically, the first follow-up is obtained at 1 month and additional follow-up occurs at 6 months, 1 year and then yearly.

CT is the test of choice to search for tumor recurrence in the postoperative period [175]. Contrast enhancement is important in detecting visceral organ metastases and local recurrence. However, the risk of nephrotoxicity from iodinated CT contrast is higher in the patients who have surgery for RCC and may have compromised renal function. In these patients MRI is often a reasonable alternative to CT.

Local recurrence after resection or ablation manifests as an enhancing mass at the resection site in the residual kidney or nephrectomy bed. In the immediate postoperative period, operative changes are significant after both partial nephrectomy and tumor ablation and should not be confused for residual disease. These include perinephric fluid or scarring and a defect at the operative site. Residual hemostatic agents such as oxidized cellulose (Surgicel, Johnson and Johnson, Arlington, TX) may be present [176]. After ablation, the mass undergoes progressive decrease in size over time (Fig. 4.19) [177, 178]. This involution is more evident after cryoablation than radiofrequency ablation [179–182]. A normal postablation CT or MRI should show no residual enhancement of the tumor with a rim of nonenhancing ablated normal renal parenchyma (Fig. 4.20). Incomplete ablation manifests as residual enhancing tumor [169, 170]. New areas of enhancement or mass-like contour change suggest recurrent disease (Fig. 4.21).

Imaging After Targeted Antiangiogenic Therapies

Antiangiogenic agents have been shown to be more effective than conventional therapies for metastatic RCC [183]. Assessment of therapeutic response is most often based on tumor size and response evaluation criteria in solid tumors (RECISTs). However, despite the substantial improvement in survival obtained with angiogenesis inhibitors, the RECIST response rate is relatively low. This primarily results from RECIST reliance on tumor size change to indicate response. Response to antiangiogenic therapy has been shown to lead to necrosis with only modest size change in other tumors such as GI stromal tumor. Criteria were developed to gauge the treatment response of GIST that are based on quantification of change in both tumor size and density on CT. A similar approach has recently been taken for RCC [184, 185]. In one series, a favorable response according to newly developed criteria had a sensitivity of 86% and specificity of 100% in identifying patients with a good clinical outcome (i.e., progression-free survival of >250 days) compared to 17% sensitivity and 100%

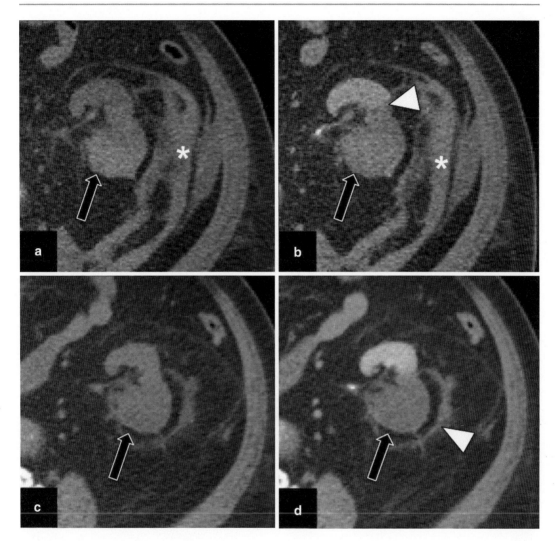

Fig. 4.19 Post cryoablation changes. Pre- and post-contrast images (**a** and **b**, respectively) 24-h after cryoablation of renal mass. The cryoablation zone (*arrow*) encompass the mass entirely and part of the normal renal parenchyma (*arrowhead*) with no contrast enhancement. Small perinephric hematoma is observed (*asterisks*). Three months follow-up CT scan before (**c**) and after (**d**) contrast administration. The ablation zone has decreased in size (tumor involution) and in attenuation. There is no enhancement to suggest residual or recurrent disease. The perinephric hematoma has nearly resolved. There is a characteristic perinephric halo (*arrowhead* on **d**) demarcating the ablation zone

specificity for the RECIST category of partial response.

Summary

With modern computed tomography and MRI, imaging serves as an accurate means to characterize, stage, and plan therapy for patients with renal tumors, and to evaluate patients after therapy for complications or disease progression. Because of developments in both imaging technology and therapies for patients with RCC, imaging is used in new ways, in particular to plan and guide therapy by depicting precise anatomical details. While there has been an increased recognition that small renal masses can be benign, the majority of solid renal masses are RCC. Imaging can distinguish some of the subtypes of RCC. Clear cell RCC, oncocytoma, and AML are the most vascular of

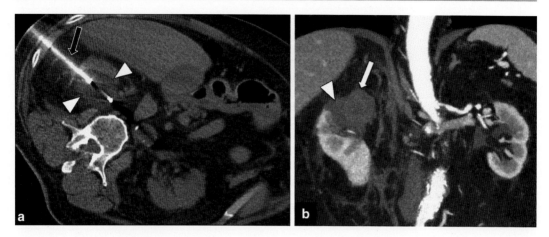

Fig. 4.20 CT-guided percutaneous cryoablation. (**a**) Axial CT scan obtained with the patient in the left lateral decubitus position during cryoablation procedure showing the cryoprobe (*black arrow*) and early ice ball formation (*arrowheads*). (**b**) Contrast-enhanced CT image on coronal plane, obtained 24-h post procedure demonstrating expected lack of enhancement of the ablation zone (*arrowhead*), with hyperdense areas related to hemorrhage (*white arrow*)

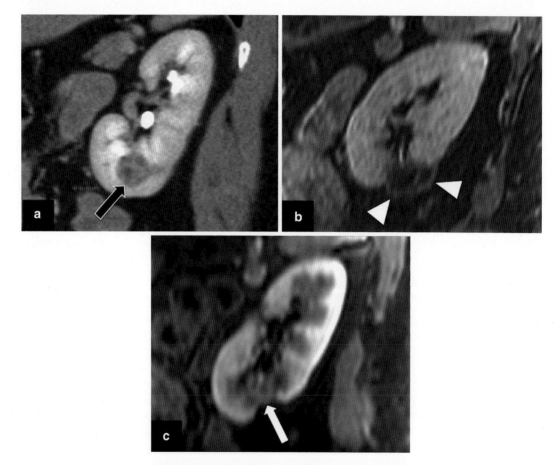

Fig. 4.21 Renal cell carcinoma recurrence post cryoablation. (**a**) Sagittal plane contrast-enhanced CT image demonstrating a left lower renal pole enhancing lesion (*arrow*). (**b**) Sagittal contrast-enhanced MR image postablation showing no enhancing lesion within the ablation zone (*arrowheads*). (**c**) Sagittal contrast-enhanced MR image over 2 years post-ablation revealing enhancing tumor at the inner margin of the ablation zone (*arrow*) consistent with recurrence

the renal primary tumors; AML can usually be distinguished from other tumors based on the presence of fat within the lesion. Papillary and chromophobe RCC are typically hypovascular and less aggressive tumors. CT, because of its ready availability, ease of use, and accuracy, is the primary imaging modality for diagnosis and staging of RCC. MR imaging has accuracy similar to CT, but in most institutions is used for patients with lesions indeterminate at CT, or who have contrast allergies or renal insufficiency.

References

1. Zagoria RJ. Imaging of small renal masses: a medical success story. Am J Roentgenol. 2000;175:945–55.
2. Konnak JW, Grossman HB. Renal cell carcinoma as an incidental finding. J Urol. 1985;134:1094–6.
3. Rodriguez-Rubio FI, Diez-Caballero F, Martin-Marquina A, Abad JI, Berian JM. Incidentally detected renal cell carcinoma. Br J Urol. 1996;78:29–32.
4. Thompson IM, Peek M. Improvement in survival of patients with renal cell carcinoma: the role of the serendipitously detected tumor. J Urol. 1988;140:487–90.
5. Chow WH, Devesa SS, Warren JL, Fraumeni Jr JF. Rising incidence of renal cell cancer in the United States. JAMA. 1999;281:1628–31.
6. Homma Y, Kawabe K, Kitamura T, et al. Increased incidental detection and reduced mortality in renal cancer: recent retrospective analysis at eight institutions. Int J Urol. 1995;2:77–80.
7. Sedjo RL, Byers T, Barrera E, et al. A midpoint assessment of the American Cancer Society challenge goal to decrease cancer incidence by 25% between 1992 and 2015. CA Cancer J Clin. 2007;57:326–40.
8. Duchene DA, Lotan Y, Cadeddu JA, Sagalowsky AI, Koeneman KS. Histopathology of surgically managed renal tumors: analysis of a contemporary series. Urology. 2003;62:827–30.
9. Ozen H, Colowick A, Freiha FS. Incidentally discovered solid renal masses: what are they? Br J Urol. 1993;72:274–6.
10. Jayson M, Sanders H. Increased incidence of serendipitously discovered renal cell carcinoma. Urology. 1998;51:203–5.
11. Luciani LG, Cestari R, Tallarigo C. Incidental renal cell carcinoma-age and stage characterization and clinical implications: study of 1092 patients (1982–1997). Urology. 2000;56:58–62.
12. Smith SJ, Bosniak MA, Megibow AJ, Hulnick Dh, Horri SC, Ragavendra BN. Renal cell carcinoma: earlier discovery and increased detection. Radiology. 1989;170:699–703.
13. Breatheau D, Lechevallier E, Eghazarian C, et al. Prognostic significance of incidental renal cell carcinoma. Eur Urol. 1995;27:319–23.
14. Silverman SG, Yu UG, Mortele KJ, Tuncali K, Cibas ES. Renal masses in the adult patient: the role of percutaneous biopsy. Radiology. 2006;240:6–22.
15. Israel GM, Bosniak MA. Renal imaging for diagnosis and staging of renal cell carcinoma. Urol Clin N Am. 2003;30:499–514.
16. Hélénon O, Correas JM, Balleyquier C, et al. Ultrasound of renal tumors. Eur Radiol. 2001;11:1890–901.
17. Kitamura H, Fujimoto H, Tobisu K, et al. Dynamic computed tomography and color Doppler ultrasound of renal parenchymal neoplasms: correlation with histopathological findings. Jpn J Clin Oncol. 2004;34: 78–81.
18. Mihara S, Kuroda K, Yoshioka R, et al. Early detection of renal cell carcinoma by ultrasonographic screening – based on 13 years screening in exam. Ultrasound Med Biol. 1999;25:1033–9.
19. Tosaka A, Ohya K, Yamada K, et al. Incidence and properties of renal masses and asymptomatic renal cell carcinoma detected by abdominal ultrasonography. J Urol. 1990;144:1097–9.
20. Park BK, Kim SH, Choi HJ. Characterization of renal cell carcinoma using agent detection imaging: comparison with gray-scale ultrasound. Korean J Radiol. 2005;6:173–8.
21. Correas J-M, Claudon M, Tranquart F, Hélénon O. The kidney: imaging with microbubble contrast agents. Ultrasound Q. 2006;22:53–66.
22. Park BK, Kim B, Kim SH, et al. Assessment of cystic renal masses based on Bosniak classification: comparison of CT and contrast-enhanced US. Eur J Radiol. 2007;61(2):310–4.
23. Quaia E, Bertolotto M, Cioffi V, et al. Comparison of contrast-enhanced sonography with unenhanced sonography and contrast-enhanced CT in the diagnosis of malignancy in complex cystic renal masses. Am J Roentgenol. 2008;191(4):1239–49.
24. Tamai H, Takiguchi Y, Oka M, et al. Contrast enhanced ultrasonography in the diagnosis of solid renal tumors. J Ultrasound Med. 2005;24(12):1635–40.
25. Cohan RH, Sherman LS, Korobkin M, et al. Renal masses: assessment of corticomedullary-phase and nephrographic-phase CT scans. Radiology. 1995;196: 445–51.
26. Herts BR, Einstein DM, Paushter DM. Spiral CT of the abdomen: artifacts and potential pitfalls. Am J Roentgenol. 1993;161:1185–90.
27. Jinzaki M, Tanimoto A, Mukai M, et al. Double-phase helical CT of small renal parenchymal neoplasms: correlation with pathological findings and tumor angiogenesis. J Comput Assist Tomogr. 2000;24: 835–42.
28. Herts BR, Coll DM, Novick AC, et al. Enhancement characteristics of papillary renal neoplasms revealed on triphasic helical CT of the kidneys. Am J Roentgenol. 2002;178:367–72.
29. Birnbaum BA, Jacobs JE, Ramchandani P. Multiphasic renal CT: comparison of renal mass

enhancement during the corticomedullary and nephrographic phases. Radiology. 1996;200:753–8.

30. Kopka L, Fischer U, Zoeller G, et al. Dual-phase
helical CT of the kidney: value of the corticomedullary and nephrographic phase for evaluation of renal
lesions and preoperative staging of renal cell carcinoma. Am J Roentgenol. 1997;169:1573–8.

31. Kauczor HU, Schwickert HC, Schweden F, et al. Bolus-
enhanced renal spiral CT: techniques, diagnostic value
and drawbacks. Eur J Radiol. 1994;18:153–7.

32. Garant M, Bonaldi VM, Taourel P, et al. Enhancement
patterns of renal masses during multiphase helical
CT acquisitions. Abdom Imaging. 1998;23:431–6.

33. Szolar DH, Kammerhuber F, Altziebler S, et al.
Multiphasic helical CT of the kidney: increased con-
spicuity for detection and characterization of small
(<3-cm) renal masses. Radiology. 1997;202:211–7.

34. Sadowski EA, Bennett LK, Chan MR, et al.
Nephrogenic systemic fibrosis: risk factors and incidence estimation. Radiology. 2007;243(1):148–57.

35. Herts BR, Coll DM, Lieber ML, et al. Triphasic helical CT of the kidneys: contribution of vascular phase
scanning in patients before urologic surgery. Am J
Roentgenol. 1999;173:1273–7.

36. Narumi Y, Hricak H, Presti Jr JC, et al. MR imaging
of renal cell carcinoma. Abdom Imaging. 1997;22:
216–25.

37. Ho VB, Allen SF, Hood MN, et al. Renal masses:
quantitative assessment of enhancement with dynamic
MR imaging. Radiology. 2002;224:695–700.

38. Kanal E, Barkovich AJ, Bell C, et al. ACR guidance
document for safe MR practices: 2007. Am J
Roentgenol. 2007;188:1447–74.

39. Walter C, Kruessell M, Gindele A, et al. Imaging of
renal lesions: evaluation of fast MRI and helical CT.
Br J Radiol. 2003;76:696–703.

40. Chung EP, Herts BR, Linnell G, et al. Analysis of
changes in attenuation of proven renal cysts on different scanning phases of triphasic MDCT. Am J
Roentgenol. 2004;182:405–10.

41. Coulam CH, Sheafor DH, Leder RA, et al. Evaluation
of pseudoenhancement of renal cysts during contrast-
enhanced CT. Am J Roentgenol. 2000;174:493–8.

42. Maki DD, Birnbaum BA, Chakraborty DP, et al. Renal
cyst pseudoenhancement: beam-hardening effects on
CT numbers. Radiology. 1999;213:468–72.

43. Coll DM, Uzzo RG, Herts BR, et al. 3-Dimensional
volume rendered computerized tomography for preoperative evaluation and intraoperative treatment of
patients undergoing nephron sparing surgery. J Urol.
1999;161:1097–102.

44. Coll DM, Herts BR, Davros WJ, et al. Preoperative
use of 3D volume rendering to demonstrate renal
tumors and renal anatomy. Radiographics. 2000;20:
431–8.

45. Choyke PL, Walther MM, Wagner JR, et al. Renal
cancer: preoperative evaluation with dual-phase
three-dimensional MR angiography. Radiology.
1997;205:767–71.

46. Catalano C, Fraioli F, Laghi A, et al. High-resolution
multidetector CT in the preoperative evaluation of
patients with renal cell carcinoma. Am J Roentgenol.
2003;180:1271–7.

47. Sheth S, Scatarige JC, Horton KM, et al. Current
concepts in the diagnosis and management of renal
cell carcinoma: role of multidetector CT and three-
dimensional CT. Radiographics. 2001;21:S237–54.

48. Wunderlich H, Reichelt O, Schubert R, et al.
Preoperative simulation of partial nephrectomy with
three-dimensional computed tomography. BJU Int.
2000;86:777–81.

49. Rofsky NM, Weinreb JC, Bosniak MA, et al. Renal
lesion characterization with gadolinium-enhanced
MR imaging: efficacy and safety in patients with
renal insufficiency. Radiology. 1991;180:85–9.

50. Broome DR, Girguis MS, Baron PW, Cottrell AC,
Kjellin I, Kirk GA. Gadodiamide-associated nephrogenic systemic fibrosis: why radiologists should be
concerned. Am J Roentgenol. 2007;188(2):586–92.

51. Altum E, Martin DR, Wertman R, Lugo-Somolinos
A, Fuller 3rd ER, Semelka RC. Nephrogenic systemic fibrosis: change in incidence following a
switch in gadolinium agents and adoption of a gadolinium policy – report from two U.S. universities.
Radiology. 2009;253:689–96.

52. Kramer LA. Magnetic resonance imaging of renal
masses. World J Urol. 1998;16:22–8.

53. Hecht EM, Israel GM, Krinsky GA, et al. Renal
masses: quantitative analysis of enhancement with
signal intensity measurements versus qualitative
analysis of enhancement with image subtraction for
diagnosing malignancy at MR imaging. Radiology.
2004;232:373–8.

54. Ho VB, Choyke PL. MR evaluation of solid renal
masses. MRI Clinics of NA. 2004;12:413–27.

55. Semelka RC, Shoenut JP, Magro CM, et al. Renal
cancer staging: comparison of contrast-enhanced CT
and gadolinium-enhanced fat-suppressed spin-echo
and gradient-echo MR imaging. J Magn Reson
Imaging. 1993;3:597–602.

56. Hallscheidt PJ, Bock M, Riedasch G, et al. Diagnostic
accuracy of staging renal cell carcinoma using mul-
tidetector-row computed tomography and magnetic
resonance imaging. J Comput Assist Tomogr.
2004;28:333–9.

57. Pretorius ES, Wickstrom L, Siegelman ES. MR
imaging of renal neoplasms. MRI Clinics of NA.
2000;8: 813–36.

58. Suh M, Coakley FV, Qayyum A, et al. Distinction of
renal cell carcinomas from high-attenuation renal
cysts at portal venous phase contrast-enhanced CT.
Radiology. 2003;228:330–4.

59. Israel GM, Bosniak MA. How I do it: evaluating
renal masses. Radiology. 2005;236:441–50.

60. Frank I, Blute ML, Cheville JC, Lohse CM, Weaver
AL, Zincke H. Solid renal tumors: an analysis of
pathological features related to tumor size. J Urol.
2003;170:2217–20.

61. Zagoria RJ, Wolfman NT, Karstaedt N, Hinn GC, Dyer RB, Chen YM. CT features of renal cell carcinoma with emphasis on relation to tumor size. Invest Radiol. 1990;25:261.

62. Jinzaki M, Tanimoto A, Narimatsu Y, et al. Angiomyolipoma: imaging findings in lesions with minimal fat. Radiology. 1997;205:497–502.

63. Simpfendorfer C, Herts BR, Motta-Ramirez GA, Lockwood DS, et al. Angiomyolipoma with minimal fat on MDCT: can pixel counts aid diagnosis? Am J Roentgenol. 2009;192:438–43.

64. Kim JK, Park SY, Shon JH, Cho KS. Angiomyolipoma with minimal fat: differentiation from renal cell carcinoma at biphasic helical CT. Radiology. 2004;230(3):677–84.

65. Davidson AJ, Hayes WJ, Hartman DS, et al. Renal oncocytoma and carcinoma: failure of differentiation with CT. Radiology. 1993;186:693–6.

66. Yamashita Y, Watanabe O, Miyazaki T, et al. Cystic renal cell carcinoma; imaging findings with pathologic correlation. Acta Radiol. 1994;35:19–24.

67. Curry NS. Atypical cystic renal masses. Abdom Imaging. 1998;23:230–6.

68. Eble JN, Bonsib SM. Extensively cystic renal neoplasms: cystic nephroma, cystic partially differentiated nephroblastoma, multilocular cystic renal cell carcinoma, and cystic hamartoma of the renal pelvis. Sem Diag Pathol. 1998;15:2–20.

69. Bosniak MA. The current radiological approach to renal cysts. Radiology. 1986;158:1–10.

70. Bosniak MA. Difficulties in classifying cystic lesions of the kidney. Urol Radiol. 1991;13:91–3.

71. Israel GM, Bosniak MA. Calcification in cystic renal masses: is it important in diagnosis? Radiology. 2003;226:47–52.

72. Israel GM, Hindman N, Bosniak MA. Evaluation of cystic renal masses: comparison of CT and MR using the Bosniak classification system. Radiology. 2004;231:365–71.

73. Siegel CL, Fisher AJ, Bennett HF. Interobserver variability in determining enhancement of renal masses on helical CT. Am J Roentgenol. 1999;172:1207–12.

74. Wilson TE, Doelle EA, Cohan RH, et al. Cystic renal masses: a reevaluation of the usefulness of the Bosniak classification system. Acad Radiol. 1996;3:564–70.

75. Jonisch AI, Rubinowitz AN, Mutalik PG, Israel GM. Can high-attenuation renal cysts be differentiated from renal cell carcinoma at unenhanced CT? Radiology. 2007;243(2):445–50.

76. Harishinghani MG, Maher MM, Gervais DA, et al. Incidence of malignancy in complex cystic renal masses (Bosniak III): should biopsy precede surgery. Am J Roentgenol. 2003;180:755–8.

77. Lang EK, Macchia RJ, Gayle B, et al. CT-guided biopsy of indeterminate renal cystic masses (Bosniak 3 and 2F): accuracy and impact on clinical management. Eur Radiol. 2002;12:2518–24.

78. Lane BR, Campbell SC, Remer EM, et al. Cystic nephroma and mixed epithelial and stromal tumor of the kidney: ideal lesions for nephron-sparing surgery. Urology. 2008;71:1142–8.

79. Pickhardt PJ, Lonergan GJ, Davis CJ, et al. Infiltrative renal lesions: radiologic–pathologic correlation. Radiographics. 2000;20:215–43.

80. Cohan RH, Dunnick NR, Leder RA. Computed tomography of renal lymphoma. J Comput Assist Tomogr. 1990;14:933–8.

81. Araki T. Leukemic involvement of the kidney in children: CT features. J Comput Assist Tomogr. 1982;6:781–4.

82. Mitnick JS, Bosniak MA, Rothberg M. Metastatic neoplasm to the kidney studied by computed tomography and sonography. J Comput Assist Tomogr. 1985;9:43–9.

83. Gattuso P, Ramzy I, Truong LD, et al. Utilization of fine-needle aspiration in the diagnosis of metastatic tumors to the kidney. Diagnostic Cytopathol. 1999;21:35–8.

84. Weiss LM, Gelb AB, Medeiros LJ. Adult renal epithelial neoplasms. Am J Clin Pathol. 1995;103:624–35.

85. Bostwick DG, Eble JN. Diagnosis and classification of renal cell carcinoma. Urol Clin North Am. 1999;26:627–35.

86. Zisman A, Chao DH, Pantuck AJ, et al. Unclassified renal cell carcinoma: clinical features and prognostic impact of a new histological subtype. J Urol. 2002;168:950–5.

87. Kim JK, Kim TK, Ahn HJ, Kim CS, Kim KR, Cho KS. Differentiation of subtypes of renal cell carcinoma on helical CT scans. Am J Roentgenol. 2002;178:1499–506.

88. Sheir KZ, El-Azab M, Mosbah A, et al. Differentiation of renal cell carcinoma subtypes by multislice computerized tomography. J Urol. 2005;174:451–5.

89. Shinmoto H, Yuasa Y, Tanimoto A, et al. Small renal cell carcinoma: MRI with pathological correlation. J Magn Reson Imaging. 1998;8:690–4.

90. Uzzo RG, Cherullo EE, Myles J, et al. Renal cell carcinoma invading the urinary collecting system: implications for staging. J Urol. 2002;167:2392–6.

91. Han K-R, Janzen JK, McWhorter VC, et al. Cystic renal cell carcinoma: biology and clinical behavior. Urol Oncol. 2004;22:410–4.

92. Delahunt B, Eble JN. Papillary renal cell carcinoma: a clinopathologic and immunohistochemical study of 105 cases. Mod Pathol. 1997;10:537–44.

93. Lager DJ, Huston BJ, Timmerman TG, Bonsib SM. Papillary renal tumors. Cancer. 1995;76:669.

94. Ruppert-Kohlmayr AJ, Uggowitzer M, Meissnitzer T, et al. Differentiation of renal clear cell carcinoma and renal papillary carcinoma using quantitative CT enhancement parameters. Am J Roentgenol. 2004;183:1387–91.

95. Roy C, Sauer B, Lindner V, Lang H, Saussine C, Jacqmin D. MR Imaging of papillary renal neoplasms: potential application for characterization of

small renal masses. Eur Radiol. 2007;17(1): 193–200.

96. Polascik TJ, Bostwick DG, Cairns P. Molecular genetics and histopathologic features of adults distal nephron tumors. Urology. 2002;60:941–6.

97. Schacter LR, Cookson MS, Chang SS, et al. Frequency of benign renal cortical tumors and histologic subtypes based on size in a contemporary series: what to tell our patients. J Endourol. 2007;21:819–23.

98. Mejean A, Hopirtean V, Bazin JP, et al. Prognostic factors for the survival of patients with papillary renal cell carcinoma: meaning of histologic typing and multifocality. J Urol. 2003;170:764–7.

99. Yamada T, Endo M, Tsuboi M, et al. Differentiation of pathologic subtypes of papillary renal cell carcinoma on CT. Am J Roentgenol. 2008;191(5): 1559–63.

100. Megumi Y, Nishimura K. Chromophobe renal cell carcinoma. Urol Int. 1998;61:172–4.

101. Kondo T, Nakazawa H, Sakai F, et al. Spoke-wheel-like enhancement as an important imaging finding of chromophobe cell renal carcinoma: a retrospective analysis on computed tomography and magnetic resonance imaging studies. Int J Urol. 2004;11: 817–24.

102. Srigley JR, Eble JN. Collecting duct carcinoma of kidney. Semin Diagn Pathol. 1998;15:54–67.

103. Fukuya T, Honda H, Goto K, et al. Computed tomographic findings of Bellini duct carcinoma of the kidney. J Comput Assist Tomogr. 1996;20:399–403.

104. Gurocak S, Sozen S, Akyurek N, et al. Cortically located collecting duct carcinoma. Urology. 2005;65:1226.

105. Pickhardt PJ, Siegel CL, McLarney JK. Collecting duct carcinoma of the kidney: are imaging findings suggestive of the diagnosis? Am J Roentgenol. 2001;176:627–33.

106. Pickhardt PJ. Collecting duct carcinoma arising in a solitary kidney: imaging findings. Clin Imaging. 1999;23:115–8.

107. Mian BM, Bhadkamkar NJ, Slaton JW, et al. Prognostic factors and survival of patients with sarcomatoid renal cell carcinoma. Urology. 2002;167:65–70.

108. Staelens L, Van Poppel H, Vanuytsel L, et al. Sarcomatoid renal cell carcinoma: case report and review of the literature. Acta Urol Belg. 1997;65:39–42.

109. Silverman SG, Herts BR, Israel GM, Ritchie JP. Management of the incidental renal mass. Radiology. 2008;249:16–31.

110. Wiatrowska BA, Zakowski MF. Fine-needle aspiration biopsy of chromophobe renal cell carcinoma and oncocytoma: comparison of cytomorphologic features. Cancer. 1999;87:161–7.

111. Liu J, Fanning CV. Can renal oncocytomas be distinguished from renal cell carcinoma on fine-needle aspiration specimens? A study of conventional

smears in conjunction with ancillary studies. Cancer. 2001;93:390–7.

112. Eble JN, Sauter G, Epstein JL, et al. Pathology and genetics of tumours of the urinary system and male genital organs, in WHO classification of tumors. Lyon: IARC; 2004.

113. Park HS, Kim SH, Kim SH, et al. Benign mixed epithelial and stromal tumor of the kidney: imaging findings. J Comput Assist Tomogr. 2005;29(6):786–9.

114. Bracken RB, Chica G, Johnson DE, et al. Secondary renal neoplasms: an autopsy study. South Med J. 1979;72:806–7.

115. Wood BJ, Khan MA, McGovern F, et al. Imaging guided biopsy of renal masses: indications, accuracy and impact on clinical management. J Urol. 1999;161:1470–4.

116. Sheeran SR, Sussman SK. Renal lymphoma: spectrum of CT findings and potential mimics. Am J Roentgenol. 1998;171:1067–72.

117. Silverman SG, Mortele KJ, Tuncali K, Jinzaki M, Cibas ES. Hyperattenuating renal masses: etiologies pathogenesis, and imaging evaluation. Radiographics. 2007;27:1131–43.

118. Kim JK, Park SY, Shon JH, et al. Angiomyolipoma with minimal fat: differentiation from renal cell carcinoma at biphasic helical CT. Radiology. 2004;230:677–84.

119. Schuster TG, Ferguson MR, Baker DE, et al. Papillary renal cell carcinoma containing fat without calcification mimicking angiomyolipoma on CT. Am J Roentgenol. 2004;183:1402–4.

120. Hammadeh MY, Thomas K, Philp T, et al. Renal cell carcinoma containing fat mimicking angiomyolipoma: demonstration with CT scan and histopathology. Eur Radiol. 1998;8:228–9.

121. Wang LJ, Wong YC, Chen CJ, et al. Computerized tomography characteristics that differentiate angiomyolipomas from liposarcomas in the perinephric space. J Urol. 2002;167:490–3.

122. Israel GM, Bosniak MA, Slywotzky CM, et al. CT differentiation of large exophytic angiomyolipomas and perirenal liposarcomas. Am J Roentgenol. 2002;179:769–73.

123. Robson CJ, Churchill BM, Anderson W, et al. The results of radical nephrectomy for renal cell carcinoma. J Urol. 1969;101:297.

124. Fleming ID, Cooper JS, Henson DE, et al., editors. American Joint Committee on Cancer (AJCC). AJCC manual for staging of cancer, 5th ed. Philadelphia: Lippincott-Raven; 1997. p. 231–4.

125. Gettman MT, Blute ML, Spotts B, et al. Pathologic staging of renal cell carcinoma. Cancer. 2001;91:354–61.

126. Guinan P, Sobin LH, Algaba F, et al. TNM staging of renal cell carcinoma. Cancer. 1997;80:992–3.

127. Sobin LH, Wittekind CH, editors. International Union Against Cancer (UICC). TNM classification of malignant tumors, 5th ed. New York: John Wiley & Sons; 1997. p. 180–2.

128. Tsui KH, Shvarts O, Smith R, et al. Prognostic indicators for renal cell carcinoma: a multivariate analysis of 643 patients using the revised 1997 TNM staging system. J Urol. 2000;163:1090–5.

129. Dinney CP, Awad SA, Gajewski J, et al. Analysis of imaging modalities, staging systems, and progostic indicators for renal cell carcinoma. Urology. 1992;39:122–9.

130. Constantinides C, Recker F, Bruehlmann W, et al. Accuracy of magnetic resonance imaging compared to computerized tomography and selective renal angiography in preoperatively staging renal cell carcinoma. Urol Int. 1991;47:181–5.

131. Bechtold RE, Zagoria RJ. Imaging approach to staging of renal cell carcinoma. Urol Clin North Am. 1997;24:507–22.

132. Johnson CD, Dunnick NR, Cohan RH, et al. Renal adenocarcinoma: CT staging of 100 tumors. Am J Roentgenol. 1987;148:59–63.

133. Cronan JJ, Zeman RK, Rosenfeld AT. Comparison of computerized tomography, ultrasound and angiography in staging renal cell carcinoma. J Urol. 1982;127:712–4.

134. Prati GF, Saggin P, Boschiero L, et al. Small renal-cell carcinomas: clinical and imaging features. Urol Int. 1993;51:19–22.

135. London NJ, Messios N, Kinder RB, et al. A prospective study oft he value of conventional CT, dynamic CT, ultrasonography and arteriography for staging renal carcinoma. Br J Urol. 1989;64:209–17.

136. Hricak H, Thoeni RF, Carroll PR, et al. Detection and staging of renal neoplasms: a reassessment of MR imaging. Radiology. 1988;166:643–9.

137. Zagoria RJ, Bechtold RE, Dyer RB. Staging of renal adenocarcinoma: role of various imaging procedures. Am J Roentgenol. 1995;164:363–70.

138. Ukimura O, Haber GP, Remer EM, Gill IS. Laparoscopic partial nephrectomy for incidental stage pT2 or worse tumors. Urology. 2006;68(5):976–82.

139. Roberts WW, Bhayani J, Allaf ME, et al. Pathological stage does not alter the prognosis for renal lesions determined to be stage T1 by computerized tomography. Urol. 2005;173:713–5.

140. Kamel IR, Hochman MG, Keogan MT, et al. Accuracy of breath-hold magnetic resonance imaging in preoperative staging of organ-confined renal cell carcinoma. J Comput Assist Tomogr. 2004;28(3):327–32.

141. Thompson RH, Leibovich BC, Cheville JC, et al. Is renal sinus fat invasion the same as perinephric fat invasion for pt3a renal cell carcinoma? J Urol. 2005;174:1218–21.

142. Hallscheidt P, Wagener N, Gholipour F, et al. Multislice computed tomography in planning nephron-sparing surgery in a prospective study with 76 patients: comparison of radiological and histopathological findings in the infiltration of renal structures. J Comput Assist Tomogr. 2006;30(6):869–74.

143. Irani J, Humbert M, Lecocq B, et al. Renal tumor size: comparison between computed tomography and surgical measurements. Eur Urol. 2001;39:300–3.

144. Yaycioglu O, Rutman MP, Balasubramaniam M, et al. Clinical and pathologic tumor size in renal cell carcinoma; difference, correlation, and analysis of influencing factors. Urology. 2002;60:33–8.

145. Herr HW, Lee CT, Sharma S, et al. Radiographic versus pathologic size of renal tumors: implications for partial nephrectomy. Urology. 2001;58:157–60.

146. Khaitan A, Gupta NP, Hemal AK, et al. Is there a need for pelvic CT scan in cases of renal cell carcinoma? Int Urol Nephrol. 2002;33:13–5.

147. Fielding JR, Aliabadi N, Renshaw AA, et al. Staging of 119 patients with renal cell carcinoma: the yield and cost-effectiveness of pelvic CT. Am J Roentgenol. 1999;172:1721–3.

148. Lim DJ, Carter F. Computerized tomography in the preoperative staging for pulmonary metastases in patients with renal cell carcinoma. J Urol. 1993;150:1112–4.

149. Tsui KH, Shvarts O, Barbaric Z, et al. Is adrenalectomy a necessary component of radical nephrectomy? UCLA experience with 511 radical nephrectomies. J Urol. 2000;163:437–41.

150. Tsui KH, Shvarts O, Smith RB, Figlin R, DeKernion JB, Belldegrun A. Renal cell carcinoma: prognostic significance of incidentally detected tumors. J Urol. 2000;163:426–30.

151. Sawai Y, Kinochi T, Mano M, et al. Ipsilateral adrenal involvement from renal cell carcinoma: retrospective study of the predictive value of computed tomography. Urology. 2002;59:28–31.

152. Gill IS, McClennan BL, Kerbi K, et al. Adrenal involvement from renal cell carcinoma: predictive value of computerized tomography. J Urol. 1994;154:1082–5.

153. Hamrahian AH, Ioachimescu AG, Remer EM, et al. Clinical utility of noncontrast computed tomography attenuation value (Hounsfield units) to differentiate adrenal adenomas/hyperplasias from nonadenomas: Cleveland Clinic experience. J Clin Endocrinol Metab. 2005;90:871–7.

154. Israel GM, Korobkin M, Wang C, et al. Comparison of unenhanced CT and chemical shift MRI in evaluating lipid-rich adrenal adenomas. Am J Roentgenol. 2004;183:215–9.

155. Hatcher PA, Anderson EE, Paulson DF, et al. Surgical management and prognosis of renal cell carcinoma invading the vena cava. J Urol. 1991;145:20–4.

156. Oto A, Herts BR, Remer EM, Novick AC. Inferior vena cava tumor thrombus in renal cell carcinoma: staging by MR imaging and impact on surgical treatment. Am J Roentgenol. 1998;171:1619–24.

157. Gupta NP, Ansari MD, Khaitan A, et al. Impact of imaging and thrombus level in management of renal cell carcinoma extending to veins. Urol Int. 2004;72:129–34.

158. Glazer A, Novick AC. Preoperative transesophageal echocardiography for assessment of venal caval tumor thrombi: a comparative study with venacavography and magnetic resonance imaging. Urology. 1997;49:32–4.

159. Lawrentschuk N, Gani J, Riordan R, et al. Multidetector computed tomography vs magnetic resonance imaging for defining the upper limit of tumour thrombus in renal cell carcinoma: a study and review. BJU Int. 2005;96:291–5.

160. Kallman DA, King BF, Hattery RR, et al. Renal vein and inferior vena cava tumor thrombus in renal cell carcinoma: CT, US, MRI and venacavography. J Comput Assist Tomogr. 1992;16:240–7.

161. Goldfarb DA, Novick AC, Lorig R, et al. Magnetic resonance imaging for assessment of vena cava tumor thrombi: a comparative study with venacavography and computerized tomography scanning. J Urol. 1990;144:1100–3.

162. Hockley NM, Foster RS, Bihrle R, et al. Use of magnetic resonance imaging to determine surgical approach to renal cell carcinoma with vena caval extension. Urology. 1990;36:55–60.

163. Motzer RJ, Bander NH, Nanus DM. Medical progress: renal cell carcinoma. N Engl J Med. 1996;335:865.

164. Ghavamian R, Klein KA, Stephens DH, et al. Renal cell carcinoma metastatic to the pancreas: clinical and radiographic features. Mayo Clin Proc. 2000;75:581–5.

165. Ng CS, Loyer EM, Iyer RB, et al. Metastases to the pancreas from renal cell carcinoma: findings on three-phase contrast-enhanced helical CT. Am J Roentgenol. 1999;172:1555–9.

166. Novick AC. Nephron-sparing surgery for renal cell carcinoma. Annu Rev Med. 2002;53:393–407.

167. Israel GM, Hecht E, Bosniak MA. CT and MR imaging of complications of partial nephrectomy. Radiographics. 2006;26(5):1419–29.

168. Sarwani NI, Motta Ramirez GA, Remer EM, Kaouk JH, Gill IS. Imaging findings after minimally invasive nephron-sparing renal therapies. Clin Radiol. 2007;62(4):333–9.

169. Albani JM, Novick AC. Renal artery pseudoaneurysm after partial nephrectomy: three case reports and a literature review. Urology. 2003;62:227–31.

170. Singh D, Gill I. Renal artery pseudoaneurysm following laparoscopic partial nephrectomy. J Urol. 2005;174:2256–9.

171. Hafez KS, Novick AC, Campbell SC. Patterns of tumor recurrence and guidelines for followup after nephron sparing surgery for sporadic renal cell carcinoma. J Urol. 1997;157:2067–70.

172. Stephenson AJ, Chetner MP, Rourke K, et al. Guidelines for the surveillance of localized renal cell carcinoma based on the patterns of relapse after nephrectomy. J Urol. 2004;172:58–62.

173. Frank I, Blute ML, Cheville JC, et al. A multifactorial postoperative surveillance model for patients with surgically treated clear cell renal cell carcinoma. J Urol. 2003;170(6):2225–32.

174. Janzen NK, Kim HL, Figlin RA, Belldegrun AS. Surveillance after radical or partial nephrectomy for localized renal cell carcinoma and management of recurrent disease. Urol Clin North Am. 2003;30:843–52.

175. Casalino DD, Francis IR, Arellano RS, et al. Follow-up of renal cell carcinoma. American College of Radiology. ACR Appropriateness Criteria. 2009; online access 14 Mar 2011.

176. Oto A, Remer EM, O'Malley CM, Tkach JA, Gill IS. MR characteristics of oxidized cellulose (surgicel). Am J Roentgenol. 1999;172:1481–4.

177. Gill IS, Novick AC, Meraney AM, et al. Laparoscopic renal cryoablation in 32 patients. Urology. 2000;56:748–53.

178. Remer EM, Weinberg EJ, Oto A, O'Malley CM, Gill IS. MR imaging of the kidneys after laparoscopic cryoablation. Am J Roentgenol. 2000;174:635–40.

179. Brady PS, Remer EM, Gill IS. MRI after renal cryoablation: findings at 1–2 year follow-up. Radiology. 2000;217(P):581.

180. Merkle EM, Nour SG, Lewin JS. MR imaging follow-up after percutaneous radiofrequency ablation of renal cell carcinoma: findings in 18 patients during first 6 months. Radiology. 2005;235:1065–71.

181. Kawamoto S, Permpongkosol S, Bluemke DA, Fishman EA, Solomon SB. Sequential changes after radiofrequency ablation and cryoablation of renal neoplasms: role of CT and MR imaging. Radiographics. 2007;27:343–55.

182. Wile GE, Leyendecker JR, Krehbiel KA, Dyer RB, Zagoria RJ. CT and MR imaging after imaging-guided thermal ablation of renal neoplasms. Radiographics. 2007;27(2):325–39.

183. Motzer RJ, Hutson TE, Tomczak P, et al. Sunitinib versus interferon alfa in metastatic renal-cell carcinoma. N Engl J Med. 2007;356:115–24.

184. Smith AD, Lieber ML, Shah SN. Assessing tumor response and detecting recurrence in metastatic renal cell carcinoma on targeted therapy: importance of size and attenuation on contrast-enhanced CT. Am J Roentgenol. 2010;194(1):157–65.

185. Smith AD, Shah SN, Rini BI, Lieber ML, Remer EM. Morphology, attenuation, size, and structure (MASS) criteria: assessing response and predicting clinical outcome in metastatic renal cell carcinoma on antiangiogenic targeted therapy. Am J Roentgenol. 2010;194:1470–8.

Prognostic Factors for Localized Renal Cell Carcinoma

5

Brian R. Lane

Introduction

Renal cell carcinoma (RCC) responds modestly to conventional systemic therapies, and when not completely removed surgically, remains the most lethal of the common genitourinary cancers [1]. Cancer-specific survival correlates strongly with tumor stage, although several other factors have been shown to be independent predictive factors as well [2–4]. Long-term survival exceeds 90% in patients with RCC up to 7 cm in size and contained within the kidney (pathologic stage T1), but is less than 5% in patients with metastatic RCC [3]. Although surgical treatment is curative for localized disease, 25% of patients present with locally advanced or disseminated disease, and 20–30% of those with localized disease at presentation will recur systemically [1]. Unfortunately, the incidence of all stages of RCC continues to increase by about 2.5% per year and RCC was responsible for more than 13,000 cancer-related deaths in the USA in

2010 [5–7]. The pressing need for more effective systemic therapies has led to the development of multiple targeted treatments for metastatic RCC that are now available for clinical use [8]. The Food and Drug Administration-approved agents fall into two main categories: multi-tyrosine kinase inhibitors that target the vascular endothelial growth factor (VEGF) pathway and those that target the mammalian target of rapamycin (mTOR) pathway [8]. These agents can provide a modest extension of survival for patients with metastatic RCC and are now being investigated in adjuvant trials for high-risk patients after complete surgical resection. However, targeted agents are very expensive and can be associated with substantial side effects.

Therefore, it is important to identify postsurgical patients at greatest risk for recurrence, for consideration for these and future adjuvant trials, and such information can also guide the intensity of surveillance. Determination of the risk of recurrence in patients without evidence of metastasis has traditionally been based on several predictive models that integrate known clinical and pathologic risk factors for disease recurrence [2, 9–20]. Some studies suggest that the addition of molecular markers to clinical risk factors may improve the predictive ability of these models [18, 21]. This chapter will highlight the predictive factors and algorithms for risk stratification for patients with localized RCC.

B.R. Lane MD, PhD (✉)
Urology Division, Spectrum Health Medical Group,
4069 Lake Drive, Suite 313, Grand Rapids,
MI 49546, USA

Michigan State University College of Human Medicine,
Grand Rapids, MI, USA

Van Andel Institute, Grand Rapids, MI, USA
e-mail: brian.lane@spectrum-health.org

S.C. Campbell and B.I. Rini (eds.), *Renal Cell Carcinoma: Clinical Management*, Current Clinical Urology, 83
DOI 10.1007/978-1-62703-062-5_5, © Springer Science+Business Media New York 2013

Table 5.1 Impact of pathologic findings and TNM stage on 5-year cancer-specific survival for patients with renal cell carcinoma

Tumor characteristics	Stage Robson	TNM (2002)	TNM (2010)	5-Year survival (%)
Organ confined (overall)	I	T1-2 N0 M0	T1-2 N0 M0	70–90
≤4.0 cm	I	T1a N0 M0	T1a N0 M0	90–100
>4.0–7.0 cm	I	T1b N0 M0	T1b N0 M0	80–90
>7.0–10.0 cm	I	T2 N0 M0	T2a N0 M0	65–80
>10.0 cm	I	T2 N0 M0	T2b N0 M0	50–70
Invasion of perinephric or renal sinus fat	II	T3a N0 M0	T3a N0 M0	50–70
Extension of tumor into renal vein or branches grossly	III-A	T3b N0 M0	T3a N0 M0	40–60
Extension of tumor into IVC below diaphragm	III-A	T3c N0 M0	T3b N0 M0	30–50
Extension of tumor into IVC above diaphragm or invasion of IVC wall	III-A	T3c N0 M0	T3c N0 M0	20–40
Direct adrenal involvement	II	T3a N0 M0	T4 N0 M0	0–30
Locally advanced (invasion beyond Gerota's fascia)	IV-A	T4 N0 M0	T4 N0 M0	0–20
Lymphatic involvement	III-B	T_{any} N1-2 M0	T_{any} N1 M0	0–20
Systemic metastases	IV-B	T_{any} N_{any} M1	T_{any} N_{any} M1	0–10

Modified from AJCC Cancer Staging Manual, 7th ed. New York: Springer-Verlag, 2009. References: [2, 12, 13, 22–46]

TNM Staging System

In the latter half of the twentieth century, Robson's radical nephrectomy and modification of the staging system proposed by Flocks and Kadesky provided the most reliable prognostic information for clinicians caring for patients with RCC [3]. RCC was often detected at advanced stage and patients had a correspondingly poor prognosis even with such "radical" surgical intervention. The most common system in current use was built upon this foundation by the Union International Contre le Cancer (UICC) and the American Joint Committee on Cancer (AJCC) (Table 5.1) [47, 48]. This TNM classification has undergone several modifications in an effort to more accurately reflect tumor biology and prognosis and to guide clinical management. The 2002 modification demonstrated better prognostic ability than the 1997 staging system [14, 49], and the 2010 staging system appears likely to provide further improvement [22, 23, 47, 49]. Although

TNM stage remains the single best prognostic indicator for RCC, it may be better viewed as an algorithm that combines several factors, each of which provides information about the risk of progression.

T stage, which is a composite of tumor size and local extension or invasion, is the foundation of the TNM system, representing a powerful and independent prognostic factor for RCC in virtually all series. Cancer-specific survival for RCC at 5 years ranges from 90% to 100% for pT1a to 0–20% for pT4 (Table 5.1) [22, 23, 47, 49]. Organ-confined cancers (pT1–2) are subclassified according to tumor size: pT1a (≤4.0 cm), pT1b (4.1–7.0 cm), pT2a (7.1–10.0 cm), and pT2b (>10.0 cm). Tumor size is an independent prognostic factor for both organ-confined and invasive RCC [2, 9, 16, 24, 25, 50, 51]. A review of 1,771 patients with organ-confined RCC showed 10-year cancer-specific survival rates of 90–95%, 80–85%, and 75% for patients with pT1a, pT1b, and pT2 tumors, respectively [13]. Larger tumors are more likely to exhibit clear cell histology and high nuclear grade, and both of these factors correlate with lower survival rates [52–54]. Many other studies have shown a particularly favorable prognosis for the unilateral pT1a tumors that are now being discovered with increased frequency. In series from the Cleveland Clinic and the Mayo Clinic, such tumors were associated with greater than 95% 5-year cancer-specific survival rates, whether they were managed with nephron-sparing surgery or radical nephrectomy [26, 27, 50, 55–57].

Several studies have documented a 15% or greater reduction in survival associated with RCC invasion through the renal capsule and into the perinephric fat [2, 22, 24]. Renal sinus involvement is now classified along with perinephric fat invasion as T3a, and several studies suggest that these patients are at even higher risk for metastasis related to increased access to the venous system [28–31, 58, 59]. Collecting system invasion has also been shown to confer poorer prognosis in otherwise organ-confined RCC, but is not a component of the current TNM staging system [58, 60].

Vascular Involvement

Although venous involvement was previously thought to be a very poor prognostic finding, several reports demonstrate that many patients with tumor thrombi can be cured with an aggressive surgical approach. These studies document 45–69% 5-year survival rates for patients with venous tumor thrombi as long as the tumor is otherwise confined to the kidney [4, 22, 32, 61–68]. Gross tumor thrombus into the inferior vena cava (IVC) above the diaphragm is pT3c, below the diaphragm is pT3b, and involvement of the renal vein or major branches has been down-staged to pT3a to reflect its relatively favorable prognosis [22, 23, 47, 69]. Patients with venous tumor thrombi and concomitant lymph node or systemic metastases have markedly decreased survival, and those with tumor extending into the perinephric fat have intermediate survival

[22, 69–76]. Patients with microscopic venous invasion may also have a reduced prognosis, but this has not been incorporated into TNM staging at present [77–79]. The most recent version of the TNM system advocates capturing all such adverse features during the staging process, but does not allow for formal integration of such features, which is a potential disadvantage of this system when compared with other predictive tools.

The prognostic significance of the cephalad extent of tumor thrombus has been controversial in part because the presence or absence of nodal and/or distant metastases has been variably recorded. In several series, the incidence of advanced locoregional or systemic disease increased with the cephalad extent of the tumor thrombus, accounting for the reduced survival associated with tumor thrombus extending into or above the level of the hepatic veins [22, 69–76]. On the other hand, other series suggest that the cephalad extent of tumor thrombus is not of prognostic significance as long as the tumor is otherwise confined [61, 63, 73, 80, 81]. Independent of the level of tumor thrombus, direct invasion of the wall of the vein is clearly an adverse predictor and is now classified as pT3c [82, 73].

The major drop in prognosis comes in patients whose tumor extends beyond the Gerota fascia to involve contiguous organs (stage T4) or has spread to lymph nodes or distant sites [2, 4, 23]. Many reports have shown that most patients with direct or metastatic ipsilateral adrenal involvement, which is found in 1–2% of patients, eventually succumb to systemic disease progression [33–37, 84]. Although previously staged as T3a, direct extension into the ipsilateral adrenal involvement is now classified as T4 and metastatic involvement of either adrenal gland as M1 to reflect the likely pattern of dissemination and similarly poor outcomes [23, 33, 47, 48].

Lymph node metastases portend a poor prognosis, with cancer-specific survival rates of 5–30% and 0–5% at 5 and 10 years, respectively [3, 38, 85]. Distant metastases to lung, bone, and other sites are associated with survival rates of 50%, 5–15%, and 0–5% at 1, 5, and 10 years, respectively [3, 39, 86, 87]. Factors predicting poorer outcomes in patients with metastatic disease include synchronous metastases, reduced performance status, larger burden of metastatic disease, bone, brain, and/or liver metastases, anemia, hypercalcemia, elevated alkaline phosphatase or lactate dehydrogenase levels, thrombocytosis, and sarcomatoid histology [3, 39, 86–96]. These factors have been used to effectively categorize patients with metastatic RCC as low, intermediate, and poor risk [3, 39, 86–91], which provide important information for determining the likelihood of benefit a patient may expect to receive after cytoreductive nephrectomy and/or resection of other metastatic disease and are discussed further in a subsequent chapter.

Patient-Related Factors

Although TNM staging facilitates communication about groups of cancer patients, it does not take into account a number of other significant predictive factors that contribute to significant heterogeneity among patients within each classification [2, 22, 23, 47, 49]. This has led investigators to explore various prognostic factors to determine whether they can add value to tumor stage alone (Table 5.2) [2, 97]. Patient characteristics have a significant impact on overall survival, with age and medical comorbidities playing a dominant role in the survival of patients with localized disease [98–100]. Hollingsworth et al. demonstrated that competing cause mortality was far greater than cancer-specific mortality for many patients with localized RCC [98]. This indicates that reduction of the impact of surgery on renal functional outcomes may have as much or greater impact on overall survival as cancer treatment. Patient factors should be given primary consideration during treatment planning for patients with localized RCC [98–100]. In fact, strong retrospective data demonstrated that surgical intervention will not lengthen survival for those with limited life expectancy [101].

Patient characteristics at presentation also impact cancer-specific survival. Those who present with systemic symptoms have a worse

Table 5.2 Prognostic factors for renal cell carcinoma

Anatomic	Clinical
Tumor size	Performance status
Venous involvement	(Karnofsky, ECOG)
Extension into contiguous organs	Systemic symptoms (cachexia, loss of greater than 10% of body weight)
Adrenal involvement (direct or metastatic)	Symptomatic vs. incidental presentation
Lymph node metastases	Anemia
Distant metastases	Hypercalcemia
Metastatic burden of disease	Elevated LDH
	Elevated erythrocyte sedimentation rate
	Elevated C-reactive protein (pre- and post-nephrectomy)
	Thrombocytosis
	Elevated alkaline phosphatase

Histologic	Molecular
Nuclear grade	Hypoxia-inducible factors:
Histological subtype	*CA-IX, IGF-1, VEGF,*
Presence of sarcomatoid features	*VEGFRs, CA-XII, CXCR3, CXCR4, HIF*
Presence of histologic necrosis	Co-stimulatory immune regulators: *B7-H1, B7-H3*
Microscopic vascular invasion	*(tumor cell/vascular), B7-H4, PD-1*
Invasion of perinephric or renal sinus fat	Cell cycle regulators: *PTEN, p53, Bcl-2, Cyclin A, p27,*
Collecting system invasion	*Skp2*
Surgical margin status	Adhesion molecules: *EpCAM, EMA, E-Cad, alpha-catenin, Cad-6*
	Other factors: *Ki-67, XIAP, Survivin, EphA2, Smac/ DIABLO, PCNA, Caveolin-1, AR, CD44, Annexin II, Gelsolin, Vimentin, CA-125), aberrant DNA methylation, Na-K ATPase α1 subunit, vitamin D receptor, retinoid X receptor*

Modified from Lane BR and Kattan MW. Prognostic models and algorithms in renal cell carcinoma. Urol Clin N Am 2008;35:613–625

prognosis then those with incidentally detected tumors [9, 11–13]. Overall health is commonly assessed using either the Karnofsky scale (0–100% function) or Eastern Cooperative Oncology Group (ECOG) performance status [102]. The presence of symptoms of cachexia, including weight loss (exceeding 10% of body weight), anorexia, or malaise, or a reduction in overall health at diagnosis, confers a poor prognosis in both localized and metastatic RCC [9, 10, 103, 104]. These symptoms may be related to circulating factors released by aggressive tumors and/or micrometastatic disease that is not clinically evident.

Paraneoplastic Syndromes

Paraneoplastic signs or symptoms have been correlated with poor outcomes for patients with RCC. Under normal circumstances, the kidney produces 1,25-dihydroxycholecalciferol, renin, erythropoietin, and various prostaglandins. RCC may produce pathologic amounts of these substances, which are normally tightly regulated. These include the substances above, as well as parathyroid hormone-like peptides, lupus-type anticoagulant, human chorionic gonadotropin, insulin, and various cytokines and inflammatory mediators [105–109]. Hypercalcemia has been reported in up to 13% of patients with RCC and can be due to either paraneoplastic phenomena or osteolytic metastatic involvement of the bone [106, 107, 110–112]. The expression of parathyroid hormone-like peptides is suppressed by the wild-type VHL protein, and these peptides may act as potent growth factors for RCC [113]. This may account in part for the observation that patients with RCC who present with hypercalcemia have a compromised prognosis, with a relative risk of death from cancer progression of 1.78 compared with patients with normal serum calcium levels [110]. Polycythemia, due to erythropoietin production by the tumor, and hypertension secondary to increased production of renin directly by the tumor; compression or encasement of the renal artery or its branches; or arteriovenous fistula within the tumor are also commonly found in patients with RCC [114]. In general, treatment of paraneoplastic syndromes associated with RCC has required surgical excision or systemic therapy and, except for hypercalcemia, medical therapies have not proved helpful. Pathologic expression of these and other

inflammatory or immunomodulatory factors by the tumor is believed to be responsible for the development of constitutional symptoms such as weight loss, fever, and anemia as well as some of the distinct paraneoplastic syndromes, thereby negatively impacting cancer-free survival [105].

Laboratory-Related Factors

Several abnormal laboratory values, even without associated signs and symptoms, have been associated with poorer outcomes in RCC patients, including anemia (hemoglobin <10 g/dL for females or <12 g/dL for males), thrombocytosis, hypercalcemia, albuminuria, and elevated serum alkaline phosphatase, C-reactive protein, lactate dehydrogenase, or erythrocyte sedimentation rate (>30 mm/h) [103, 104, 110, 115–120]. Some of these abnormalities, including hypercalcemia, anemia, and elevated erythrocyte sedimentation rate, are independent predictors of cancer-specific mortality in patients with localized clear cell RCC [110]. Each is present more commonly in patients with advanced RCC and some are predictive in this population as well. The most promising of these laboratory values appears to be C-reactive protein, which is predictive of metastasis when obtained preoperatively and during surveillance after nephrectomy [105, 117, 121–123].

Histopathologic Factors

Other tumor features that are routinely captured at histopathologic analysis are strong predictors of cancer-related outcomes and provide independent and additional predictive ability when combined with TNM stage. Several factors have been studied; the most critical being nuclear grade, presence of sarcomatoid features, and histologic subtype.

Nuclear Grade

Several grading systems for RCC have been proposed on the basis of nuclear size, nuclear configuration, and presence of nucleoli. Although interobserver variability is common in the assignment of nuclear grade, almost all proposed grading systems have provided independent prognostic information when subjected to multivariable analysis [2, 9, 17, 124–126]. In Fuhrman and colleagues' original report (1982), the 5-year survival rates for grades 1–4 were 64%, 34%, 31%, and 10%, respectively [127]. Nuclear grade also proved to be the most significant prognostic factor for organ-confined tumors in this study [127]. Fuhrman's classification scheme remains the most commonly used system and subsequent reports have demonstrated correlations between Fuhrman's nuclear grade and tumor stage, tumor size, venous tumor thrombi, and lymph node and systemic metastases [124, 125, 128, 129]. Significant differences have been consistently observed between low-grade (grades 1/2) and high-grade (grade 3/4) tumors, leading some to suggest a two-tier grading system [124]. Other investigators have proposed a three-tier system because of interobserver variability and the difficulty distinguishing the intermediate grades, but this has not gained wide support [124, 130]. In addition, although significant differences according to nuclear grade have been reported in series of patients with clear cell RCC alone or RCC of all subtypes combined, the value of Fuhrman grade in other subtypes of RCC is not entirely clear. Subclassification of papillary RCC into type 1 and type 2 takes nuclear features into account, and appears to better stratify patients into higher-risk and low-risk groups than does nuclear grade [131–133]. Chromophobe RCC is a generally indolent tumor that is now recognized to be more similar genetically to hybrid oncocytic tumors and oncocytomas than to other RCC subtypes [134–136]. Only chromophobe with aggressive histologic features such as sarcomatoid differentiation and/or advanced pathologic stage portend poorer outcomes [135, 136]. Therefore, papillary RCC may be better subgrouped into type 1 and type 2, and oncocytic neoplasms may be better classified as chromophobe RCC, hybrid oncocytic tumors, and oncocytomas, without reference to nuclear grade, but this requires further investigation [137].

Sarcomatoid Differentiation

RCC displaying sarcomatoid differentiation is characterized by spindle cell histology, positive staining for vimentin, infiltrative growth pattern, aggressive local and metastatic behavior, and poor prognosis [137–141]. Sarcomatoid differentiation is found in 1–5% of RCCs, most commonly in association with clear cell RCC or chromophobe RCC, but variants of most other subtypes of RCC have been described [130, 142–147]. Sarcomatoid lesions almost certainly represent poorly differentiated regions of other histologic subtypes of RCC rather than independently derived tumors. Thorough examination of a predominantly sarcomatoid tumor almost always yields some epithelial-derived components [144]. For this reason, this entity is no longer recognized as a distinct histologic subtype of RCC [145]. Invasion of adjacent organs is common, and median survival has been less than 1 year in most series [137, 138, 140, 148–151]. Optimal management of patients with resected sarcomatoid RCC remains controversial, but multimodal approaches should be considered if the patient's overall health allows based on the extremely poor prognosis with surgery alone. Selected reports have demonstrated modestly improved response rates in patients receiving IL-2-based immunotherapy, chemotherapy, or targeted molecular therapy after nephrectomy [8, 140, 162, 153].

Other Histopathologic Factors

Invasion of the renal sinus is now established as an adverse feature, with similar (or potentially worse) outcome compared with perinephric fat invasion [28–31, 58, 59]. Likewise, collecting system invasion is a poor prognostic feature, at least for low-stage tumors [58, 60]. Histologic tumor necrosis has been shown to be a negative prognostic indicator for clear cell RCC [17, 121, 154, 155] and has been incorporated into some algorithms. There is controversy, however, regarding the value of macroscopic (vs. microscopic) tumor necrosis and the importance of the amount of necrosis as prognostic factors. Further research may clarify this debate, but the lack of uniform coding will likely limit its universal applicability as a predictive factor. Although the presence of multiple renal tumors may complicate surgical management, multifocality has been demonstrated to confer either a neutral or positive influence on cancer-specific outcomes, which appear to be driven by the tumor of highest T stage [156–161].

Histologic Subtype

RCC is now known to be a heterogeneous malignancy with several subtypes that exhibit distinct clinical and pathological features [162, 163]. Several histologic subtypes of RCC have been described, which most experts believe have their origins from distinct portions of the nephron. The three most common RCC subtypes are clear cell RCC, papillary RCC, and chromophobe RCC. Several studies now suggest that clear cell RCC may have a worse prognosis on average compared with papillary RCC and chromophobe RCC, although there are clearly poorly differentiated tumors in each of these subcategories that can be lethal [2, 9, 128, 162–172]. Papillary RCC and chromophobe RCC account for about 15–25% of RCC, and patients with these subtypes generally present at lower stage and have a better long-term disease-free survival than those with clear cell RCC [9, 121, 162–165, 167]. Several less common subtypes denote poor prognosis, including collecting duct carcinoma, renal medullary carcinoma, and the unclassified RCC histologic subtype [130, 147, 148, 150, 151, 173–179]. Finally, several subtypes of RCC are predictably indolent, including multiloculated cystic clear cell RCC and mucinous tubular and spindle cell carcinoma [180–182].

Consistent clinical behavior is not observed within each of the major subtypes, suggesting that genetic heterogeneity exists within each RCC subtype. The unique molecular defects that are pathognomonic for familial and sporadic occurrences of each subtype are becoming defined [183]. For example, the von Hippel–Lindau (VHL) gene on chromosome 3p25 has

been implicated in VHL disease, a condition in which patients often develop multiple, bilateral clear cell RCC. Mutations in the VHL gene or hypermethylation of the VHL gene promoter region have been identified in 57–70% of patients with sporadic RCC [184]. More recent work indicates, however, that the presence of a detectable VHL mutation does not affect survival in patients with localized clear cell RCC [185]. Moreover, a gene dysregulated in 30% of sporadic RCC has now been identified and may play a role downstream of VHL [186]. Dysregulation of hypoxia-inducible factors (HIFs) by alterations in VHL creates a vasculogenic environment favoring tumor growth. Genes linked to the development of RCC have also been identified in individuals with hereditary papillary RCC syndrome, Birt–Hogg–Dubé syndrome, and hereditary leiomyomatosis and RCC syndrome [183]. However, only 4% of patients with RCC develop the disease within the context of these familial syndromes, suggesting that there are many other genes and pathways yet to be implicated in the pathogenesis of RCC. A number of molecular factors have been found to further subclassify RCC and, in some cases, to serve as independent prognostic factors for RCC [187].

Molecular Factors

A large number of genes that may have prognostic and therapeutic significance in RCC have been identified using high-throughput technologies (Table 5.2) [188–196]. The list includes hypoxia-induced factors, co-stimulatory immunoregulatory molecules, cell cycle regulators, adhesion molecules, and other factors that play a variety of known and/or unknown functions in the cancer microenvironment. Several studies demonstrate that each histologic subtype of RCC can be differentiated by gene expression profiling of renal tumors [188–200]. Correlation of changes in gene expression with location of their gene products can be analyzed using immunohistochemical staining of individual tissue samples. Construction of tissue microarrays can facilitate the screening of a larger number of pathologic samples, but interpretation of results from these and other high-throughput analyses can be difficult [201, 202].

The two molecules that have been most rigorously evaluated at present are carbonic anhydrase IX (CA-IX), the hypoxia-induced protein product of MN-9 gene, and the co-stimulatory molecule B7-H1. Although initial studies indicated that decreased CA-IX expression is independently associated with poor survival in patients with advanced clear cell RCC [21, 203], the same may not be true in patients with localized disease [204]. CA-IX is expressed in the vast majority of clear cell RCC (97%) and only rarely in other histologic subtypes, making it an attractive marker for diagnostic evaluation of renal masses [204, 205]. In addition, CA-IX may serve as a marker for response to systemic therapy, making CA-IX immunostaining potentially of value in advanced RCC as well. One study reported that all complete responders to immunotherapy with IL-2 had high CA-IX expression [206]. Some clinicians have advocated using CA-IX expression and other histopathologic information to select patients with characteristics predicting the highest chance of benefit from high-dose IL-2 [207, 208]. However, a recent clinical trial testing this hypothesis was negative. In addition, other recent trials indicate that CA-IX expression does not appear to reliably predict for response to sunitinib or temsirolimus [209, 210].

B7-H1 expression in clear cell RCC was initially found to be associated with a 4.5-fold greater risk of cancer-specific mortality [211]. This finding has been internally validated [212], with the additional finding that high Survivin and B7-H1 expression together were associated with a 2.8-fold higher risk of cancer-specific death [213]. In addition to serving as a tumor marker for progression, B7-H1 is an attractive therapeutic target in patients with advanced RCC. Since B7-H1 may function as an inhibitor of T-cell-mediated antitumoral immunity, blockade of its activity with a humanized neutralizing antibody has been postulated to facilitate immunotherapeutic responses in patients with clear cell RCC and clinical trials are anticipated [214].

Many experts believe that the best prognostic tools will incorporate both clinical and molecular factors. Proof-of-principle has been illustrated by groups at UCLA and Mayo Clinic, which demonstrated that a clinical and molecular model can outperform models that rely only on clinical predictors [18, 21, 201]. Kim and colleagues demonstrated that the addition of expression data from five markers, including CA-IX, Ki-67, gelsolin, vimentin, and p53 improved the discriminating ability of the UISS for localized RCC [201]. A second integrative tool was developed by Parker and colleagues based on expression of B7-H1, survivin, and Ki-67 [18]. The BioScore provided improvements in predictive accuracy above UISS and SSIGN score, particularly in patients at intermediate-to-high risk for recurrence [18]. The authors hypothesized that BioScore could therefore play a role selectively in these subsets of patients [18].

Prior to the incorporation of any new marker into routine use, molecular or otherwise, it must be evaluated after considering the contribution of established clinical and pathologic factors. In other words, a new marker should improve the ability to predict a given outcome beyond what can already be achieved with existing markers. For example, the initial finding that high Ki-67 expression predicted for disease recurrence was called into question by data indicating that it was simply a surrogate for histologic necrosis [155]. More recent evidence seems to indicate that Ki-67 and necrosis have independent prognostic information [215]. In order to validate the cost of obtaining molecular data in the current clinical landscape, studies must evaluate the predictive ability of a new marker in this manner. A new marker that merely replaces an existing marker is not particularly helpful and certainly not cost effective [97].

Integrative Predictive Tools

As discussed above, there are several factors that are independently associated with various outcomes, such as cancer-specific and overall survival. The value of any individual predictor is established by its ability to improve the predictive ability beyond other known predictors.

The most helpful tools are those that integrate the most important factors into a single prediction for each individual patient. Several predictive algorithms, or nomograms, have been developed for patients with localized RCC (Table 5.3). Most predict cancer-specific survival, but likelihood of malignancy, competing-cause survival and post-operative renal function have also been evaluated [53, 216, 217]. Paper versions can provide a visual aid to clinicians for use during patient counseling. Online versions of many of these are available, and most have been compiled at a website organized by Fox Chase Cancer Center (labs.fcc.edu/nomograms).

Table 5.3 Integrated predictive tools for renal cell carcinoma

Institution, author	Year	Setting	Tumor subtype	Prognostic indicators	Prognostic information	Format
Preoperative						
Cleveland Clinic, Lane	2008	Localized, amenable to PN	All	Tumor size, symptoms, gender, age, smoking	Histology	Nomogram
MSK/Mayo Clinic, Raj	2008	Localized	All	Tumor size, symptoms, gender, lymphadenopathy, necrosis on imaging	Recurrence	Nomogram
Keio (Japan), Kanao,	2009	Localized, metastatic	All	TNM stage	Survival	Nomogram
Postoperative						
MSK, Kattan	2001	Localized	All	TNM stage, tumor size, histology, symptoms	Recurrence	Nomogram
UCLA, Zisman	2001	Localized	All	TNM stage, nuclear grade, performance status	Survival	Algorithm, decision boxes
UCLA, Zisman	2002	Localized, metastatic	All	TNM stage, nuclear grade, performance status, metastasis (UISS)	Survival	Algorithm, decision boxes
Mayo Clinic, Frank	2002	Localized, metastatic	Clear cell	TNM stage, tumor size, nuclear grade, histological necrosis (SSIGN)	Survival	Algorithm
Mayo Clinic, Leibovich	2003	Localized	Clear cell	TN stage, tumor size, nuclear grade, histological necrosis	Recurrence	Algorithm
UCLA, Kim	2004	Localized, metastatic	All	TNM stage, performance status, metastasis, expression of p53, vimentin, CA-IX in metastatic patients	Survival	Nomogram
MSK, Sorbellini	2005	Localized	Clear cell	TNM stage, tumor size, nuclear grade, histological necrosis, microvascular invasion, symptoms	Recurrence	Nomogram
Multi-institutional, Karakiewicz	2007	Localized	All	TNM stage, tumor size, nuclear grade, histologic subtype, local symptoms, age, gender	Survival	Nomogram
Mayo Clinic, Parker	2009	Localized	Clear cell	Expression of B7-H1, survivin, Ki-67 (BioScore)	Survival	Algorithm
UCLA, Klatte	2009	Localized	Clear cell	Expression of Ki-67, p53, endothelial VEGFR-1, epithelial VEGFR-1, epithelial VEGF-D	Survival	Nomogram

(continued)

Table 5.3 (continued)

Institution, author	Year	Setting	Tumor subtype	Prognostic indicators	Prognostic information	Format
Other (renal function/competing cause mortality)						
MSK, Sorbellini	2006	Localized, metastatic	All	Preoperative creatinine, age, gender, ASA score, percent change in kidney volume	Renal insufficiency	Nomogram
Fox Chase, Kutikov	2010	Localized, metastatic	All	Tumor size, age, gender, race	Survival (Non-cancer, kidney cancer, other cancer)	Nomogram

MSK Memorial Sloan Kettering Cancer Center, *Keio* Keio University School of Medicine, Tokyo, Japan

Preoperative Nomograms for Suspected Renal Malignancy

Prior to intervention for a suspected RCC, clinical and radiographic features can be used to determine the likelihood of benign or malignant pathology and cancer-specific survival. Based on pathologic data obtained during 862 partial nephrectomies in patients with a single enhancing renal neoplasm amenable to partial nephrectomy, the predicted probability of benign disease ranged from 5% to 50% [53]. Overall, 20% of suspected renal malignancies had benign histology and the likelihood for a given patient was based on readily identifiable preoperative factors (tumor size, age, gender, symptoms at presentation, and smoking history). This information may be particularly applicable when active surveillance or tumor ablation is being considered for smaller tumors in more infirm patients; especially given recent evidence that active treatment may not increase life expectancy in such individuals [101, 218].

Several additional preoperative nomograms for recurrence-free survival have been developed [219–223], but none perform as well as algorithms that incorporate data obtained during nephrectomy [15]. Using the nomogram developed by Raj et al., the 12-year recurrence free survival for an incidentally detected 3, 5, or 7 cm RCC is about 95%, 88%, or 75%, respectively. This information may be particularly useful in counseling patients in whom non-extirpative options are being considered. However, for other patients, we feel that estimation of this endpoint is more useful in the postoperative setting, when this information might affect subsequent decision-making (e.g., surveillance protocol, adjuvant treatment). If additional information is needed prior to a decision regarding treatment, molecular characterization by either renal mass biopsy or advanced imaging techniques can be performed [205, 224]. Certainly, the ultimate utility of such an approach is as yet to be fully realized.

Postoperative Prognostic Algorithms for Localized RCC

Using pathologic information obtained at nephrectomy, several groups have developed postoperative prognostic algorithms. In 2001, Memorial Sloan-Kettering Cancer Center (MSKCC) researchers proposed a nomogram for patients with localized clear cell, papillary, or chromophobe RCC [9]. Predictive factors included tumor stage, tumor size, histologic subtype, and symptoms at presentation [9]. Subsequently, the same group produced a second nomogram for patients with clear cell RCC based on tumor stage, tumor size, nuclear grade, necrosis, vascular invasion, and symptoms at presentation [9].

Researchers at other institutions also published postoperative prognostic systems incorporating a slightly different set of predictors. The UCLA integrated staging system (UISS) as proposed in 2001 initially divided patients into five groups shown to have statistically significant differences in disease-specific survival [10].

Although the UCLA group evaluated many potential prognostic parameters, the UISS was reduced to include only tumor stage, nuclear grade, and ECOG performance status for simplification [10]. In a subsequent report, the UISS was modified to identify patients with nonmetastatic or metastatic disease at low, intermediate, or high risk of disease progression [225]. This modified UISS has been validated in larger series of patients both internally and externally, but was found to be out-performed by other nomograms (each of which included tumor size) [225, 226]. One significant drawback of the UISS (and the TNM staging system) is that it does not predict a probability of failure for an individual patient, and instead places individuals into low, intermediate, and high risk groups that have heterogeneous outcomes.

In 2002, the group at the Mayo Clinic devised the SSIGN score, in which patients with clear cell RCC are assigned a score based on tumor stage, tumor size, nuclear grade, and the presence of histologic necrosis [17]. The estimated cancer-specific survival for an individual patient at 1–10 years is then provided based on the total of the SSIGN score. The SSIGN score was developed based on data from over 1,800 patients and has been validated internally and externally against additional datasets [17, 125, 126, 227, 228].

Many statistical methods can be employed in order to evaluate predictive models [97]. The concordance index (c-index) is a measure of the predictive accuracy of prognostic algorithms, in which the algorithm is asked to predict which of two patients will experience clinical failure first. Comparison with the actual outcome in a large series of patient pairs determines the c-index. Perfect predictive accuracy yields a highest possible value of 1.0 (100%), while random chance provides a baseline value of 0.5 (50%). Although the predictive accuracy of these integrative algorithms improves upon individual factors, such as tumor size and nuclear grade and TNM stage, each has been reported to have a c-index substantially less than 1.0, indicating further room for improvement.

Comparative evaluation of prognostic algorithms should be performed with care and statistical rigor. First, and most importantly, any tool to be used in clinical practice should be subjected to external validation. Second, because the c-index is a measure of the ranking of outcomes and does not address the absolute predictive accuracy, calibration of a particular predicted probability should also be performed. This is usually accomplished by plotting predicted vs. actual probabilities. Third, predictive accuracy cannot be compared directly across datasets, so a conclusion about the "best" nomogram cannot be made by comparing c-index values in two reports using two distinct patient populations. Far more accurate information is obtained from head-to-head comparisons on the same dataset.

Several examples of such work now exist, including a comparison of the 1997 and 2002 TNM staging systems and two reports that directly compared prognostic algorithms using the same dataset [15, 19, 49, 125]. Benefiting from earlier work, Karakiewicz and colleagues developed a nomogram for use in RCC patients of any histology and TNM stage using data from 2,530 patients with median follow-up of 39 months [19]. The reduced model included T stage, N stage, M stage, tumor size, Fuhrman grade, and symptom classification (none, local, systemic) and was externally validated using 1,422 patients' data from other institutions (Fig. 5.1) [19]. The model was found to outperform the UISS, with a c-index of 86.7% vs. 83.9% for predicting survival at 5 years ($p = 0.02$) [19]. While direct comparison with the other nomograms mentioned above has not been performed, this nomogram benefits from relying solely on the strongest and commonly available predictors (stage, size, and grade) and omitting histopathologic features that can be variably collected across institutions (vascular invasion and necrosis). In addition, the use of symptom classification which has been shown previously to improve accuracy over TNM stage alone also improves predictive accuracy in the published model [12, 13, 19]. Further studies comparing each of the prognostic models on the same datasets will help to identify the most practical and accurate nomograms for use in patients with localized RCC.

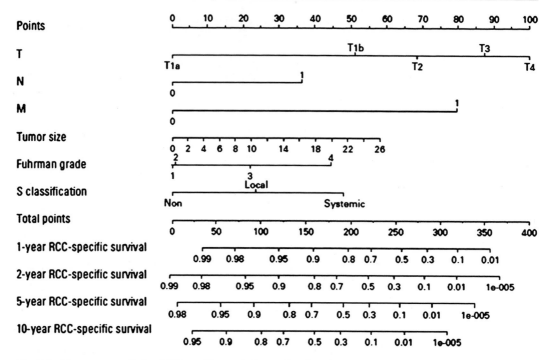

Fig. 5.1 Nomogram predicting RCC-specific survival at 1, 2, 5, and 10 years after nephrectomy. *T* T stage, *N* N stage, *M* M stage, *S classification* symptoms at presenta- tion. Reprinted with permission from Karakiewicz et al.: J Clin Oncol 2007;25(11):1316–1322. © 2008 American Society of Clinical Oncology. All rights reserved

Other Predictive Algorithms

Additional nomograms have been developed to predict outcomes that impact the overall survival of patients with localized RCC, including non-RCC-related mortality and renal function after surgery [216, 217]. Based on review of over 30,000 cases of localized RCC contained within the SEER database, Kutikov and colleagues calculated 5-year probabilities of kidney cancer death, other cancer death, and non-cancer death to be 4%, 7%, and 11%, respectively [217]. This tool may be particularly helpful in elderly patients because quantifying the risk of death unrelated to RCC may greatly impact treatment selection. Based on the excellent recurrence-free survival outcomes following surgical treatment of organ-confined RCC, renal functional outcomes also contribute to overall survival, as chronic kidney disease has been associated with increased cardiovascular morbidity [229]. Compared with radical nephrectomy, partial nephrectomy better preserves renal function and a nomogram predicting renal function after either approach can facilitate discussions about surgical options [216, 230].

Conclusions

Patients should be provided with the most accurate information about their likely individual disease course currently available to expert clinicians. Many patient and tumor characteristics have been associated with cancer outcomes for those with localized RCC. Combination of these predictors into integrated predictive tools provides more accurate assessments than any single predictor alone. A preoperative nomogram can predict the likelihood that a suspected malignancy is a cancer and estimate survival after definitive treatment. At least five postoperative predictive algorithms exist for localized RCC, each of which improves upon predictions based on the TNM staging system. Refinement of the existing tools, with corresponding increases in accuracy, allows physicians to better counsel patients regarding their likely clinical course, assists in the planning and tailoring of follow-up, and identifies patients who are more likely to benefit from additional treatments. Future algorithms predicting disease outcomes or response to treatment will likely incorporate molecular factors with the potential to provide information of even greater quality.

References

1. Janzen NK, Kim HL, Figlin RA, Belldegrun AS. Surveillance after radical or partial nephrectomy for localized renal cell carcinoma and management of recurrent disease. Urol Clin North Am. 2003;30(4): 843–52.
2. Lane BR, Kattan MW. Prognostic models and algorithms in renal cell carcinoma. Urol Clin North Am. 2008;35(4):613–25.
3. Campbell SC, Novick AC, Bukowski RM. Renal tumors. In: Wein AJ, Kavoussi LR, Novick AC, Partin AW, Peters CA, editors. Campbell-Walsh urology, 9th ed., vol 4. Philadelphia: Saunders; 2007. p. 2672–731.
4. Thrasher JB, Paulson DF. Prognostic factors in renal cancer. Urol Clin North Am. 1993;20(2):247–62.
5. Chow WH, Devesa SS, Warren JL, Fraumeni Jr JF. Rising incidence of renal cell cancer in the United States. JAMA. 1999;281(17):1628–31.
6. Chow WH, Devesa SS. Contemporary epidemiology of renal cell cancer. Cancer J. 2008;14(5):288–301.
7. Jemal A, Siegel R, Xu J, Ward E. Cancer statistics, 2010. CA Cancer J Clin. 2010;60(5):277–300.
8. Rini BI. Metastatic renal cell carcinoma: many treatment options, one patient. J Clin Oncol. 2009;27(19): 3225–34.
9. Kattan MW, Reuter V, Motzer RJ, Katz J, Russo P. A postoperative prognostic nomogram for renal cell carcinoma. J Urol. 2001;166(1):63–7.
10. Zisman A, Pantuck AJ, Dorey F, et al. Improved prognostication of renal cell carcinoma using an integrated staging system. J Clin Oncol. 2001; 19(6):1649–57.
11. Pantuck AJ, Zisman A, Belldegrun AS. The changing natural history of renal cell carcinoma. J Urol. 2001;166(5):1611–23.
12. Patard JJ, Leray E, Cindolo L, et al. Multi-institutional validation of a symptom based classification for renal cell carcinoma. J Urol. 2004; 172(3):858–62.
13. Patard JJ, Dorey FJ, Cindolo L, et al. Symptoms as well as tumor size provide prognostic information on patients with localized renal tumors. J Urol. 2004; 172(6, Part 1 of 2):2167–71.
14. Ficarra V, Schips L, Guille F, et al. Multiinstitutional European validation of the 2002 TNM staging system in conventional and papillary localized renal cell carcinoma. Cancer. 2005;104(5):968–74.
15. Cindolo L, Patard JJ, Chiodini P, et al. Comparison of predictive accuracy of four prognostic models for nonmetastatic renal cell carcinoma after nephrectomy. Cancer. 2005;104(7):1362–71.
16. Sorbellini M, Kattan MW, Snyder ME, et al. A postoperative prognostic nomogram predicting recurrence for patients with conventional clear cell renal cell carcinoma. J Urol. 2005;173(1):48–51.
17. Frank I, Blute ML, Cheville JC, Lohse CM, Weaver AL, Zincke H. An outcome prediction model for patients with clear cell renal cell carcinoma treated with radical nephrectomy based on tumor stage, size, grade and necrosis: the SSIGN score. J Urol. 2002; 168(6):2395–400.
18. Parker AS, Leibovich BC, Lohse CM, et al. Development and evaluation of BioScore: a biomarker panel to enhance prognostic algorithms for clear cell renal cell carcinoma. Cancer. 2009;115: 2092–103.
19. Karakiewicz PI, Briganti A, Chun FK, et al. Multi-institutional validation of a new renal cancer-specific survival nomogram. J Clin Oncol. 2007;25(11): 1316–22.
20. Isbarn H, Karakiewicz PI. Predicting cancer-control outcomes in patients with renal cell carcinoma. Curr Opin Urol. 2009;19(3):247–57.
21. Kim HL, Seligson D, Liu X, et al. Using tumor markers to predict the survival of patients with metastatic renal cell carcinoma. J Urol. 2005;173(5): 1496–501.
22. Leibovich BC, Cheville JC, Lohse CM, et al. Cancer specific survival for patients with pT3 renal cell carcinoma – can the 2002 primary tumor classification be improved? J Urol. 2005;173(3):716–9.
23. Thompson RH, Cheville JC, Lohse CM, et al. Reclassification of patients with pT3 and pT4 renal cell carcinoma improves prognostic accuracy. Cancer. 2005;104(1):53–60.
24. Kontak JA, Campbell SC. Prognostic factors in renal cell carcinoma. Urol Clin North Am. 2003;30(3): 467–80.
25. Guinan P, Saffrin R, Stuhldreher D, Frank W, Rubenstein M. Renal cell carcinoma: comparison of the TNM and Robson stage groupings. J Surg Oncol. 1995;59(3):186–9.
26. Butler BP, Novick AC, Miller DP, Campbell SA, Licht MR. Management of small unilateral renal cell carcinomas: radical versus nephron-sparing surgery. Urology. 1995;45(1):34–40. discussion 40–1.
27. Lerner SE, Hawkins CA, Blute ML, et al. Disease outcome in patients with low stage renal cell carcinoma treated with nephron sparing or radical surgery. J Urol. 1996;155(6):1868–73.
28. Thompson RH, Leibovich BC, Cheville JC, et al. Is renal sinus fat invasion the same as perinephric fat invasion for pT3a renal cell carcinoma? J Urol. 2005;174(4 Pt 1):1218–21.

29. Margulis V, Tamboli P, Matin SF, Meisner M, Swanson DA, Wood CG. Location of extrarenal tumor extension does not impact survival of patients with pT3a renal cell carcinoma. J Urol. 2007;178(5):1878–82.

30. Bedke J, Buse S, Pritsch M, et al. Perinephric and renal sinus fat infiltration in pT3a renal cell carcinoma: possible prognostic differences. BJU Int. 2009;103(10):1349–54.

31. Bertini R, Roscigno M, Freschi M, et al. Renal sinus fat invasion in pT3a clear cell renal cell carcinoma affects outcomes of patients without nodal involvement or distant metastases. J Urol. 2009;181(5):2027–32.

32. Wotkowicz C, Wszolek MF, Libertino JA. Resection of renal tumors invading the vena cava. Urol Clin North Am. 2008;35(4):657–71. viii.

33. Sagalowsky AI, Kadesky KT, Ewalt DM, Kennedy TJ. Factors influencing adrenal metastasis in renal cell carcinoma. J Urol. 1994;151(5):1181–4.

34. Sandock DS, Seftel AD, Resnick MI. Adrenal metastases from renal cell carcinoma: role of ipsilateral adrenalectomy and definition of stage. Urology. 1997;49(1):28–31.

35. Paul R, Mordhorst J, Leyh H, Hartung R. Incidence and outcome of patients with adrenal metastases of renal cell cancer. Urology. 2001;57(5):878–82.

36. Siemer S, Lehmann J, Loch A, et al. Current TNM classification of renal cell carcinoma evaluated: revising stage T3a. J Urol. 2005;173(1):33–7.

37. Thompson RH, Leibovich BC, Cheville JC, et al. Should direct ipsilateral adrenal invasion from renal cell carcinoma be classified as pT3a? J Urol. 2005;173(3):918–21.

38. Phillips CK, Taneja SS. The role of lymphadenectomy in the surgical management of renal cell carcinoma. Urol Oncol. 2004;22(3):214–23. discussion 223–4.

39. Motzer RJ, Mazumdar M, Bacik J, Berg W, Amsterdam A, Ferrara J. Survival and prognostic stratification of 670 patients with advanced renal cell carcinoma. J Clin Oncol. 1999;17(8):2530–40.

40. Targonski PV, Frank W, Stuhldreher D, et al. Value of tumor size in predicting survival from renal cell carcinoma among tumors, nodes and metastases stage 1 and stage 2 patients. J Urol. 1994;152:1389–92.

41. Hafez KS, Fergany AF, Novick AC: Nephron sparing surgery for localized renal cell carcinoma: impact of tumor size on patient survival, tumor recurrence and TNM staging. J Urol. 1999;162:1930.

42. Igarashi T, Tobe T, Nakatsu HO, et al. The impact of a 4 cm. cutoff point for stratification of T1N0M0 renal cell carcinoma after radical nephrectomy. J Urol. 2001;165:1103.

43. Vasselli JR, Yang JC, Linehan WM, et al. Lack of retroperitoneal lymphadenopathy predicts survival of patients with metastatic renal cell carcinoma. J Urol. 2001;166:68.

44. Von Knobloch R, Varga Z, Schrader AJ, et al. All patients with adrenal metastasis from RCC will eventually die in tumor progression: there is no cure

or benefit from simultaneous adrenalectomy. J Urol. 2004;171:115.

45. Kanao K, Mizuno R, Kikuchi E et al: Preoperative prognostic nomogram (probability table) for renal cell carcinoma based on TNM classification. J Urol. 2009;181:480.

46. Campbell SC, Novick AC, Belldegrun A, et al. Guideline for management of the clinical T1 renal mass. J Urol. 2009;182:1971–9.

47. AJCC cancer staging manual, 7th ed. New York: Springer; 2010.

48. Guinan P, Sobin LH, Algaba F, et al. TNM staging of renal cell carcinoma: Workgroup No. 3. Union International Contre le Cancer (UICC) and the American Joint Committee on Cancer (AJCC). Cancer. 1997;80(5):992–3.

49. Frank I, Blute ML, Leibovich BC, Cheville JC, Lohse CM, Zincke H. Independent validation of the 2002 American Joint Committee on cancer primary tumor classification for renal cell carcinoma using a large, single institution cohort. J Urol. 2005;173(6):1889–92.

50. Crispen PL, Boorjian SA, Lohse CM, et al. Outcomes following partial nephrectomy by tumor size. J Urol. 2008;180(5):1912–7.

51. Nguyen MM, Gill IS. Effect of renal cancer size on the prevalence of metastasis at diagnosis and mortality. J Urol. 2009;181(3):1020–7. discussion 1027.

52. Frank I, Blute ML, Cheville JC, Lohse CM, Weaver AL, Zincke H. Solid renal tumors: an analysis of pathological features related to tumor size. J Urol. 2003;170(6 Pt 1):2217–20.

53. Lane BR, Babineau D, Kattan MW, et al. A preoperative prognostic nomogram for solid enhancing renal tumors 7 cm or less amenable to partial nephrectomy. J Urol. 2007;178(2):429–34.

54. Thompson RH, Kurta JM, Kaag M, et al. Tumor size is associated with malignant potential in renal cell carcinoma cases. J Urol. 2009;181(5):2033–6.

55. Gill IS, Kavoussi LR, Lane BR, et al. Comparison of 1,800 laparoscopic and open partial nephrectomies for single renal tumors. J Urol. 2007;178(1):41–6.

56. Lane BR, Gill IS. 7-Year oncological outcomes after laparoscopic and open partial nephrectomy. J Urol. 2010;183(2):473–9.

57. Cheville JC, Blute ML, Zincke H, Lohse CM, Weaver AL. Stage pT1 conventional (clear cell) renal cell carcinmoa: pathological features associated with cancer specific survival. J Urol. 2001;166(2):453–6.

58. Uzzo RG, Cherullo EE, Myles J, Novick AC. Renal cell carcinoma invading the urinary collecting system: implications for staging. J Urol. 2002;167(6):2392–6.

59. Bonsib SM, Gibson D, Mhoon M, Greene GF. Renal sinus involvement in renal cell carcinomas. Am J Surg Pathol. 2000;24(3):451–8.

60. Klatte T, Chung J, Leppert JT, et al. Prognostic relevance of capsular involvement and collecting system invasion in stage I and II renal cell carcinoma. BJU Int. 2007;99(4):821–4.

61. Blute ML, Boorjian SA, Leibovich BC, Lohse CM, Frank I, Karnes RJ. Results of inferior vena caval interruption by greenfield filter, ligation or resection during radical nephrectomy and tumor thrombectomy. J Urol. 2007;178(2):440–5.

62. Haferkamp A, Bastian PJ, Jakobi H, et al. Renal cell carcinoma with tumor thrombus extension into the vena cava: prospective long-term followup. J Urol. 2007;177(5):1703–8.

63. Staehler G, Brkovic D. The role of radical surgery for renal cell carcinoma with extension into the vena cava. J Urol. 2000;163(6):1671–5.

64. Quek ML, Stein JP, Skinner DG. Surgical approaches to venous tumor thrombus. Semin Urol Oncol. 2001;19(2):88–97.

65. Zisman A, Wieder JA, Pantuck AJ, et al. Renal cell carcinoma with tumor thrombus extension: biology, role of nephrectomy and response to immunotherapy. J Urol. 2003;169(3):909–16.

66. Parekh DJ, Cookson MS, Chapman W, et al. Renal cell carcinoma with renal vein and inferior vena caval involvement: clinicopathological features, surgical techniques and outcomes. J Urol. 2005;173(6):1897–902.

67. Klatte T, Pantuck AJ, Riggs SB, et al. Prognostic factors for renal cell carcinoma with tumor thrombus extension. J Urol. 2007;178(4 Pt 1):1189–95. discussion 1195.

68. Subramanian VS, Stephenson AJ, Goldfarb DA, Fergany AF, Novick AC, Krishnamurthi V. Utility of preoperative renal artery embolization for management of renal tumors with inferior vena caval thrombi. Urology. 2009;74(1):154–9.

69. Moinzadeh A, Libertino JA. Prognostic significance of tumor thrombus level in patients with renal cell carcinoma and venous tumor thrombus extension. Is all T3b the same? J Urol. 2004;171(2 Pt 1):598–601.

70. Gettman MT, Boelter CW, Cheville JC, Zincke H, Bryant SC, Blute ML. Charlson co-morbidity index as a predictor of outcome after surgery for renal cell carcinoma with renal vein, vena cava or right atrium extension. J Urol. 2003;169(4):1282–6.

71. Kim HL, Zisman A, Han KR, Figlin RA, Belldegrun AS. Prognostic significance of venous thrombus in renal cell carcinoma. Are renal vein and inferior vena cava involvement different? J Urol. 2004;171 (2 Pt 1):588–91.

72. Montie JE, el Ammar R, Pontes JE, et al. Renal cell carcinoma with inferior vena cava tumor thrombi. Surg Gynecol Obstet. 1991;173(2):107–15.

73. Glazer AA, Novick AC. Long-term followup after surgical treatment for renal cell carcinoma extending into the right atrium. J Urol. 1996;155(2):448–50.

74. Naitoh J, Kaplan A, Dorey F, Figlin R, Belldegrun A. Metastatic renal cell carcinoma with concurrent inferior vena caval invasion: long-term survival after combination therapy with radical nephrectomy, vena caval thrombectomy and postoperative immunotherapy. J Urol. 1999;162(1):46–50.

75. Sweeney P, Wood CG, Pisters LL, et al. Surgical management of renal cell carcinoma associated with

76. Bissada NK, Yakout HH, Babanouri A, et al. Long-term experience with management of renal cell carcinoma involving the inferior vena cava. Urology. 2003;61(1):89–92.

77. Lang H, Lindner V, Letourneux H, Martin M, Saussine C, Jacqmin D. Prognostic value of microscopic venous invasion in renal cell carcinoma: long-term follow-up. Eur Urol. 2004;46(3):331–5.

78. Ishimura T, Sakai I, Hara I, Eto H, Miyake H. Microscopic venous invasion in renal cell carcinoma as a predictor of recurrence after radical surgery. Int J Urol. 2004;11(5):264–8.

79. Dall'Oglio MF, Antunes AA, Sarkis AS, et al. Microvascular tumour invasion in renal cell carcinoma: the most important prognostic factor. BJU Int. 2007;100(3):552–5.

80. Libertino JA, Zinman L, Watkins Jr E. Long-term results of resection of renal cell cancer with extension into inferior vena cava. J Urol. 1987;137(1):21–4.

81. Martinez-Salamanca JI, Huang WC, Millan I, et al. Prognostic impact of the 2009 UICC/AJCC TNM staging system for renal cell carcinoma with venous extension. Eur Urol. 2011;59(1):120–7.

82. Hatcher PA, Anderson EE, Paulson DF, Carson CC, Robertson JE. Surgical management and prognosis of renal cell carcinoma invading the vena cava. J Urol. 1991;145(1):20–3. discussion 23–4.

83. Zini L, Destrieux-Garnier L, Leroy X, et al. Renal vein ostium wall invasion of renal cell carcinoma with an inferior vena cava tumor thrombus: prediction by renal and vena caval vein diameters and prognostic significance. J Urol. 2008;179(2):450–4.

84. von Knobloch R, Schrader AJ, Walthers EM, Hofmann R. Simultaneous adrenalectomy during radical nephrectomy for renal cell carcinoma will not cure patients with adrenal metastasis. Urology. 2009;73(2):333–6.

85. Bassil B, Dosoretz DE, Prout Jr GR. Validation of the tumor, nodes and metastasis classification of renal cell carcinoma. J Urol. 1985;134(3):450–4.

86. Motzer RJ, Bacik J, Schwartz LH, et al. Prognostic factors for survival in previously treated patients with metastatic renal cell carcinoma. J Clin Oncol. 2004;22(3):454–63.

87. Mekhail TM, Abou-Jawde RM, Boumerhi G, et al. Validation and extension of the Memorial Sloan-Kettering prognostic factors model for survival in patients with previously untreated metastatic renal cell carcinoma. J Clin Oncol. 2005;23(4):832–41.

88. Boumerhi G, Mekhail TM, Abou-Jawde RM, Malhi S, Olencki T, Leschinsky A. Prognostic factors for survival in previously treated patients with metastatic renal cell cancer. J Clin Oncol 2003;22(16s): abstract 1647

89. Choueiri TK, Xie W, Kollmannsberger C, et al. The impact of cytoreductive nephrectomy on survival of patients with metastatic renal cell carcinoma receiv-

ing vascular endothelial growth factor targeted therapy. J Urol. 2011;185(1):60–6.

90. Choueiri TK, Garcia JA, Elson P, et al. Clinical factors associated with outcome in patients with metastatic clear-cell renal cell carcinoma treated with vascular endothelial growth factor-targeted therapy. Cancer. 2007;110(3):543–50.

91. Escudier B, Choueiri TK, Oudard S, et al. Prognostic factors of metastatic renal cell carcinoma after failure of immunotherapy: new paradigm from a large phase III trial with shark cartilage extract AE 941. J Urol. 2007;178(5):1901–5.

92. Maldazys JD, de Kernion JB. Prognostic factors in metastatic renal carcinoma. J Urol. 1986;136(2):376–9.

93. Motzer RJ, Russo P. Systemic therapy for renal cell carcinoma. J Urol. 2000;163(2):408–17.

94. Leibovich BC, Cheville JC, Lohse CM, et al. A scoring algorithm to predict survival for patients with metastatic clear cell renal cell carcinoma: a stratification tool for prospective clinical trials. J Urol. 2005;174(5):1759–63. discussion 1763.

95. Leibovich BC, Han KR, Bui MH, et al. Scoring algorithm to predict survival after nephrectomy and immunotherapy in patients with metastatic renal cell carcinoma: a stratification tool for prospective clinical trials. Cancer. 2003;98(12):2566–75.

96. Negrier S, Escudier B, Gomez F, et al. Prognostic factors of survival and rapid progression in 782 patients with metastatic renal carcinomas treated by cytokines: a report from the Groupe Francais d'Immunotherapie. Ann Oncol. 2002;13(9):1460–8.

97. Kattan MW. Evaluating a new marker's predictive contribution. Clin Cancer Res. 2004;10(3):822–4.

98. Hollingsworth JM, Miller DC, Daignault S, Hollenbeck BK. Rising incidence of small renal masses: a need to reassess treatment effect. J Natl Cancer Inst. 2006;98(18):1331–4.

99. Pettus JA, Jang TL, Thompson RH, Yossepowitch O, Kagiwada M, Russo P. Effect of baseline glomerular filtration rate on survival in patients undergoing partial or radical nephrectomy for renal cortical tumors. Mayo Clin Proc. 2008;83(10):1101–6.

100. Berger DA, Megwalu II, Vlahiotis A, et al. Impact of comorbidity on overall survival in patients surgically treated for renal cell carcinoma. Urology. 2008;72(2):359–63.

101. Lane BR, Abouassaly R, Gao T, et al. Active treatment of localized renal tumors may not impact overall survival in patients aged 75 years or older. Cancer. 2010;116(13):3119–26.

102. Oken MM, Creech RH, Tormey DC, et al. Toxicity and response criteria of the Eastern Cooperative Oncology Group. Am J Clin Oncol. 1982;5(6):649–55.

103. Gelb AB. Renal cell carcinoma: current prognostic factors. Union Internationale Contre le Cancer (UICC) and the American Joint Committee on Cancer (AJCC). Cancer. 1997;80(5):981–6.

104. Srigley JR, Hutter RV, Gelb AB, et al. Current prognostic factors – renal cell carcinoma: Workgroup No. 4. Union Internationale Contre le Cancer (UICC) and the American Joint Committee on Cancer (AJCC). Cancer. 1997;80(5):994–6.

105. Altundag O, Altundag K, Gunduz E. Interleukin-6 and C-reactive protein in metastatic renal cell carcinoma. J Clin Oncol. 2005;23(5):1044. author reply 1044–5.

106. Sufrin G, Chasan S, Golio A, Murphy GP. Paraneoplastic and serologic syndromes of renal adenocarcinoma. Semin Urol. 1989;7(3):158–71.

107. Gold PJ, Fefer A, Thompson JA. Paraneoplastic manifestations of renal cell carcinoma. Semin Urol Oncol. 1996;14(4):216–22.

108. Ather MH, Mithani S, Bhutto S, Adil S. Lupus type anticoagulant in a patient with renal cell carcinoma: an autoimmune paraneoplastic syndrome. J Urol. 2002;167(5):2129.

109. Elias AN. New-onset insulinopenic diabetes mellitus in a patient with an incidentally discovered renal cell carcinoma. Am J Med. 2005;118(9):1047–8.

110. Magera Jr JS, Leibovich BC, Lohse CM, et al. Association of abnormal preoperative laboratory values with survival after radical nephrectomy for clinically confined clear cell renal cell carcinoma. Urology. 2008;71(2):278–82.

111. Pepper K, Jaowattana U, Starsiak MD, et al. Renal cell carcinoma presenting with paraneoplastic hypercalcemic coma: a case report and review of the literature. J Gen Intern Med. 2007;22(7):1042–6.

112. Klatte T, Said JW, Belldegrun AS, Pantuck AJ. Differential diagnosis of hypercalcemia in renal malignancy. Urology 2007;70(1):179.e7–8.

113. Massfelder T, Lang H, Schordan E, et al. Parathyroid hormone-related protein is an essential growth factor for human clear cell renal carcinoma and a target for the von Hippel–Lindau tumor suppressor gene. Cancer Res. 2004;64(1):180–8.

114. Moein MR, Dehghani VO. Hypertension: a rare presentation of renal cell carcinoma. J Urol. 2000;164(6):2019.

115. Ljungberg B, Grankvist K, Rasmuson T. Serum acute phase reactants and prognosis in renal cell carcinoma. Cancer. 1995;76(8):1435–9.

116. O'Keefe SC, Marshall FF, Issa MM, Harmon MP, Petros JA. Thrombocytosis is associated with a significant increase in the cancer specific death rate after radical nephrectomy. J Urol. 2002;168(4 Pt 1):1378–80.

117. Karakiewicz PI, Hutterer GC, Trinh QD, et al. C-reactive protein is an informative predictor of renal cell carcinoma-specific mortality: a European study of 313 patients. Cancer. 2007;110(6):1241–7.

118. Jacobsen J, Grankvist K, Rasmuson T, Ljungberg B. Prognostic importance of serum vascular endothelial growth factor in relation to platelet and leukocyte counts in human renal cell carcinoma. Eur J Cancer Prev. 2002;11(3):245–52.

119. Vaglio A, Buzio L, Cravedi P, Pavone L, Garini G, Buzio C. Prognostic significance of albuminuria in patients with renal cell cancer. J Urol. 2003;170(4 Pt 1):1135–7.

120. Symbas NP, Townsend MF, El-Galley R, Keane TE, Graham SD, Petros JA. Poor prognosis associated with thrombocytosis in patients with renal cell carcinoma. BJU Int. 2000;86(3):203–7.

121. Komai Y, Saito K, Sakai K, Morimoto S. Increased preoperative serum C-reactive protein level predicts a poor prognosis in patients with localized renal cell carcinoma. BJU Int. 2007;99(1):77–80.

122. Johnson TV, Abbasi A, Owen-Smith A, et al. Absolute preoperative C-reactive protein predicts metastasis and mortality in the first year following potentially curative nephrectomy for clear cell renal cell carcinoma. J Urol. 2010;183(2):480–5.

123. Johnson TV, Abbasi A, Owen-Smith A, et al. Postoperative better than preoperative C-reactive protein at predicting outcome after potentially curative nephrectomy for renal cell carcinoma. Urology 2010;76(3):766.e1–5.

124. Lang H, Lindner V, de Fromont M, et al. Multicenter determination of optimal interobserver agreement using the Fuhrman grading system for renal cell carcinoma: assessment of 241 patients with >15-year follow-up. Cancer. 2005;103(3):625–9.

125. Ficarra V, Novara G, Galfano A, et al. The 'stage, size, grade and necrosis' score is more accurate than the University of California Los Angeles integrated staging system for predicting cancer-specific survival in patients with clear cell renal cell carcinoma. BJU Int. 2009;103(2):165–70.

126. Ficarra V, Martignoni G, Lohse C, et al. External validation of the Mayo Clinic stage, size, grade and necrosis (SSIGN) score to predict cancer specific survival using a European series of conventional renal cell carcinoma. J Urol. 2006;175(4):1235–9.

127. Fuhrman SA, Lasky LC, Limas C. Prognostic significance of morphologic parameters in renal cell carcinoma. Am J Surg Pathol. 1982;6(7):655–63.

128. Lohse CM, Cheville JC. A review of prognostic pathologic features and algorithms for patients treated surgically for renal cell carcinoma. Clin Lab Med. 2005;25(2):433–64.

129. Bretheau D, Lechevallier E, de Fromont M, Sault MC, Rampal M, Coulange C. Prognostic value of nuclear grade of renal cell carcinoma. Cancer. 1995;76(12):2543–9.

130. Medeiros LJ, Jones EC, Aizawa S, et al. Grading of renal cell carcinoma: Workgroup No. 2. Union Internationale Contre le Cancer and the American Joint Committee on Cancer (AJCC). Cancer. 1997;80(5):990–1.

131. Klatte T, Remzi M, Zigeuner RE, et al. Development and external validation of a nomogram predicting disease specific survival after nephrectomy for papillary renal cell carcinoma. J Urol. 2010;184(1):53–8.

132. Klatte T, Pantuck AJ, Said JW, et al. Cytogenetic and molecular tumor profiling for type 1 and type 2 papillary renal cell carcinoma. Clin Cancer Res. 2009;15(4):1162–9.

133. Pignot G, Elie C, Conquy S, et al. Survival analysis of 130 patients with papillary renal cell carcinoma: prognostic utility of type 1 and type 2 subclassification. Urology. 2007;69(2):230–5.

134. Tan MH, Wong CF, Tan HL, et al. Genomic expression and single-nucleotide polymorphism profiling discriminates chromophobe renal cell carcinoma and oncocytoma. BMC Cancer. 2010;10:196.

135. Klatte T, Han KR, Said JW, et al. Pathobiology and prognosis of chromophobe renal cell carcinoma. Urol Oncol. 2008;26(6):604–9.

136. Cindolo L, de la Taille A, Schips L, et al. Chromophobe renal cell carcinoma: comprehensive analysis of 104 cases from multicenter European database. Urology. 2005;65(4):681–6.

137. Zhou M. Pathology of renal cell carcinomas. In: Campbell SC, Rini BI, editors. Renal cell carcinoma. 1st ed. Shelton: People's Medical Publishing House; 2009. p. 1–14.

138. Ro JY, Ayala AG, Sella A, Samuels ML, Swanson DA. Sarcomatoid renal cell carcinoma: clinicopathologic. A study of 42 cases. Cancer. 1987;59(3):516–26.

139. DeLong W, Grignon DJ, Eberwein P, Shum DT, Wyatt JK. Sarcomatoid renal cell carcinoma. An immunohistochemical study of 18 cases. Arch Pathol Lab Med. 1993;117(6):636–40.

140. Cangiano T, Liao J, Naitoh J, Dorey F, Figlin R, Belldegrun A. Sarcomatoid renal cell carcinoma: biologic behavior, prognosis, and response to combined surgical resection and immunotherapy. J Clin Oncol. 1999;17(2):523–8.

141. Eble JN, Sauter G, Epstein JI, Sesterhenn IA. Pathology and genetics of tumours of the urinary system and male genital organs. In: WHO classification of tumors, vol 7. Lyon: IARC Press; 2004.

142. Weiss LM, Gelb AB, Medeiros LJ. Adult renal epithelial neoplasms. Am J Clin Pathol. 1995;103(5):624–35.

143. Storkel S, Eble JN, Adlakha K, et al. Classification of renal cell carcinoma: Workgroup No. 1. Union Internationale Contre le Cancer (UICC) and the American Joint Committee on Cancer (AJCC). Cancer. 1997;80(5):987–9.

144. Delahunt B. Sarcomatoid renal carcinoma: the final common dedifferentiation pathway of renal epithelial malignancies. Pathology. 1999;31(3):185–90.

145. de Peralta-Venturina M, Moch H, Amin M, et al. Sarcomatoid differentiation in renal cell carcinoma: a study of 101 cases. Am J Surg Pathol. 2001;25(3):275–84.

146. Kuroda N, Toi M, Hiroi M, Enzan H. Review of sarcomatoid renal cell carcinoma with focus on clinical and pathobiological aspects. Histol Histopathol. 2003;18(2):551–5.

147. Cheville JC, Lohse CM, Zincke H, et al. Sarcomatoid renal cell carcinoma: an examination of underlying

histologic subtype and an analysis of associations with patient outcome. Am J Surg Pathol. 2004;28(4): 435–41.

148. Mian BM, Bhadkamkar N, Slaton JW, et al. Prognostic factors and survival of patients with sarcomatoid renal cell carcinoma. J Urol. 2002;167(1):65–70.

149. Dall'Oglio MF, Lieberknecht M, Gouveia V, Sant'Anna AC, Leite KR, Srougi M. Sarcomatoid differentiation in renal cell carcinoma: prognostic implications. Int Braz J Urol. 2005;31(1):10–6.

150. Escudier B, Droz JP, Rolland F, et al. Doxorubicin and ifosfamide in patients with metastatic sarcomatoid renal cell carcinoma: a phase II study of the Genitourinary Group of the French Federation of Cancer Centers. J Urol. 2002;168(3):959–61.

151. Nanus DM, Garino A, Milowsky MI, Larkin M, Dutcher JP. Active chemotherapy for sarcomatoid and rapidly progressing renal cell carcinoma. Cancer. 2004;101(7):1545–51.

152. Fujiwara Y, Kiura K, Tabata M, et al. Remarkable shrinkage of sarcomatoid renal cell carcinoma with single-agent gemcitabine. Anticancer Drugs. 2008; 19(4):431–3.

153. Bangalore N, Bhargava P, Hawkins MJ, Bhargava P. Sustained response of sarcomatoid renal-cell carcinoma to MAID chemotherapy: case report and review of the literature. Ann Oncol. 2001;12(2):271–4.

154. Sengupta S, Lohse CM, Leibovich BC, et al. Histologic coagulative tumor necrosis as a prognostic indicator of renal cell carcinoma aggressiveness. Cancer. 2005;104(3):511–20.

155. Lam JS, Shvarts O, Said JW, et al. Clinicopathologic and molecular correlations of necrosis in the primary tumor of patients with renal cell carcinoma. Cancer. 2005;103(12):2517–25.

156. Steinbach F, Stockle M, Griesinger A, et al. Multifocal renal cell tumors: a retrospective analysis of 56 patients treated with radical nephrectomy. J Urol. 1994;152(5 Pt 1):1393–6.

157. Baltaci S, Orhan D, Soyupek S, Beduk Y, Tulunay O, Gogus O. Influence of tumor stage, size, grade, vascular involvement, histological cell type and histological pattern on multifocality of renal cell carcinoma. J Urol. 2000;164(1):36–9.

158. Lang H, Lindner V, Martin M, et al. Prognostic value of multifocality on progression and survival in localized renal cell carcinoma. Eur Urol. 2004;45(6): 749–53.

159. Dimarco DS, Lohse CM, Zincke H, Cheville JC, Blute ML. Long-term survival of patients with unilateral sporadic multifocal renal cell carcinoma according to histologic subtype compared with patients with solitary tumors after radical nephrectomy. Urology. 2004;64(3):462–7.

160. Richstone L, Scherr DS, Reuter VR, et al. Multifocal renal cortical tumors: frequency, associated clinicopathological features and impact on survival. J Urol. 2004;171(2 Pt 1):615–20.

161. Blute ML, Thibault GP, Leibovich BC, Cheville JC, Lohse CM, Zincke H. Multiple ipsilateral renal tumors discovered at planned nephron sparing surgery: importance of tumor histology and risk of metachronous recurrence. J Urol. 2003;170(3):760–3.

162. Cheville JC, Lohse CM, Zincke H, Weaver AL, Blute ML. Comparisons of outcome and prognostic features among histologic subtypes of renal cell carcinoma. Am J Surg Pathol. 2003;27(5): 612–24.

163. Lau WK, Cheville JC, Blute ML, Weaver AL, Zincke H. Prognostic features of pathologic stage T1 renal cell carcinoma after radical nephrectomy. Urology. 2002;59(4):532–7.

164. Moch H, Gasser T, Amin MB, Torhorst J, Sauter G, Mihatsch MJ. Prognostic utility of the recently recommended histologic classification and revised TNM staging system of renal cell carcinoma: a Swiss experience with 588 tumors. Cancer. 2000;89(3): 604–14.

165. Amin MB, Tamboli P, Javidan J, et al. Prognostic impact of histologic subtyping of adult renal epithelial neoplasms: an experience of 405 cases. Am J Surg Pathol. 2002;26(3):281–91.

166. Krejci KG, Blute ML, Cheville JC, Sebo TJ, Lohse CM, Zincke H. Nephron-sparing surgery for renal cell carcinoma: clinicopathologic features predictive of patient outcome. Urology. 2003;62(4):641–6.

167. Beck SD, Patel MI, Snyder ME, et al. Effect of papillary and chromophobe cell type on disease-free survival after nephrectomy for renal cell carcinoma. Ann Surg Oncol. 2004;11(1):71–7.

168. Patard JJ, Leray E, Rioux-Leclercq N, et al. Prognostic value of histologic subtypes in renal cell carcinoma: a multicenter experience. J Clin Oncol. 2005;23(12):2763–71.

169. Crispen PL, Boorjian SA, Lohse CM, Leibovich BC, Kwon ED. Predicting disease progression after nephrectomy for localized renal cell carcinoma: the utility of prognostic models and molecular biomarkers. Cancer. 2008;113(3):450–60.

170. Dall'Oglio MF, Antunes AA, Pompeo AC, Mosconi A, Leite KR, Srougi M. Prognostic relevance of the histological subtype of renal cell carcinoma. Int Braz J Urol. 2008;34(1):3–8.

171. Margulis V, Tamboli P, Matin SF, Swanson DA, Wood CG. Analysis of clinicopathologic predictors of oncologic outcome provides insight into the natural history of surgically managed papillary renal cell carcinoma. Cancer. 2008;112(7):1480–8.

172. Rothman J, Egleston B, Wong YN, Iffrig K, Lebovitch S, Uzzo RG. Histopathological characteristics of localized renal cell carcinoma correlate with tumor size: a SEER analysis. J Urol. 2009;181(1): 29–33. discussion 33–4.

173. Carter MD, Tha S, McLoughlin MG, Owen DA. Collecting duct carcinoma of the kidney: a case report and review of the literature. J Urol. 1992; 147(4):1096–8.

174. Chao D, Zisman A, Pantuck AJ, et al. Collecting duct renal cell carcinoma: clinical study of a rare tumor. J Urol. 2002;167(1):71–4.

175. Mejean A, Roupret M, Larousserie F, Hopirtean V, Thiounn N, Dufour B. Is there a place for radical nephrectomy in the presence of metastatic collecting duct (Bellini) carcinoma? J Urol. 2003;169(4):1287–90.

176. Polascik TJ, Bostwick DG, Cairns P. Molecular genetics and histopathologic features of adult distal nephron tumors. Urology. 2002;60(6):941–6.

177. Tokuda N, Naito S, Matsuzaki O, et al. Collecting duct (Bellini duct) renal cell carcinoma: a nationwide survey in Japan. J Urol. 2006;176(1):40–3. discussion 43.

178. Kobayashi N, Matsuzaki O, Shirai S, Aoki I, Yao M, Nagashima Y. Collecting duct carcinoma of the kidney: an immunohistochemical evaluation of the use of antibodies for differential diagnosis. Hum Pathol. 2008;39(9):1350–9.

179. Davis Jr CJ, Mostofi FK, Sesterhenn IA. Renal medullary carcinoma. The seventh sickle cell nephropathy. Am J Surg Pathol. 1995;19(1):1–11.

180. Lane BR, Campbell SC, Remer EM, et al. Adult cystic nephroma and mixed epithelial and stromal tumor of the kidney: clinical, radiographic, and pathologic characteristics. Urology. 2008;71(6):1142–8.

181. Gong K, Zhang N, He Z, Zhou L, Lin G, Na Y. Multilocular cystic renal cell carcinoma: an experience of clinical management for 31 cases. J Cancer Res Clin Oncol. 2008;134(4):433–7.

182. Ferlicot S, Allory Y, Comperat E, et al. Mucinous tubular and spindle cell carcinoma: a report of 15 cases and a review of the literature. Virchows Archiv. 2005;447(6):978–83.

183. Linehan WM, Pinto PA, Srinivasan R, et al. Identification of the genes for kidney cancer: opportunity for disease-specific targeted therapeutics. Clin Cancer Res. 2007;13(2 Pt 2):671s–9.

184. Yao M, Yoshida M, Kishida T, et al. VHL tumor suppressor gene alterations associated with good prognosis in sporadic clear-cell renal cell carcinoma. J Natl Cancer Inst. 2002;94(20):1569–75.

185. Smits KM, Schouten LJ, van Dijk BA, et al. Genetic and epigenetic alterations in the von Hippel–Landau gene: the influence on renal cancer prognosis. Clin Cancer Res. 2008;14(3):782–7.

186. Varela I, Tarpey P, Raine K, et al. Exome sequencing identifies frequent mutation of the SWI/SNF complex gene PBRM1 in renal carcinoma. Nature. 2011;469(7331):539–42.

187. Zhao H, Ljungberg B, Grankvist K, Rasmuson T, Tibshirani R, Brooks JD. Gene expression profiling predicts survival in conventional renal cell carcinoma. PLoS Med. 2006;3(1):e13.

188. Takahashi M, Rhodes DR, Furge KA, et al. Gene expression profiling of clear cell renal cell carcinoma: gene identification and prognostic classification. Proc Natl Acad Sci U S A. 2001;98(17):9754–9.

189. Higgins JP. Gene array studies in renal neoplasia. Sci World J. 2006;6:502–11.

190. Young AN, Master VA, Paner GP, Wang MD, Amin MB. Renal epithelial neoplasms: diagnostic applications of gene expression profiling. Adv Anat Pathol. 2008;15(1):28–38.

191. Gieseg MA, Cody T, Man MZ, Madore SJ, Rubin MA, Kaldjian EP. Expression profiling of human renal carcinomas with functional taxonomic analysis. BMC Bioinformatics. 2002;3(1):26.

192. Boer JM, Huber WK, Sultmann H, et al. Identification and classification of differentially expressed genes in renal cell carcinoma by expression profiling on a global human 31,500-element cDNA array. Genome Res. 2001;11(11):1861–70.

193. Moch H, Schraml P, Bubendorf L, et al. High-throughput tissue microarray analysis to evaluate genes uncovered by cDNA microarray screening in renal cell carcinoma. Am J Pathol. 1999;154(4):981–6.

194. Yao M, Tabuchi H, Nagashima Y, et al. Gene expression analysis of renal carcinoma: adipose differentiation-related protein as a potential diagnostic and prognostic biomarker for clear-cell renal carcinoma. J Pathol. 2005;205(3):377–87.

195. Vasselli JR, Shih JH, Iyengar SR, et al. Predicting survival in patients with metastatic kidney cancer by gene-expression profiling in the primary tumor. Proc Natl Acad Sci U S A. 2003;100(12):6958–63.

196. Skubitz KM, Skubitz AP. Differential gene expression in renal-cell cancer. J Lab Clin Med. 2002;140(1):52–64.

197. Huo L, Sugimura J, Tretiakova MS, et al. C-kit expression in renal oncocytomas and chromophobe renal cell carcinomas. Hum Pathol. 2005;36(3):262–8.

198. Junker K, Hindermann W, von Eggeling F, Diegmann J, Haessler K, Schubert J. CD70: a new tumor specific biomarker for renal cell carcinoma. J Urol. 2005;173(6):2150–3.

199. Tretiakova MS, Sahoo S, Takahashi M, et al. Expression of alpha-methylacyl-CoA racemase in papillary renal cell carcinoma. Am J Surg Pathol. 2004;28(1):69–76.

200. Yang XJ, Tan MH, Kim HL, et al. A molecular classification of papillary renal cell carcinoma. Cancer Res. 2005;65(13):5628–37.

201. Kim HL, Seligson D, Liu X, et al. Using protein expressions to predict survival in clear cell renal carcinoma. Clin Cancer Res. 2004;10(16):5464–71.

202. Liu X, Minin V, Huang Y, Seligson DB, Horvath S. Statistical methods for analyzing tissue microarray data. J Biopharm Stat. 2004;14(3):671–85.

203. Bui MH, Seligson D, Han KR, et al. Carbonic anhydrase IX is an independent predictor of survival in advanced renal clear cell carcinoma: implications for prognosis and therapy. Clin Cancer Res. 2003;9(2):802–11.

204. Leibovich BC, Sheinin Y, Lohse CM, et al. Carbonic anhydrase IX is not an independent predictor of outcome for patients with clear cell renal cell carcinoma. J Clin Oncol. 2007;25(30):4757–64.

205. Divgi CR, Pandit-Taskar N, Jungbluth AA, et al. Preoperative characterisation of clear-cell renal car-

cinoma using iodine-124-labelled antibody chimeric G250 (124I-cG250) and PET in patients with renal masses: a phase I trial. Lancet Oncol. 2007;8(4): 304–10.

206. Bui MH, Visapaa H, Seligson D, et al. Prognostic value of carbonic anhydrase IX and KI67 as predictors of survival for renal clear cell carcinoma. J Urol. 2004;171(6 Pt 1):2461–6.

207. Atkins MB, Choueiri TK, Cho D, Regan M, Signoretti S. Treatment selection for patients with metastatic renal cell carcinoma. Cancer. 2009;115 (10 Suppl):2327–33.

208. Dudek AZ, Yee RT, Manivel JC, Isaksson R, Yee HO. Carbonic anhydrase IX expression is associated with improved outcome of high-dose interleukin-2 therapy for metastatic renal cell carcinoma. Anticancer Res. 2010;30(3):987–92.

209. Choueiri TK, Regan MM, Rosenberg JE, et al. Carbonic anhydrase IX and pathological features as predictors of outcome in patients with metastatic clear-cell renal cell carcinoma receiving vascular endothelial growth factor-targeted therapy. BJU Int. 2010;106(6):772–8.

210. Cho D, Signoretti S, Dabora S, et al. Potential histologic and molecular predictors of response to temsirolimus in patients with advanced renal cell carcinoma. Clin Genitourin Cancer. 2007;5(6): 379–85.

211. Thompson RH, Gillett MD, Cheville JC, et al. Costimulatory B7-H1 in renal cell carcinoma patients: indicator of tumor aggressiveness and potential therapeutic target. Proc Natl Acad Sci U S A. 2004;101(49):17174–9.

212. Thompson RH, Kuntz SM, Leibovich BC, et al. Tumor B7-H1 is associated with poor prognosis in renal cell carcinoma patients with long-term follow-up. Cancer Res. 2006;66(7):3381–5.

213. Krambeck AE, Dong H, Thompson RH, et al. Survivin and b7-h1 are collaborative predictors of survival and represent potential therapeutic targets for patients with renal cell carcinoma. Clin Cancer Res. 2007;13(6):1749–56.

214. Thompson RH, Dong H, Kwon ED. Implications of B7-H1 expression in clear cell carcinoma of the kidney for prognostication and therapy. Clin Cancer Res. 2007;13(2 Pt 2):709s–15.

215. Tollefson MK, Thompson RH, Sheinin Y, et al. Ki-67 and coagulative tumor necrosis are independent predictors of poor outcome for patients with clear cell renal cell carcinoma and not surrogates for each other. Cancer. 2007;110(4):783–90.

216. Sorbellini M, Kattan MW, Snyder ME, Hakimi AA, Sarasohn DM, Russo P. Prognostic nomogram for renal insufficiency after radical or partial nephrectomy. J Urol. 2006;176(2):472–6. discussion 476.

217. Kutikov A, Egleston BL, Wong YN, Uzzo RG. Evaluating overall survival and competing risks of death in patients with localized renal cell carcinoma using a comprehensive nomogram. J Clin Oncol. 2010;28(2):311–7.

218. Hollingsworth JM, Miller DC, Daignault S, Hollenbeck BK. Five-year survival after surgical treatment for kidney cancer: a population-based competing risk analysis. Cancer. 2007;109(9):1763–8.

219. Raj GV, Thompson RH, Leibovich BC, Blute ML, Russo P, Kattan MW. Preoperative nomogram predicting 12-year probability of metastatic renal cancer. J Urol. 2008;179(6):2146–51. discussion 2151.

220. Yaycioglu O, Rutman MP, Balasubramaniam M, Peters KM, Gonzalez JA. Clinical and pathologic tumor size in renal cell carcinoma; difference, correlation, and analysis of the influencing factors. Urology. 2002;60(1):33–8.

221. Cindolo L, de la Taille A, Messina G, et al. A preoperative clinical prognostic model for non-metastatic renal cell carcinoma. BJU Int. 2003;92(9):901–5.

222. Jeldres C, Sun M, Liberman D, et al. Can renal mass biopsy assessment of tumor grade be safely substituted for by a predictive model? J Urol. 2009;182(6): 2585–9.

223. Karakiewicz PI, Suardi N, Capitanio U, et al. A preoperative prognostic model for patients treated with nephrectomy for renal cell carcinoma. Eur Urol. 2009;55(2):287–95.

224. Lane BR, Samplaski MK, Herts BR, Zhou M, Novick AC, Campbell SC. Renal mass biopsy – a renaissance? J Urol. 2008;179(1):20–7.

225. Zisman A, Pantuck AJ, Wieder J, et al. Risk group assessment and clinical outcome algorithm to predict the natural history of patients with surgically resected renal cell carcinoma. J Clin Oncol. 2002;20(23):4559–66.

226. Patard JJ, Kim HL, Lam JS, et al. Use of the University of California Los Angeles integrated staging system to predict survival in renal cell carcinoma: an international multicenter study. J Clin Oncol. 2004;22(16):3316–22.

227. Zigeuner R, Hutterer G, Chromecki T, et al. External validation of the Mayo Clinic stage, size, grade, and necrosis (SSIGN) score for clear-cell renal cell carcinoma in a single European centre applying routine pathology. Eur Urol. 2010;57:102–9.

228. Thompson RH, Leibovich BC, Lohse CM, et al. Dynamic outcome prediction in patients with clear cell renal cell carcinoma treated with radical nephrectomy: the D-SSIGN score. J Urol. 2007;177(2): 477–80.

229. Lane BR, Poggio ED, Herts BR, Novick AC, Campbell SC. Renal function assessment in the era of chronic kidney disease: renewed emphasis on renal function centered patient care. J Urol. 2009; 182(2):435–43. discussion 443–4.

230. Lane BR, Fergany AF, Weight CJ, Campbell SC. Renal functional outcomes after partial nephrectomy with extended ischemic intervals are better than after radical nephrectomy. J Urol. 2010;184(4):1286–90.

Part II

Management of Localized RCC

Assessment of Oncologic Risk for Clinical Stage T1 Renal Tumors and the Emerging Role of Renal Mass Biopsy

Matthew N. Simmons and Steven C. Campbell

Introduction

The incidence of RCC has been rising steadily over the past several decades, and aggressive surgical treatment of RCC has increased in parallel. However RCC mortality rates have not declined and some studies show an increase in mortality in patients with localized disease [1–3]. This alarming trend has prompted reexamination of long-held beliefs regarding aggressive treatment of localized RCC, particularly the overutilization of radical nephrectomy. Prior to the CT era most patients presented with symptomatic high-grade tumors. Since the 1980s there has been a steady downward stage migration due to an increased rate of incidental tumor detection, such that 50–70% of patients currently present with asymptomatic stage T1 (cT1) tumors [4, 5]. One would expect RCC mortality rates to decrease as a result of early detection and the increased proportion of low-risk tumors, yet this has not happened.

Survival in patients who undergo surgery for RCC is impacted by two major factors, namely cancer-related death and death due to non-oncologic causes, some of which may be treatment related. One potential cause of non-oncologic mortality in these patients is postoperative chronic kidney disease (CKD) and its harmful sequelae. Specific subsets of patients including the elderly and those with baseline CKD are at elevated risk for non-oncologic mortality after kidney surgery [6, 7]. These patient subsets comprise up to 35% of all RCC patients and this percentage is expected to increase [8]. More intelligent and selective utilization of surgery has the potential to significantly reduce non-oncologic mortality in these patients. Individualized treatment of patients with cT1 tumors depends on the ability to accurately assess the relative contributions of oncologic and non-oncologic risk. Non-oncologic risk assessment is currently feasible and relatively straightforward. Factors such as general health status and baseline kidney function can be objectified using Charlson comorbidity score, ECOG performance score, and the K/DOQI CKD classification system. Oncological risk analysis is more of a challenge, especially for cT1 tumors. Emerging data demonstrate that the majority of cT1 tumors are at low risk for metastatic progression. The role of renal mass biopsy (RMB) to evaluate cT1 tumors is evolving to allow for improved oncologic risk stratification. This chapter will focus on recent advances in RMB biopsy and ongoing efforts to provide a more rational and balanced approach to the management of patients with clinical T1 renal tumors.

M.N. Simmons MD, PhD • S.C. Campbell MD, PhD (✉)
Center for Urologic Oncology,
Glickman Urological and Kidney Institute,
Cleveland Clinic, 9500 Euclid Avenue, Suite Q10-1,
Cleveland, OH 44195, USA
e-mail: campbes3@ccf.org

S.C. Campbell and B.I. Rini (eds.), *Renal Cell Carcinoma: Clinical Management*, Current Clinical Urology,
DOI 10.1007/978-1-62703-062-5_6, © Springer Science+Business Media New York 2013

Table 6.1 Contemporary SRM pathology data

Author	n	Percent benign (%)	Percent indolent (%)	Percent aggressive (%)	Percent metastatic	Aggressiveness criteria
Frank et al. [9]	947	23	64	13	NA	FG ≥3
Remzi et al. [54]	287	20	58	22	5%	Stage ≥T3a or metastatic
Schlomer et al. [55]	206	23	52	25	NA	FG ≥3
Pahernik et al. [56]	663	17	70	13	3%	FG ≥3, stage ≥T3a or metastatic
Lane et al. [10]	862	20	56	24	NA	FG ≥3 or stage ≥T3a
Mean values		20	60	20		

FG Fuhrman grade, *NA* not available

Fig. 6.1 Pathologic distribution of cT1 tumors. Large contemporary pathology studies have revealed that for contrast-enhancing solid cT1 kidney tumors, 20% are benign, 60% are RCC with low-risk features, and 20% are RCC with high-risk features

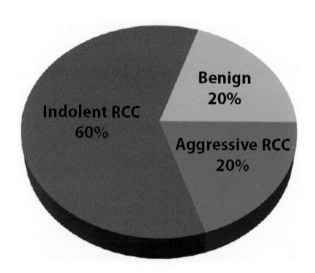

Pathologic Features of T1 Tumors

Contemporary pathological studies of solid contrast-enhancing cT1 tumors are summarized in Table 6.1. Two of the largest independent studies reviewed cT1 tumor pathology in nearly 2,000 patients [9, 10]. In general it was found that approximately 20% of incidental cT1 tumors were benign, 50–60% were RCC tumors with low-risk features, and only 20–25% were RCC tumors with high-risk features (Fig. 6.1). High-risk features in contemporary pathology studies include Fuhrman nuclear grade ≥3 pattern, presence of type II papillary, medullary, sarcomatoid or collecting duct histology; presence

of invasion into sinus fat or vascular structures (pT3 disease); and presence of extrarenal extension.

There are several issues with pathology studies that limit their clinical relevance. Definitions of high-risk criteria are not standardized among studies, and as a result there is variability in the reported percentages of high-risk tumor rates ranging from 13% to 25%. Pathological studies are also limited because they cannot definitively assess the relationship between tumor risk features and clinical behavior. It is assumed that RCC tumors with low-risk features follow an indolent clinical course, but this has not been proven in controlled prospective studies. Nonetheless, pathologic data illustrate the

Table 6.2 SRM active surveillance and natural history

Author	N	Mean cm tumor size	Mean cm/year growth rate	Mean months follow-up	Metastatic progression (%)
Kato et al. [57]	18	2	0.42	26.9	0
Lamb et al. [13]	36	7.2	0.39	27.7	1 (2.8%)
Volpe and Jewett [58]	32	2.48	0.1	38.9	0
Wehle et al. [59]	29	1.83	0.12	32	0
Abouassaly et al. [60]	110	2.5[a]	0.26	24[a]	0
Kouba et al. [61]	46	2.92	0.7	35.8	0
Kunkle et al. [11]	106	2.0[a]	0.19[a]	29[a]	1 (1.1%)
Youssif et al. [62]	41	2.2	0.21	47.6	2 (5.7%)
Crispen et al. [63]	173	2.45	0.29	31	2 (1.3%)
Rosales et al. [26]	223	2.8[a]	0.34[a]	35[a]	4 (1.9%)
Mean values		2.7	0.31	33	1.2%

[a]Median values

important concept that approximately 80% of cT1 tumors pose relatively low oncologic risk.

Natural History of cT1 Tumors

Investigation of the natural history of untreated cT1 tumors is an area of active research. Observational studies provide a basis for risk assessment in patients who have elected to undergo AS. Contemporary AS studies have established parameters that define "normal" and "abnormal" cT1 tumor growth rates, and they have characterized cT1 tumor metastatic progression rates. A data summary of contemporary studies is presented in Table 6.2.

AS studies show that cT1 tumors grow slowly at an average rate of 3 mm/year with a low risk of metastatic progression. There is a general assumption that tumors with faster growth pose higher risk for malignancy and metastatic progression but these relationships remain incompletely characterized. For example, Kunkle et al. performed a systematic pathologic study in 106 cT1a tumors that were observed over a median of 12 months [11]. Zero net growth was observed in 33% of tumors while growth was observed in the remainder. There was no difference in the percentage of tumors with malignant pathology in fast- versus slow-growing tumors. Zhang et al. examined

growth rates in 53 patients and found that the proportion of clear cell RCC was 31% in the 1st quartile growth rate group versus 62% in the 4th quartile growth rate group [12]. This study also compared specific tumor types under observation, finding no significant difference in growth rates, and there was a wide range of growth rates within each histological group. Similarly, Kato et al. examined 18 cT1a tumors and also found no difference in the proportion of RCC in fast- versus slow-growing tumors. However this study did find that tumors with faster growth rate were more likely to have higher Fuhrman nuclear grade (FG). Tumors with FG 3/4 grew at an average rate of 9 mm/year compared to 3 mm/year for tumors with FG 1/2. Larger prospective studies are required to validate the data obtained from these more limited cohorts.

In addition to analysis of growth rates, AS studies have examined cT1 tumor metastatic progression rates. Mean incidence of de novo metastasis over a 2- to 3-year period in these studies has ranged from 0% to 5% [13–16]. For instance, Haramis et al. reported clinical behavior of 51 cT1 tumors followed for >5 years [17]. RMB was conducted in 39% of patients, and RCC was identified in 100% of those biopsies. Tumor growth rate for the biopsied specimens was 2.5 mm/year, and none of the patients with biopsy required treatment during the study period.

No patients exhibited metastatic progression or died from RCC. A report by Zini et al. examined cancer-specific mortality (CSM) rates of surgically treated ($n = 9,858$) versus untreated ($n = 433$) T1a RCC tumors. CSM in the surgically treated group at 1, 2, and 5 years was 1%, 1.6%, and 3%, respectively. In comparison the CSM at 1, 2, and 5 years in the untreated group was 6%, 8%, and 12%, respectively. Age and tumor size were independently associated with CSM.

AS study data imply that cT1 tumors pose low risk for metastasis; however, the studies are limited and the data may not be generalized to all cT1 tumors. A major issue with these studies is selection bias. Assignment of patients to AS protocols was predicated on small tumor size, absence of adverse radiologic features and slow growth rate. In this regard the data represent only this highly selected low risk subset of cT1 tumors. In addition, in most studies only a small percentage of patients underwent biopsy at the initiation of the observation period, therefore the ability to correlate pathologic findings with clinical behavior remains limited.

Contemporary cT1 Risk Assessment

Preoperative oncologic risk assessment of kidney tumors is currently based primarily on radiologic tumor size, morphology, and staging. There is a clear gradation of risk among tumors of different stage. However, comparison of oncologic risk for tumors of a single stage is considerably more difficult, particularly for cT1 tumors. In these patients analysis must rely on additional nuanced risk features. Demographic factors that may augment oncologic risk analysis include age, performance status, comorbidity status, and presence of tumor-related symptomatology. Radiologic features that impact risk analysis include size, morphology, contrast enhancement, and growth pattern. In isolation these adjunct features have low diagnostic and prognostic sensitivity and specificity and are not relied upon to guide clinical management. However, when considered collectively they may enhance standard risk analysis.

Patient Demographic Factors

Patient factors of primary importance in determining oncologic risk include presence of symptoms, baseline performance status, and comorbidity score. Local and systemic symptoms are more common in patients with large tumors, but their presence in the context of cT1 tumors is associated with increased malignancy rates and poorer outcomes. Lee et al. reported oncologic outcomes according to symptomatology in 633 patients who underwent nephrectomy for RCC [18]. In this study 23% of stage cT1 tumors were symptomatic and this subgroup exhibited an increased incidence of clear cell histology and high Fuhrman nuclear grade.

Comorbidity and performance status have been established as independent predictors of disease-specific survival, and as such are integral components of two widely used oncologic risk prediction nomograms [19, 20]. These features are unique in that they are important for assessment of both oncologic and non-oncologic risk. In terms of oncologic risk, studies have shown that there is an association of ECOG performance status with presence of tumor necrosis and decreased cancer-specific survival [21]. There is no definitive data to support a causal relationship between the two, but it is reasonable to suspect that patients with major comorbidities and poor performance status are more likely to have higher risk tumors.

Epidemiologic data suggest that specific demographic factors such as age and gender are associated with malignancy rates. Benign tumors tend to be more commonly encountered in younger women <50 years of age. In this demographic the rate of malignancy is on the order of 50%, because a variety of benign histological subtypes such as atypical angiomyolipoma and metanephric adenoma are more common in this population, suggesting an important role of the hormonal milieu [10]. DeRoche et al. reported that males have a 12% higher likelihood of malignancy than females for all age groups [22]. They also found that in patients <68 years of age with tumors ≤3.5 cm malignancy was present in 87% of males versus 69% of females. Verhoest et al.

examined pathologic features as they relate to patient age in 4,774 patients [23]. They found that patients ≤40 years of age were more likely to have papillary or chromophobe RCC than clear cell RCC. These demographic and clinical correlates associate with likelihood of malignancy, but in a nonspecific manner. Use of patient demographics in risk assessment can augment tumor evaluation but should not be relied upon independently to guide clinical management.

In a small subset of patients there exist specific tumor presentations that are nearly pathognomonic for certain malignancies. Patients who present with small, multifocal bilateral kidney tumors should be suspected to have a heritable syndrome such as Von Hippel–Lindau (VHL). VHL tumors measuring <3 cm pose low risk for metastasis, and routine observation of these tumors is accepted practice. Medullary RCC, while very rare, occurs primarily in young African males with sickle cell trait. Medullary RCC is an aggressive tumor; therefore, it is advisable to manage incidentally detected SRMs in this demographic aggressively.

Radiologic Risk Assessment

The majority of information pertaining to tumor risk analysis is obtained from cross-sectional CT and MRI imaging. Key anatomical features include tumor size, location, and appearance. In patients who have had serial imaging studies measurement of tumor growth rate may also be possible. As discussed previously, tumor size and tumor growth rate are potential indicators of oncological risk. In order to assess risk differential among tumors with similar size and growth rate we must rely on more subtle features.

Tumor Size

At present the best indicator of tumor malignancy and high nuclear grade is tumor size [9, 24]. Most data pertaining to this relationship compared tumors of different stages over a wide size range from stage T1a through T2. How tumor size

relates to aggressiveness within a narrower range, particularly 1–4 cm, has only recently been characterized. For T1 tumors every 1 cm increase in tumor diameter is associated with a 16–17% increase in the odds of malignancy [9, 24]. In two major studies 38–46% of tumors measuring ≤1 cm were benign compared to 6–7% of tumors ≥7 cm. The risk of high nuclear grade (i.e., Fuhrman nuclear grade ≥3) disease was also related to tumor size. Each 1 cm increase in tumor size increased the odds of high-grade disease by 32% in clear cell stage T1 RCC [24].

These data ideally would answer the question of what size is "safe" for AS. One group has described surveillance outcomes in patients with T1a versus T1b–T2 masses [17, 25]. Failure of surveillance was defined as progression to metastatic disease or conversion from surveillance to delayed treatment. Of 41 patients with pT1a tumors, only one failed surveillance (2%), and none progressed to metastasis. In contrast, of 42 patients with T1b–T2 tumors 14% failed surveillance and 6% progressed to metastasis disease. No study has adequately assessed risk differential across a 0–4 cm size range; however, associations between tumor size and failure of surveillance have been reported. Rosales et al. observed 223 tumors over a median time period of 35 months [26]. Failure of surveillance defined as metastatic progression or requirement for intervention occurred in 9% of patients. Median tumor size of tumors in the failed group was 3.6 cm compared to 2.6 cm in the success group. Final tumor size at the end of the surveillance period in failed and success groups was 5.2 cm versus 3.6 cm, respectively. These data suggest that tumors ≤3 cm are less likely to behave aggressively. Large systematic studies are required to validate these findings.

Contrast Enhancement

A critical radiologic feature of RCC is the presence of contrast enhancement, defined as an increase of 15–20 Hounsfield units (HU). Presence of contrast enhancement has a positive predictive value for detection of malignancy of approximately 80–90%. Several studies have examined the relationships between the magnitude of contrast enhancement and pathology. In general, contrast enhancement is relatively higher in clear cell carcinomas and lower in papillary RCC. This is an important distinction in that clear cell RCC has a greater tendency to metastasize than papillary RCC. One caveat to this is type II papillary RCC which comprises 20–40% of all papillary tumors. Type II papillary RCC can behave aggressively with 5-year CSM rates double that of type I papillary RCC [27]. Alshumrani et al. examined 46 cT1 tumors and found that the degree of contrast enhancement in clear cell RCC, oncocytoma, and papillary RCC tumors was 65, 80, and 16 HU, respectively [28]. Herts et al. reported that low tumor-to-aorta and tumor-to-parenchyma enhancement ratios correlated with papillary RCC [29]. These enhancement characteristics can also be observed with MRI imaging. Sun et al. examined 122 patients and found a >200% increase in signal intensity in clear cell RCC versus a 32–96% increase for papillary RCC [30]. However, the sensitivity and specificity of enhancement features are low, and findings must be interpreted with caution.

A recently reported MRI imaging parameter termed apparent diffusion coefficient (ADC) has also shown potential to distinguish low versus high Fuhrman grade [31]. Measurements conducted in 57 clear cell RCC tumors demonstrated a significantly lower ADC in high-grade tumors compared to low-grade ones. Two different ADC mapping protocols were capable of 89% sensitivity and 96% specificity to detect high-grade pathology. These performance characteristics were determined by correlating preoperative MRI study data to surgical pathology. These data illustrate the potential for cross-sectional imaging to extend beyond gross evaluation into the microscopic realm.

Specialized Tumor Features

Specialized tumor features that can gauge oncologic risk include morphology, growth pattern, location, and internal organization. Tumor morphology refers to the overall appearance of the tumor in terms of the uniformity of its peripheral edge. Birnbaum correlated CT findings with pathologic features in 100 surgically resected clear cell RCC tumors [32]. They found that well circumscribed spherical tumors were more likely to have Fuhrman grades 1–2 compared to tumors with irregular borders. Soyer et al. reported data from a similar study in 35 clear cell RCC tumors and found that radiographically apparent complete encapsulation of the tumor was observed in 40% of tumors with Fuhrman grades 1–2, but in no tumors with Fuhrman grades 3–4 [33]. Tumor growth pattern can be classified as expansive or infiltrative. Expansive tumors are typically well circumscribed and appear to displace adjacent tissues. In contrast, infiltrative tumors have indistinct edges and appear to replace adjacent tissue. An infiltrative appearance is strongly associated with high grade or sarcomatoid differentiation and poor prognosis [32]. Similarly, the internal organization of tumors can also provide an indication of the degree of tumor differentiation. A homogeneous appearance suggests preservation of tissue organization, uniform histology, and ordered vascularity. Heterogeneous organization suggests poor differentiation, loss of organization, central necrosis, and aberrant vascularization. Zhang et al. examined 193 tumors and found that 79–88% of tumors with heterogeneous enhancement patterns had clear cell RCC pathology [34]. In contrast papillary and chromophobe tumors tended to have more homogenous appearance. As with other radiologic tumor features, these findings are nonspecific and must be interpreted with caution.

Renal Mass Biopsy

Tumor biopsy forms the foundation for diagnosis and management of many cancer types. Breast and prostate tissues are relatively easy to sample, and protocols for biopsy in these tissues are firmly established. RBM has not been routinely utilized due to several key obstacles. First, these tumors are deep within the body and often adjacent to large blood vessels or major organs. Safe and accurate guidance of biopsy needle to these tumors relies heavily upon high-resolution image guidance and technical expertise. Second, sampling of tumor tissue is complicated by the presence of tumor heterogeneity, regions of focal necrosis, and shared eosinophilic histological features of certain benign and malignant tumors. The historical noninformative rate of RMB was on the order of 20–40%, and its accuracy to obtain the correct pathologic diagnosis ranged from 70% to 80% [35–37]. Over the past decade the accuracy and informative rate of RMB has increased significantly due to advances in CT and US technology that have enabled high-resolution tumor imaging and precise stereotactic needle placement [38]. Additional improvements include optimization of sampling techniques and standardization of pathologic analysis and interpretation. As a result the contemporary noninformative rate has decreased to approximately 10–15%, and accuracy to distinguish between benign and malignant disease has increased to 97% for informative biopsies [39–43].

RMB Techniques

Techniques for percutaneous RMB include core needle biopsy and fine needle aspiration (FNA). Core biopsy involves sampling of the tumor with an 18-guage core biopsy needle. Core specimens can be preserved, sectioned, stained, and evaluated using standard surgical pathology protocols. FNA is conducted by using multiple passes through the tissue of interest using a small bore needle under negative pressure. This collection method results in the collection of cellular aspirates which are best suited for cytology, immunohistology, flow cytometry, and fluorescence in situ hybridization (FISH). The technique of FNA may be better suited to situations in which the biopsy tract must traverse bowel or adjacent organs.

A summary of contemporary core and FNA biopsy data is presented in Table 6.3. Core biopsy is equivalent to FNA in terms of informative rate, and superior in terms of diagnostic accuracy. The informative rate for both biopsy techniques

Table 6.3 Contemporary renal mass biopsy data summary

Author	n	Informative rate (%)	Benign/malignant accuracy (%)	Histological accuracy	Nuclear grade accuracy	Complication rate
FNA studies						
Lechevallier et al. [49]	63	79	97	89%	79%	0%
Neuzillet et al. [43]	88	91	92	92%	70%	0%
Schmidbauer et al. [41]	44	91	83	86%	28%	1%
Masoom et al. [64]	31	100	97	97%	NA	NA
Veltri et al. [65]	26	92	88	NA	NA	3%
Mean values		91	91	91%	59%	1%
Core biopsy studies						
Lebret et al. [66]	119	79	92	86%	46%	0%
Maturen et al. [67]	152	96	97	NA	NA	2%
Somani et al. [68]	70	87	100	100%	NA	1%
Schmidbauer et al. [41]	78	97	96	98%	76%	1%
Shannon et al. [42]	235	78	100	98%	98%	1%
Volpe et al. [46]	100	84	100	93%	68%	3%
Wang et al. [69]	110	91	100	NA	NA	7%
Blumenfeld et al. [40]	81	98	97	88%	43%	NA
Veltri et al. [65]	45	92	91	93%	NA	6%
Mean values		89	97	94%	66%	3%

Informative rate refers to percent of biopsies providing diagnostic information; accuracy refers to percent correlation of biopsy with definitive surgical pathology results for informative biopsies; complication rate includes both minor and major events
NA not available

is 89–91% on average. The accuracy of core RMB to correctly distinguish malignant versus benign pathology is 97% for informative biopsies, and accuracy to correctly diagnose histology and nuclear grade are 94% and 66%, respectively. FNA is heavily dependent on consistency of cytological preparation and pathologic analysis. As a result there can be considerable variability of results among institutions. Current data demonstrate that FNA has an average informative rate of 91%. Mean accuracies of FNA to properly diagnose malignancy, histology, and Fuhrman nuclear grade were 91%, 91%, and 59%, respectively [41, 43–45].

Several groups have reported improved results using a combination of both FNA and core biopsy. In one of the earliest studies, Wood et al. reported sensitivity and specificity of combined FNA and core biopsy to be 95% and 93%, respectively. Volpe et al. showed that the combination of FNA and core biopsy resulted in a 22% increase in informative rate [46]. A recent side-by-side evaluation of core versus FNA versus combined core + FNA biopsy accuracy has been reported by Veltri et al. The histological diagnostic accuracies of FNA and core biopsy were 76% and 93%, respectively. The combination of core biopsy and FNA resulted in a 23% increase in histological diagnostic accuracy.

RMB Limitations

In the past noninformative RMBs were often classified as false-negative results; however, this was misleading. By definition, a false-negative biopsy occurs when benign disease is diagnosed in the biopsy specimen and malignant disease is subsequently confirmed. Fortunately this event occurs rarely at an incidence of approximately 1%. The term "noninformative" refers to several scenarios and is encountered in 10–15% of cases. "Failed" noninformative biopsies refer to cases in which insufficient tissue was obtained for analysis. "Indeterminant" noninformative biopsies refer to cases in which tumor tissue was obtained but a definitive pathological diagnosis could not be made. Commonly encountered indeterminant

biopsies include those that report oncocytic tumor features. These features reflecting an eosinophilic staining pattern can be observed in oncocytoma, eosinophilic variants of conventional RCC, chromophobe RCC, papillary RCC, and even epithelioid AML tumors. At one extreme, Liu et al. reported detection of oncocytic features in ten biopsies (56%) from 18 patients [47]. On final pathology of these oncocytic neoplasms, eight proved to be benign oncocytomas, while the remaining two were chromophobe RCC and eosinophilic papillary RCC. In cases where the first biopsy renders noninformative results, a second biopsy has been advocated, and has a reported success rate of 75–100% [48].

Informative rates are influenced by sampling technique and tumor size. Sampling error is affected by two major variables—accuracy of stereotactic needle placement and adequate sampling of tumor subcomponents. Noninformative biopsy rates have been reported to be higher for tumors <3 cm on average (37% versus 9%, $P=0.006$) [49]. This is likely because it is more difficult to guide biopsy needles to these small tumors, and also because the sampling tract for small masses is short. In smaller pT1a tumors 1–3 biopsies from central and peripheral regions should be obtained [44]. In larger tumors, adequate sampling can be hindered by the presence of central tumor necrosis. In larger pT1b tumors it is recommended that two or three cores from the periphery of the tumor be acquired due to the high prevalence of central necrosis. A recent study published by Rybickowski et al. illustrates these effects of tumor size on informative rates. In this study noninformative rates were higher for masses <3 and >6 cm (60% and 44%, respectively) versus those between 4 and 6 cm (NPV of 89%) [50]. As protocols and imaging technologies improve, sampling error will become less prevalent, and the limitations of RMB will diminish.

Complications of RMB

Potential complications of RMB include hemorrhage, pseudoaneurysm formation, infection, adjacent organ injury, pneumothorax, and tract seeding. Average minor and major complication rates in contemporary studies are 5% and 1%, respectively. Hemorrhage is a primary concern given the highly vascular nature of the kidney. Bleeding complications are typically managed with conservative measures including bed rest and transfusion. Angioembolization or surgery is rarely necessary. It is important that patients stop coumadin, aspirin, or IIa/IIIb inhibitors 7–10 days prior to biopsy to allow for normalization of coagulation parameters. Cessation of the medications and bridging with short-acting agents such as heparin or eptifibadtide may be necessary in some cases, and coordination of this process should be made in conjunction with the patient's cardiologist or vascular medicine specialist. In patients who do not require bridging, the risk of cessation of anticoagulation medications must be balanced by the potential benefit of the proposed biopsy. Tumor seeding of the biopsy tract appears to occur very rarely such that incidents have been documented only in isolated case report studies. Current practice is to conduct RMB via a coaxial dilator to minimize the risk of needle tract seeding.

Evolving Role for RMB

At present RMB yields histological information including RCC subtype and Fuhrman nuclear grade. These phenotypic descriptions of cancers cells are limited indicators of the pathobiology of the tumor. Large pan-genomic studies have shown that clear cell RCC tumors with indistinguishable histology have substantial genotypic heterogeneity [51]. Molecular analysis is able to characterize tumor pathobiology at a level of resolution that is orders of magnitude greater than standard histological analysis. In this regard molecular analysis may facilitate a shift to routine use of RMB to diagnose and evaluate kidney tumors.

The emergence of technologies that allow for genome-wide and proteome-wide analysis are allowing for comprehensive characterization of mutation patterns that occur in RCC tumors. Genetic "signatures" have been identified for specific RCC subtypes. Study is ongoing to assess the association between specific signatures and clinical behavior and response to targeted therapy. One of the most comprehensive array studies conducted to date was conducted by Rini et al. [52]. In this study expression of 732 genes were examined in samples from 931 patients who were followed for a median duration of 5.6 years. Ultimately 16 genes were identified that were associated with recurrence after definitive treatment. Development of rapid and cost-effective genome-wide expression analysis has the potential to replace histopathology as the primary means by which tumors are characterized.

Pan-genomic mutational analysis has been a primary focus of active investigation. Array-based comparative genomic hybridization (CGH) allows for detection of microdeletions and copy number changes at a resolution of 5–10 kilobases. One of the most comprehensive CGH studies to date was published by Beroukhim et al. in which 90 clear cell RCC specimens were analyzed [53]. The study identified specific regions of the genome that were commonly mutated and allowed for classification of sporadic clear cell RCC tumors into those with or without biallelic VHL inactivation. The study has identified new categorization criteria that may have significant clinical implications in terms of prognosis and response to targeted therapy.

Basic science studies are rapidly identifying key molecules and processes involved in RCC tumorigenesis. Translational studies are in great demand in order to define the relationships between these biomarkers and clinical tumor behavior. It is likely that surgical intervention will remain the mainstay for high stage RCC tumors. However, for lower risk cT1 tumors the use of RMB-based molecular analysis may dictate management. If molecular analysis revealed indolent RCC pathology, then surveillance or minimally invasive ablative therapies may be validated as safe options. Molecular analysis may also allow for assessment of sensitivity to targeted therapy. In this manner appropriate combinations of targeted therapy and surgery can be initiated to optimally treat these tumors.

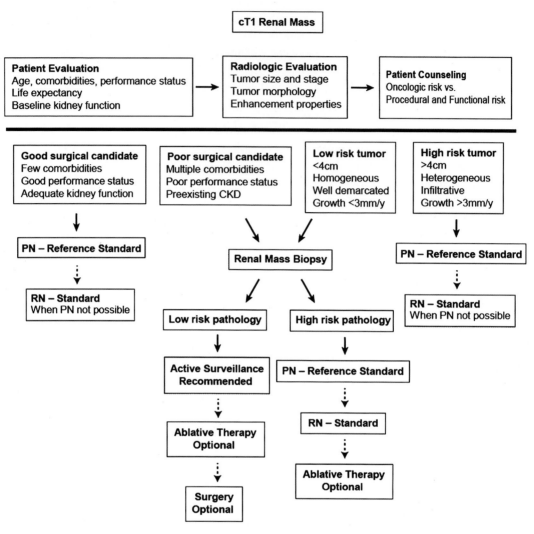

Fig. 6.2 Stage T1 RCC management options. Management of patients with cT1 RCC tumors should factor in patient and radiologic tumor features and should include a balanced discussion of oncologic risk versus procedural benefit. In healthy patients with normal kidney function and in patients with high-risk tumors, partial nephrectomy is the reference standard. In poor surgical candidates or in patients with tumors suspected to pose low risk, renal mass biopsy may alter management and improve survival rates by averting low-risk patients away from surgical management

Contemporary Management of the cT1 Kidney Tumor

The management of patients with cT1 tumors involves assessment of oncologic risk, technical feasibility of surgery, baseline patient health status, and baseline kidney functional status. An outline for cT1 RCC management options is shown in Fig. 6.2. Radical and partial nephrectomy com-

prise the primary treatment modalities for cT1 tumors, but we are now recognizing that in select patients survival may actually be decreased as a result of intervention, particularly for radical nephrectomy. In 2009 the AUA convened a panel to establish recommendations regarding management of T1 renal masses, and one of the main take home points of this document related to a strong preference for nephron-sparing modalities whenever feasible [36]. Key elements of preoperative evaluation include age, performance status, and presence of major comorbidities including atherosclerosis, hypertension, diabetes, and cardiac disease. Other important considerations include smoking history, level of daily activity, and estimation of physical ability needed for recovery. Key laboratory factors include presence of anemia of chronic disease as well as serum creatinine. Radiologic evaluation should consist of a high-resolution CT or MRI with and without contrast to assess tumor anatomy and enhancement features. Key aspects of radiologic evaluation include tumor size, location, and morphology, amenability to partial nephrectomy, and feasibility of laparoscopic intervention.

Counseling of patients should consist of a balanced discussion regarding the risks and benefits of treatment. Available management options include partial nephrectomy, radical nephrectomy, thermal ablation, and AS. Each of these interventions will be discussed in detail in the upcoming chapters. Each management type is unique in terms of oncological efficacy, functional preservation, and treatment-related morbidity, and mortality. In general, PN is now defined as the reference standard for T1 tumors, and RN should be reserved as an alternate standard of care when tumor anatomy precludes a nephron-sparing approach, a situation that is now relatively uncommon. RN is associated with the highest degree of functional decline, and should be avoided if possible. Thermal ablation is a less invasive treatment option compared to PN and RN and poses a relatively lower risk for post-treatment renal functional decline. However, TA is associated with decreased oncologic efficacy, and as such is primarily reserved for high operative risk patients who desire proactive treatment. Percutaneous RMB should be performed in all patients undergoing ablation therapy to define histology. AS is currently reserved as an option primarily for patients with limited life expectancy.

The current absolute indications for RMB are for assessment of tumors which are suspicious for lymphoma, abscess or metastatic involvement of the kidney. RMB should also be conducted if it is anticipated that the results may alter clinical management, a utility-based approach. There is an emerging role for RMB in patients who are at elevated operative risk, who have limited life expectancy, or in those who are at high risk of developing CKD as a result of intervention. An example would be an active 74-year-old man with a 2.5 cm exophytic, contrast-enhancing renal tumor with a baseline estimated glomerular filtration rate of 48 ml/min/1.73 m [2], and comorbidities including diabetes and a history of coronary artery disease. In this patient PN, ablation or surveillance would all be reasonable options, and RMB can stratify oncologist risk and guide counseling and management. For instance if RMB indicated a potentially high-grade clear cell RCC, PN would be considered, while RMB suggesting an oncocytic tumor might prompt more conservative management. A shift in practice toward use of this approach has the potential to significantly improve survival in this subset of patients. With the development of reliable molecular diagnostics, we may eventually be able to predict clinical tumor behavior with a much higher degree of accuracy. In this event we would expect that the role for RMB-based analysis would be extended to all kidney tumors.

Conclusions

Contemporary data indicate that only about 20–30% of stage cT1 kidney tumors exhibit aggressive clinical behavior, therefore surgery for all tumors, particularly smaller ones, may constitute overtreatment. Demographics of patients with stage cT1 tumors are trending toward increasing age and decreasing preoperative kidney function, and traditional surgery can be associated with significant increases in morbidity and risk for non-oncologic mortality in these vulnerable patients. This is especially true for radical nephrectomy, which should be avoided whenever feasible. There has been renewed interest in the use of RMB to differentiate patients with indolent versus aggressive disease prior to surgery. In this manner, patients with indolent disease could be identified and observed, or managed less aggressively. Advances in imaging resolution and ability to reliably sample tumor tissue have allowed for dramatic increases in accuracy and sensitivity of the procedure. Emerging data are allowing for identification of novel biomarkers that have the potential to identify tumors with potentially aggressive biology.

References

1. Hock LM, Lynch J, Balaji KC. Increasing incidence of all stages of kidney cancer in the last 2 decades in the United States: an analysis of surveillance, epidemiology and end results program data. J Urol. 2002; 167(1):57–60.

2. Hollingsworth JM, Miller DC, Daignault S, et al. Rising incidence of small renal masses: a need to reassess treatment effect. J Natl Cancer Inst. 2006;98(18): 1331–4.

3. Sun M, Thuret R, Abdollah F, et al. Age-adjusted incidence, mortality, and survival rates of stage-specific renal cell carcinoma in North America: a trend analysis. Eur Urol. 2011;59:135–41.

4. Chow WH, Devesa SS, Warren JL, et al. Rising incidence of renal cell cancer in the United States. JAMA. 1999;281(17):1628–31.

5. Nguyen CT, Campbell SC. Staging of renal cell carcinoma: past, present, and future. Clin Genitourin Cancer. 2006;5(3):190–7.

6. Huang WC. Impact of nephron sparing on kidney function and non-oncologic mortality. Urol Oncol. 2010;28(5):568–74.

7. Weight CJ, Larson BT, Fergany AF, et al. Nephrectomy induced chronic renal insufficiency is associated with increased risk of cardiovascular death and death from any cause in patients with localized cT1b renal masses. J Urol. 2010;183(4):1317–23.

8. Chow WH, Dong LM, Devesa SS. Epidemiology and risk factors for kidney cancer. Nat Rev Urol. 2010; 7(5):245–57.

9. Frank I, Blute ML, Cheville JC, et al. Solid renal tumors: an analysis of pathological features related to tumor size. J Urol. 2003;170(6 Pt 1):2217–20.

10. Lane BR, Babineau D, Kattan MW, et al. A preoperative prognostic nomogram for solid enhancing renal tumors 7 cm or less amenable to partial nephrectomy. J Urol. 2007;178(2):429–34.

11. Kunkle DA, Crispen PL, Chen DY, et al. Enhancing renal masses with zero net growth during active surveillance. J Urol. 2007;177(3):849–53 [discussion 53–4].

12. Zhang J, Kang SK, Wang L, et al. Distribution of renal tumor growth rates determined by using serial volumetric CT measurements. Radiology. 2009;250(1): 137–44.

13. Lamb GW, Bromwich EJ, Vasey P, et al. Management of renal masses in patients medically unsuitable for nephrectomy – natural history, complications, and outcome. Urology. 2004;64(5):909–13.

14. Sowery RD, Siemens DR. Growth characteristics of renal cortical tumors in patients managed by watchful waiting. Can J Urol. 2004;11(5):2407–10.

15. Volpe A, Panzarella T, Rendon RA, et al. The natural history of incidentally detected small renal masses. Cancer. 2004;100(4):738–45.

16. Crispen PL, Viterbo R, Fox EB, et al. Delayed intervention of sporadic renal masses undergoing active surveillance. Cancer. 2008;112(5):1051–7.

17. Haramis G, Mues AC, Rosales JC, et al. Natural history of renal cortical neoplasms during active surveillance with follow-up longer than 5 years. Urology. 2011;77:787–91.

18. Lee CT, Katz J, Fearn PA, et al. Mode of presentation of renal cell carcinoma provides prognostic information. Urol Oncol. 2002;7(4):135–40.

19. Zisman A, Pantuck AJ, Wieder J, et al. Risk group assessment and clinical outcome algorithm to predict the natural history of patients with surgically resected renal cell carcinoma. J Clin Oncol. 2002;20(23): 4559–66.

20. Sorbellini M, Kattan MW, Snyder ME, et al. A postoperative prognostic nomogram predicting recurrence for patients with conventional clear cell renal cell carcinoma. J Urol. 2005;173(1):48–51.

21. Lam JS, Shvarts O, Said JW, et al. Clinicopathologic and molecular correlations of necrosis in the primary tumor of patients with renal cell carcinoma. Cancer. 2005;103(12):2517–25.

22. DeRoche T, Walker E, Magi-Galluzzi C, et al. Pathologic characteristics of solitary small renal masses: can they be predicted by preoperative clinical parameters? Am J Clin Pathol. 2008;130(4):560–4.

23. Verhoest G, Veillard D, Guille F, et al. Relationship between age at diagnosis and clinicopathologic features of renal cell carcinoma. Eur Urol. 2007;51(5):1298–304 [discussion 304–5].

24. Thompson RH, Kurta JM, Kaag M, et al. Tumor size is associated with malignant potential in renal cell carcinoma cases. J Urol. 2009;181(5):2033–6. PMCID: 2734327.

25. Mues AC, Haramis G, Badani K, et al. Active surveillance for larger (cT1bN0M0 and cT2N0M0) renal cortical neoplasms. Urology. 2010;76(3):620–3.

26. Rosales JC, Haramis G, Moreno J, et al. Active surveillance for renal cortical neoplasms. J Urol. 2010; 183(5):1698–702.

27. Pignot G, Elie C, Conquy S, et al. Survival analysis of 130 patients with papillary renal cell carcinoma: prognostic utility of type 1 and type 2 subclassification. Urology. 2007;69(2):230–5.

28. Alshumrani G, O'Malley M, Ghai S, et al. Small (< or = 4 cm) cortical renal tumors: characterization with multidetector CT. Abdom Imaging. 2010;35(4):488–93.

29. Herts BR, Coll DM, Novick AC, et al. Enhancement characteristics of papillary renal neoplasms revealed on triphasic helical CT of the kidneys. Am J Roentgenol. 2002;178(2):367–72.

30. Sun MR, Ngo L, Genega EM, et al. Renal cell carcinoma: dynamic contrast-enhanced MR imaging for

differentiation of tumor subtypes – correlation with pathologic findings. Radiology. 2009;250(3):793–802.

31. Rosenkrantz AB, Niver BE, Fitzgerald EF, et al. Utility of the apparent diffusion coefficient for distinguishing clear cell renal cell carcinoma of low and high nuclear grade. Am J Roentgenol. 2010;195(5): W344–51.

32. Birnbaum BA, Bosniak MA, Krinsky GA, et al. Renal cell carcinoma: correlation of CT findings with nuclear morphologic grading in 100 tumors. Abdom Imaging. 1994;19(3):262–6.

33. Soyer P, Dufresne A, Klein I, et al. Renal cell carcinoma of clear type: correlation of CT features with tumor size, architectural patterns, and pathologic staging. Eur Radiol. 1997;7(2):224–9.

34. Zhang J, Lefkowitz RA, Ishill NM, et al. Solid renal cortical tumors: differentiation with CT. Radiology. 2007;244(2):494–504.

35. Torp-Pedersen S, Juul N, Larsen T, et al. US-guided fine needle biopsy of solid renal masses – comparison of histology and cytology. Scand J Urol Nephrol Suppl. 1991;137:41–3.

36. Dechet CB, Sebo T, Farrow G, et al. Prospective analysis of intraoperative frozen needle biopsy of solid renal masses in adults. J Urol. 1999;162(4):1282–4. PMCID: 2734327.

37. Richter F, Kasabian NG, Irwin Jr RJ, et al. Accuracy of diagnosis by guided biopsy of renal mass lesions classified indeterminate by imaging studies. Urology. 2000;55(3):348–52.

38. Skenazy JF, Mirabile G, Hruby GW, et al. Comparison of manual and computer assisted ultrasonic guidance for transparenchymal percutaneous renal needle placement. J Urol. 2009;181(2):867–71.

39. Renshaw AA, Lee KR, Madge R, et al. Accuracy of fine needle aspiration in distinguishing subtypes of renal cell carcinoma. Acta Cytol. 1997;41(4): 987–94.

40. Blumenfeld AJ, Guru K, Fuchs GJ, et al. Percutaneous biopsy of renal cell carcinoma underestimates nuclear grade. Urology. 2010;76(3):610–3.

41. Schmidbauer J, Remzi M, Memarsadeghi M, et al. Diagnostic accuracy of computed tomography-guided percutaneous biopsy of renal masses. Eur Urol. 2008;53(5):1003–11.

42. Shannon BA, Cohen RJ, de Bruto H, et al. The value of preoperative needle core biopsy for diagnosing benign lesions among small, incidentally detected renal masses. J Urol. 2008;180(4):1257–61 [discussion 61].

43. Neuzillet Y, Lechevallier E, Andre M, et al. Accuracy and clinical role of fine needle percutaneous biopsy with computerized tomography guidance of small (less than 4.0 cm) renal masses. J Urol. 2004; 171(5):1802–5.

44. Wunderlich H, Hindermann W, Al Mustafa AM, et al. The accuracy of 250 fine needle biopsies of renal tumors. J Urol. 2005;174(1):44–6.

45. Jaff A, Molinie V, Mellot F, et al. Evaluation of imaging-guided fine-needle percutaneous biopsy of renal masses. Eur Radiol. 2005;15(8):1721–6.

46. Volpe A, Mattar K, Finelli A, et al. Contemporary results of percutaneous biopsy of 100 small renal masses: a single center experience. J Urol. 2008; 180(6):2333–7.

47. Liu J, Fanning CV. Can renal oncocytomas be distinguished from renal cell carcinoma on fine-needle aspiration specimens? A study of conventional smears in conjunction with ancillary studies. Cancer. 2001;93(6):390–7.

48. Samplaski MK, Zhou M, Lane BR, et al. Renal mass sampling: an enlightened perspective. Int J Urol. 2011;18:5–19.

49. Lechevallier E, Andre M, Barriol D, et al. Fine-needle percutaneous biopsy of renal masses with helical CT guidance. Radiology. 2000;216(2):506–10.

50. Rybicki FJ, Shu KM, Cibas ES, et al. Percutaneous biopsy of renal masses: sensitivity and negative predictive value stratified by clinical setting and size of masses. Am J Roentgenol. 2003;180(5):1281–7.

51. Dalgliesh GL, Furge K, Greenman C, et al. Systematic sequencing of renal carcinoma reveals inactivation of histone modifying genes. Nature. 2010;463(7279): 360–3. PMCID: 2820242.

52. Rini BI, Zhou M, Aydin H. Identification of prognostic genomic markers in patients with localized clear cell renal cell carcinoma. J Clin Oncol. 2010;28 Suppl 15:4501.

53. Beroukhim R, Brunet JP, Di Napoli A, et al. Patterns of gene expression and copy-number alterations in von-Hippel Lindau disease-associated and sporadic clear cell carcinoma of the kidney. Cancer Res. 2009;69(11):4674–81. PMCID: 2745239.

54. Remzi M, Ozsoy M, Klingler HC, et al. Are small renal tumors harmless? Analysis of histopathological features according to tumors 4 cm or less in diameter. J Urol. 2006;176(3):896–9.

55. Schlomer B, Figenshau RS, Yan Y, et al. Pathological features of renal neoplasms classified by size and symptomatology. J Urol. 2006;176(4 Pt 1):1317–20 [discussion 20].

56. Pahernik S, Ziegler S, Roos F, et al. Small renal tumors: correlation of clinical and pathological features with tumor size. J Urol. 2007;178(2):414–7 [discussion 6–7].

57. Kato M, Suzuki T, Suzuki Y, et al. Natural history of small renal cell carcinoma: evaluation of growth rate, histological grade, cell proliferation and apoptosis. J Urol. 2004;172(3):863–6.

58. Volpe A, Jewett MA. The natural history of small renal masses. Nat Clin Pract Urol. 2005;2(8):384–90.

59. Wehle MJ, Thiel DD, Petrou SP, et al. Conservative management of incidental contrast-enhancing renal masses as safe alternative to invasive therapy. Urology. 2004;64(1):49–52.

60. Abouassaly R, Lane BR, Novick AC. Active surveillance of renal masses in elderly patients. J Urol. 2008;180(2):505–8 [discussion 8–9].

61. Kouba E, Smith A, McRackan D, et al. Watchful waiting for solid renal masses: insight into the natural history and results of delayed intervention. J Urol. 2007;177(2):466–70 [discussion 70].

62. Abou Youssif T, Kassouf W, Steinberg J, et al. Active surveillance for selected patients with renal masses: updated results with long-term follow-up. Cancer. 2007;110(5):1010–4.

63. Crispen PL, Wong YN, Greenberg RE, et al. Predicting growth of solid renal masses under active surveillance. Urol Oncol. 2008;26(5):555–9. PMCID: 2720098.

64. Masoom S, Venkataraman G, Jensen J, et al. Renal FNA-based typing of renal masses remains a useful adjunctive modality: evaluation of 31 renal masses with correlative histology. Cytopathology. 2009; 20(1):50–5.

65. Veltri A, Garetto I, Tosetti I, et al. Diagnostic accuracy and clinical impact of imaging-guided needle biopsy of renal masses. Retrospective analysis on 150 cases. Eur Radiol. 2011;21:393–401.

66. Lebret T, Poulain JE, Molinie V, et al. Percutaneous core biopsy for renal masses: indications, accuracy and results. J Urol. 2007;178(4 Pt 1):1184–8 [discussion 8].

67. Maturen KE, Nghiem HV, Caoili EM, et al. Renal mass core biopsy: accuracy and impact on clinical management. Am J Roentgenol. 2007;188(2): 563–70.

68. Somani BK, Nabi G, Thorpe P, et al. Image-guided biopsy-diagnosed renal cell carcinoma: critical appraisal of technique and long-term follow-up. Eur Urol. 2007;51(5):1289–95 [discussion 96–7].

69. Wang R, Wolf Jr JS, Wood Jr DP, et al. Accuracy of percutaneous core biopsy in management of small renal masses. Urology. 2009;73(3):586–90 [discussion 90–1].

Radical Nephrectomy for Localized Renal Tumors: Optimum Oncological and Renal Functional Considerations

7

Paul Russo

Introduction

There will be an estimated 58,240 new cases and 13,040 deaths from kidney cancer in the USA in 2010 [1]. Compared to 1971, this represents a fivefold increase in the incidence and twofold increase in the mortality of renal cancer. Associated risk factors for kidney cancer include hypertension, obesity, and African American race. Epidemiological evidence suggests an increase in all stages of renal cancer, including the advanced and metastatic cases. It is now understood that renal cortical tumors are a family of distinct tumors with variable histology, cytogenetic defects, and metastatic potential [2]. Approximately 90% of the tumors that metastasize are the conventional clear cell carcinoma [3]; however, they account for only 54% of the total number of resected tumors. Approximately 30–40% of renal tumor patients will either present with or later develop metastatic disease. The widespread use of the modern abdominal imaging techniques (CT, MRI, and abdominal ultrasound) over the last two decades, usually ordered to evaluate nonspecific abdominal and musculoskeletal complaints or during unrelated cancer care, has changed the profile of the typical renal tumor patient from one with a massive, symptomatic tumor at presentation to one with a small, asymptomatic, renal mass (<4 cm) incidentally discovered in 70% of the cases [4]. A survival rate of 90% or greater, depending on the tumor histology, is expected for these small tumors if partial (PN) or radical nephrectomy (RN) is performed.

RN was once considered the "gold standard" and utilized to treat all tumors, small and large, and even to solve diagnostic dilemmas when an uncertain renal mass was encountered. PN was only utilized in restricted conditions such as tumor in a solitary kidney or in patients with conditions which compromised renal function. New concerns that RN could cause or worsen preexisting chronic kidney disease (CKD) has lead to recommendations for more restricted use of RN, whether performed by open or minimally invasive techniques, for the resection of large renal tumors, including those which destroy the majority of the kidney, invade the renal sinus, invade branched or main renal veins or extend into the inferior vena cava, and/or are associated with regional adenopathy or metastatic disease. The increased treatment and cure of small, incidentally discovered renal tumors, most of which are nonlethal in nature, does not appear to offset the increased mortality caused by the advanced and metastatic tumors. This "treatment disconnect" may result from unaccounted etiological factors

P. Russo MD, FACS (✉)
Department of Surgery, Urology Service,
Memorial Sloan Kettering Cancer Center,
New York, NY, 10021, USA

Weill Medical College, Cornell University,
1275 York Avenue, New York, NY, 10021, USA
e-mail: RussoP@MSKCC.org

increasing the incidence of all renal cortical tumors and their virulence. In this chapter, the optimum contemporary utilization of RN in the management of localized renal tumors and its impact on renal function will be discussed.

Radical Nephrectomy: Historical Considerations

Successful attempts to surgically cure renal tumors were reported widely after World War 2 with surgical strategies designed to address the renal capsular and perinephric fat infiltration observed in up to 70% of the tumors [5]. Using a thoracoabdominal incision, Mortensen [6] reported the first radical nephrectomy, an operation that removed all of the contents of Gerota's fascia. Radical nephrectomy was popularized in the 1960s by Robson who described this operation as the perifascial resection of the tumor-bearing kidney and perirenal fat, regional lymph nodes, and ipsilateral adrenal gland [7]. In 1969 Robson reported RN results in a series of 88 patients and described a 65% survival for tumors confined within Gerota's fascia (Robson stages 1 and 2), but the finding of regional nodal metastases led to less than 30% 5-year survival rate [8].

En bloc RN, ipsilateral adrenalectomy, and extensive regional lymphadenectomy, usually through large abdominal or transthoracic incisions, became the standard approach to the renal tumors for the next 20 years as major centers began reporting favorable results [9, 10]. In this era, the imaging studies used to diagnose a patient, who was generally symptomatic with a large renal tumor, was intravenous urograms, retrograde pyelograms, and arteriograms. These techniques were unable to detect small tumors and the incidental tumor detection rate was <5%. Despite this acceptance of RN by urologic surgeons, convincing data did not exist establishing the therapeutic impact of the component parts of the operation (i.e., the need for adrenalectomy [11] or the need for and extent of lymph node dissection [12, 13]). Historical series were subjected to selection biases, and the virtues of randomized trials in clinical investigation to address the many

questions in kidney tumor surgery were not yet realized. Although a subsequent report with longer follow-up from Robson in 1982 projected declining long-term survival rates in the range of 40% [14], there was no doubt that the surgical techniques associated with the safe removal of large renal tumors were established, well described, and reproducible making RN the only effective treatment for renal cortical tumors. Today, at major centers with a commitment to renal tumor surgery, despite the above-described imaging-induced stage and tumor size migration, RN is still required in approximately 20–30% of patients with renal tumors not amenable to kidney sparing approaches (Fig. 7.1).

Radical Nephrectomy: Patient Selection and Preoperative Evaluation

To a large extent, the modern imaging studies of CT, ultrasound, and MRI that have been so effective in creating the era of the "incidentaloma" and the associated tumor size and stage migration also provide the surgeon with an accurate description of the extent of disease prior to operation. At MSKCC, tumors routinely selected for RN include those large and centrally localized tumors that have effectively replaced the majority of the normal renal parenchyma, often associated with regional adenopathy, inferior vena cava, or right atrial extension, none of which are amenable to a PN [15]. In addition, RN is performed on patients with metastatic disease referred by medical oncology for cytoreductive nephrectomy prior to the initiation of systemic therapy [16–18]. Patients with extensive metastatic disease and a poor Karnofsky performance status are advised to undergo percutaneous needle biopsy of the primary tumor or a metastatic site and subsequently referred for systemic therapy. Patients with small incidentally discovered or exophytic tumors amenable to PN are asked to also sign consent for radical nephrectomy if operative findings or technical problems arise making PN unsafe or unwise. Over the last 3 years at our center, 1,030 surgical nephrectomies have been

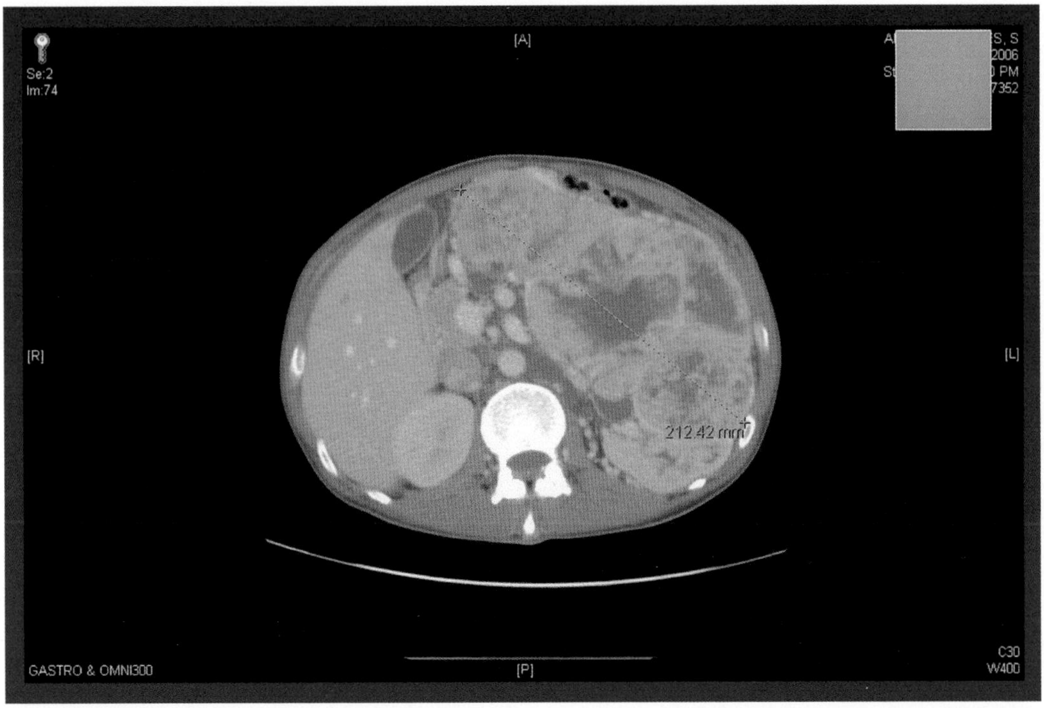

Fig. 7.1 CT of the abdomen of a 44-year-old male with massive left renal tumor (21 cm × 15 cm × 12 cm) completely replacing the kidney. He subsequently underwent left radical nephrectomy, regional lymph node dissection, and ipsilateral adrenalectomy

performed with 21% RN and 79% PN, reflecting our center's commitment to kidney sparing approaches whenever possible.

Prior to operation, routine serum chemistries, coagulation profile, type and cross match (or autologous blood donation), and chest X-ray are obtained. Routine brain imaging and bone scanning are not performed unless site-specific abnormalities in the history, physical, or routine preoperative laboratory examination are discovered. For patients with significant comorbid conditions, particularly cardiac and pulmonary related, appropriate consultations are obtained with an effort made to optimize patients for operation whenever possible. Patients with significant coronary or carotid artery disease may require revascularization prior to RN. For patients with compromised pulmonary status, consultation with anesthesiology is requested for consideration of epidural postoperative analgesia.

Open Radical Nephrectomy: Surgical Anatomy, Choice of Incisions, and Operative Considerations

The kidneys are retroperitoneal organs located in the lumbar fossa. They are covered with a variable amount of perinephric fat and Gerota's fascia and lay in proximity to the psoas major and quadratus lumborum muscles, and diaphragm. The right kidney abuts the right adrenal gland; liver, hepatic flexure of the colon, and second portion of the duodenum cover the renal hilum. The left kidney is in proximity to the left adrenal whose main vein drains into the left renal vein, pancreatic tail, and spleen superiorly and the left colon medially. Depending on the surgeon's preference, relating mainly to patient's body habitus, the tumor size and location, the RN can be performed through an eleventh rib flank incision, a transperitoneal midline or subcostal incision, or a transthoracic incision or a miniflank supra eleventh rib incision rib miniflank incision [15]. The "miniflank incision" (Fig. 7.2) has the advantage of speedy entry into the retroperitoneum and avoidance of the rib resection with a decreased likelihood (<5%) of subsequent atony of the flank muscles and bulge [19]. For large tumors with any question of liver, pancreatic, splenic, or IVC extension optimum exposure with bilateral subcostal (chevron) or thoracoabdominal incision is preferred and leaves options open for gaining control over the renal hilum particularly when there is regional adenopathy and parasitic veins to contend with. In the retroperitoneal approach to RN, the peritoneum and pleura are dissected off Gerota's fascia exposing the kidney and ipsilateral great vessel.

During transabdominal RN, the colon is reflected medially along the white line of Toldt. We commonly employ self-retaining retractors to provide maximum exposure with care taken to pad organs prone to iatrogenic injury such as the spleen, liver, and pancreas. On the right side, mobilization of the duodenum (Kocher maneuver) medially provides clear exposure of the inferior vena cava and renal hilum. Peritoneal attachments to the liver and ligamentous attachments to the spleen are carefully divided with care taken not to tear liver and splenic capsules. Inferiorly, the ureter is identified, ligated, and divided. The gonadal vessels are identified coursing through the retroperitoneal soft tissues entering either the left renal vein or inferior vena cava on the right where it is ligated and divided. Split and roll techniques are used along the ipsilateral great vessel until the renal vein is identified. All lymphatic attachments overlying the renal vein are carefully divided. On the left side, the adrenal and gonadal veins are identified as they drain into the renal vein, ligated and divided. Using blunt dissection, a vessel loop is placed around the renal vein allowing for upward traction and identification of the renal artery. Care is taken not to tear a posterior lumbar vein which often also drains into the renal vein. The renal vein should be palpated and inspected to exclude the possibility of a tumor thrombus. As soon as is possible, the renal artery is identified beneath the renal

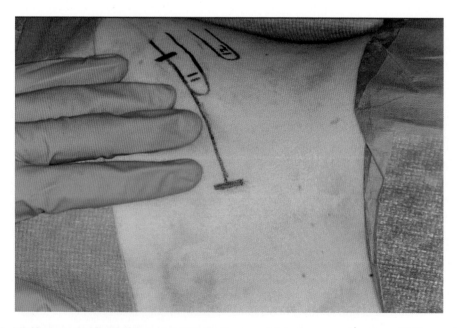

Fig. 7.2 Miniflank surgical incision is a quick and effective approach to the retroperitoneum and kidney and can be utilized both for partial and radical nephrectomy [19]

vein at its aortic ostium, ligated, suture ligated, and divided. The arterial decompression that ensues renders the kidney more mobile and deflates the many fragile and distended parasitic vessels along the surface of the kidney that often bleed during this mobilization process. Lack of renal vein decompression indicates an accessory renal artery often emanating from the aorta either superior or inferior to the level of the renal vein. The surgeon should avoid the renal vein ligation prior to complete arterial decompression which will cause marked venous congestion and hemorrhage from the tumor and parasitic vessels.

It is our practice to perform ipsilateral adrenalectomy and regional node dissection to maximize local tumor control, decrease the chance of local recurrence if these tissues are harboring micrometastatic disease, and provide maximum pathological staging to allow entry into ongoing adjuvant clinical trials. Little evidence currently exists that the resection of tumor-bearing lymph nodes or ipsilateral adrenal gland provides a therapeutic effect [20]. Care is taken not to traumatize the tail of the pancreas or the splenic vein during this portion of the dissection. Dissection continues along the aorta clipping and ligating arterial and venous supply to the adrenal. Following removal of the kidney and surrounding perinephric soft tissues and adrenal, the operative bed is thoroughly irrigated and inspected for any bleeding vessels. The spleen and pancreas are thoroughly inspected. Drains are not used unless a laceration of the pancreas is suspected or documented.

Once the tumor resection is accomplished, postoperative nomograms are available that incorporate clinical presentation, tumor histological subtype, size, and stage to provide and provide a clinical prognosis. Results for our center indicate 5-year survival rates following resection of non-metastatic tumors ranging from 30% to 98% depending on the above-mentioned clinical and pathological features. These postoperative nomograms have been extremely useful in patient counseling, tailoring cost-effective follow-up strategies, and designing clinical trials [3, 21].

Minimally Invasive Radical Nephrectomy

Following its introduction in 1991 by Clayman et al. [22], laparoscopic radical nephrectomy (LRN) offered a minimally invasive alternative to the classical open RN with dividends of less wound pain and morbidity, decreased analgesic requirement, decreased hospitalization, more rapid convalescence, and faster return to normal activities. Survival rates were directly comparable to those achieved with open RN [23–28]. At the time of its introduction, RN in general was the preferred treatment for all renal masses and PN was largely reserved for only essential cases where RN would put a patient at risk for dialysis. The choice of which procedure to offer the patient with the small renal tumor, LRN or open PN, posed a dilemma for surgical groups possessing both capabilities as the literature in each respective field developed in parallel over the last decade. A 9-year experience compared LRN ($N=61$) to open RN ($N=33$) for suspected renal cancer [23] and found advantages for the laparoscopic operation which included less estimated blood loss (172 ml vs.451 ml), shorter hospital stay (3.4 days vs. 5.2 days), and quicker return to normal activity (3.6 weeks vs.8.1 weeks), but disadvantages for the laparoscopic operation were longer operating time (5.5 h vs. 2.8 h) and greater costs ($15,816 vs. $13,672.45). Interestingly, 23% of patients in the LRN group had benign disease versus 9% for the ORN group perhaps indicating a willingness of both surgeon and patient to accept a minimally invasive solution to a renal mass of uncertain nature.

Other centers also described their initial experiences in similar terms and readily concluded that LRN should supplant ORN particularly in cases with small renal tumors which remained well within the technical capabilities of the early laparoscopic surgeons [24, 25]. Many of the initial laparoscopic studies described renal cortical tumors in a historical context as a single tumor type (renal cell carcinoma) with a single metastatic potential and did not utilize the 1997

Heidelberg classification of renal tumors [2], did not discuss the uncertainties of preoperative radiological diagnosis, and did not discuss the deleterious impact of RN (by whatever means) on renal function. Often patients who underwent LRN and were found to have benign conditions were not included in the outcomes analysis. These articles argued strongly that LRN should be the new "gold standard" for all small, T1 renal tumors.

A study comparing open PN ($N = 82$) and LRN ($N = 35$) for small T1a renal tumors (<4 cm) discussed similar advantages of LRN described in other papers but noted a deleterious impact on renal function in the patients undergoing LRN [26]. In this study too, 20% of the patients in each treatment group had lesions that were not renal cell carcinoma. The question beginning to face the urology community was this; was the price of a future of renal insufficiency for a speedy recovery, lesser surgical incisions, and faster return to normal activities after LRN potentially too great?

Evidence for intra-institutional differences in the treatment of small renal masses since the availability of laparoscopy was reported in a series of 194 patients Cornell Medical Center. Of the operations performed, 63 (33%, mean tumor size 3.6 cm) were open partial nephrectomies, 51 (26%, mean tumor size 7.6 cm) were ORN, and 80 (41%, mean tumor size 4.6 cm) were LRN. When analyzed over time, in the latter half of 2000, 89% of the LRN were performed on tumors of 4 cm or less. In 2002, the number of LRN performed for tumors 4 cm or less had decreased to 42%. The experience with OPN during the same time frame was more consistent; 30% for tumors of 4 cm or greater from 1997 to 2000 and 26% from 2000 to 2002. For OPN tumors of 4 cm or less, 70% from the years 1997–2000 and 73% from 2000 to 2002 were performed. During the same period, the number of ORN performed for tumors of 4 cm or less continued to decrease to 2.9% in 2001 and 0% in 2002 [28]. A recent study demonstrated the negative impact of LRN vs. LPN on renal function. The investigators compared 93 patients undergoing an LPN to 171 patients undergoing an LRN for a unilateral, sporadic renal tumor with a normal contra lateral kidney and a serum creatinine <1.5 mg/dl. Tumors treated by LPN were smaller than LRN (2.4 cm vs. 5.4 cm), whereas age, BMI, serum creatinine, gender, and tumor location were similar between the two groups. The mean 6-month serum creatinine was greater in the LRN group vs. the LPN group (1.4 mg/dl vs. 1.0 mg/dl) and 36% of the LRN developed renal insufficiency (defined as serum creatinine >1.5 mg/dl) vs. 0% of the patients undergoing LPN [29].

Considerable effort was spent in the urology literature introducing and evaluating laparoscopic techniques for RN and comparing these approaches to historical surgical approaches (i.e., thoracoabdominal, chevron, or rib resecting flank incisions from the 1960s and 1970s) but not to the recently described min-flank surgical incisions which do not require rib resection and can be widely adopted and practiced without elaborate laparoscopic training [19]. Not discussed in the laparoscopic literature was the role of adrenalectomy and regional node dissections or issues related to training or learning curves. Laparoscopic studies focused on comparing oncological outcomes to open RN (no apparent differences), length of stay (LOS) in the hospital, analgesic requirements, time to return to work and normal activities (better than open RN), and complications. At the same time, improvements in perioperative care and the use of clinical pathways were reducing LOS for all urological procedures, including open and laparoscopic kidney surgery. Other reports detailing technical concerns such as surgical approach (transperitoneal vs. retroperitoneal vs. hand assisted) [30], intact tumor extraction vs. morcellation [31], the impact of prior operations [32], and concerns for LRN in obese and comorbidly ill patients were published [33]. It would appear that morcellation procedures are rarely done today due to loss of pathological clarity and concerns for intra-abdominal contamination during the morcellation process. Descriptions of laparoscopic extraction incisions would indicate that they did not adversely affect LOS and patient recovery. These extraction incisions were in the range of 7 cm, not much smaller than the described miniflank incisions (8–10 cm), raising the question, as in other laparoscopic procedures such as cholecystectomy, whether patient expectations play a significant role in many of the laparoscopic outcomes. Surgeons have also used robotic-assisted techniques to perform RN, and the recent literature has compared outcomes to classical laparoscopic techniques with similar perioperative outcomes such as EBL and complications but not surprisingly, at the front end of any new approach, operating time and costs were significantly greater in the robotic-assisted cases [34].

Complications of Radical Nephrectomy

In a review of 688 RN from 1995 to 2002, 112 patients (16%) experienced a perioperative complication [35]. Complications were graded using a five-tiered scale based on the severity of impact or the intensity of treatment required to address the complication. There were 21 (3%) complications that were directly attributed to the procedure (*procedure related*) including three patients with acute renal failure, one patient with a retroperitoneal hemorrhage, seven patients with an adjacent organ injury, four patients with a bowel obstruction, and six patients with a pneumothorax. Four patients required surgical re-exploration, three for decompression of bowel obstruction, and one for delayed splenic rupture (grade 4, $N = 3$). There were three postoperative deaths (grade 5), two due to myocardial infarction, and one due to pulmonary embolism. The remainder of the complications was grade 1–3 and was managed by oral medication or bedside care (grade 1, $N = 78$), intravenous therapy or thoracostomy tube (grade 2, $N = 43$), or intubation, interventional radiology, endoscopy, or reoperation (grade 3, $N = 11$). The grading scale employed correlated with mean hospital LOS as follows: no complications, 5.2 days; grade 1 complications, 6.8 days; grade 2 complications, 7.4 days; and grades 3–5 complications, 9.3 days. Grading complications provide an effective means of describing the severity of complications although its current use in the literature is limited.

Complications unique to LRN in particular and laparoscopy in general have been reported from individual centers and are more likely to occur earlier in a center's experience (initial 50 cases). In one series, when the initial 50 LRN cases are compared to the subsequent 50 cases, surgical time decreased from 2.9 to 2.7 h while the mean tumor size increased from 4.8 to 5.4 cm. Major complications were 14%, minor complications were 11%, and two patients required open conversion in one series [27]. Intra-operative events occur in approximately 4% of cases and include adjacent organ injury (spleen, bowel), vascular stapler malfunction with open conversion occurring in approximately 1–2% of cases [36–41]. Minimally invasive surgical (MIS) training has gradually been integrated into more residency training programs, and, despite this, a stable complication rate over the last 5 years in centers with a major commitment to MIS has been observed which is attributed by some to the passage of more relatively inexperienced surgeons through the learning curve [23].

Radical Nephrectomy: Adverse Renal Medical Impact

A historical misconception exists that RN can cause a permanent rise in serum creatinine due to the sacrifice of normal renal parenchyma not involved by tumor but will not cause serious long-term side effects as long as the patient has a normal contralateral kidney. The renal transplant literature is cited as the clinical evidence to support this view since patients undergoing donor nephrectomy have not been reported to have higher rates of kidney failure requiring dialysis or death [42]. However, distinct differences between kidney donors and kidney tumor patients exist. Donors tend to be carefully screened for medical comorbidities and are generally young (age 45 or less) [43, 44]. In contrast, renal tumor patients are not screened, are older (mean age 61 years), and many have significant comorbidities affecting baseline kidney function including metabolic syndrome, hypertension, coronary artery disease, obesity, vascular disease, and diabetes. In addition, as patients age, particularly beyond 60 years, nephrons atrophy and glomerular filtration rate progressively decreases [45]. A study of 110 nephrectomy specimens in which the non-tumor-bearing kidney was examined demonstrated extensive and unsuspected underlying renal disease including vascular sclerosis, diabetic nephropathy, glomerular hypertrophy, mesangial expansion, and diffuse glomerulosclerosis [46]. Only 10% of patients had completely normal renal tissue adjacent to the tumor.

Evidence that RN could cause a significant rise in the serum creatinine when compared to PN in patients with renal cortical tumors of 4 cm or less was published by investigators from Mayo Clinic and MSKCC in 2000 and 2002, respectively. RN patients were more likely to have elevated serum creatinine levels to >2.0 ng/ml and proteinuria (Mayo Study) [47], a persistent finding even when study patients were carefully matched for associated risk factors (MSKCC study) including diabetes, smoking history, preoperative serum creatinine, and ASA score [48]. In both studies, oncological outcomes were highly favorable (>90% survival rates) whether PN or RN was done.

CKD, defined as an estimated glomerular filtration rate (eGFR) of less than 60 min/min/1.73 m^2, is increasingly viewed as a major public health problem in the USA and since 2003 is considered an independent cardiovascular risk factor [49–53]. An estimated 19 million adults in the USA have CKD, and by the year 2030, two million will be in need of chronic dialysis or renal transplantation [54]. Traditional risk factors for CKD include age greater than 60, hypertension, diabetes, cardiovascular disease, and family history of renal disease, factors also common in the population of patients that develop renal cortical tumors. A study involving 1,120,295 patients demonstrated a direct correlation between CKD and rates of hospitalization, cardiovascular events, and death, which occurred before overt renal failure requiring dialysis or renal transplantation [55]. As kidney function deteriorated, the percentage of patients with two associated cardiovascular risk factors increased from 34.7% (stages 1 and 2 CKD) to 83.6% (for stage 3) to 100% for stages 4 and 5 subjects. Patients with CKD are more likely to require medical interventions to treat cardiovascular disease than those with normal renal function. The low prevalence of patients with stage 4 or 5 CKD is attributable to their 5-year survival rates of only 30% [56].

A concern that the overzealous use of RN, particularly in patients with small renal masses and common comorbidities that can affect renal function, could be causing or worsening preexisting CKD became a focus of intense research. MSKCC investigators used a widely available formula, the Modification in Diet and Renal Disease (MDRD) equation [57] (http://www.nephron.com/MDRD_GFR.cgi), to estimate the glomerular filtration rate (eGFR) in a retrospective cohort study of 662 patients with a normal serum creatinine and two healthy kidneys that underwent either elective PN or RN for an RCT 4 cm or less in diameter. To their surprise, 171 patients (26%) had preexisting CKD (GFR <60) prior to operation. Data were analyzed using two threshold definitions of CKD, a GFR<60 ml/min/1.73 m^2 or a GFR<45 ml/min/1.73 m^2. After surgery, the 3-year probability of freedom from new onset of GFR<60 was 80% after PN but only 35% after RN. Corresponding values for 3-year probability of freedom from a GFR<45, a more severe level of CKD, was 95% for PN and 64% for RN. Multivariable analysis indicated that RN was an independent risk factor for the development of new onset CKD (Fig. 7.3) [58]. Mayo Clinic investigators identified 648 patients from 1989 to 2003 treated with RN or PN for a solitary renal tumor less than or equal to 4 cm with a normal contralateral kidney. In 327 patients younger than 65, it was found that RN was significantly associated with an increased risk of death which persisted after adjusting for year of surgery, diabetes, Charlson–Romano index, and tumor histology [59]. Using the surveillance, epidemiology and end results (SEER) cancer registry data linked with Medicare claims, MSKCC investigators studied 2,991 patients older than 65 years for resected renal tumors of 4 cm or less from 1995 to 2002. A total of 254 patients (81%) underwent RN and 556 patients underwent PN. During a median follow-up of 4 years, 609 patients experienced a cardiovascular event and

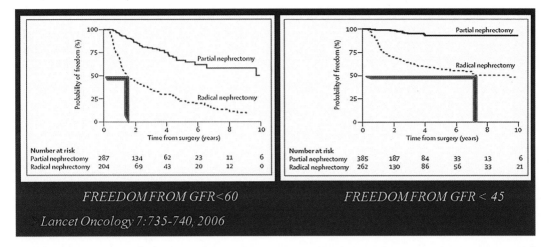

Fig. 7.3 Impact of radical vs. partial nephrectomy on renal function after management of T1a renal tumors. Radical nephrectomy is associated with a 3-year probability of freedom from new onset of GFR <60 ml/min/1.73 m² of only 35% (vs. 80% after PN) and a 3-year probability of freedom from a GFR <45 ml/min/1.73 m², a more severe level of CKD, of 64% (vs. 95% for PN) [58]

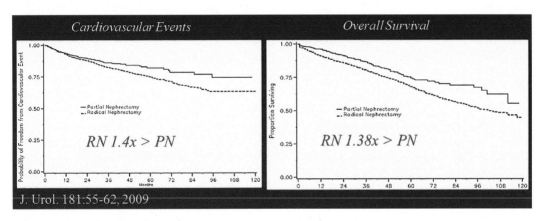

Fig. 7.4 Data from the SEER linked to Medicare database indicates that radical nephrectomy is associated with a 1.38 times increased risk of overall mortality and a 1.4 times greater number of cardiovascular events when compared to partial nephrectomy [60]

892 patients died. After adjusting for preoperative demographic and comorbidity variables, RN was associated with a 1.38 times increased risk of overall mortality and a 1.4 times greater number of cardiovascular events (Fig. 7.4) [60]. Tan and colleagues recently confirmed these findings in an updated report which utilized the same SEER linked with Medicare data between 1992 and 2007 in 7,138 patients of whom 1,925 (27%) patients underwent PN and 5,213 (73%) underwent RN for T1a renal tumors. In this study, patients undergoing PN had a significantly decreased risk of all cause mortality compared to those undergoing RN (HR 0.54), whereas no significant difference was noted in kidney cancer-specific survival [61]. A recent pooled analysis of 51 studies involving 31,728 patients from the world's literature was published by Kim and colleagues. The authors reported that PN was associated with a 19% risk reduction in all cause mortality, a 29% risk reduction in cancer-specific mortality, and a 61% risk reduction in severe CKD. Despite these findings, the authors pointed out that the data obtained were observational and subject to selection biases and

statistical heterogeneity [62]. Similar results were reported in patients undergoing laparoscopic RN and PN [63].

Confusing matters to some extent was a recently published randomized clinical trial from Europe comparing PN (N=268) to RN (N=273) for tumors of 5 cm or less (T1a, T1b) operated upon from 1992 to 2003. After a median follow-up of 9.3 years, oncologic events were uncommon with only 12 of 117 deaths due to RCC (8 in the PN group, 4 in the RN group). Tumor progression was also uncommon (12 in the PN group, 9 in the RN group). In this study the PN patients did not experience better overall survival (76% vs. 81% in the RN group). The most common cause of death was cardiovascular, but again there was no advantage for PN (25 cardiovascular deaths in the PN group vs. 20 in the RN group). This study had significant limitations, including accrual difficulties leading to premature closure, inclusion of some tumors >4 cm, the fact that some patients (10.2%) switched treatment groups after randomization, the fact that the trial was conducted at many centers and occurred during a treatment era when elective PN was not common, and the oncological efficacy was questioned by many. Despite these factors, the study was randomized and raises the possibility that within the contemporary pool of patients undergoing PN or RN for T1 renal tumors, other preexisting medical factors, including those that could adversely affect renal function such as diabetes and hypertension, could be to some extent responsible for the apparent advantage to PN in the more vulnerable patient, whereas patients with excellent baseline renal function my not suffer the same ill consequence of RN despite a reduced eGFR. Also unknown is to what degree the solitary healthy kidney can recover and compensate follow RN. Further investigation to clarify this important issue is ongoing [64]. The effect of these reports has made urologists increasingly aware that preexisting CKD can be significantly worsened by the liberal use of RN for the treatment of the small renal mass [65]. Short-term end points, including length of hospital stay, analgesic requirements, and cosmetic elements viewed by many as the reason to elect laparoscopic RN

over the more challenging PN, must now be tempered by these new concerns regarding CKD and overall survival. The most recent AUA guidelines for the management of the small renal tumor emphasize these points and strongly support the use of PN whenever technically feasible [66].

Radical Nephrectomy Is Overutilized

Despite the above well-described oncological and medical arguments in the contemporary literature supporting PN as an ideal treatment for such small renal masses, the urological oncology community continues to use RN as the predominant treatment of the T1a renal mass. A cross-sectional view of clinical practice using the Nationwide Inpatient Sample revealed that only 7.5% of kidney tumor operations in the USA from 1988 to 2002 were PN [67]. Using the SEER database, investigators from the University of Michigan reported from 2001, only 20% of all renal cortical tumors between 2 and 4 cm were treated by PN [68] and using the SEER database linked with Medicare claims, Huang and colleagues from MSKCC reported a utilization rate of only 19% for T1a tumors (4 cm or less) [58]. Interestingly and for uncertain reasons, women and elderly patients are more likely to be treated with RN [69]. Many urologists believe that a "quick" RN in an elderly patient would expose the patient to fewer postoperative complications than would a PN. However, MSKCC investigators evaluated age and type of procedure performed in 1,712 patients with kidney tumors found the interactive term was not significant indicating a lack of statistical evidence that the risk of complications associated with PN increased with advancing age. Furthermore, no evidence was reported linking age with estimated blood loss or operative time. Given the advantages of renal functional preservation, the authors concluded that elderly patients should be perfectly eligible for PN [70].

Although the urology literature has many great articles written concerning the use of laparoscopic techniques to resect kidney tumors, the penetrence of laparoscopic RN according to the

National Inpatient Sample from 1991 to 2003 was only 4.6% with a peak incidence of 16% in 2003. These data indicate that the bulk of "kidney wasting operations" are being done by traditional open surgical approaches [71]. In England, a similar under-utilization of PN was reported in 2002 with only 108 (4%) PN out of 2,671 nephrectomies performed [72]. Investigators at MSKCC tracked nephrectomy use in 1,533 patients between 2000 and 2007 excluding patients with bilateral tumors and tumors in a solitary kidney and including only patients with an eGFR of greater than 45 ml/min/1.73 m². Overall 854 (56%) patients underwent PN and 679 (44%) underwent RN. In the 820 patients with a renal tumor of 4 cm or less, the frequency of PN increased from 69% in 2000 to 89% in 2007. In the 365 patients with a renal tumor from 4 to 7 cm, the frequency of PN increased from 20% in 2000 to 60% in 2007. Despite a commitment to kidney sparing operations during this time frame by the MSKCC group, multivariate analysis indicated that PN was a significantly favored approach for males, younger patients, smaller tumors, and open surgeons [73].

Conclusions

Modern imaging capabilities has created a renal tumor stage and size migration with approximately 70% of patients today detected incidentally with a median tumor size of 4 cm or less. In addition, our current understanding indicates that renal cortical tumors are a family of neoplasms with distinct histopathological and cytogenetic features and variable metastatic potential. The conventional clear cell tumor has a malignant potential and accounts for only 54% of the total renal cortical tumors but 90% of those that metastasize. RN nephrectomy, whether performed by open or MIS technique, plays an important role in the management of massive renal tumors that have replaced the normal renal parenchyma, invade the renal vein, and have associated regional lymphadenopathy or metastatic disease. For patients with smaller tumors amenable to PN, RN should not be performed since it is associated with the causation or worsening of preexisting CKD which may cause an increased likelihood of cardiovascular morbidity and mortality. Despite a wealth of evidence supporting the more restricted indications for RN, strong evidence exists that it remains overutilized in the USA. Widespread education and training in kidney preserving surgical strategies is essential going forward.

References

1. Jemal A, Siegel R, Xu J, Ward E. Cancer statistics 2010. CA Cancer J Clin. 2010;60(5):277–300.
2. Linehan WM, Walther MM, Zbar B. The genetic basis of cancer of the kidney. J Urol. 2003;170:2163–72.
3. Kattan MW, Reuter VE, Motzer RJ, Russo P. A postoperative prognostic nomogram for renal cell carcinoma. J Urol. 2001;166:63.
4. Russo P. Renal cell carcinoma: presentation, staging, and surgical treatment. Semin Oncol. 2000;27:160–76.
5. Beare JB, McDonald JR. Involvement of renal capsule in surgically removed hypernephroma: gross and histopathological study. J Urol. 1949;61:857–61.
6. Mortensen H. Transthoracic nephrectomy. J Urol. 1948;60:855.
7. Robson CJ. Radical nephrectomy for renal cell carcinoma. J Urol. 1963;89:37.
8. Robson CJ, Churchill BM, Andersen W. The results of radical nephrectomy for renal cell carcinoma. J Urol. 1969;101:297.
9. Skinner DG, Colvin RB, Vermillion CD, Pfister RC, Leadbetter WF. Diagnosis and management of renal cell carcinoma: a clinical and pathological study of 309 cases. Cancer. 1971;28:1165–77.
10. Patel NP, Lavengood RW. Renal cell carcinoma: natural history and results of treatment. J Urol. 1978;119:722.
11. Sagalowsky AI, Kadesky KT, Ewalt DM, Kennedy TJ. Factors influencing adrenal metastases in renal cell carcinoma. J Urol. 1994;151:1181–4.
12. Herrlinger JA, Schrott KM, Schott G, et al. What are the benefits of extended dissection of the regional lymph nodes in the therapy of renal cell carcinoma? J Urol. 1991;146:1224.
13. Ditonno P, Traficante A, Battaglia M, et al. Role of lymphadenectomy in renal cell carcinoma. Prog Clin Biol Res. 1992;378:169.
14. Robson CJ. Results of radical thoraco-abdominal nephrectomy in the treatment of renal cell carcinoma. Prog Clin Biol Res. 1982;100:481–8.
15. Russo P. Open radical nephrectomy for localized renal cell carcinoma. In: Vogelzang NJ, editor. Genitourinary oncology. 3rd ed. Philadelphia: Lippincott Williams and Wilkins; 2006. p. 725–31.
16. Flanigan RC, Salmon SE, Blumenstein BA, et al. Nephrectomy followed by interferon alfa-2b compared

with interferon alfa-2b alone for metastatic renal-cell cancer. NEJM. 2001;23:1655–9.

17. Russo P, O'Brien MF. Surgical intervention in patients with metastatic renal cancer: metastasectomy and cytoreductive nephrectomy. Urol Clin North Am. 2008;35:679–86.

18. Russo P. Multi-modal treatment for metastatic renal cancer – the role of surgery. World J Urol. 2010;28: 295–301.

19. Diblasio CJ, Snyder ME, Russo P. Mini flank supra-eleventh incision for open partial or radical nephrectomy. BJU Int. 2006;97(1):149–56.

20. Vasselli JR, Yang JC, Linehan WM, White DE, Rosenberg SA, Walther MM. Lack of retroperitoneal lymphadenopathy predicts survival of patients with metastatic renal cell carcinoma. J Urol. 2001;166:68.

21. Sorbellini M, Kattan MW, Snyder ME, et al. A post-operative prognostic nomogram predicting recurrence for patients with conventional clear cell renal cell carcinoma. J Urol. 2005;173:48–51.

22. Clayman RV, Kavoussi LR, Soper NJ, et al. Laparoscopic nephrectomy: initial case report. J Urol. 1991;146:278.

23. Dunn MD, Portis AJ, Shalhav AL, et al. Laparoscopic versus open radical nephrectomy: 9-year experience. J Urol. 2000;164:1153–9.

24. Chan DY, Cadeddu JA, Jarrett TW, et al. Laparoscopic radical nephrectomy: cancer control for renal cell carcinoma. J Urol. 2001;166:2095–100.

25. Makhoul B, De La Taille A, Vordos D, et al. Laparoscopic radical nephrectomy for T1 renal cancer: the gold standard? A comparison of laparoscopic vs. open nephrectomy. BJU Int. 2004;93:67–70.

26. Matin S, Gill I, Worley S, Novick AC. Outcome of laparoscopic radical nephrectomy for sporadic 4 cm or less renal tumor with a normal contra lateral kidney. J Urol. 2002;168:1356–60.

27. Gill IS, Meraney AM, Schweizer DK, et al. Laparoscopic radical nephrectomy in 100 patients. Cancer. 2001;92:1843–55.

28. Scherr DS, Ng C, Munver R, Sosa ER, Vaughan ED, Del Pizzo J. Practice patterns among urologic surgeons treating localized renal cell carcinoma in the laparoscopic age: technology vs. oncology. Urology. 2003;62:1007–11.

29. Zorn KC, Gong EM, Orvieto MA, et al. Comparison of laparoscopic radical and partial nephrectomy: effects on long-term serum creatinine. Urology. 2007;69:1035–40.

30. Nadler RB, Loeb S, Clemens JQ, et al. A prospective study of laparoscopic radical nephrectomy for T1 tumors – is transperitoneal, retroperitoneal, or hand assisted the best approach? J Urol. 2006;4:1230–3.

31. Hernandez F, Rha KH, Pinto PA, et al. Laparoscopic nephrectomy: assessment of morcellation versus intact specimen extraction of postoperative status. J Urol. 2003;170:412–5.

32. Viterbo R, Greenberg RE, Al-Saleem T, et al. Prior abdominal surgery and radiation do not complicate the retroperitoneoscopic approach to the kidney or adrenal gland. J Urol. 2005;174:57–60.

33. Fugita OE, Chan DY, Roberts WW, et al. Laparoscopic radical nephrectomy in obese patients: outcomes and technical considerations. Urology. 2004;63:247–52.

34. Hemal AK, Kumar A. A prospective comparison of laparoscopic and robotic radical nephrectomy for T1-2N0M0 renal cell carcinoma. World J Urol. 2009;27:89–94.

35. Stephanson A, Hakimian A, Snyder ME, Russo P. Complications of radical and partial nephrectomy in a large contemporary cohort. J Urol. 2004;171:130–4.

36. Soulie M, Seguin P, Richeux L, et al. Urological complications of laparoscopic surgery: experience with 350 procedure at a single center. J Urol. 2000; 165:1960.

37. Vallancien G, Cathelineau X, Baumert H, et al. Complications of transperitoneal laparoscopic surgery in urology. Review of 1311 procedures at a single center. J Urol. 2002;168:23–6.

38. Wile AH, Roigas J, Degor S, et al. Laparoscopic radical nephrectomy: techniques, results, and oncological outcome in 125 consecutive cases. Eur Urol. 2004; 45:483–8.

39. Meraney AM, Samee AA, Gill IS. Vascular and bowel complications during retroperitoneal laparoscopic surgery. J Urol. 2002;168:1941–4.

40. Kim FJ, Rha KH, Hernandez F, Jarrett TW, Pinto P, Kavoussi L. Laparoscopic radical versus partial nephrectomy: assessment of complications. J Urol. 2003; 170:408–11.

41. Simon SD, Castle EP, Ferrigni RG, et al. Complications of laparoscopic nephrectomy: the Mayo Clinic experience. J Urol. 2004;171:1447–50.

42. Segev DL, Muzaale AD, Caffo BS, et al. Perioperative mortality and long-term survival following live kidney donation. JAMA. 2010;503:959–66.

43. Fehrman-Ekholm I, Duner F, Brink B, et al. No evidence of loss of kidney function in living kidney donors from cross sectional follow up. Transplantation. 2001;72:444–9.

44. Goldfarb DA, Matin SF, Braun WE, et al. Renal outcome 25 years after donor nephrectomy. J Urol. 2001;166:2043.

45. Kaplan C, Pasternack B, Shah H, et al. Age-related incidence of sclerotic glomeruli in human kidneys. Am J Pathol. 1975;80:227.

46. Bijol V, Mendez GP, Hurwitz S, Rennke HG, Nosé V. Evaluation of the nonneoplastic pathology in tumor nephrectomy specimens. Am J Surg Pathol. 2006; 30:575.

47. Lau WK, Blute ML, Weaver AL, et al. Matched comparison of radical nephrectomy vs. nephron-sparing surgery in patients with unilateral renal cell carcinoma and a normal contra lateral kidney. Mayo Clin Proc. 2000;75:1236–42.

48. McKiernan J, Simmons R, Katz J, Russo P. Natural history of chronic renal insufficiency after partial and radical nephrectomy. Urology. 2002;59:816–20.

49. Sarnak M, Levey AS, Schoolwerth AC, et al. Kidney disease as a risk factor for the development of cardiovascular disease: a statement from the American Heart Association Council on kidney in cardiovascular disease. High blood pressure research, clinical cardiology, and epidemiology and prevention. Circulation. 2003;108:2154–69.

50. Chobanian AV, Bakris GL, Black HR, et al. The seventh report of the Joint National Committee on TN prevention, detection, evaluation, and treatment of high blood pressure: the JNC 7 report. JAMA. 2003;289:2560–72.

51. Kidney Disease Outcome Quality Imitative. K/DOQI clinical guideline for chronic kidney disease evaluation, classification, stratification. Am J Kidney Dis. 2002;39 Suppl 2:51:5246.

52. Ritz E, McClellan WW. Overview: increased cardiovascular risk in patients with minor renal dysfunction: an emerging issue with far-reaching consequences. J Am Soc Nephrol. 2004;15:513–6.

53. Shlipak MG, Fried LF, Cushman M, et al. Cardiovascular mortality risk in chronic kidney disease. JAMA. 2005;293:1737–45.

54. Coresh J, Selvin E, Stevens LA, et al. Prevalence of chronic kidney disease in the United States. JAMA. 2007;298:2038–47.

55. Go AS, Chertow GM, Fan D, et al. Chronic kidney disease and the risks of death, cardiovascular events, and hospitalization. N Engl J Med. 2004;35:1296–305.

56. Foley RN, Wang C, Collins AJ. Cardiovascular risk factor profiles and kidney function stage in the US general population: the NHANES 3 study. Mayo Clin Proc. 2005;80:1270–7.

57. Stevens LA, Coresh J, Green T, Levey AS. Assessing kidney function – measured and estimated glomerular filtration rate. N Engl J Med. 2006;354:2473–83.

58. Huang WC, Levey AS, Serio AM, et al. Chronic kidney disease after nephrectomy in patients with renal cortical tumors: a retrospective cohort study. Lancet Oncol. 2006;7:735–40.

59. Thompson HR, Boorjian SA, Lohse CM, et al. Radical nephrectomy for pT1a renal masses may be associated with decreased overall survival compared to partial nephrectomy. J Urol. 2008;179:468–73.

60. Huang WC, Elkin EB, Levey AS, Jang TL, Russo P. Partial nephrectomy versus radical nephrectomy in patients with small renal tumors – is there a difference in mortality and cardiovascular outcomes. J Urol. 2009;181:55–62.

61. Tan HJ, Norton EC, Ye Z, Hafez K, Gore JL, Miller DC. Long-term survival following partial vs radical nephrectomy among older patients with early-stage kidney cancer. JAMA. 2012;207:1629–35.

62. Kim SP, Thompson H, Boorjian SA, et al. Comparative effectiveness for survival and renal function of partial and radical nephrectomy for localized renal tumors: a systematic review and meta-analysis. J Urol. 2012;188:51–7.

63. Foyil KV, Ames CD, Ferguson GG, et al. Long-term changes in creatinine clearance after laparoscopic renal surgery. J Am Coll Surg. 2008;206:511–5.

64. Van Poppel H, Da Pozzo L, Albrecht W, et al. A prospective, randomized EORTC intergroup phase 3 study comparing the oncologic outcome of elective nephron-sparing surgery and radical nephrectomy for low-stage renal cell carcinoma. Eur Urol. 2011;59:543–52.

65. Lane BR, Poggio ED, Herts BR, Novick AC, Campbell SC. Renal function assessment in the era of chronic kidney disease: renewed emphasis on renal function centered patient care. J Urol. 2009;182:436–44.

66. Campbell SC, Novick AC, Belldegrun A, et al. Guideline for management of the clinical T1 renal mass. J Urol. 2009;182:1271–9.

67. Hollenback BK, Tash DA, Miller DC, et al. National utilization trends of partial nephrectomy for renal cell carcinoma: a case of underutilization? Urology. 2006;67:254–9.

68. Miller DC, Hollingsworth JM, Hafez KS, et al. Partial nephrectomy for small renal masses. An emerging quality of care concern? J Urol. 2006;175:853–7.

69. Dulabon LM, Lowrance WT, Russo P, Huang WC. Trends in renal tumor surgery delivery within the United States. Cancer. 2010;116:2316–21.

70. Lowrance WT, Yee DS, Savage C, et al. Complications after radical and partial nephrectomy as a function of age. J Urol. 2010;183:1725–30.

71. Miller DC, Taub DA, Dunn RL, Wei JT, Hollenbeck BK. Laparoscopy for renal cell carcinoma: diffusion versus regionalization? J Urol. 2006;176:1102–6.

72. Nuttail M, Cathcart P, van der Meulen J, et al. A description of radical nephrectomy practice and outcomes in England: 1995–2002. BJU Int. 2005;96:58–61.

73. Thompson HR, Kaag M, Vickers A, et al. Contemporary use of partial nephrectomy at a tertiary care center in the United States. J Urol. 2009;181:993–7.

Nephron-Sparing Surgery for Renal Cancer

8

Alon Z. Weizer, Jeffery S. Montgomery, and Khaled S. Hafez

History of Nephron-Sparing Surgery

Renal cell carcinoma (RCC) is a relatively rare tumor that accounts for approximately 3% of adult malignancies. In 2010 approximately 58,240 new cases developed, with close to 13,000 patients dying of the disease [1]. Over the last century the incidence and mortality of RCC has increased for both clinical T1 and T2 disease [2]. Although radical surgery remains the mainstay of treatment for locally advanced disease, recent guidelines encourage the use of nephron-sparing approaches for T1 disease whenever feasible [3].

The first partial nephrectomy (PN) was performed in 1884 by Wells for removal of a perirenal fibrolipoma [4]. In 1887, Czerny was the first to use PN for excision of a renal neoplasm when he successfully removed an angiosarcoma from the upper third of the right kidney of a gardener [5]. At this time, however, PN was associated with significant complications, including renal bleeding, urinary fistula, and death as compared with total nephrectomy, which had a lower operative morbidity and satisfactory long-term results. In 1950, Vermooten published his techniques and indications for PN and suggested that this procedure could be performed, even in the presence of a normal contralateral kidney. Vermooten suggested that peripheral encapsulated renal neoplasms could be excised locally while leaving a margin of normal parenchyma around the tumor [6]. In the early 1960s, however, Robson et al., established radical nephrectomy (RN) as the treatment of choice for localized RCC, reporting a 66% and 64% overall survival for stage I and II tumors, respectively [7]. These results represented a significant improvement in survival rates when compared with patients treated with simple nephrectomy, and this therapy became the treatment of choice for localized RCC.

Over the last two decades, advances in renal imaging, renal and vascular surgery (such as improved methods for prevention of ischemic renal damage), and the significant increase in the rate of incidentally discovered small renal masses have all driven the renewed enthusiasm for nephron-sparing surgery (NSS). The fact that NSS can be performed safely with low morbidity, good preservation of renal function and sound oncologic outcomes is not debated, however, recent data suggests that NSS continues to be underutilized [8, 9]. This is largely driven by surgeon practice pattern; competing approaches, such as laparoscopic RN, are often favored because of decreased morbidity and lower technical complexity. This chapter outlines the indications, techniques, and outcomes that support NSS as the treatment of choice for localized renal masses.

A.Z. Weizer, MD, MS • J.S. Montgomery, MD, MHSA • K.S. Hafez, MD (✉)
Division of Urologic Oncology,
Department of Urology, University of Michigan,
3875 Taubman Center SPC 5330, 1500 East Medical Center Drive, Ann Arbor, MI, 48109, USA
e-mail: khafez@umich.edu

S.C. Campbell and B.I. Rini (eds.), *Renal Cell Carcinoma: Clinical Management*, Current Clinical Urology,
DOI 10.1007/978-1-62703-062-5_8, © Springer Science+Business Media New York 2013

Indications for Nephron-Sparing Surgery

NSS is the preferred treatment for localized renal masses, particularly in patients at risk of renal dysfunction. Potential indications for this approach include:

(a) Bilateral synchronous renal masses
(b) Mass in an anatomically or functionally solitary kidney
(c) Unilateral mass with a functioning contralateral kidney and any concomitant condition with the potential to adversely impact renal function
(d) Renal masses in familial and hereditary disease
(e) Unilateral mass <7 cm with a normal contralateral kidney
(f) Advanced renal cancer

Bilateral Renal Masses

Early experience with PN was gained in patients with bilateral, synchronous RCC, where the need for preservation of at least a portion of one kidney was obvious [10]. Bilateral renal tumors are reported in 1–5% of patients [11]. In a study from Memorial Sloan-Kettering Cancer Center (MSKCC), investigators identified 46 patients with bilateral tumors (4%) of which 33 (72%) were synchronous and 13 (28%) were asynchronous. The second tumor in the asynchronous group occurred at a median time of 84.5 (28–240) months after diagnosis of the incident tumor. The histological concordance rate was 76% between tumors [12]. In these patients, it is crucial to preserve as much functioning renal tissue as possible. This entails performing bilateral partial nephrectomies whenever possible, usually as staged procedures beginning with the kidney that seems most amenable to PN. When a large tumor on one side precludes PN, the operative sequence is usually to perform the PN first, thereby obviating the need for temporary dialysis in the immediate postoperative period if acute renal injury occurs. Occasionally a partial rather than RN on the second side is necessary to avoid chronic

kidney disease (CKD) when the initial procedure results in a renal remnant of borderline size or function.

Unilateral Renal Mass with Impaired or Absent Contralateral Kidney or Concomitant Disease Processes that Can Adversely Affect Renal Function

Renal tumors in a functionally or anatomically solitary kidney also necessitate a nephron-sparing approach. In these circumstances, it is crucial to counsel patients that temporary or permanent renal replacement therapy may be necessary postoperatively. Generally, a renal remnant with the function of at least 20% is necessary to avoid permanent renal failure. A report from the Cleveland Clinic that represents the largest published experience of renal tumors in solitary kidneys showed that in 323/400 total patients (81%) the absent kidney had been surgically removed and 77 (19%) had a congenitally solitary kidney. In 46% of these patients, evidence of renal insufficiency was present at baseline. Renal hilar clamping was used in 96% of the cases, with a mean tumor size of 4.18 cm. Interestingly, 36% of these patients had multifocal disease and 92% of the tumors were malignant. Postoperatively, 95% had satisfactory long-term renal function [13]. Authors from the same institution compared outcomes of laparoscopic ($n=30$) and open PN ($n=169$) in solitary kidneys and reported that the laparoscopic cases required longer ischemia times, a greater need for postoperative dialysis, and experienced twice the complication rate than the open approach. They concluded that open PN is safer in these patients at high risk of CKD [14].

The presence of a unilateral renal tumor with a functionally impaired contralateral kidney is another common indication for NSS. Contralateral functional impairment may be due to a variety of systemic or urologic diseases, including diabetes mellitus, nephrosclerosis, renal artery stenosis, hydronephrosis, chronic pyelonephritis, and vesicoureteral reflux. The clinical and operative considerations in these patients are similar to those with true solitary kidneys.

Unrecognized medical renal disease is another challenge in renal cancer patients. A study from the Harvard Medical School examined the non-tumor-bearing kidney of patients undergoing surgery for renal tumors, and reported that only 10% of patients had completely normal tissue adjacent to the tumor, and 90% were found to have vascular sclerotic changes, diabetic nephropathy, glomerular hypertrophy, and diffuse glomerulosclerosis [15]. In these patients, it is crucial to evaluate pre-operative renal function not solely based on serum creatinine but also instead with the measurement of urine albumin and estimated glomerular filtration rate (GFR) using equations based on the level of serum creatinine, age, sex and race [16].

Another indication for NSS is in patients with unilateral tumors and a normally functioning contralateral kidney but with a condition that might threaten future renal function. This includes renal calculi, diabetes mellitus, hypertension, or renal artery disease. The decision to perform a partial rather than an RN in these patients depends on the feasibility of partial resection. However, current guidelines indicate that PN is the default approach whenever feasible.

Renal Masses in Familial/ Hereditary Disease

Multifocal and bilateral tumors are common in hereditary and familial tumor syndromes such as von Hippel–Lindau (VHL) disease, hereditary papillary renal cancer, and the Birt–Hogg–Dube syndrome, and can account for 3–5% of all renal cancers [17]. RCC occurs in approximately 45% of patients with VHL [18]. The rationale for a nephron-sparing approach in patients with this disease is based on a younger average age of presentation than sporadic RCC and the propensity for renal tumors in VHL to be multifocal, bilateral, and recurrent. However, because of the multifocal nature of renal tumors in VHL, these patients are at increased risk for developing local recurrences over the long term. In the era of advanced abdominal imaging and genetic screening, most patients are diagnosed with small, asymptomatic renal tumors. Intervention is generally recommended before an individual

tumor exceeds 3 cm in diameter, after which point there is a risk for developing metastatic disease [19].

Unilateral Renal Cell Carcinoma with Normal Contralateral Kidney

Refinements in imaging techniques have enhanced the detection of early stage, incidental renal masses and have contributed to an increasing role of NSS in patients with localized disease and a contralateral normal kidney [20, 21]. Extended experience has established that NSS can be performed safely with minimal morbidity, preservation of renal function, and long-term survival in patients with small, incidental renal masses [22]. Multiple reports have shown that PN results in survival rates equivalent to those achieved after RN for T1 disease [23, 24].

The more recent expansion of the indications for NSS includes patients with renal masses 4–7 cm in diameter in anatomically favorable locations. A recently published study which combined patients from the Mayo Clinic and MSKCC evaluated 1,159 patients with renal tumors 4–7 cm in size. There was no significant difference in survival between patients treated with RN or NSS. A more recent study from MSKCC reported on the use of NSS in tumors >7 cm in diameter with favorable outcomes. This study confirmed that tumor size should not restrict the use of NSS, but rather tumor location, careful case selection, and tumor biology are more critical factors [25]. In addition, the amount of remaining functional renal tissue should guide the use of NSS in patients with renal masses greater than 7 cm.

Advanced Renal Cell Carcinoma

The use of PN in the setting of advanced RCC has not been extensively addressed. Angermeier et al. reported on nine patients who underwent PN for RCC with venous involvement in a solitary functioning kidney. Complete tumor resection and preservation of renal function was achieved in all cases, although recurrence rates were significantly higher than for low-stage disease [26]. Currently, surgical resection after systemic therapy (e.g., mTOR and tyrosine kinase inhibitors) can be considered as part of a multimodal approach. Cleveland Clinic researchers reported on 19 patients treated with systemic targeted therapies (sunitinib, bevacizumab/interleukin-2) followed by surgical resection in cases of stable disease or a partial clinical response. In the subset of patients who subsequently underwent PN after tumor downsizing, no substantial complications were encountered despite the potential impact of these agents on wound healing and vascular integrity [27]. These clinical scenarios will be encountered more frequently as the use of systemic therapy in locally advanced disease expands.

Techniques of Nephron-Sparing Surgery for Renal Cell Carcinoma

Although RN is considered optimum curative therapy for patients with locally advanced RCC, PN is the treatment of choice for T1 carcinomas. In such patients, PN allows complete surgical excision of the primary tumor while preserving sufficient renal parenchyma to avoid future renal dysfunction. A variety of surgical techniques are available for performing PN in patients with RCC. All of these techniques require adherence to basic principles of early vascular control, avoidance of ischemic renal damage, complete tumor excision with negative margins, precise closure of the collecting system, careful hemostasis, and bolstering of the renal defect with adjacent fat, peritoneum, or hemostatic agents. At its origin, laparoscopic PN was developed to replicate the open surgical approach, so as a result these techniques share several similarities. We describe the common characteristics below.

Selection of Open Versus Minimally Invasive Nephron-Sparing Surgery

The first report of laparoscopic PN for malignancy was only 2 years after the original description of laparoscopic nephrectomy by Clayman [28, 29]. Widespread adoption of minimally invasive PN, though, has been hindered by competition from laparoscopic RN and ablative therapies as well as the increased technical expertise required for the often complex intracorporeal reconstruction necessary during laparoscopic PN [30]. Recent data suggests that robotic assistance may lower this barrier, making laparoscopic management of small renal masses more accessible to urologists and their patients [31]. However, a solid laparoscopic foundation is important to the adoption of robotic-assisted PN. Surgeons must determine which approach to PN in their hands will provide the best oncologic and functional outcomes for their patients based on the preoperative patient and tumor characteristics. Surgeons with experience performing both open and minimally invasive NSS can select the best approach for individual patients and tumors on a case-by-case basis. Surgeons with a greater comfort level with one approach over another must consider whether their skills match the needs of their patient.

Patient Characteristics

In our experience, minimally invasive NSS (e.g., laparoscopic or robotic PN) is the default approach for most patients. However, there are important factors to consider as possible contraindications for minimally invasive approaches:

- Prior open renal surgery such as open stone surgery, upper tract reconstructive procedures or prior open PN.
- Prior minimally invasive NSS or ablative procedures (laparoscopic or percutaneous).
- Inability to tolerate insufflation due to chronic obstructive pulmonary disease or other conditions.
- Limitations on access or instrumentation due to patient body habitus, although multiple reports describe safe and effective minimally invasive NSS in patients with morbid obesity who may benefit most by avoiding a flank incision [32].
- Prior extensive intra-abdominal surgery, although a retroperitoneal approach can be utilized in many circumstances as long as the retroperitoneal space can be developed safely.
- Patients with advanced CKD particularly those with complex tumors requiring prolonged renal ischemia time during resection.

Tumor Characteristics

The majority of patients with sporadic small renal masses <4 cm in diameter and select patients with tumors <7 cm should be considered for robotic-assisted or laparoscopic PN. In patients with solitary kidney (anatomically or functionally) and those with impaired renal function, the surgeon must determine whether a minimally invasive approach will expose the patient's kidney to undue additional ischemia time that would be minimized by the open surgical approach and use of cold ischemia. While a significant number of methods have been described to cool the kidney during minimally invasive NSS, none have been widely adopted due to the lack of obvious benefit or cumbersome application [33]. The patient may derive greater long-term benefit from an open PN, promoting the preservation of renal function instead of shorter incision length and short-term convalescence advantages. When minimally invasive NSS is considered for endophytic tumors, it is crucial that the surgeon has access to and is proficient in performing laparoscopic ultrasound.

At our institution where the majority of surgeons offer both minimally invasive and open NSS, we review all complex cases and offer a consensus opinion regarding proper approach. If the patient's initial surgeon does not offer a particular approach, the patient is referred to another surgeon in our group who is capable of offering the approach to the patient.

Selecting Approach to Laparoscopic and Robotic Assisted Partial Nephrectomy

The best approach to minimally invasive NSS depends on patient and tumor characteristics. We have previously published our approach algorithm and herein present a modification based on the flexibility of NSS using the robotic platform [34]. The patient characteristics that most affect surgical approach are prior abdominal surgery and body habitus. In patients with extensive previous intra-abdominal surgery, a retroperitoneal (RP) approach can be used if the tumor is posterior or anterior in the lower or interpolar region.

Upper pole tumors are challenging to access via an RP approach in our experience. An RP approach is contraindicated if the RP space has been violated by previous surgery, such as prior kidney surgery, some vascular procedures, and colectomy. A hand-assisted laparoscopic approach can be considered for patients with extensive intra-abdominal adhesions and tumors involving the upper pole. The hand port incision (usually 6–8 inches in length) can be used for initial lysis of adhesions until additional laparoscopic ports can be placed safely to then complete the remainder of the adhesiolysis laparoscopically. Alternatively, the surgeon can elect to perform the procedure via an open flank incision.

Body habitus can also limit minimally invasive NSS approaches. While there is no established body mass index (BMI) limit in choosing a transperitoneal or RP approach, it is crucial to assess the location and distribution of body fat preoperatively to determine the best approach. Review of the three-dimensional axial imaging is also important to determine the distribution of body fat. A significant amount of cutaneous and RP body fat can make a retroperitoneal laparoscopic approach difficult because of limitations of space and instrument mobility.

For most patients, the proper approach rests with the location of the tumor and its proximity to the renal hilum. Historically, we used a hand-assisted laparoscopic approach to manage upper pole tumors. Our current preference is to use a robotic-assisted approach to manage these tumors to avoid the small yet real risk of port site hernia associated with hand ports (3.5%) [35]. In addition, we also prefer to use a robotic-assisted approach for anterior and posterior hilar tumors because of the greater flexibility in dissecting and suturing with the robot. The remainder of the anterior and posterior kidney can be approached via either a robotic-assisted or laparoscopic approach, with posterior tumors accessed retroperitoneally.

Several recent publications have proposed more specific methods to describe the location and complexity of a renal tumor such as the R.E.N.A.L. Nephrometry Score, PADUA classification, and C-Index [36–38]. This can be used as another variable in the surgical approach selection equation. We currently utilize an algorithm to guide the decision to clamp the renal hilum and suture the renal defect after minimally invasive NSS based on tumor depth of penetration and proximity to the renal sinus. This technique has performed well when compared to R.E.N.A.L. Nephrometry Score in avoiding adverse perioperative outcomes [36, 39].

Patients referred for a renal mass have often already undergone cross-sectional imaging with CT or MRI. If the patient is diagnosed based on ultrasound or the renal anatomy is not adequately defined on the initial imaging, a renal mass protocol study should be obtained. To minimize blood loss and ischemic damage to adjacent parenchyma, knowledge of the number and location of renal vessels is crucial. There are important distinctions between the arterial and venous blood supply of the kidney that must be kept in mind when performing these operations. All segmental renal arteries are end-arteries with no collateral circulation; therefore, all branches supplying tumor-free parenchyma must be preserved to avoid devitalizing functioning renal tissue. In contrast, intrarenal venous branches communicate among the various renal segments. Ligation of a branch of the renal vein, therefore, will not result in segmental congestion because collateral veins will provide adequate drainage. Tumors in the renal hilum therefore can be accessed by ligating and dividing small, adjacent or overlying venous branches as needed. Major venous branches can then be mobilized completely and retracted freely to expose the tumor with no vascular compromise of uninvolved parenchyma.

In addition, given the low yet real risk of metastasis in patients with tumors <4 cm in diameter (3%) [40], additional preoperative staging studies needed include a chest radiograph, complete blood count, and comprehensive metabolic panel with estimation of GFR. The utility and need of nuclear medicine bone scan and other imaging, such as head CT, depends on the patient's symptoms or the finding of elevated serum alkaline phosphatase or calcium levels on initial laboratory evaluations.

The basic surgical principles of a PN include:

(a) Mobilization of the kidney with early vascular control
(b) Preservation of renal function by limiting hilar clamping
(c) Complete tumor excision with negative surgical margins
(d) Hemostasis
(e) Watertight closure of the collecting system
(f) Closure of the renal defect

The retroperitoneal approach avoids entry of the peritoneal cavity which limits morbidity should a postoperative hemorrhage or urine leak develop. In addition, postoperative recovery is often hastened as early return of bowel function is the norm. All approaches to NSS follow similar principles. The only difference between robotic-assisted, laparoscopic, and open surgery is the tools used to accomplish the same goals; the goals of the surgery are the same no matter the approach. The surgeon must pick the right set of tools in their hands to accomplish the procedure to the benefit of the patient.

Kidney Mobilization and Vascular Control

Open Approach

After the incision has been made, the retroperitoneal space is entered, the psoas muscle is exposed and the peritoneum is mobilized medially. The kidney is then mobilized outside of Gerota's fascia, first freeing the upper pole of the kidney, dissecting the medial upper pole from the adrenal gland. The lower pole is then mobilized, identifying the ureter with a vessel loop as needed. The gonadal vein can then be followed cephalad to the renal vein on the left side and inferior vena cava on the right side. Once the renal vein is isolated, further mobilization of the kidney posteriorly is often necessary to identify the renal artery. Alternatively, the renal artery can be identified by freeing the upper pole completely and lifting it laterally. Kidney mobilization should be sufficient to clamp the renal hilum if necessary, resect the renal mass with negative margins, and reconstruct the kidney (Fig. 8.1).

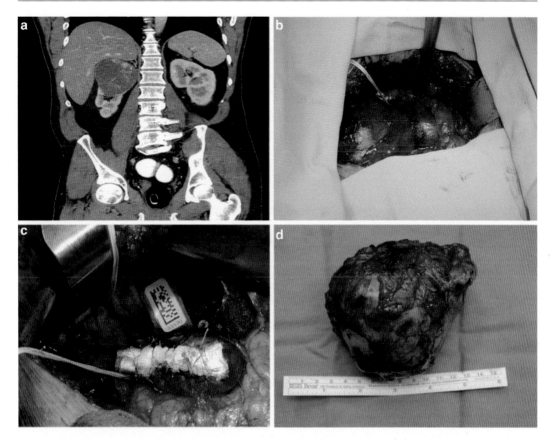

Fig. 8.1 Open partial nephrectomy in a 48-year-old man with a symptomatic 9.2 cm mass. (**a**) Coronal computed tomography image demonstrates an exophytic right upper pole renal mass. (**b**) Exposure of the renal mass via an open flank incision. (**c**) Surgical resection of renal mass with closure of defect over a bolster. No evidence of bleeding after hilar clamp was released. (**d**) Excised renal mass. Final pathology was classic clear cell renal carcinoma, Fuhrman grade 2/4 with negative margins

Minimally Invasive Transperitoneal Approach

Whether using a conventional, hand-assisted or robotic-assisted laparoscopic approach, we take the same approach for kidney mobilization. For left-sided tumors, the colon is mobilized medially and the lower pole of the kidney is identified. The ureter and gonadal vein are identified, and the lower pole of the kidney is bluntly mobilized off of the psoas muscle, and the lower pole of the kidney and ureters are lifted anteriorly. For the robotic-assisted approach, the third robotic arm is useful at this point to maintain anterior elevation of the kidney. For the hand-assisted and conventional laparoscopic approaches, a laparoscopic kitner or suction/irrigator device through an assistant port provides lift. The medial dissection is carried cephalad following the gonadal vein to identify the renal vein. If exposure is not ideal, the upper pole of the kidney can be mobilized, further releasing attachments of the pancreas, spleen, and colon. In general, even if we do not intend to clamp the hilum, we isolate the renal vein and artery to be able to clamp the hilum *en bloc*, artery only, or artery and vein separately. For hilar tumors, further dissection of more distal branches of the artery and vein can be carried out to allow for clamping of segmental branches or ligation of individual vessels entering the tumor (Fig. 8.2).

For right-sided tumors, we begin the dissection by incising the peritoneum over the right

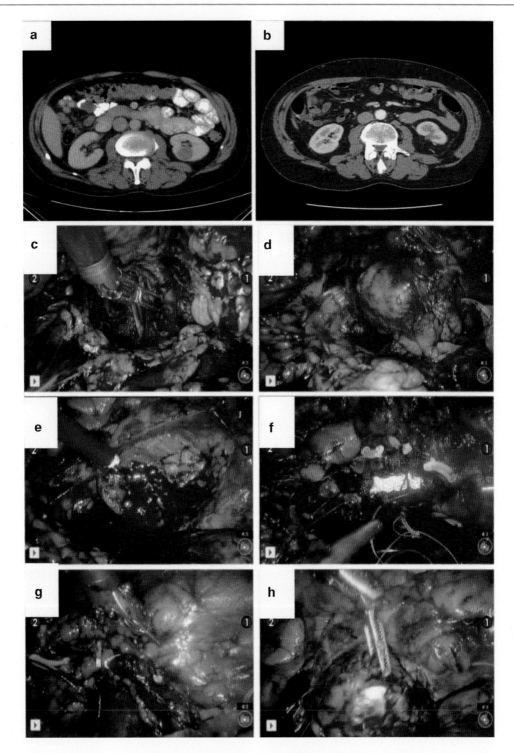

Fig. 8.2 Robotic-assisted partial nephrectomy in a 59-year-old woman with biopsy-proven renal cell carcinoma. (**a**) Computed tomography image demonstrates an endophytic left lower pole renal mass. (**b**) Postoperative CT demonstrating good perfusion and complete excision. (**c**) Exposed renal hilum. (**d**) Tumor exposed. (**e**) Resection bed. (**f**) Repaired defect using nitrocellulose bolster. (**g**) Closure of Gerota's fascia over defect using clips. (**h**) Resected tumor ready for removal. Final pathology was clear cell renal carcinoma, Fuhrman grade 3/4 with negative margins

kidney and mobilizing to medially until the duodenum is identified. The duodenum is then Kocherized and further dissection is carried cephalad so that the peritoneum between the upper pole of the kidney and liver is incised. From that point, the dissection progresses as described for the left-sided procedure.

Further dissection depends on the location of the tumor. For upper pole tumors it is often necessary to mobilize the entire kidney so that the upper pole can be lifted anteriorly. The surgeon must judge whether this mobilization is best performed with Gerota's fascia intact or within Gerota's.

The assistant role in aiding exposure is critical in both the laparoscopic and robotic-assisted approaches. One advantage of the robotic approach is that once the lower pole and ureter are mobilized and elevated by the third arm, the console surgeon is less reliant on retraction from the bedside assistant.

Minimally Invasive Retroperitoneal Approach

As initial access to the kidney is posterior and interpolar in this approach, the renal hilum is mobilized and isolated first. The hilum is typically in line with the port placed at the costovertebral angle. If the thoracolumbar fascia has not been incised when obtaining access, the hilum may be obscured. It is useful to identify the ureter, gonadal vein, and psoas muscle to maintain proper orientation. For most cases, the renal artery is encountered first when dissecting the renal hilum. The vein, which is usually behind the artery in this approach, can also be isolated if the surgeon intends to clamp it as well.

Tumor Localization

High quality preoperative cross-sectional imaging is crucial as a guide to tumor location. For open PN, the tumor may be identified and isolated early in the dissection if mobilization is performed within Gerota's fascia. However, for minimally invasive approaches, Gerota's is entered and the tumor is isolated after mobiliza-

tion of the hilum so that the perinephric fat will not obscure the hilum during dissection. We enter Gerota's fascia at a point away from the tumor and identify the capsule of the normal kidney first. Ideally, Gerota's is mobilized in such a way that flaps of perinephric fat remain intact to re-approximate over the site of resection at the conclusion of the case. The fat covering the tumor is left in place to send with the specimen to pathology, but it is important to expose the kidney capsule circumferentially around the tumor in preparation for the renorrhaphy after the tumor is excised.

Several reports have established intraoperative ultrasonography (US) as a useful adjunct when performing PN. Intraoperative US is particularly useful for patients with intrarenal tumors that are not visible or palpable even after the perinephric fat has been removed. The topographical information obtained from intraoperative US is also useful in patients with tumors that extend deep into the kidney [41, 42]. In such instances US is useful for defining the appropriate margins of resection and for allowing preservation of as much uninvolved parenchyma as possible while still obtaining negative surgical margins. Ultrasound is also useful for locating multicentric tumors, venous extension, and the presence of other renal lesions. Advances in laparoscopic US have greatly aided the management of increasingly complex tumors through a minimally invasive approach. We advocate its use on every NSS to provide "real time" information about tumor dimensions to assist in surgical dissection and to improve the surgeon's US skill for assessing and managing more complex tumors. The incorporation of ultrasound for robotic NSS has been greatly aided by TilePro, which allows the console surgeon to visualize the operative field and US image at the same time [43].

Prevention of Ischemic Injury

A number of steps can be taken to minimize ischemic injury during PN. Some of these options are available to both the open and minimally invasive surgeon and depend largely on the depth of the tumor, proximity to the renal sinus, location of the tumor in the kidney and its blood supply.

Depth of Tumor

For laparoscopic and robotic-assisted procedures, we have created an algorithm to determine when it is advisable to clamp the renal hilum [31]. If the tumor has less than 5 mm of penetration into the kidney and is greater than 5 mm from the renal sinus, it is often unnecessary to clamp the hilum, although the hilum should still be isolated in the event that the need to clamp arises during dissection. It is important to confirm the superficial nature of the tumor with intraoperative ultrasound. Hemostasis can frequently be achieved with a combination of argon beam coagulation and hemostatic agents. For those tumors with >5 mm but <10 mm of penetration into the parenchyma, we typically clamp the hilum but unclamp once adequate hemostasis of the base of the resection has been obtained, either with a running absorbable suture or application of hemostatic agents. This is often referred to as "early unclamping" in the recent literature; however, this technique has been practiced for some time and can be used in any approach.

Proximity to Sinus

For those tumors within 5 mm of the renal sinus/hilum, the hilum should be clamped. Again, if the base of the tumor can be controlled with a running absorbable suture, early hilar unclamping can minimize ischemia time. Early unclamping is not recommended for large, central tumors where large segmental vessel can result in significant blood loss or result in the need for complex reconstruction. In this scenario, the use of cold ischemia may be more appropriate.

Segmental artery clamping can be used in any approach. When the tumor is supplied by a distinct artery, ligation of this artery can provide hemostasis without ischemia to the remainder of the kidney. Not clamping the renal vein also helps to minimize ischemic injury [44].

If the anticipated renal hilum clamp time exceeds 20 min, additional protection from ischemic renal injury is necessary. Local hypothermia currently offers the most effective means for this. Ice slush packed around the kidney is a common method for renal cooling. A wide variety of alternative approaches have been presented without obvious advantage over ice slush. To date, there is no compelling evidence that cold ischemia offers a significant advantage over warm ischemia as long as hilar clamp time is minimized. A recent multi-institutional study of 660 patients with solitary kidneys undergoing PN demonstrated no significant difference in long-term renal function between warm and cold ischemia. The most critical determinants of renal function were the quality and quantity of the renal remnant [45]. Cold ischemia allows up to 40–60 min of clamp time without permanent kidney damage. It is important to cover the entire kidney with ice for at least 5–10 min immediately after occluding the renal artery before beginning the PN. This allows the kidney core temperature to reach 15–20°C, optimizing renal preservation. Administration of intravenous mannitol (12.5 g) 15–30 min before clamping the renal artery induces diereses, reduces renal tubule swelling and protects against ischemic renal damage. Careful attention to perioperative fluid status is crucial, particularly for patients with a solitary kidney.

Other Considerations Related to Ischemia

We have found that it is valuable in all cases to be prepared prior to tumor resection to clamp the renal hilum and suture the base of resection. There is considerable literature touting the resection of renal masses without hilar clamping for minimally invasive approaches. The most commonly reported technique is to utilize a radiofrequency energy device such as the Habib. While this has been demonstrated to be effective [46], our concern is that the tissue char created by the device makes visualizing the resection margin difficult, destroys surrounding benign parenchyma, and can result in delayed bleeding or urine leak. Other techniques described to limit ischemia include pre-placement of hemostatic sutures under the tumor with ultrasound guidance [47] and relative hypotension [48]. While reducing kidney ischemia is important, this must be balanced with sound oncologic principles. We believe that cold resection in a bloodless field achieved with renal artery clamping best achieves this.

A second related issue is the decision to clamp the renal artery alone, both the artery and vein, or segmental arteries alone. The literature suggests that clamping the artery alone is safe and likely limits renal damage [44]. However, if the tumor is deep and/or central in location, it is often helpful to clamp the renal artery and vein to achieve the best visualization. The choice of clamp (bulldog or Satinsky) depends on the anatomy of the renal hilum and patient. Every effort should be made to isolate the renal artery separately from the renal vein, but in the case of a complex hilum with multiple renal vessels, using a Satinsky clamp across the entire hilum is often safer and more expedient. For minimally invasive approaches, laparoscopic bulldog or Satinsky clamps are available. Extra care must be taken when using a laparoscopic Satinsky clamp with a robotic approach as the robotic arms can clash with the clamp externally and cause major vascular injury. Segmental clamping with a bulldog clamp is appropriate when there is clearly a discrete artery branch supplying the tumor. Preoperative imaging can aid in defining the renal vasculature, but the ultimate decision on how to proceed with hilar clamping is made intraoperatively once the hilum and tumor have been exposed. Caution should be exercised in segmental clamping of posterior polar tumors as these tumors are often supplied by both the polar artery and the posterior branch. It is important to prepare the hilum to clamp the main renal artery and vein even when segmental clamping is employed in the event that vascular control is insufficient, and the main artery and/or vein need to be clamped during tumor excision.

Tumor Excision

Excision of the tumor with a conservative margin (2–3 mm) of normal parenchyma is the preferred technique for PN. This can best be accomplished by wedge resection for centrally or peripherally located tumors, or by transverse heminephrectomy for large polar tumors. Frozen sections of the base of resection to confirm negative surgical margins can be obtained if needed. The perinephric fat overlying the tumor should be left undisturbed to ensure en bloc removal of the malignancy. Patients with multifocal disease can be managed by PN if possible, but they are at increased risk for local recurrence after NSS [49]. Regardless of the approach used, cold excision allows for optimal visualization to discern malignant from benign renal tissue.

Simple Enucleation

Renal masses are often completely enveloped by a pseudocapsule of fibrous tissue that can allow relatively avascular tumor removal by enucleation. The technique of enucleation involves circumferentially incising of the parenchyma around the tumor, identifying the plane between the pseudocapsule and adjacent uninvolved parenchyma, and then gently mobilizing the lesion with a blunt instrument. During enucleation of peripheral tumors, it is generally unnecessary to occlude the renal artery, and the few transected blood vessels at the base of the enucleation can simply be ligated with suture. The argon beam coagulator can be used to treat the resection base, fat or oxycel can be placed into the cavity, and the resection edges can be sutured together to further assure hemostasis.

While enucleation has typically been reserved for patients with a peripheral, well-encapsulated tumor or hereditary renal cancer syndromes, growing data suggests that oncologic outcomes of enucleation are similar to wedge resection. A retrospective cohort study of 982 patients undergoing standard PN and 537 patients undergoing enucleation showed no significant difference in progression-free or cancer-specific survival after adjusting for other meaningful variables [50]. The advantage of enucleation is maximal preservation of renal function and improved hemostasis without apparent loss of oncologic efficacy. Ultimately, the surgeon must judge whether enucleation is appropriate on a case-by-case basis.

Hemostasis

Obtaining early vascular control and occluding the renal artery when necessary are essential maneuvers to minimize intraoperative blood loss during NSS. Temporary occlusion of both the renal artery and vein also provides improved operative visualization which can be invaluable during challenging cases. The renal vein clamp is removed first and the parenchyma is carefully inspected during deep forced inspiration to identify additional bleeding sites that are not otherwise apparent. For minimally invasive procedures, decreasing the insufflation pressure to 5 mm Hg at the end of the procedure helps to determine it adequate hemostasis has been achieved.

When excising the tumor during an open surgical approach, vessels can be suture ligated or clipped when they are encountered as they can retract into the parenchyma and become more difficult to control after the tumor is removed. Larger vessels tend to be located medially within or near the renal sinus. Residual bleeding vessels should be ligated with absorbable suture once the tumor is excised. The use of Argon beam coagulator, fibrin glue, and other hemostatic agents is also helpful for obtaining hemostasis. Reapproximation of the capsule with absorbable suture tied over a nitrocellulose bolster or perinephric fat aides in hemostasis, but this should not be done until the parenchymal bleeding has been adequately controlled. Other energy sources, such as radiofrequency devices or laser, have been described to aid in hemostasis.

For minimally invasive approaches, we have found that using a running suture at the base of the resection (2–0 absorbable suture) can improve hemostasis and does not add significantly to the warm ischemia time. However, larger transected veins or arteries should be individually controlled with absorbable suture first. Better visualization in the case of venous bleeding can be achieved by increasing the insufflation pressure to 20 mm Hg for short periods of time without detrimental effects on renal function.

For tumors within 5 mm of the renal sinus or collecting system, our preference is to resect the tumor with cold scissors while the hilum is clamped, close the renal sinus or collecting system with an absorbable suture, re-approximate the base of the resection bed with an absorbable suture, and then unclamp the kidney. Following that, a bolster composed of rolled nitrocellulose sheets with pre-attached 0-vicryl sutures on CT-1

needles is placed and secured in on position using Hem-O-Lok clips using a sliding renorrhaphy technique [51]. Additional sutures of 0-vicryl on CT 1 needles with a Hem-O-Lok pre-tied in place at the end can be used to further secure the bolster in place after tightening the suture with a second Hem-O-Lok clip.

Closure of the Collecting System

Watertight closure of the collecting system is essential to prevent urinary fistula formation. Surgeons should look for entries into the collecting system centrally as the renal tumor is excised. If possible, the collecting system should be closed with absorbable suture before it has been completely transected. Calices and infundibula are often more difficult to locate if they have been allowed to retract into the parenchyma or perisinus fat. For minimally invasive approaches, entries into the collecting system can be closed with a running absorbable suture which can be secured using Lapry-Ty clips to save ischemia time.

The perspective regarding ureteral stenting at the time of PN has evolved as experience with NSS has accumulated [22]. Initially, stents were placed whenever a significant opening in the collecting system was identified, regardless of the location of the defect or the complexity of the reconstruction. More recently, stents are placed only when major reconstruction of the collecting system is required. With any entry into the collecting system, a drain should be placed at the conclusion of the case.

Outcomes of Nephron-Sparing Surgery for Renal Cell Carcinoma

Perhaps the best way to judge the various approaches for extirpative management of small renal masses is to directly compare their outcomes. More robust, long-term data exit for open PN than for the laparoscopic or robotic-assisted approaches. In addition, there is also appropriate selection bias among the approaches making direct comparison difficult. The focus of the following literature review is on contemporary series. While we report the mean results here, they are not weighted by the number of patients in the individual study included, and therefore may not be representative of all patients undergoing the various approaches. The table references are included in the reference section [34, 46, 52–95].

Demographic/Perioperative Factors

Table 8.1 summarizes general demographic information and perioperative outcomes of patients undergoing NSS. Patient age was similar across all series with a larger percentage of patients with solitary kidneys treated with an open surgical approach. Only a small number series report results for the retroperitoneal laparoscopic or robotic approaches. We did not include data for the hand-assisted approach because of the small number of cases reported in the literature.

Mean tumor size was larger on average for the open surgical approach. The shortest operative times were reported for the retroperitoneoscopic approach, reflecting the direct access to the renal hilum and tumor with this approach and the

advantage of avoiding an open flank incision. On average, though, the open surgical approach took less time than robotic or laparoscopic transperitoneal approaches. There was variable reporting of hilar clamp time, with the shortest ischemia times reported for the robotic-assisted approach. Hospital stays were shortest for the laparoscopic and robotic-assisted approaches; however, this is based on only a few series for the retroperitoneoscopic approach and may not reflect the true advantage of the retroperitoneoscopic PN in terms of convalescence and recovery. We recently reported our experience with robotic-assisted retroperitoneal PN with a mean length of hospital stay of 1 day [96]. Estimated blood loss was consistently less for minimally invasive than the open approach.

Complications

Table 8.2 summarizes the complications of NSS by approach. The literature is plagued by a lack of standardization in defining and reporting complications. However, recent literature has adopted more standardized complication reporting methods, such as the National Cancer Institute Common Terminology Criteria for Adverse

Table 8.1 Demographic and perioperative outcomes by surgical approach [34, 46, 52–94]

| Variable | Partial nephrectomy approach | | | |
	Laparoscopic	Laparoscopic-RP	Robotic	Open
N[a]	11,505	255	1,055	9,947
Mean age (range)	59.4 (55–62.6)	60.4 (59–62)	60 (55–68)	60.4 (56–63)
% Solitary kidney (range)	0–5.9	Not reported	Not reported	23 (11–30)
% Retroperitoneoscopic	0–63	–	18[b]	–
Mean tumor size cm (range)	2.6 (2–3.9)	2.8 (2.4–3.5)	2.8 (2.5–3.5)	3.4 (2.5–4.1)
Operative time in minutes(range)	202 (85–293)	124 (84–200)	217 (140–373)	187 (150–266)
% Unclamped	29 (0–100)	Not reported	16[b]	20 (0–50)
Mean ischemia time in minutes (range)	28 (0–39)	24 (22–25)	18.6 (0–25.5)	28.9 (11–40)
Mean length of hospital stay in days (range)	3.1 (1–7)	5.5 (2.6–9)	3.3 (2.4–4.3)	5.7 (5–7)
Mean estimated blood loss in cc (range)	237 (100–437)	227 (194–260)	200 (127–337)	358 (294–397)

[a]Numbers may not represent mutually exclusive cases
[b]Based on single series

Table 8.2 Complications by surgical approach [34, 46, 52, 55–57, 59, 61, 62, 64, 66, 67, 70–77, 79–84, 86–93, 95]

Variable	Partial nephrectomy approach			
Mean % (range)	Laparoscopic	Laparoscopic-RP	Robotic	Open
N	11,505	255	1,055	9,947
Acute kidney injury	0.7 (0.6–0.9)	Not reported	0	3.5 (0.5–13)
Death	0.3[a]	Not reported	0	0.5[a]
Conversion to open partial	2.4 (0.6–5.4)	1.8[a]	1.6 (0–4)	–
Nephrectomy	1.8 (0.5–4)	Not reported	3.6 (1.6–7.7)	0
Clavien 3 or higher complication	11 (0–36)	4.5[a]	4.9 (0–8.2)	5 (4–6.7)
Pseudoaneurysm/embolization	1.7 (0.5–4)	0.9[a]	1.7 (1–2.6)	3[a]
Urine leak	3.4 (1–8)	0–1.8	3.9 (1–16.8)[b]	2.5 (0.6–5.5)
Hemorrhage	4.7 (0.8–11.1)	2.7–4.3	2.2 (0.7–4.8)	2 (0.9–4)
Blood transfusion	6.3 (1.6–12.5)	2.7–5.1	4.2 (0–7.1)	8.2 (5.1–11)
Cardiovascular	1.7 (0.8–2.5)	Not reported	1.4 (0.5–3.7)	4.3[a]
Neuro	0[a]	Not reported	Not reported	2[a]
Infection	2.2 (1–5.3)	0.9[a]	3.2 (0.4–7.4)	2.1 (0.5–4)
Pulmonary	1.7 (0–2.7)	5.7[a]	0.7–2.4	2–5.5
Thromboembolic	1 (1–3)	0.9[a]	1.5–2.6	1.2–2
Hernia	3 (0.5–5)	0–3.6	Not reported	Not reported
Readmission	11 (10.4–11.1)[a]	Not reported	11.9[a]	Not reported

[a]Based on single series
[b]Based on two series

Events (CTCAE) or the more surgically oriented Clavien Classification. The emphasis in this section will be the diagnosis, management, and clinical significance of the more common complications of NSS.

Urinary Fistula Formation

Urinary fistula formation is the most commonly reported complication of NSS. The mean rate for most series we reviewed is 3–4%, with fewer patients experiencing urine leak with the open approach. There is significant variability in urine fistula rates for the laparoscopic and robotic-assisted approaches. This possibly reflects the early experience of surgeons with these approaches and the more frequent use of energy sources to perform the tumor resection, potentially obscuring the renal anatomy. Urinary fistula is defined as persistent (>7 days) drainage of fluid (>50 cm³/day) with a drainage fluid to serum creatinine ratio of greater than 2 mg/dl.

Risk factors for urinary fistula formation in both the open and minimally invasive approaches include large tumor size (>4.0 cm), the need for extensive reconstruction of the collecting system

and central tumor location [97]. Urine fistulas often resolve spontaneously with conservative management. If urine fistulas persist, endoscopic manipulation, including retrograde pyelography and placement of a temporary ureteral stent to encourage the flow of urine down the ureter, may be necessary [22]. The surgical drain is left in place until the fistula resolves, and the drain fluid creatinine level should be reassessed before removing the drain. If a normal pyelocalyceal system is identified on retrograde pyelogram yet drain output persists, a renal papilla that was excluded from the remaining collecting system during the rhenorraphy is the likely source. In this circumstance, it may take several months until that papilla no longer functions and the urine leak resolves. Alternatively, variable success has been reported with ureteroscopic division of suture obstructing infundibula using the holmium laser [98].

Acute Kidney Injury

Acute renal failure (ARF) requiring renal replacement therapy is the second most common complication of NSS. The low rates of this complication reported for minimally invasive approaches suggest either under-reporting or that tumors managed by these approaches are consistently less complex than those managed with the open approach. Ischemic renal injury from hilar clamping and reduced parenchymal mass after PN are the primary causes of ARF. Perinephric urinoma and vascular thrombosis can also lead to ARF after NSS [22]. The most significant predisposing factor for the development of ARF in this series was the presence of a solitary kidney. Novick et al. found that ARF only occurred in 2% patients with a normal contralateral kidney. In contrast, ARF developed in 26% of patients with a solitary kidney. In the solitary kidney cohort, additional risk factors for ARF included large tumor size (>7 cm), greater than 50% parenchymal excision, and greater than 60 min of cold ischemia time. ARF rates after elective PN should be relatively low as these patients have normal contralateral kidneys which can maintain perioperative renal function. The management of ARF after NSS should include careful attention to volume status, appropriate adjustment of medication doses, and dialysis as needed. More recently, the same group evaluated factors that determine renal function after PN in solitary kidneys. In multivariable analyses, increasing age, larger tumor size, lower preoperative GFR, and longer ischemia time were associated with decreased postoperative GFR ($p < 0.05$). On multivariable analysis, the percentage of renal parenchyma spared and the preoperative GFR proved to be the primary determinants of ultimate renal function, and time of intraoperative renal ischemia lost statistical significance. Long-term renal function after PN was determined primarily by the quantity and quality of renal parenchyma preserved [45]. It is important to emphasize that these results were obtained in a series notable for short warm ischemic times and liberal use of hypothermia and will likely not apply to cases with longer warm ischemia. Indeed, when this was evaluated in a more homogenous group of patients with solitary kidneys managed only with warm ischemia, the ischemic interval proved to be a significant predictor of ARF, and when extended beyond 25 min, it served as an independent predictor of new onset severe CKD.

Other Complications

Other complications of NSS include postoperative hemorrhage, perinephric abscess formation, and renal vessel thrombosis. Hemorrhage is more frequently reported in laparoscopic series and occurs at a similar rate in open and robotic-assisted series (Table 8.2). Most studies defined hemorrhage as intraoperative bleeding requiring resuscitation. Pseudoaneurysm or arteriovenous fistula form when suture thrown in the base of the tumor resection bed fuses arteries and veins, resulting in direct communication between the two. This is more frequently reported in open surgical series, likely reflecting the greater complexity of these tumors. Delayed postoperative bleeding with perinephric hematoma can present with pain, gross hematuria, hypotension, flank mass, or bruising, and occurs more frequently with the open than minimally invasive approaches. After initial resuscitation and stabilization of the patient, a CT scan of the abdomen and pelvis is useful in making the diagnosis. Delayed bleeding can frequently be treated in interventional radiology with selective renal artery angiography and coil embolization. Avoiding deep passes with large needles into the renal sinus intraoperatively diminishes the risk of this complication.

Although complications of NSS are not uncommon, most can be managed conservatively and associated morbidity is often minimal. The rate of major complications (Clavien 3 or higher) is approximately 5% for most approaches. For the conventional laparoscopic approach, the rate is 11%, potentially reflecting its inherent technical challenges, especially early in a surgeon's experience. Table 8.2 also summarizes complications by system. Complication rates in most series are likely under-reported. Standardized reporting of complications and meticulous patient follow-up is essential to better compare the approaches for NSS. Mortality rates after NSS compare favorably with those for RN (1–2%).Taken together; these results suggest that NSS can be performed safely and with minimal morbidity. Of course, individual outcomes depend greatly on surgeon experience and tumor complexity.

The rate of conversion to open PN is similar for the different minimally invasive approaches.

Table 8.3 Oncologic and renal function outcomes [34, 46, 54–56, 58–62, 64–67, 69–73, 75–85, 87, 88, 93]

| Variable | Partial nephrectomy approach | | | |
Mean % (range)	Laparoscopic	Laparoscopic-RP	Robotic	Open
N	11,505	255	1,055	9,947
Positive margin	2.4 (0–12)	0–4.7	3.1 (0–7.7)	2.3 (0–7)
Recurrence	1.2 (0–4.2)	0–0.9	0.2–2.9	0.8–5.9
Mean follow-up (months)	26 (10–44)	15–23	7.8–26	25
Change in creatinine from baseline	0.13	Not reported	0.13	0.16
Change GFR from baseline	6.3–18	22[a]	6.3–23	Not reported
Disease-specific survival	3 years: 99.3%	Not reported	Not reported	3 years: 99–100
	5 years: 97.6%			5 years: 82–100
				10 years: 77–100

[a]Based on single series

Conversion to nephrectomy was reported more commonly with robotic-assisted NSS, reflecting the early experience with this approach and issues with patient and tumor selection.

Functional and Oncologic Outcomes Following Nephron-Sparing Surgery

Preservation of Renal Function

Table 8.3 summarizes the renal function and oncologic outcomes of NSS by approach. A fundamental issue with such a comparison is the lack of standardized methods or timeframe for reporting renal function, as well as the absence of this data in many series. Several series report the change in creatinine from baseline, but newer series more often report the change in GFR which better assess the level of CKD and the need for renal replacement therapy. Most approaches demonstrate similar renal function outcomes. It must be kept in mind, though, that most open series represent larger, more complex tumors. The use of R.E.N.A.L. Nephrometry Score may allow future series to compare results in patients with similar tumor size and complexity.

Novick et al. reported on the long-term renal function in 14 patients with solitary kidneys who underwent PN for localized tumors with no preoperative clinical or histopathologic evidence of primary renal disease. Postoperative renal func-

tion remained stable in 12 patients, whereas two developed end-stage renal failure. Nine patients developed proteinuria: low grade in four (<750 mg/24 h) and moderate to severe in five (930–6,740 mg/24 h). A statistically significant inverse association was found between the degree of proteinuria and amount of residual renal tissue. Renal biopsy performed in four patients with moderate to severe proteinuria showed focal segmental or global glomerulosclerosis [99].

These data suggest that patients with solitary kidneys with more than a 50% reduction in renal mass after PN are at increased risk for developing a hyperfiltration injury, manifested by proteinuria, glomerulopathy, and progressive azotemia. The development of significant proteinuria usually preceded detectable renal deterioration [99]. These observations suggest that patients with solitary kidneys who undergo PN should be followed with serial 24-h urinary protein evaluations in addition to serum creatinine levels and calculated GFR. A low-protein diet should be instituted in patients who develop proteinuria of >150 mg/24 h, and treatment with angiotensin-converting enzyme inhibitors should be considered.

Oncologic Outcomes

As there is less robust, long-term data with some of the newer minimally invasive approaches, surgical margin status is often used to assess oncologic efficacy. Recent reports, though, suggest that focal positive margins have minimal adverse oncologic impact following PN [100]. Positive margin rates for most approaches are reported to be 2–3%. However, there is considerable variability in this rate, suggesting the impact of surgeon experience. The rates of local recurrence, another short-term oncologic endpoint, are consistently low regardless of the approach, further strengthening the argument that focal positive margins likely have minimal oncologic impact.

A recent report of a randomized controlled trial of radical versus NSS demonstrated a 10-year overall survival of 81.1% for RN and 75.7% for PN, with a statistically significant difference in favor of RN ($p = 0.03$). When the authors limited the analysis to patients with RCC only, there was no significant difference found between these approaches. The fundamental limitation of this multicenter randomized-controlled study was poor accrual which limits its power to detect a difference between the approaches. Another major issue was the less than expected number of events seen in the study, with only 12/117 patients dying from RCC and 21 patients developing disease progression after a median follow-up of 9.3 years [101].

Several recent reports have documented long-term disease-specific survival rates for most of the surgical approaches to NSS. Ten-year disease-specific survival for open PN ranges from 77% to 100% in the series reporting this endpoint. While this data is not available for the robotic-assisted approaches as of yet, a 5-year disease-specific survival of 97.6% has been reported for the conventional laparoscopic approach, suggesting that in well-selected patients, it can offer comparable cancer control to the open approach (Table 8.3). Reviewing the outcome of NSS in 216 patients with sporadic RCC treated at the Cleveland Clinic Foundation, disease-specific survival was associated with pathologic stage, tumor size, multiplicity, unilaterality, and whether the tumor was discovered incidentally or on the basis of clinical symptoms [102]. Another study reported the outcome of NSS in 241 patients. The mean disease-specific survival rate was 95% at 3 years, and there were only two cases of local tumor recur-

rence. The development of renal failure after PN also has a significant impact on quality of life and mortality. The 1-, 2-, and 5-year survival rates for patients aged 55–64 years while on dialysis following RN for RCC in a solitary kidney are 84%, 67%, and 33%, respectively, and fall to 73%, 51%, and 16% in patients older than 64 years [20]. Currently, these patients have to survive disease free on dialysis for 12–24 months before renal transplantation is considered.

Patterns of Tumor Recurrence and Guidelines for Follow-Up After NSS

The surveillance schedule after NSS for RCC receives relatively little attention in the literature. There is a higher risk of local tumor recurrence after NSS compared to RN, with larger studies suggesting an incidence of up to 10% [22]. Data concerning the occurrence of metastatic disease after NSS for RCC has also been lacking, although it is presumed that rates are not markedly different from those observed after RN. The incidence of both local and metastatic tumor recurrences after NSS for RCC varies according to the pathologic tumor stage. In designing an appropriate strategy for postoperative surveillance after NSS for RCC, a balance must be established between detecting recurrent disease early and overly aggressive follow-up. The cost of postoperative monitoring studies is an additional issue. The available data indicates that surveillance after NSS can be tailored according to the pathologic tumor stage and can perhaps be more limited than the current practice in many centers.

The recommended postoperative surveillance scheme after NSS for sporadic localized RCC is as follows: all patients should be evaluated with a medical history, physical examination and selected blood studies, including serum calcium, alkaline phosphatase, liver function tests, blood urea nitrogen, serum creatinine, and electrolytes on a yearly basis. A 24-h urinary protein measurement should also be obtained in patients with a solitary remnant kidney to screen for hyperfiltration nephropathy [96]. The need

Table 8.4 Surveillance regimen after partial nephrectomy for localized RCC

Risk category	Low risk (T1/grades 1–2)	Intermediate risk (T1/grades 3–4; any T2; T3/grades 1)	High risk (T3/grades 2–4, any T4)
Return visit interval	Every year to 5 years, then every other year	6, 12, 18, 24 months, then annually	6, 12, 18, 24 months, then annually
History and physical examination	Every visit	Every visit	Every visit
Complete blood count	Every visit	Every visit	Every visit
Comprehensive panel	Every visit	Every visit	Every visit
Chest X-ray	Every visit	Every visit	Every visit
Three-dimensional axial abdominal imaging	Years 1 and 3, then as needed	Every other visit starting at 12 months	Every visit

for postoperative radiographic surveillance studies varies by stage. A yearly chest X-ray is recommended after NSS for all stages since the lung is the most common site of postoperative metastasis. We recommend obtaining abdominal CT scans based on modified risk criteria. (Table 8.4).

Conclusions

Despite the clinical research supporting NSS for the treatment of small renal masses, this procedure remains underutilized. Further education and awareness of treatment outcomes associated with NSS is essential. Whether an open or minimally invasive technique is used, it is important for surgeons to have a firm grasp on the concepts unique to NSS, including kidney mobilization, techniques for clamping the renal hilum, and management of postoperative complications, such as bleeding, infection, and urinary fistula. It is now clear that, despite the technical challenges associated with NSS, excellent oncologic control and preservation of renal function make PN the preferred approach for the treatment of small renal masses. All patients with tumors <7 cm in greatest diameter should be considered for a nephron-sparing procedure whenever possible. Only once this is decided should the surgeon select the appropriate surgical approach: open or minimally invasive.

References

1. Jemal A, Siegel R, Xu J, Ward E. Cancer statistics, 2010. CA Cancer J Clin. 2010;60(5):277–300.
2. Hollingsworth JM, Miller DC, Daignault S, Hollenbeck BK. Rising incidence of small renal masses: a need to reassess treatment effect. J Natl Cancer Inst. 2006;98(18):1331–4.
3. Campbell SC, Novick AC, Belldegrun A, et al. Guideline for management of the clinical T1 renal mass. J Urol. 2009;182(4):1271–9.
4. Wells S. Successful removal of two solid circum renal tumours. Br Med J. 1884;1:758–9.
5. Czerny V. Reported by Herczel E: Uber Nierenexsirpation. Beitr Z Klinik Chir. 1890;6:485.
6. Vermooten V. Indications for conservative surgery in certain renal tumors: a study based on the growth pattern of clear cell carcinoma. J Urol. 1950;64:200–8.
7. Robson CJ, Churchill BM, Anderson W. The results of radical nephrectomy for renal cell carcinoma. J Urol. 1969;101(3):297–301.
8. Miller DC, Hollingsworth JM, Hafez KS, Daignault S, Hollenbeck BK. Partial nephrectomy for small renal masses: an emerging quality of care concern? J Urol. 2006;175(3 Pt 1):853–7. discussion 858.
9. Huang WC, Elkin EB, Levey AS, Jang TL, Russo P. Partial nephrectomy versus radical nephrectomy in patients with small renal tumors – is there a difference in mortality and cardiovascular outcomes? J Urol. 2009;181(1):55–61. discussion 61–52.
10. Novick AC, Streem S, Montie JE, et al. Conservative surgery for renal cell carcinoma: a single-center experience with 100 patients. J Urol. 1989;141(4):835–9.
11. Marshall FF, Stewart AK, Menck HR. The national cancer data base: report on kidney cancers. The American College of Surgeons Commission on Cancer and the American Cancer Society. Cancer. 1997;80(11):2167–74.

12. Patel MI, Simmons R, Kattan MW, Motzer RJ, Reuter VE, Russo P. Long-term follow-up of bilateral sporadic renal tumors. Urology. 2003;61(5):921–5.

13. Fergany AF, Saad IR, Woo L, Novick AC. Open partial nephrectomy for tumor in a solitary kidney: experience with 400 cases. J Urol. 2006;175(5):1630–3. discussion 1633.

14. Lane BR, Novick AC, Babineau D, Fergany AF, Kaouk JH, Gill IS. Comparison of laparoscopic and open partial nephrectomy for tumor in a solitary kidney. J Urol. 2008;179(3):847–51. discussion 852.

15. Bijol V, Mendez GP, Hurwitz S, Rennke HG, Nose V. Evaluation of the nonneoplastic pathology in tumor nephrectomy specimens: predicting the risk of progressive renal failure. Am J Surg Pathol. 2006;30(5):575–84.

16. Stevens LA, Coresh J, Greene T, Levey AS. Assessing kidney function – measured and estimated glomerular filtration rate. N Engl J Med. 2006;354(23):2473–83.

17. Coleman JA, Russo P. Hereditary and familial kidney cancer. Curr Opin Urol. 2009;19(5):478–85.

18. Novick AC, Streem SB. Long-term followup after nephron sparing surgery for renal cell carcinoma in von Hippel–Lindau disease. J Urol. 1992;147(6):1488–90.

19. Grubb 3rd RL, Choyke PL, Pinto PA, Linehan WM, Walther MM. Management of von Hippel–Lindau-associated kidney cancer. Nat Clin Pract Urol. 2005;2(5):248–55.

20. Licht MR, Novick AC. Nephron sparing surgery for renal cell carcinoma. J Urol. 1993;149(1):1–7.

21. Herr HW. Partial nephrectomy for unilateral renal carcinoma and a normal contralateral kidney: 10-year followup. J Urol. 1999;161(1):33–4. discussion 34–35.

22. Campbell SC, Novick AC, Streem SB, Klein E, Licht M. Complications of nephron sparing surgery for renal tumors. J Urol. 1994;151(5):1177–80.

23. Lee CT, Katz J, Shi W, Thaler HT, Reuter VE, Russo P. Surgical management of renal tumors 4 cm or less in a contemporary cohort. J Urol. 2000;163(3):730–6.

24. Lesage K, Joniau S, Fransis K, Van Poppel H. Comparison between open partial and radical nephrectomy for renal tumours: perioperative outcome and health-related quality of life. Eur Urol. 2007;51(3):614–20.

25. Karellas ME, O'Brien MF, Jang TL, Bernstein M, Russo P. Partial nephrectomy for selected renal cortical tumours of >/=7 cm. BJU Int. 2010;106(10):1484–7.

26. Angermeier KW, Novick AC, Streem SB, Montie JE. Nephron-sparing surgery for renal cell carcinoma with venous involvement. J Urol. 1990;144(6):1352–5.

27. Thomas AA, Rini BI, Stephenson AJ, et al. Surgical resection of renal cell carcinoma after targeted therapy. J Urol. 2009;182(3):881–6.

28. Clayman RV, Kavoussi LR, Figenshau RS, Chandhoke PS, Albala DM. Laparoscopic nephroureterectomy: initial clinical case report. J Laparoendosc Surg. 1991;1(6):343–9.

29. McDougall EM, Clayman RV, Anderson K. Laparoscopic wedge resection of a renal tumor: initial experience. J Laparoendosc Surg. 1993;3(6):577–81.

30. Breau RH, Crispen PL, Jenkins SM, Blute ML, Leibovich BC. Treatment of patients with small renal masses: a survey of the American Urological Association. J Urol. 2011;185(2):407–13.

31. Rogers C, Sukumar S, Gill IS. Robotic partial nephrectomy: the real benefit. Curr Opin Urol. 2011;21(1):60–4.

32. Romero FR, Rais-Bahrami S, Muntener M, Brito FA, Jarrett TW, Kavoussi LR. Laparoscopic partial nephrectomy in obese and non-obese patients: comparison with open surgery. Urology. 2008;71(5):806–9.

33. Ramani AP, Ryndin I, Lynch AC, Veetil RT. Current concepts in achieving renal hypothermia during laparoscopic partial nephrectomy. BJU Int. 2006;97(2):342–4.

34. Weizer AZ, Gilbert SM, Roberts WW, Hollenbeck BK, Wolf Jr JS. Tailoring technique of laparoscopic partial nephrectomy to tumor characteristics. J Urol. 2008;180(4):1273–8.

35. Montgomery JS, Johnston 3rd WK, Wolf Jr JS. Wound complications after hand assisted laparoscopic surgery. J Urol. 2005;174(6):2226–30.

36. Kutikov A, Uzzo RG. The R.E.N.A.L. nephrometry score: a comprehensive standardized system for quantitating renal tumor size, location and depth. J Urol. 2009;182(3):844–53.

37. Ficarra V, Novara G, Secco S, et al. Preoperative aspects and dimensions used for an anatomical (PADUA) classification of renal tumours in patients who are candidates for nephron-sparing surgery. Eur Urol. 2009;56(5):786–93.

38. Simmons MN, Ching CB, Samplaski MK, Park CH, Gill IS. Kidney tumor location measurement using the C index method. J Urol. 2010;183(5):1708–13.

39. Ellison J, Montgomery J, Hafez K, et al. Effect of R.E.N.A.L. Nephrometry score on peri-operative outcomes in minumally invasive partial nephrectomy. Paper presented at American Urologic Association Annual Meeting 2011, Washington.

40. Kunkle DA, Crispen PL, Li T, Uzzo RG. Tumor size predicts synchronous metastatic renal cell carcinoma: implications for surveillance of small renal masses. J Urol. 2007;177(5):1692–6. discussion 1697.

41. Assimos DG, Boyce H, Woodruff RD, Harrison LH, McCullough DL, Kroovand RL. Intraoperative renal ultrasonography: a useful adjunct to partial nephrectomy. J Urol. 1991;146(5):1218–20.

42. Marshall FF, Holdford SS, Hamper UM. Intraoperative sonography of renal tumors. J Urol. 1992;148(5):1393–6.

43. Rogers CG, Laungani R, Bhandari A, et al. Maximizing console surgeon independence during robot-assisted renal surgery by using the Fourth Arm and TilePro. J Endourol. 2009;23(1):115–21.

44. Gong EM, Zorn KC, Orvieto MA, Lucioni A, Msezane LP, Shalhav AL. Artery-only occlusion may provide superior renal preservation during laparoscopic partial nephrectomy. Urology. 2008;72(4): 843–6.

45. Lane BR, Russo P, Uzzo RG, et al. Comparison of cold and warm ischemia during partial nephrectomy in 660 solitary kidneys reveals predominant role of nonmodifiable factors in determining ultimate renal function. J Urol. 2011;185(2):421–7.

46. Wu SD, Viprakasit DP, Cashy J, Smith ND, Perry KT, Nadler RB. Radiofrequency ablation-assisted robotic laparoscopic partial nephrectomy without renal hilar vessel clamping versus laparoscopic partial nephrectomy: a comparison of perioperative outcomes. J Endourol. 2010;24(3):385–91.

47. Abaza R, Picard J. A novel technique for laparoscopic or robotic partial nephrectomy: feasibility study. J Endourol. 2008;22(8):1715–9.

48. Gill IS, Eisenberg MS, Aron M, et al. "Zero ischemia" partial nephrectomy: novel laparoscopic and robotic technique. Eur Urol. 2011;59(1):128–34.

49. Steinbach F, Stockle M, Muller SC, et al. Conservative surgery of renal cell tumors in 140 patients: 21 years of experience. J Urol. 1992;148(1):24–9. discussion 29–30.

50. Minervini A, Ficarra V, Rocco F, et al. Simple enucleation is equivalent to traditional partial nephrectomy for renal cell carcinoma: results of a nonrandomized, retrospective, comparative study. J Urol. 2011;185(5):1604–10.

51. Benway BM, Wang AJ, Cabello JM, Bhayani SB. Robotic partial nephrectomy with sliding-clip renorrhaphy: technique and outcomes. Eur Urol. 2009; 55(3):592–9.

52. Abukora F, Nambirajan T, Albqami N, et al. Laparoscopic nephron sparing surgery: evolution in a decade. Eur Urol. 2005;47(4):488–93. discussion 493.

53. Adamy A, Favaretto RL, Nogueira L, et al. Recovery of renal function after open and laparoscopic partial nephrectomy. Eur Urol. 2010;58(4):596–601.

54. Allaf ME, Bhayani SB, Rogers C, et al. Laparoscopic partial nephrectomy: evaluation of long-term oncological outcome. J Urol. 2004;172(3):871–3.

55. Benway BM, Bhayani SB, Rogers CG, et al. Robot assisted partial nephrectomy versus laparoscopic partial nephrectomy for renal tumors: a multi-institutional analysis of perioperative outcomes. J Urol. 2009;182(3):866–72.

56. Benway BM, Bhayani SB, Rogers CG, et al. Robot-assisted partial nephrectomy: an international experience. Eur Urol. 2010;57(5):815–20.

57. Breda A, Stepanian SV, Lam JS, et al. Use of haemostatic agents and glues during laparoscopic partial nephrectomy: a multi-institutional survey from the United States and Europe of 1347 cases. Eur Urol. 2007;52(3):798–803.

58. Breda A, Stepanian SV, Liao J, et al. Positive margins in laparoscopic partial nephrectomy in 855 cases: a multi-institutional survey from the United States and Europe. J Urol. 2007;178(1):47–50. discussion 50.

59. Dulabon LM, Kaouk JH, Haber GP, et al. Multi-institutional analysis of robotic partial nephrectomy for hilar versus nonhilar lesions in 446 consecutive cases. Eur Urol. 2011;59(3):325–30.

60. Gettman MT, Blute ML, Chow GK, Neururer R, Bartsch G, Peschel R. Robotic-assisted laparoscopic partial nephrectomy: technique and initial clinical experience with DaVinci robotic system. Urology. 2004;64(5):914–8.

61. Gill IS, Kamoi K, Aron M, Desai MM. 800 Laparoscopic partial nephrectomies: a single surgeon series. J Urol. 2010;183(1):34–41.

62. Gill IS, Kavoussi LR, Lane BR, et al. Comparison of 1,800 laparoscopic and open partial nephrectomies for single renal tumors. J Urol. 2007;178(1):41–6.

63. Godoy G, Ramanathan V, Kanofsky JA, et al. Effect of warm ischemia time during laparoscopic partial nephrectomy on early postoperative glomerular filtration rate. J Urol. 2009;181(6):2438–43. discussion 2443–2435.

64. Haber GP, White WM, Crouzet S, et al. Robotic versus laparoscopic partial nephrectomy: single-surgeon matched cohort study of 150 patients. Urology. 2010;76(3):754–8.

65. Jeldres C, Bensalah K, Capitanio U, et al. Baseline renal function, ischaemia time and blood loss predict the rate of renal failure after partial nephrectomy. BJU Int. 2009;103(12):1632–5.

66. Jeschke K, Peschel R, Wakonig J, Schellander L, Bartsch G, Henning K. Laparoscopic nephron-sparing surgery for renal tumors. Urology. 2001;58(5): 688–92.

67. Kava BR, De Los Santos R, Ayyathurai R, et al. Contemporary open partial nephrectomy is associated with diminished procedure-specific morbidity despite increasing technical challenges: a single institutional experience. World J Urol. 2010;28(4):507–12.

68. Kim FJ, Rha KH, Hernandez F, Jarrett TW, Pinto PA, Kavoussi LR. Laparoscopic radical versus partial nephrectomy: assessment of complications. J Urol. 2003;170(2 Pt 1):408–11.

69. Lane BR, Gill IS. 7-Year oncological outcomes after laparoscopic and open partial nephrectomy. J Urol. 2010;183(2):473–9.

70. Lifshitz DA, Shikanov SA, Deklaj T, et al. Laparoscopic partial nephrectomy: a single-center evolving experience. Urology. 2010;75(2):282–7.

71. Link RE, Bhayani SB, Allaf ME, et al. Exploring the learning curve, pathological outcomes and perioperative morbidity of laparoscopic partial nephrectomy performed for renal mass. J Urol. 2005;173(5): 1690–4.

72. Marszalek M, Chromecki T, Al-Ali BM, et al. Laparoscopic partial nephrectomy: a matched-pair comparison of the transperitoneal versus the retroperitoneal approach. Urology. 2011;77(1):109–13.

73. Marszalek M, Meixl H, Polajnar M, Rauchenwald M, Jeschke K, Madersbacher S. Laparoscopic and open partial nephrectomy: a matched-pair comparison of 200 patients. Eur Urol. 2009;55(5):1171–8.

74. Moore NW, Nakada SY, Hedican SP, Moon TD. Complications of hand-assisted laparoscopic renal surgery: single-center ten-year experience. Urology. 2011;77:1353–8.

75. Nadu A, Mor Y, Laufer M, et al. Laparoscopic partial nephrectomy: single center experience with 140 patients – evolution of the surgical technique and its impact on patient outcomes. J Urol. 2007;178(2): 435–9. discussion 438–439.

76. Nogueira L, Katz D, Pinochet R, et al. Critical evaluation of perioperative complications in laparoscopic partial nephrectomy. Urology. 2010;75(2):288–94.

77. Permpongkosol S, Bagga HS, Romero FR, Sroka M, Jarrett TW, Kavoussi LR. Laparoscopic versus open partial nephrectomy for the treatment of pathological T1N0M0 renal cell carcinoma: a 5-year survival rate. J Urol. 2006;176(5):1984–8. discussion 1988–1989.

78. Permpongkosol S, Colombo Jr JR, Gill IS, Kavoussi LR. Positive surgical parenchymal margin after laparoscopic partial nephrectomy for renal cell carcinoma: oncological outcomes. J Urol. 2006;176(6 Pt 1):2401–4.

79. Porpiglia F, Volpe A, Billia M, Scarpa RM. Laparoscopic versus open partial nephrectomy: analysis of the current literature. Eur Urol. 2008; 53(4):732–42. discussion 742–733.

80. Pyo P, Chen A, Grasso M. Retroperitoneal laparoscopic partial nephrectomy: surgical experience and outcomes. J Urol. 2008;180(4):1279–83.

81. Ray ER, Turney BW, Singh R, Chandra A, Cranston DW, O'Brien TS. Open partial nephrectomy: outcomes from two UK centres. BJU Int. 2006;97(6): 1211–5.

82. Scoll BJ, Uzzo RG, Chen DY, et al. Robot-assisted partial nephrectomy: a large single-institutional experience. Urology. 2010;75(6):1328–34.

83. Shah SK, Matin SF, Singer EA, Eichel L, Kim HL. Outcomes of laparoscopic partial nephrectomy after fellowship training. JSLS. 2009;13(2):154–9.

84. Shao P, Qin C, Yin C, et al. Laparoscopic partial nephrectomy with segmental renal artery clamping: technique and clinical outcomes. Eur Urol. 2011; 59(5):849–55.

85. Shikanov S, Lifshitz D, Chan AA, et al. Impact of ischemia on renal function after laparoscopic partial nephrectomy: a multicenter study. J Urol. 2010; 183(5):1714–8.

86. Stephenson AJ, Hakimi AA, Snyder ME, Russo P. Complications of radical and partial nephrectomy in a large contemporary cohort. J Urol. 2004;171(1): 130–4.

87. Thompson RH, Leibovich BC, Lohse CM, Zincke H, Blute ML. Complications of contemporary open nephron sparing surgery: a single institution experience. J Urol. 2005;174(3):855–8.

88. Tsivian A, Tsivian M, Benjamin S, Sidi AA. Laparoscopic partial nephrectomy for multiple tumours: feasibility and analysis of peri-operative outcomes. BJU Int. 2011;108:1330–4.

89. Turna B, Frota R, Kamoi K, et al. Risk factor analysis of postoperative complications in laparoscopic partial nephrectomy. J Urol. 2008;179(4):1289–94. discussion 1294–1285.

90. Wang AJ, Bhayani SB. Robotic partial nephrectomy versus laparoscopic partial nephrectomy for renal cell carcinoma: single-surgeon analysis of >100 consecutive procedures. Urology. 2009;73(2):306–10.

91. Weld KJ, Ames CD, Hruby G, Humphrey PA, Landman J. Evaluation of a novel knotless self-anchoring suture material for urinary tract reconstruction. Urology. 2006;67(6):1133–7.

92. Wille AH, Tullmann M, Roigas J, Loening SA, Deger S. Laparoscopic partial nephrectomy in renal cell cancer – results and reproducibility by different surgeons in a high volume laparoscopic center. Eur Urol. 2006;49(2):337–42. discussion 342–333.

93. Williams SB, Kacker R, Alemozaffar M, Francisco IS, Mechaber J, Wagner AA. Robotic partial nephrectomy versus laparoscopic partial nephrectomy: a single laparoscopic trained surgeon's experience in the development of a robotic partial nephrectomy program. World J Urol. 2011.

94. Wright JL, Porter JR. Laparoscopic partial nephrectomy: comparison of transperitoneal and retroperitoneal approaches. J Urol. 2005;174(3):841–5.

95. Zimmermann R, Janetschek G. Complications of laparoscopic partial nephrectomy. World J Urol. 2008;26(6):531–7.

96. Weizer AZ, Palella GV, Montgomery JS, Miller DC, Hafez KS. Robot-assisted retroperitoneal partial nephrectomy: technique and perioperative results(*). J Endourol. 2011;25(4):553–7.

97. Wheat J, Weizer AZ, Wolf JS. Tumor size and depth are associated with complications of laparoscopic partial nephrectomy. J Urol. 2009;181(4):536.

98. Mues AC, Landman J, Gupta M. Endoscopic management of completely excluded calices: a single institution experience. J Endourol. 2010;24(8):1241–5.

99. Novick AC, Gephardt G, Guz B, Steinmuller D, Tubbs RR. Long-term follow-up after partial removal of a solitary kidney. N Engl J Med. 1991;325(15): 1058–62.

100. Bensalah K, Pantuck AJ, Rioux-Leclercq N, et al. Positive surgical margin appears to have negligible impact on survival of renal cell carcinomas treated by nephron-sparing surgery. Eur Urol. 2010;57(3):466–71.

101. Van Poppel H, Da Pozzo L, Albrecht W, et al. A prospective, randomised EORTC intergroup phase 3 study comparing the oncologic outcome of elective nephron-sparing surgery and radical nephrectomy for low-stage renal cell carcinoma. Eur Urol. 2011;59(4):543–52.

102. Licht MR, Novick AC, Goormastic M. Nephron sparing surgery in incidental versus suspected renal cell carcinoma. J Urol. 1994;152(1):39–42.

Thermal Ablation

Surena F. Matin and Kamran Ahrar

Introduction

With the increasing acceptance of partial nephrectomy as the standard of care for small renal cell carcinomas (RCCs), as well as its endorsement by groups such as the American Urological Association (AUA), nephron-sparing surgery will be increasingly employed [1, 2]. Partial nephrectomy has been shown to provide equivalent cancer control to that of radical nephrectomy, but with the additional advantage of renal preservation, which has important long-term health benefits [1]. Nevertheless, there are some patients with small RCCs, particularly elderly patients, those with severe renal dysfunction, and those with competing comorbidities, who may be poor candidates for surgical excision. Many of these patients are good candidates for thermal ablation, either by radiofrequency ablation (RFA) or by cryoablation. Recently published AUA

S.F. Matin, MD, FACS (✉)
Department of Urology, Minimally Invasive New Technology in Oncologic Surgery (MINTOS), The University of Texas MD Anderson Cancer Center, 1515 Holcombe Boulevard, Unit 1373, Houston, TX, 77030, USA
e-mail: surmatin@MDanderson.org

K. Ahrar, MD
Department of Diagnostic Radiology, Section of Interventional Radiology, The University of Texas MD Anderson Cancer Center, Houston, TX, USA
e-mail: kahrar@mdanderson.org

guidelines list ablative therapies as options for the management of patients with small renal masses [1].

Cytotoxic Mechanisms of Thermal Ablation

In RFA, friction of water molecules reacting to radiofrequencies generates heat which destroys tumor tissue. Under light microscopy chromatin blurring, increased cytoplasmic eosinophilia, loss of cell membrane integrity, and interstitial hemorrhage are the earliest changes seen in renal parenchyma [3]. Later, extensive coagulative necrosis with early infiltration of fibroblasts and acute inflammatory elements at the border of the RFA can be seen. Nuclear degeneration and acute inflammation becomes more pronounced after 1 week. Cell death occurs within minutes of exposure to temperatures at or above 50°C. Temperatures in the 50–100°C range are maintained homogeneously throughout the target area for optimal therapy [4]. High temperatures (greater than 100°C) can actually compromise treatment because tissue carbonization occurs, which limits heat conduction and thus the efficacy of RFA.

Cryoablation directly kills tumor cells by causing osmotic dehydration that damages enzymatic pathways, organelles, and the cell membrane and by causing intracellular ice formation that supercools the cytoplasmic contents [5, 6].

Small blood vessels are injured and in time become thrombotic resulting in a hypoxic tumor microenvironment that adds to the cytotoxicity [6, 7]. Four parameters determine the rate of cellular cytotoxicity: cooling rate, minimum temperature reached, time maintained at the minimum temperature, and thawing rate [5]. A temperature of −40°C must be achieved throughout the tumor; this typically occurs when the ice ball extends 0.5–1 cm beyond the tumor margins [8]. Faster cooling and slower thawing also improve cytotoxicity.

The Role of Diagnostic Biopsy in Patients Undergoing Thermal Ablation

If a patient has a small renal mass suspected to be RCC and is a candidate for ablative therapy, a biopsy is performed for histologic confirmation of malignancy. At our institution, we perform these biopsies as a separate and preliminary step before deciding whether to pursue aggressive therapy, because a substantial number of tumors will prove to be benign and not require treatment [9]. Thus, patients at high risk of complications with benign lesions are spared unnecessary procedures and anesthetics, as these have an indolent behavior that is unlikely to cause morbidity or shorten survival. The argument to not biopsy because of high non-diagnostic rates is no longer fully valid. The false-negative and non-diagnostic rates of percutaneous biopsy of renal masses have significantly improved in recent years as a result of improved techniques (such as core sampling in addition to fine-needle aspiration) and improved pathologic immunostaining panels [10–13]. Patients confirmed to have RCC should be counseled about therapeutic alternatives, such as the reference standard of partial nephrectomy and the possible appropriateness of active surveillance.

In addition to pretreatment biopsies, in some cases postablation biopsies may be needed, as evidence suggests that imaging by itself may not be not sufficient to confirm treatment success in all cases, as outlined below [14, 15].

Patient Selection and Preparation

The single most important requirement for the appropriate selection of patients for ablative therapy is the availability of good-quality imaging with a renal-protocol computed tomography (CT) or magnetic resonance imaging (MRI) examination. Thermal ablative treatments are all primarily guided by such imaging. The most ideal candidates for ablative therapy are patients with small (<3.5 cm) renal masses that are relatively exophytic and accessible percutaneously. In reality, many patients have variations of anatomy that present less ideal situations. Examples include tumors larger than 3.5 cm, tumors that are deeper and more central, and tumors in locations such as the anterior upper pole, which may be difficult to access percutaneously [16–18]. In particular, larger tumors and deeper tumors have a lower success rate with ablative therapies, as has been shown in multiple studies [17–19]. For example, Zagoria et al. showed that with each 1-cm increase in tumor diameter over 3.6 cm, the likelihood of recurrence-free survival decreased by a factor of 2.19 [18]. To enhance the effectiveness of ablation for larger tumors, some investigators have advocated embolization of the tumor prior to ablation [20]. Renal angiography and selective embolization of the tumor-feeding arteries can reduce perfusion-mediated cooling of the tissue (i.e., a heat-sink effect) during RFA, allowing a larger volume of tissue to attain a cytotoxic temperature.

Although tumor factors are important in determining the adequacy of an ablative therapy approach, patient-related factors are just as important and sometimes trump less than ideal indications for ablation. For example, we now often see patients who cannot be taken off anticoagulation agents, such as those with drug-eluting coronary stents; these patients have a very high risk of coronary thrombosis if the anticoagulants are acutely discontinued. Because ablative therapy minimizes the time off such compounds, it may represent the best form of treatment for these patients, even if they have less favorable tumor factors such as a central location or large size. Table 9.1 outlines our current indications for ablative therapy.

Table 9.1 Factors considered when evaluating patients for ablative therapy

Tumor factors
Tumor size: <3.5 cm most ideal
Tumor depth: peripheral more favorable than central
Tumor location: determination for percutaneous or laparoscopic access
Patient factors
Elderly physiologic age or health status unfit for major surgery
Major medical comorbidities or another primary malignancy that requires active therapy
Enlargement of renal mass to 3 cm in size during active surveillance
Need to minimize time off anticoagulation or antiplatelet compounds
Prior ipsilateral partial nephrectomy or other major renal surgery
Chronic kidney disease

The potential for complications still exists despite the minimally invasive nature of thermal ablative therapies. Also, given the lack of knowledge about the long-term results of these novel treatments, strict imaging surveillance is imperative for an indefinite period. Patients who are unable to meet these follow-up criteria—imaging surveillance and possible postablation biopsies—should not, in our opinion, be considered for ablative therapy.

Patients also must be medically cleared for delivery of general anesthesia. Although some centers perform ablative therapy with moderate sedation [21], our philosophy is that the likelihood for a single successful treatment depends on the ability to control respiratory excursion of the kidney, resulting in better targeting, and on allowing for treatment as long as is needed during the case. These two factors are critical for complete tumor ablation in a single procedure.

Techniques

Radiofrequency Ablation

After a needle biopsy confirms malignant histology, patients are referred to an interventional radiologist to assess whether the tumor is accessible percutaneously under CT or MRI guidance. On occasion repositioning the patient in the prone or oblique-prone position will shift some of the structures such as the spleen or colon away from the zone of treatment, allowing percutaneous therapy. Other adjunctive maneuvers, described below, may also be performed to mobilize or protect structures from heat injury. Tumors that remain in a difficult location or close to bowel or the ureter may require a laparoscopic approach, which allows mobilization of these structures away from the tumor and the intended zone of ablation. In the laparoscopic approach, initial electrode placement is performed under laparoscopic ultrasound guidance.

Our RFA technique has been previously described [22, 23]. Briefly, percutaneous RFA is performed with the patient under general anesthesia in prone position. RFA is delivered using a 200 W impedance-based device. One or more electrodes (depending on tumor size) are positioned into the tumor under CT guidance, and sequential overlapping ablations are then performed, depending on the size and location of the tumor, until it is completely ablated, along with a margin of surrounding normal tissue. Some interventional radiologists withdraw the electrode into the subcutaneous tissues and ablate the tract, although it is not clear that this is required. In cases in which the tumor may remain adjacent to critical structures such as the intestine, nonionic fluid (5% dextrose in water or sterile water) may be injected and hydrodissection performed, allowing displacement of the critical structures away from the area of intense heat [24]. Additional measures for protecting normal tissues from heat injury include irrigating cooled saline in a retrograde fashion through a ureteral catheter to protect the collecting system, rotating the RFA electrode to displace the kidney, and strategically placing an angioplasty balloon [25, 26]. Immediately after RFA treatment, contrast material is given intravenously to assess the ablation zone and confirm adequate treatment. Contrast-enhanced CT images taken immediately after ablation demonstrate a sharp boundary between the zone of ablation and the normal renal parenchyma. Mild, diffuse enhancement within

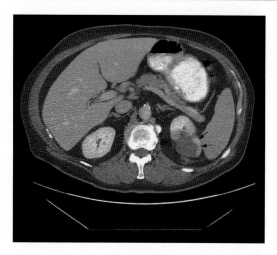

Fig. 9.1 Computed tomography scan 1 month after RFA of a left renal mass showing an enhancing crescent shaped area of unablated tumor (*arrows*). Repeat ablation was guided by this imaging, specifically targeting these areas. Copyright S.F. Matin 2011

the zone of ablation is expected with delayed images [27], but any nodular or crescent areas of intense enhancement are considered unablated (Fig. 9.1) [26]. Under these circumstances or when the margin of ablation is close to the tumor boundary, an RFA electrode can be placed directly into the area of concern, and an overlapping ablation can be performed. With this strategy, most renal tumors can be completely ablated in a single session.

Tumors that require laparoscopic RFA (such as anterior or medial tumors or those close to the renal hilum or ureter) are treated using a transperitoneal laparoscopic approach. The patient is placed in modified flank position, and access is gained using a Veress needle. A standard three-port approach is performed; the colon is mobilized, as are other critical structures, such as the ureter, as dictated by tumor location, and the area around the tumor is exposed. The perinephric fat is mobilized, except that overlying the tumor, which may either be left in place or sent for pathologic evaluation to confirm the absence of fat invasion. Intraoperative ultrasonography is then performed to evaluate the location of the tumor and its depth. At this point, small cautery marks are placed on the renal capsule at the margin of intended treatment to serve as visual

landmarks, as there will be significant shrinkage and distortion of anatomic landmarks during treatment. The RFA electrode is then placed into the tumor under ultrasound guidance until the tip is at the deepest tumor margin. This initial targeting is absolutely critical because visualization of this margin is most optimal *before* treatment. After RFA starts, the resulting vaporization and cavitation cause gas and microbubbles to form in the parenchyma, significantly degrading the ultrasound image and limiting accurate targeting. Once the deep margin is treated, the electrode is withdrawn partially and the process repeated. In addition to facilitating visualization, this maneuver actually achieves a vascular amputation of the more superficial untreated levels, such that the overlapping superficial ablations proceed more quickly. The electrode can also be repositioned as necessary into the more peripheral aspects of the zone of intended ablation, again treating from deepest to more superficial levels, until the entire tumor and margin are treated.

Cryoablation

Cryoablation has been described using a variety of access methods, including open, laparoscopic, and percutaneous. The open approach is now largely historical, although there are occasional cases of multifocal disease in which open partial nephrectomy can be combined with thermal ablation of additional lesions to minimize the ischemic interval [28]. The most common approach is laparoscopic, although an increasing number of publications report percutaneous route [29–31]. The laparoscopic approach is similar to that described for RFA, with a notable exception: during cryoablation, laparoscopic ultrasound guidance is utilized throughout the entire treatment process. The ice-ball edge is seen in excellent detail as an advancing hyperechoic rim with postacoustic shadowing. This ability to monitor the treatment probably is cryoablation's single greatest advantage. However, such monitoring requires significant mobilization of the kidney, because the postacoustic shadowing prevents visualization of the treatment edge opposite the ultrasound transducer. Therefore, the ultrasound probe needs to be navigated around the kidney at multiple locations in order to circumferentially visualize the advancing margin of treatment. This amount of renal mobilization and perinephric dissection is probably also the reason why surgical salvage of laparoscopic cases is rendered so difficult compared to salvage of percutaneous therapy, as discussed below.

Percutaneous cryoablation is also performed similarly to percutaneous RFA, as described above. Percutaneous cryoprobes are now smaller (17 gauge to 2.4 mm in diameter) than prior generation probes. As such, percutaneous cryoablation of most renal tumors requires strategic placement of more than one probe. A major advantage of percutaneous cryoablation over RFA is that growth of the ice ball can be carefully monitored using CT or MRI, allowing for optimal targeting. The ice ball appears as an area of low density on CT images, so the interface of the ice ball and the normal kidney is very well delineated. However, the boundary of the ice ball against the retroperitoneal fat, which also appears as low density on CT images, is less well defined. When percutaneous cryoablation is performed under MRI guidance, the ice ball can be imaged in multiple planes. It appears as an area of markedly low signal intensity on all pulse sequences (T1 or T2 weighted). Careful monitoring of the ice ball allows for modulation of cryogenic gases in different probes to prevent growth of the ice ball in one or more dimensions. This modulation provides an additional safety measure that is not possible with RFA. The inability to visualize beyond the advancing ice ball is the main reason that using solely ultrasound monitoring during percutaneous cryoablation cases is not recommended, as the medial (most inner) edges of the advancing ice ball cannot be adequately seen.

Whether cryoablation is done percutaneously or laparoscopically, two freeze/thaw cycles are performed, which optimizes tumor cytotoxicity. A margin of normal tissue of at least 0.5 cm beyond the tumor is treated; the ice-ball edge has been shown to represent a 0°C gradient, while 0.5 cm within the ball the temperature is −20°C, the minimum temperature required to achieve adequate tumor cytotoxicity [32]. The recent availability of thinner probes allows placement of multiple probes for ablation of larger tumors [33]. However, one concern is that the routine use of multiple probes may increase the risk of ice-ball related fracture, a complication unique to cryoablation that can predispose to significant hemorrhage during thawing [31]. In fact, in a recent analysis by Vricella and colleagues, the only significant predictors of complications after cryoablation were the number of cryoprobes used and comorbidity index [34].

Follow-Up and Outcomes After Thermal Ablative Therapy

Patients are seen 4–6 weeks after treatment for a renal-protocol CT or MRI examination, and if the initial imaging findings are favorable, patients return every 6 months for 2 years. After 2 years, depending on the findings of imaging and biopsy (if performed), semiannual, annual, or biannual follow-up is recommended. This follow-up schedule was recommended in a prior multi-institutional study and consensus statement [35].

Confirmatory biopsies after ablation are generally not performed in the first 6 months, as data suggest that in some cases, particularly after RFA, tumor and cellular architecture is preserved, possibly leading to false-positive biopsy findings [3, 36]. A postablative biopsy is considered, however, after 6 months, for any enlarging lesions or when there is a concern regarding recurrence, as discussed below.

Defining "Success"

Treatment has traditionally been considered successful on the basis of two findings on imaging studies, absence of enhancement and involution of the tumor. However, there can be confusion when thermally ablated lesions, in the absence of enhancement, do not involute. This scenario, which is common, complicates the traditional definition of success. Matsumoto and colleagues described the natural radiological history of

RFA-treated kidney tumors and showed that many tumors retained an appearance similar to that of the original tumor, but with absence of enhancement and involution [37]. There are reports showing viable cancer cells on percutaneous biopsies of ablated lesions in the absence of contrast enhancement [15]. As well, we have found that viable cancer cells are seen on biopsy in the absence of enhancement and tumor involution in approximately 8–10% of cases, at an average time of 23 months after ablation [38]. These cases essentially represent false-negative imaging findings.

As well, the potential exists for false-positive imaging findings, wherein there appears to be recurrence and progression of tumor as noted by new enhancement, enlargement, and infiltrative changes around the zone of ablation [14, 39]. Biopsies or resection in some of these cases have shown inflammation but no viable tumor despite extensive sampling [39, 40]. It is unknown what causes these de novo massive inflammatory reactions that frequently, if observed over time, lead to significant involution of the ablation zone [40]. Undoubtedly, however, these false-positive imaging scenarios complicate the clinical picture and can lead to unnecessary interventions or patient anxiety about cancer recurrence.

Biopsy samples should be obtained from any areas of nodular enhancement. In absence of any abnormal enhancement in the zone of ablation, a question arises as to the potential sampling bias of postablation biopsies. The zone of ablation is frequently larger initially than the original tumor because of treatment of a normal margin and, in some cases, tissue edema. Thus, needle biopsies, if not thoughtfully considered, may easily miss small foci of recurrence.

To address these concerns, our technique includes obtaining multi-quadrant core biopsy specimens (Fig. 9.2). A guide needle is inserted under CT or real-time CT fluoroscopic guidance into the center of the tumor. An automated, side-cutting core biopsy needle is inserted in coaxial fashion to obtain at least three biopsy samples. When the zone of ablation is large enough (at least 2 cm), the guide needle is then repositioned to obtain biopsy samples from the medial, lateral, superior, and inferior margins of the ablation zone. Samples from different areas of the ablation zone are labeled accordingly and submitted separately for pathologic analysis.

Functional Outcomes

In general, ablative therapies appear to cause less renal dysfunction than do partial nephrectomy and radical nephrectomy, although the data are likely subject to retrospective and selection biases. Lucas and colleagues compared renal function using estimated glomerular filtration rates in patients who underwent RFA, partial nephrectomy, or radical nephrectomy [41]. The investigators found that patients who underwent RFA maintained greater kidney function and were less likely to develop stage 3 chronic kidney disease than those who underwent partial nephrectomy or radical nephrectomy. In addition, Raman and colleagues evaluated patients with solitary kidneys and reported that those who underwent open partial nephrectomy with cold ischemia had a greater decline in kidney function than those who underwent RFA [42]. Another report of patients with solitary kidneys by Weisbrod and colleagues showed a large cohort treated by cryoablation with minimal change in renal function [43]. Jacobsohn et al. and Hoffmann et al., reporting on ablative therapy in patients with solitary kidneys, showed minimal reduction in kidney function in this high-risk cohort [23, 44]. While these retrospective reports may be biased by selection factors such as tumor size and tumor location, the weight of the data to date supports ablative therapy as a viable nephron-sparing approach.

Oncological Outcomes

It should be noted that there are significant differences among various studies with respect to definitions of local recurrence and the quality of reporting, complicating comparative analysis of this literature. This variability results from a multitude of limitations in the published literature.

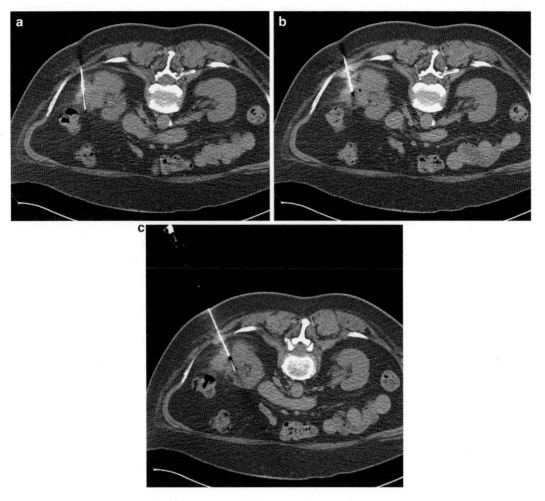

Fig. 9.2 (**a–c**) Figures showing multisite-directed CT-guided biopsy using an automated, side-cutting core biopsy needle, in order to maximize sampling of the zone of ablation. Copyright S.F. Matin 2011

For example, diagnostic pretreatment biopsies were not performed in most studies; thus, as a substantial portion of renal tumors prove to be benign, reports of survival and recurrence may be skewed. Additionally, it appears that the natural history of small RCCs is generally toward an indolent pattern of growth, thus the short follow-up of these lesions after ablative therapy has little significance [45]. Many investigators describe success as tumor eradication after a certain number of planned or unplanned treatments, and the published reports may not include this information. Variable definitions of success may also not clarify whether reported recurrences include

recurrence within the zone of ablation, in a separate area of the kidney that was not treated, and/or in an extrarenal site. These limitations in the literature were categorically described in the recent meta-analysis conducted by the AUA guidelines panel [2].

The AUA meta-analysis provides the most current summary of outcomes of various treatments for the small renal mass, including ablative therapies. Cryoablation and RFA were associated with significantly lower local recurrence-free survival (local RFS) rates (87–91%) than were surgical treatments (≥98%) [2]. This difference is made more pronounced by the fact that the follow-up period after ablative therapies was much shorter than that for open partial nephrectomy and other surgical treatments (median 18.2–19.4 months vs. 46.9 months for partial nephrectomy), suggesting that the local RFS rate seen after ablation may be even lower with longer follow-up. Metastatic RFS was high regardless of approach, but this finding may reflect the indolent nature of small renal tumors. This analysis provides valuable information that should be shared with patients during counseling.

Complications

Generally, complications related to ablation are secondary to local effects and less likely due to systemic adverse events [16, 22, 23, 46, 47]. Pain, paresthesia, neuromuscular complications, pneumothorax, and other adverse events have been reported [46, 48]. For example, Johnson et al. documented morbidity rates in a multi-institutional study from four centers involving 271 patients [48]. Complications were reported in 11.1% of patients, with the overwhelming majority of the complications classified as minor (9.2% of patients), largely consisting of pain or paresthesia at the site of probe insertion [48]. A recent meta-analysis of the published data reported major non-urological complication incidence rates in the 3–7% range and major urological complication incidence rates in the 3–8% range [2]. The rate of conversion to a more invasive or escalated procedure during cryoablation (3.5%) was nearly twice as high as during RFA (1.6%) [2].

Bleeding is generally uncommon after RFA relative to cryoablation. Small hematomas may be seen during imaging but may not be clinically evident. Transfusion incidence rates are reported in the 1–5% range [2]. Higher rates are seen with cryoablation, however, which is associated with the specific complication of ice-ball fracture as discussed previously. This complication may be caused by inadvertent torquing of the probe while the ice ball is formed, or possibly by the creation of larger cryolesions. The fracture may be hairline in size initially and not readily apparent during the freeze cycle, but during thawing, as

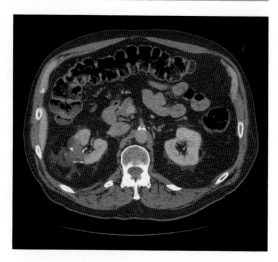

Fig. 9.3 Computed tomography scan 6 months after RFA of a right renal mass showing a small amount of urine extravasation into and around the zone of ablation. The patient was asymptomatic and observed. Copyright S.F. Matin 2011

vascularity is reestablished, sudden and significant hemorrhage can occur.

Hematuria and clot obstruction can occur with treatment of a more central tumor, and in cases of solitary kidneys, this complication can result in acute renal failure, which may require stent placement [23]. Concerns have been expressed about treatment of the urinary collecting system and formation of a urinary fistula, but animal and clinical evidence suggests that as long as the collecting system is not mechanically punctured, this adverse event is unlikely to result in a clinically meaningful adverse event [26]. Rarely, we have incidentally seen wisps of urine tracking within or just outside the ablation zone (Fig. 9.3). These patients are monitored and treated conservatively, with nearly every case showing resolution over time. Tract seeding of a tumor is exceedingly rare and is generally avoided with careful technique.

Ablation for Salvage of Previously Treated Kidneys

Repeat surgery in patients who have had prior partial nephrectomy or other renal procedures is much more difficult. The retroperitoneal and perinephric desmoplastic reaction can add significantly to the complexity of the case [49, 50]. Repeat partial nephrectomy is associated with significant rates of blood loss and morbidity and with a quantifiably higher mortality rate in some series [49]. In this setting, percutaneous ablative therapy may offer a viable, less morbid alternative to repeat partial nephrectomy, prompting some to recommend ablation as a primary option in those at high risk for reintervention, such as patients with von Hippel–Lindau syndrome [51–53].

A significant proportion of reported patients with a solitary kidney who are treated with ablative therapies had a prior partial nephrectomy. The results of such series indicate generally favorable outcomes despite the risks and challenges involved [23, 42–44]. For instance, Raman and colleagues published a multi-institutional study of patients with a solitary kidney treated with either partial nephrectomy or RFA; preservation of renal function favored RFA, possibly as a result of avoiding ischemic insults, although patient selection may have also contributed [42]. Similarly, Weisbrod and colleagues reported on cryoablation in 31 patients with a solitary kidney—the majority of whom had had prior ipsilateral renal procedures—and showed a 92% local tumor control rate, 1 day hospitalization, and a 20% major complication rate. In comparison, one can evaluate outcomes after repeat partial nephrectomy to appreciate the context of these outcomes. Liu and colleagues reported their experience with 25 patients undergoing repeat partial nephrectomy in a solitary kidney, showing an average of 2,400 ml blood loss, 8.5 h mean operative time, and a 52% major complication rate, which included one (4%) death and a 12% rate of renal loss requiring long-term hemodialysis [49]. Although the groups from these separate institutions likely have notable baseline differences, the dramatic difference in outcomes highlights the potentially important role of ablative therapy in the salvage setting, particularly if it can be delivered percutaneously.

However, surgical salvage of recurrence in previously ablated kidneys may also represent a surgical challenge. Nguyen et al. reported their experience with surgical salvage of RCC recurrence after thermal ablation, showing that cryoablation in particular can lead to extensive perinephric fibrosis, which can complicate or preclude attempted surgical salvage [54]. Of ten patients in whom partial nephrectomy was attempted, only two were able to have it done, and in most cases a laparoscopic approach was not feasible. Kowalczyk and colleagues reported their experience with partial nephrectomy in 13 patients after RFA, with no cases converted to radical nephrectomy [55]. The majority of patients had significant fibrosis present in the operative field, however, and operative times were long (7.8 h).

If one looks more critically at these studies, it appears that cases involving initial laparoscopic ablation, which were performed more frequently using cryoablation, are the ones in which the greatest difficulty is encountered and in which adverse events are most likely to occur. Cases treated percutaneously, which until recently were reported more frequently using RFA, are much easier to salvage, as the area of desmoplastic reaction is confined to the area of treatment and not throughout the entire perinephric space. To the point, when evaluating the data from Nguyen and colleagues, patients undergoing surgical salvage after RFA procedures (which were nearly all done percutaneously) had no intraoperative or postoperative complications, minimal blood loss, and no need for intraoperative blood transfusions [54].

The Future of Ablative Therapies

Other Ablative Therapies

Nearly every promising energy source has been investigated for invasive and noninvasive ablation of small renal tumors, including laser thermoablation [56, 57], photodynamic therapy [58], microwave thermotherapy [59, 60], high-intensity focused ultrasound (HIFU) [61, 62], and robotic four-dimensional radiotherapy [63]. To date, all these approaches have been associated with either: (1) technical challenges limiting their clinical application (e.g., laser, photodynamic therapy, microwaves); (2) inferior clinical outcomes (e.g., HIFU); or (3) only very preliminary experience that represents inadequate assessment of clinical potential (e.g., radiotherapy). Laser and microwave ablative therapy in particular have multiple parameters that have not been systematically studied, such as ideal wavelengths, power outputs, duration of treatment, or applicator size and type. Cryoablation and RFA thus remain the two most studied and clinically applied thermal ablative technologies to date.

Thermal Ablation as Part of an Immunotherapeutic Strategy

A novel aspect of thermal ablative therapy is its in situ treatment of malignancy, which not only destroys tissue but also initiates a local inflammatory cascade. Nonspecific inflammation has been linked as a key initial step in the development of specific immunologic events, such as rejection of transplanted organs and ischemia/reperfusion injury [64]. This potential ability of ablation to act as an in situ initiator of tumor-specific immune responses represents a potential new paradigm in the treatment of RCC and other cancers [65–67]. Case reports after cryoablation and RFA document tumor regression after ablation, even in cases of biopsy-proven metastatic disease [68]. In the majority of cases, however, such phenomena are not seen, leading to the conclusion that establishment of a nonspecific immune reaction may be insufficient by itself to trigger antitumor immune responses. There is therefore great interest in combining ablation with immune-modulating agents [65, 67]. This "combinatorial" therapy is yet to be investigated or clinically applied, but several investigators are actively researching this very interesting and novel aspect of ablation.

Summary

Thermal ablative therapy with RFA and cryoablation has gained a foothold in the armamentarium of treatments of the small renal mass. Rather than panacea, thermal ablation appears to be best suited for patients with difficult medical, anes-

thetic, or anatomic situations in whom the lower efficacy rates are balanced by the reduced risk of serious adverse events. Elderly patients with an enlarging mass, with extensive comorbidities, or those with a recurrence after prior partial nephrectomy represent situations where thermal ablation therapies may have their best roles. While newer energy modalities and delivery devices continue to be investigated, RFA and cryoablation continue to have the largest clinical experience and available data.

References

1. Campbell SC, Novick AC, Belldegrun A, et al. Guideline for management of the clinical T1 renal mass. J Urol. 2009;182(4):1271–9.
2. American Urological Association. Guideline for management of the clinical stage 1 renal mass; 2009. Available at http://wwwauanet.org. Accessed 11 Feb 2011.
3. Hsu TH, Fidler ME, Gill IS. Radiofrequency ablation of the kidney: acute and chronic histology in porcine model. Urology. 2000;56(5):872–5.
4. Goldberg SN, Gazelle GS, Mueller PR. Thermal ablation therapy for focal malignancy: a unified approach to underlying principles, techniques, and diagnostic imaging guidance. Am J Roentgenol. 2000;174(2):323–31.
5. Hoffmann NE, Bischof JC. The cryobiology of cryosurgical injury. Urology. 2002;60(2 Suppl 1):40–9.
6. Daum PS, Bowers Jr WD, Tejada J, Hamlet MP. Vascular casts demonstrate microcirculatory insufficiency in acute frostbite. Cryobiology. 1987;24(1):65–73.
7. Hoffmann NE, Bischof JC. Cryosurgery of normal and tumor tissue in the dorsal skin flap chamber: Part II – injury response. J Biomech Eng. 2001;123(4):310–6.
8. Finelli A, Rewcastle JC, Jewett MA. Cryotherapy and radiofrequency ablation: pathophysiologic basis and laboratory studies. Curr Opin Urol. 2003;13(3):187–91.
9. Tuncali K, van Sonnenberg E, Shankar S, Mortele KJ, Cibas ES, Silverman SG. Evaluation of patients referred for percutaneous ablation of renal tumors: importance of a preprocedural diagnosis. Am J Roentgenol. 2004;183(3):575–82.
10. Lebret T, Poulain JE, Molinie V, et al. Percutaneous core biopsy for renal masses: indications, accuracy and results. J Urol. 2007;178(4 Pt 1):1184–8 [discussion 8].
11. Liu J, Fanning CV. Can renal oncocytomas be distinguished from renal cell carcinoma on fine-needle aspiration specimens? A study of conventional smears

in conjunction with ancillary studies. Cancer. 2001;93(6):390–7.

12. Volpe A, Kachura JR, Geddie WR, et al. Techniques, safety and accuracy of sampling of renal tumors by fine needle aspiration and core biopsy. J Urol. 2007;178(2):379–86.

13. Kummerlin I, ten Kate F, Smedts F, et al. Core biopsies of renal tumors: a study on diagnostic accuracy, interobserver, and intraobserver variability. Eur Urol. 2008;53(6):1219–25.

14. Matin SF. Determining failure after renal ablative therapy for renal cell carcinoma: false-negative and false-positive imaging findings. Urology. 2010;75(6):1254–7.

15. Weight CJ, Kaouk JH, Hegarty NJ, et al. Correlation of radiographic imaging and histopathology following cryoablation and radio frequency ablation for renal tumors. J Urol. 2008;179(4):1277–81 [discussion 81–3].

16. Gervais DA, McGovern FJ, Arellano RS, McDougal WS, Mueller PR. Radiofrequency ablation of renal cell carcinoma: part 1, Indications, results, and role in patient management over a 6-year period and ablation of 100 tumors. Am J Roentgenol. 2005;185(1):64–71.

17. Tsivian M, Lyne JC, Mayes JM, Mouraviev V, Kimura M, Polascik TJ. Tumor size and endophytic growth pattern affect recurrence rates after laparoscopic renal cryoablation. Urology. 2010;75(2):307–10.

18. Zagoria RJ, Traver MA, Werle DM, Perini M, Hayasaka S, Clark PE. Oncologic efficacy of CT-guided percutaneous radiofrequency ablation of renal cell carcinomas. Am J Roentgenol. 2007;189(2):429–36.

19. Yoost TR, Clarke HS, Savage SJ. Laparoscopic cryoablation of renal masses: which lesions fail? Urology. 2010;75(2):311–4.

20. Yamakado K, Nakatsuka A, Kobayashi S, et al. Radiofrequency ablation combined with renal arterial embolization for the treatment of unresectable renal cell carcinoma larger than 3.5 cm: initial experience. Cardiovasc Intervent Radiol. 2006;29(3):389–94.

21. Gupta A, Allaf ME, Kavoussi LR, et al. Computerized tomography guided percutaneous renal cryoablation with the patient under conscious sedation: initial clinical experience. J Urol. 2006;175(2):447–52 [discussion 52–3].

22. Ahrar K, Matin S, Wood CG, et al. Percutaneous radiofrequency ablation of renal tumors: technique, complications, and outcomes. J Vasc Interv Radiol. 2005;16(5):679–88.

23. Jacobsohn KM, Ahrar K, Wood CG, Matin SF. Is radiofrequency ablation safe for solitary kidneys? Urology. 2007;69(5):819–23 [discussion 23].

24. Farrell MA, Charboneau JW, Callstrom MR, Reading CC, Engen DE, Blute ML. Paranephric water instillation: a technique to prevent bowel injury during percutaneous renal radiofrequency ablation. Am J Roentgenol. 2003;181(5):1315–7.

25. Cantwell CP, Wah TM, Gervais DA, et al. Protecting the ureter during radiofrequency ablation of renal cell cancer: a pilot study of retrograde pyeloperfusion with cooled dextrose 5% in water. J Vasc Interv Radiol. 2008;19(7):1034–40.

26. Gervais DA, Arellano RS, McGovern FJ, McDougal WS, Mueller PR. Radiofrequency ablation of renal cell carcinoma: part 2, lessons learned with ablation of 100 tumors. Am J Roentgenol. 2005;185(1):72–80.

27. Javadi S, Ahrar JU, Ninan E, Gupta S, Matin SF, Ahrar K. Characterization of contrast enhancement in the ablation zone immediately after radiofrequency ablation of renal tumors. J Vasc Interv Radiol. 2010;21(5):690–5.

28. Delworth MG, Pisters LL, Fornage BD, von Eschenbach AC. Cryotherapy for renal cell carcinoma and angiomyolipoma. J Urol. 1996;155(1):252–4.

29. Permpongkosol S, Nielsen ME, Solomon SB. Percutaneous renal cryoablation. Urology. 2006;68(1 Suppl):19–25.

30. Malcolm JB, Berry TT, Williams MB, et al. Single center experience with percutaneous and laparoscopic cryoablation of small renal masses. J Endourol. 2009;23(6):907–11.

31. Schmit GD, Atwell TD, Callstrom MR, et al. Percutaneous cryoablation of renal masses >/=3 cm: efficacy and safety in treatment of 108 patients. J Endourol. 2010;24:1255–62.

32. Campbell SC, Krishnamurthi V, Chow G, Hale J, Myles J, Novick AC. Renal cryosurgery: experimental evaluation of treatment parameters. Urology. 1998;52(1):29–33.

33. Atwell TD, Farrell MA, Callstrom MR, et al. Percutaneous cryoablation of 40 solid renal tumors with US guidance and CT monitoring: initial experience. Radiology. 2007;243(1):276–83.

34. Vricella GJ, Haaga JR, Adler BL, et al. Percutaneous cryoablation of renal masses: impact of patient selection and treatment parameters on outcomes. Urology. 2011;77(3):649–54.

35. Matin SF, Ahrar K, Cadeddu JA, et al. Residual and recurrent disease following renal energy ablative therapy: a multi-institutional study. J Urol. 2006;176(5):1973–7.

36. Raman JD, Stern JM, Zeltser I, Kabbani W, Cadeddu JA. Absence of viable renal carcinoma in biopsies performed more than 1 year following radio frequency ablation confirms reliability of axial imaging. J Urol. 2008;179(6):2142–5.

37. Matsumoto ED, Watumull L, Johnson DB, et al. The radiographic evolution of radio frequency ablated renal tumors. J Urol. 2004;172(1):45–8.

38. Karam JA, Ahrar K, Jonasch E, et al. Radiofrequency ablation (RFA) of renal tumors: clinical, radiographic, and pathologic results from a Tertiary Cancer Center. In: Genitourinary cancers symposium, San Francisco; 2010.

39. Lokken RP, Gervais DA, Arellano RS, et al. Inflammatory nodules mimic applicator track seeding

after percutaneous ablation of renal tumors. Am J Roentgenol. 2007;189(4):845–8.

40. Javadi S, Matin SF, Tamboli P, Ahrar K. Unexpected atypical findings on CT after radiofrequency ablation for small renal-cell carcinoma and the role of percutaneous biopsy. J Vasc Interv Radiol. 2007;18: 1186–91.

41. Lucas SM, Stern JM, Adibi M, Zeltser IS, Cadeddu JA, Raj GV. Renal function outcomes in patients treated for renal masses smaller than 4 cm by ablative and extirpative techniques. J Urol. 2008;179(1):75–9 [discussion 79–80].

42. Raman JD, Raj GV, Lucas SM, et al. Renal functional outcomes for tumours in a solitary kidney managed by ablative or extirpative techniques. BJU Int. 2010;105(4):496–500.

43. Weisbrod AJ, Atwell TD, Frank I, et al. Percutaneous cryoablation of masses in a solitary kidney. Am J Roentgenol. 2010;194(6):1620–5.

44. Hoffmann RT, Jakobs TF, Kubisch CH, et al. Renal cell carcinoma in patients with a solitary kidney after nephrectomy treated with radiofrequency ablation: mid term results. Eur J Radiol. 2010;73(3):652–6.

45. Chawla SN, Crispen PL, Hanlon AL, Greenberg RE, Chen DY, Uzzo RG. The natural history of observed enhancing renal masses: meta-analysis and review of the world literature. J Urol. 2006;175(2):425–31.

46. Bhayani SB, Allaf ME, Su LM, Solomon SB. Neuromuscular complications after percutaneous radiofrequency ablation of renal tumors. Urology. 2005;65(3):592.

47. Weizer AZ, Raj GV, O'Connell M, Robertson CN, Nelson RC, Polascik TJ. Complications after percutaneous radiofrequency ablation of renal tumors. Urology. 2005;66(6):1176–80.

48. Johnson DB, Solomon SB, Su LM, et al. Defining the complications of cryoablation and radio frequency ablation of small renal tumors: a multi-institutional review. J Urol. 2004;172(3):874–7.

49. Liu NW, Khurana K, Sudarshan S, Pinto PA, Linehan WM, Bratslavsky G. Repeat partial nephrectomy on the solitary kidney: surgical, functional and oncological outcomes. J Urol. 2010;183(5):1719–24.

50. Bratslavsky G, Liu JJ, Johnson AD, et al. Salvage partial nephrectomy for hereditary renal cancer: feasibility and outcomes. J Urol. 2008;179(1):67–70.

51. Matin SF, Ahrar K, Wood CG, Daniels M, Jonasch E. Patterns of intervention for renal lesions in von Hippel–Lindau disease. BJU Int. 2008;102(8):940–5.

52. Pautler SE, Pavlovich CP, Mikityansky I, et al. Retroperitoneoscopic-guided radiofrequency ablation of renal tumors. Can J Urol. 2001;8(4):1330–3.

53. Shingleton WB, Sewell Jr PE. Percutaneous renal cryoablation of renal tumors in patients with von Hippel–Lindau disease. J Urol. 2002;167(3):1268–70.

54. Nguyen CT, Lane BR, Kaouk JH, et al. Surgical salvage of renal cell carcinoma recurrence after thermal ablative therapy. J Urol. 2008;180(1):104–9 [discussion 9].

55. Kowalczyk KJ, Hooper HB, Linehan WM, Pinto PA, Wood BJ, Bratslavsky G. Partial nephrectomy after previous radio frequency ablation: the National Cancer Institute experience. J Urol. 2009;182(5): 2158–63.

56. Dick EA, Wragg P, Joarder R, et al. Feasibility of abdomino-pelvic T1-weighted real-time thermal mapping of laser ablation. J Magn Reson Imaging. 2003;17(2):197–205.

57. Gettman MT, Lotan Y, Lindberg G, et al. Laparoscopic interstitial laser coagulation of renal tissue with and without hilar occlusion in the porcine model. J Endourol. 2002;16(8):565–70.

58. Matin SF, Tinkey PT, Borne AT, Stephens LC, Sherz A, Swanson DA. A pilot trial of vascular targeted photodynamic therapy for renal tissue. J Urol. 2008;180(1): 338–42.

59. Murota T, Kawakita M, Oguchi N, et al. Retroperitoneoscopic partial nephrectomy using microwave coagulation for small renal tumors. Eur Urol. 2002;41(5):540–5.

60. Terai A, Ito N, Yoshimura K, et al. Laparoscopic partial nephrectomy using microwave tissue coagulator for small renal tumors: usefulness and complications. Eur Urol. 2004;45(6):744–8.

61. Illing RO, Kennedy JE, Wu F, et al. The safety and feasibility of extracorporeal high-intensity focused ultrasound (HIFU) for the treatment of liver and kidney tumours in a Western population. Br J Cancer. 2005;93(8):890–5.

62. Hacker A, Michel MS, Marlinghaus E, Kohrmann KU, Alken P. Extracorporeally induced ablation of renal tissue by high-intensity focused ultrasound. BJU Int. 2006;97(4):779–85.

63. Ponsky LE, Crownover RL, Rosen MJ, et al. Initial evaluation of Cyberknife technology for extracorporeal renal tissue ablation. Urology. 2003;61(3):498–501.

64. Lieberthal W. Biology of ischemic and toxic renal tubular cell injury: role of nitric oxide and the inflammatory response. Curr Opin Nephrol Hypertens. 1998;7:289–95.

65. Sidana A, Chowdhury WH, Fuchs EJ, Rodriguez R. Cryoimmunotherapy in urologic oncology. Urology. 2010;75(5):1009–14.

66. Staren ED, Sabel MS, Gianakakis LM, et al. Cryosurgery of breast cancer. Arch Surg. 1997;132(1):28–33.

67. Matin SF, Sharma P, Gill IS, et al. Immunological response to renal cryoablation in an in vivo orthotopic renal cell carcinoma murine model. J Urol. 2010;183(1):333–8.

68. Sanchez-Ortiz RF, Tannir N, Ahrar K, Wood CG. Spontaneous regression of pulmonary metastases from renal cell carcinoma after radio frequency ablation of primary tumor: an in situ tumor vaccine? J Urol. 2003;170(1):178–9.

Active Surveillance of the Small Renal Mass

10

Marc C. Smaldone, Daniel Canter,
Alexander Kutikov, and Robert G. Uzzo

Introduction

Kidney cancer, predominantly renal cell carcinoma (RCC), is among the most lethal of urologic malignancies. In 2010, approximately 58,240 men and women were diagnosed with cancer of the kidney or renal pelvis, and 13,040 (22.4%) will ultimately succumb to their disease [1]. Due to increased utilization of cross-sectional abdominal imaging over the past several decades [2, 3], a stage and size migration towards the detection of smaller localized renal tumors (<4 cm) has been observed in large population-based cohorts. Likewise, mean tumor size at diagnosis has decreased over time, and in 2004 tumors <3 cm represented 43.4% of all stage I tumors detected (Fig. 10.1) [4, 5]. As a result incidental detection of asymptomatic lesions now accounts for more than half of all renal masses

discovered [6]. Radiographic stage I small renal masses (SRMs) represent a heterogenous entity, with as many as 20% being benign [7] and an estimated 20–30% being potentially aggressive [8, 9]. As the incidence of SRM diagnoses has risen, an increase in the median age at RCC diagnosis has also been observed, with the most significant rise demonstrated in patients between 70 and 90 years of age [10]. However, while the rates of renal surgery have risen in conjunction with increased tumor detection, mortality rates have paradoxically risen as well [3]. These findings indicate that a proportion of SRMs represent indolent disease that may not require surgical excision and have led to the reassessment of contemporary practice patterns for incidentally diagnosed lesions.

Traditionally, clinical stage I renal masses have been treated with surgical excision, most commonly by radical nephrectomy [11]. However, concern that radical nephrectomy may predispose patients to the sequelae of chronic kidney disease (CKD) [12, 13], including increased cardiovascular risk and shortened overall survival [14–16], has led to the increased utilization of nephron sparing procedures with the goal of preserving long-term renal function without affecting cancer control [17]. With technological advances, laparoscopic [18] and robotic [19] platforms have now become well established in the armamentarium of nephron-sparing techniques, resulting in contemporary management of SRMs which is substantially less radical and less invasive.

M.C. Smaldone
123 Winchester Road, Merion Station, PA 19066, USA

Division of Urologic Oncology,
Department of Surgical Oncology,
Fox Chase Cancer Center,
333 Cottman Avenue, Philadelphia, PA 19111, USA
e-mail: marc.smaldone@fccc.edu

D. Canter • A. Kutikov • R.G. Uzzo (✉)
Division of Urologic Oncology,
Department of Surgical Oncology,
Fox Chase Cancer Center, 333 Cottman Avenue,
Philadelphia, PA 19111, USA
e-mail: Robert.Uzzo@fccc.edu

S.C. Campbell and B.I. Rini (eds.), *Renal Cell Carcinoma: Clinical Management*, Current Clinical Urology,
DOI 10.1007/978-1-62703-062-5_10, © Springer Science+Business Media New York 2013

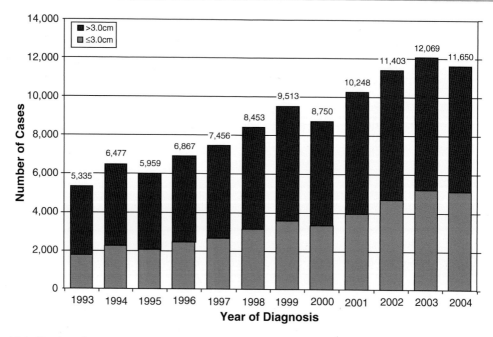

Fig. 10.1 Number of stage I renal cell carcinoma cases by diagnosis year (1993–2004) stratified by tumor size (<3 cm or ≥3 cm). (Reproduced with permission from "Cooperberg et al. Decreasing size at diagnosis of stage 1 renal cell carcinoma: Analysis from the national cancer database, 1993 to 2004. The Journal of Urology (2008); 179(6):2132"; American Urological Association by Elsevier, Inc.)

Beyond excision, tumor ablation has been broadly applied, despite a lack of meaningful published endpoints and short median follow-up periods, thereby confounding treatment decisions [20, 21]. Whereas 5-year cancer-specific survival of surgically treated stage I SRMs remains in excess of 95% [20], the formidability of RCC tumor biology has been questioned as no treatment data have been compared to lesions managed expectantly [22]. Moreover, there is a growing recognition that competing risks to longevity from comorbidities may outweigh the benefit of intervention in elderly and infirmed patients [23].

Over diagnosis of malignancy, along with receipt of unneeded treatment as well as its attendant risks, is arguably the most important harm associated with early cancer detection [24]. Conceptually, the practice of observing documented malignancies has precedence in the urologic and oncologic communities. "Watchful waiting" of elderly men with prostate cancer and substantial comorbidity has become a standard option, with definitive androgen deprivation therapy held until documentation of metastatic

disease. This management strategy has evolved and has been extended to younger and healthier men with low-volume, low-risk prostate cancer. Coined "active surveillance (AS) with delayed curative intent," immediate intervention is deferred to avoid the potential morbidities of treatment. These men are closely followed with serial PSAs, physical exams, and repeat prostate biopsies at defined intervals with the intention of undergoing active treatment if there is evidence for clinical progression of disease [25]. Although this management strategy is still in the early phases of investigation in men with prostate cancer [26], AS has recently been applied in select patients with SRMs and significant competing risks with intriguing results. Although limited by small cohorts and retrospective methodology, the current AS in SRM data represents perhaps the most comprehensive observational data for any solid organ malignancy to date. In this chapter we aim to define the malignant potential of the SRM based on preoperative radiographic characteristics, describe contemporary AS protocols, summarize the existing body of evidence

Fig. 10.2 Probability of high-grade disease vs. tumor size in localized renal cell carcinoma. (Reproduced with permission from "Rothman et al. Histopathological characteristics of localized renal cell carcinoma correlate with tumor size: A SEER analysis. The Journal of Urology (2009); 181(1):32"; American Urological Association by Elsevier, Inc.)

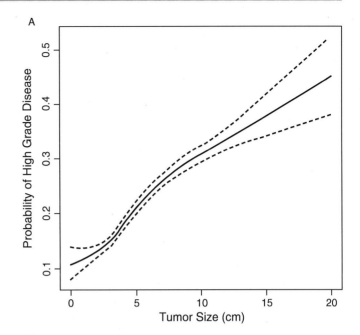

investigating the natural history of SRMs under AS, and identify which clinical and radiographic characteristics are associated with progression to metastatic disease while under AS.

Assessing the Malignant and Metastatic Potential of the Small Renal Mass

Considerable effort has been undertaken to identify preoperative radiographic characteristics of renal masses associated with malignant potential and disease progression. Currently, the most reproducible imaging characteristic on cross-sectional imaging is tumor size, and recent large series have demonstrated that as maximal linear tumor diameter increases, there is increased risk of malignant vs. benign pathology [27, 28], high-grade vs. low-grade disease [27–29], clear cell vs. more indolent histology [28, 29], and presence of synchronous metastases [30–32]. In a cohort of 2,770 patients with sporadic, unilateral, localized renal masses, Frank et al. reported that increasing tumor diameter was associated with malignant pathology [OR 1.17 (CI 1.08–1.26); $p<0.001$], clear cell vs. papillary histology [OR 1.17 (CI 1.11–1.23); $p<0.001$], and high-grade

nuclear features [stratified by clear cell, OR 1.32 (CI 1.27–1.37); $p<0.001$ or papillary, OR 1.12 (CI 1.06–1.19); $p<0.001$; histology] [27]. In a smaller retrospective series comparing 168 renal tumors ≤3 cm with 119 renal tumors >3–4 cm, Remzi et al. reported decreased rates of local extension (pT3a 19.1% vs. 35.7%, $p<0.05$), high grade (Fuhrman grades 3–4) disease (9.2% vs. 25.5%, $p<0.05$), and synchronous metastasis (M+2.4% vs. 8.4%, $p=0.05$) in patients with smaller lesions [9]. In a large single institution cohort of 2,675 renal tumors treated surgically, Thompson et al. reported similar risks of malignant pathology [OR 1.16 (CI 1.11–1.22); $p<0.001$] and high-grade disease [OR 1.25 (CI 1.21–1.30); $p<0.001$]. In fact, in this subset the incidence of high-grade lesions increased from 0% for tumors <1 cm to 59% for tumors >7 cm [28]. Using data from SEER, Rothman et al. investigated the relationship between primary tumor size at presentation and histopathological features in 19,932 patients with localized renal tumors. Findings of this study demonstrate that for each 1 cm increase in size, the probability of a high-grade tumor increased by 13% (OR 1.13, $p<0.001$) [29] (Fig. 10.2). Interestingly, while almost 85% of RCCs <4 cm were low grade, 70% of lesions >7 cm were also low-grade lesions, suggesting that a large proportion of localized renal tumors can grow quite large without acquiring metastatic potential.

While it is clear from available data that a significant proportion of SRMs are more indolent whereas only a small minority represent high-grade lesions, the biology of these lesions must be distinguished from the infrequent case of a small renal mass with aggressive malignant characteristics and synchronous metastatic disease. Using data from a single institution tumor registry, Kunkle et al. compared 110 patients with biopsy-proven synchronous metastatic disease at presentation to 250 controls with clinically localized RCC. Study findings revealed that tumors associated with synchronous metastasis were significantly larger compared to clinically localized lesions (median 8.0 cm vs. 4.5 cm, $p < 0.0001$), and the odds of synchronous metastasis increased by 22% for each 1 cm increase in tumor size ($p < 0.0001$) [30]. Importantly, no patients with tumors 2 cm or smaller presented with biopsy-proven metastatic disease, and less than 5% of all systemic metastases occurred in patients with tumors <3 cm. Although a clear association between tumor size and risk of metastasis has not been determined, most current reports utilize a 3 cm threshold that has been extrapolated from clinical data in patients with von Hippel–Lindau syndrome [33]. Using SEER data from 24,000 patients, Nguyen et al. estimated the risk of synchronous metastases to be <5% for patients with a primary tumor size ≤3 cm [31], thereby substantiating this threshold. Similarly, in a large single institution cohort of 2,691 patients with sporadic renal tumors, Thompson et al. demonstrated an association between tumor size and metastasis-free survival (HR 1.24, $p < 0.001$) and reported that only 1 in 781 (0.1%) patients with tumors <3 cm presented with synchronous metastatic disease [32].

Competing Risk Assessment in Patients with Localized Renal Masses

While surgical resection of SRMs in young, healthy patients is currently the accepted standard of care [20], management of localized RCC in elderly or infirmed patients in which comorbid medical conditions compete with RCC malignant potential as primary causes of death represents a unique set of challenges. Most contemporary RCC predictive models combine pathologic characteristics such as tumor grade, presence of tumor necrosis, vascular invasion, and, in some cases, molecular markers in attempts to predict disease recurrence following definitive therapy [34–43]. While these existing models are useful to help guide postoperative management, their utility is limited in the preoperative setting as clinical metrics such as comorbid indices or performance status [44] are not incorporated. As a result, new tools are needed to quantitate survival differences and improve effective decision-making in the preoperative setting. In an effort to predict disease recurrence following nephrectomy, Cindolo et al. included clinical presentation as well as tumor size on preoperative imaging in an analysis of pooled multi-institutional data of patients undergoing treatment for localized RCC. However, the utility of this instrument for preoperative assessment is also limited by inclusion of pathologic features to determine risk stratification [45]. Similarly, nomograms purely based on preoperative clinical and imaging characteristics have been developed to predict disease recurrence and metastasis , However, since these predictive models do not address competing health risks or survival, their clinical utility in the pre operative setting is limited [46, 47].

Recent reports have highlighted the discrepancy between cancer-specific risk of death and competing risk from comorbidity. Data from an EORTC trial comparing oncologic efficacy of radical and partial nephrectomy for localized tumors ≤5 cm revealed that, of 117 deaths over a median follow-up period of 9.3 years, 10.3% were a result of RCC compared to 89.7% from other cause [48]. In an institutional series of 537 patient >75 years of age with renal masses <7 cm, Lane et al. reported that over a median follow-up period of 3.9 years, the most common cause of death was cardiovascular (29%) compared to cancer progression (4%) [49]. Two contemporary studies have attempted to quantitate competing risks of death in patients with RCC utilizing the Charlson comorbidity index (CCI). Santos Arrontes et al. reported the results of a retrospective competing risk analysis in 192 patients with clear cell RCC. With a median follow-up of less than 4 years, there were a total of 72 patient deaths, 45 of which (63%) were attributed to RCC. Patients with clinically localized RCC and a CCI >2 demonstrated significantly reduced overall survival compared to patients with a CCI ≤2, whereas there were no significant differences in survival between CCI stratified groups with locally advanced or metastatic RCC. Interpreting these findings, the authors concluded that patients with CCI scores >2 do not gain a survival advantage from the surgical treatment of localized RCC [50]. Using the SEER database, Hollingsworth et al. performed a competing risks analysis in 26,618 patients undergoing surgical treatment of RCC. Stratified into 20 groups by tumor size and age at presentation, 5-year mortal-ity estimates were generated for cancer-specific and competing cause mortality [51]. Not surprisingly, they found that patients with the smallest tumors had the lowest cancer-specific survival, and that competing cause mortality increased with age. The authors reported that irrespective of tumor size, 5-year competing cause mortality was 28.2% in patients ≥70 years, and concluded that reevaluation of initial management strategy was necessary in select patients with SRMs.

In an effort to refine a clinical tool to stratify the competing risks of comorbidity and tumor malignant potential, Kutikov et al. developed a comprehensive nomogram to predict 5-year risk of kidney cancer death, death from other malignancy, and noncancer death utilizing select preoperative clinical and demographic variables (Fig. 10.3) [23]. In this large cohort of 30,000

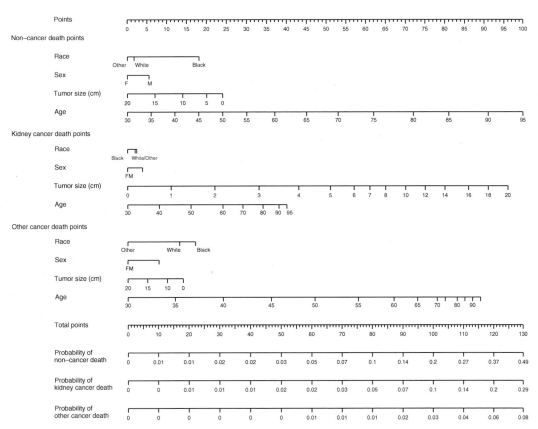

Fig. 10.3 Nomogram evaluating 5-year competing risks of death in patients with localized renal cell carcinoma. Total point values are independently calculated for each cause of death and then applied to the corresponding probability scale at the bottom of the figure. (Reproduced with permission from "Kutikov et al. Evaluating Overall Survival and Competing Risks of Death in Patients With Localized Renal Cell Carcinoma Using a Comprehensive Nomogram. The Journal of Clinical Oncology (2010); 28(2):315"; American Society of Clinical Oncology.)

patients with localized RCC identified from the SEER database, age ($p<0.001$), race ($p<0.001$), gender ($p<0.002$), and tumor size ($p<0.001$) were associated with mortality, while histologic subtype was not significantly associated with mortality and was excluded from the model. For example, utilizing this nomogram, a 75-year-old white male with a 4 cm tumor would have a 5-year predicted disease specific mortality of 5% vs. 4.5% from other malignancies and 14% from noncancerous causes. Although externally validated in another large SEER cohort [52], specific comorbidity information was not available for inclusion in this initial analysis, thereby limiting the nomogram's clinical utility. In an effort to address these limitations, our institution is currently working to enhance the nomogram by incorporating comorbidity data [53].

Role of Percutaneous Biopsy, Molecular Markers, and Non-extirpative Prediction of Malignant Potential

When an incidental renal mass is identified, a diagnosis of malignancy is presumed based on enhancement with contrast on cross-sectional imaging [20]. Preoperative counseling and treatment planning are often made in the context of this uncertainty despite the fact that 20–30% of these lesions ultimately prove benign while less than 30% are found to be potentially aggressive [7, 27]. The ability to match renal mass biology with an appropriate treatment strategy remains an elusive goal of modern urologic oncology [54]. While efforts have been made to predict malignant potential using preoperative clinical and radiographic variables [55, 56], to date the clinical utility of non-extirpative diagnostic strategies including percutaneous biopsy and pathological predictive models remains limited [57].

Percutaneous Biopsy

Traditionally, non-extirpative assessment of enhancing renal mass pathology has been largely restricted to percutaneous biopsy. Biopsy of the enhancing renal mass has been limited due to risks, sampling error and clinically irrelevant data obtained and historically was reserved only for cases where lymphoma, infection, or a metastasis from another organ to the kidney was suspected [58]. Using pooled data from a large systematic review of the literature, Lane et al. reported that prior to 2001, renal biopsy exhibited an 81% accuracy rate with four out of five biopsies correctly predicting the tumor's pathology [58]. Recently, the utility of percutaneous renal biopsy has been reexamined in select patients, and modern series utilizing 18 gauge core biopsies and improved immunohistological characterization techniques have reported improved accuracy in differentiating benign from malignant histologic types (>90%) with minimal procedure-related complications [59]. When a malignancy is found on biopsy, the positive predictive value is reported to be over 95%, and reported risks of minor complications (<5%) or tumor seeding (<0.01%) are exceedingly low [58]. Meanwhile, negative predictive value appears to be over 80% with most contemporary series reporting false negative rates less than 5% [59, 60]. Despite these improvements, small tumor size has been associated with a "nondiagnostic" biopsy, with a recent series reporting presence of insufficient tissue for diagnosis in 37% of tumors <3 cm compared to only 9% of tumors ≥3 cm [61]. While the accuracy of renal biopsy in determining histologic subtype has substantially increased, most modern series do not assess tumor grade [58] which has established prognostic implications for cancer-specific survival [62]. In fact, contemporary series utilizing modern core biopsy techniques have reported distinction of tumor grading in only 62.7% of patients undergoing biopsy as part of an active surveillance protocols [63], and underestimation of nuclear grade has been noted in more than half (55%) of patients undergoing biopsy prior to surgical resection [64].

While there is renewed interest in the utility of percutaneous biopsy in the management of the SRM, its role remains controversial in the urologic community [57]. In a recent national survey of consultant urologists in the United Kingdom, 34% reported always using biopsy in the treatment algorithm of small indeterminate renal masses; however, the majority of the sample reported either selectively (23%) or never using biopsy (43%) to inform their management decisions [65]. What remains to be determined is what precise impact does information from a biopsy have on treatment decisions, and does it justify associated procedural risks and costs? In an early retrospective review of 79 image-guided renal mass biopsies in 73 patients, clinical management was altered in 41% of cases managed nonoperatively [66]. In a contemporary series of 152 biopsies using 18 gauge core biopsy technique, Maturen et al. reported highly accurate sensitivity (97.7%), specificity (100%), positive predictive value (100%), and negative predictive values (100%) for malignancy, stating that biopsy results significantly impacted clinical management in 60.5% of cases [67]. Although these results are limited by selection bias, these findings have led some authors to change their practice to recommend a CT-guided biopsy of all SRMs before treatment to confirm malignancy, classify histologic subtype, and establish tumor grade [68]. While use of biopsy has evolved and gained traction, it has yet not been accepted as an alternative to resection in young or otherwise healthy candidates for excision, and it is currently utilized on a selective basis in patients with absolute or relative indications, or specific circumstances such as synchronous bilateral lesions [69].

Molecular Markers

Molecular biomarkers obtained from percutaneous biopsy specimens that could accurately predict aggressive RCC phenotypic features would be an ideal means of matching treatment strategy to tumor biology on an individual patient level [54]. Although a discussion of the many biomarkers currently being studied in RCC (primarily to predict disease recurrence following surgical resection) is beyond the scope of this chapter, molecular markers of cellular proliferation and apoptosis currently under investigation include Ki-67 (a nuclear antigen

that is a marker of active cellular proliferation) [70, 71], p53 (marker of apoptosis) [72, 73], HER-2 (epidermal growth factor) [74], vascular endothelial growth factor (VEGF) [75], bcl-2 (apoptotic inhibitor) [76], cyclin-D1 (cell-cycle regulatory molecule) [77], vimentin (epithelial cell adhesion molecule) [78], C-reactive inflammatory protein [79], carbonic anhydrase IX (cell surface transmembrane enzyme upregulated by hypoxia-inducible factor in low oxygen environments) [80], among others [81]. Unfortunately, although many show promise, few, if any, of these preliminary data can be considered robust enough to be relevant or even applicable in determining which patients with SRMs require immediate intervention and which can be safely observed [54].

For the purpose of this review, we focus on the current body of evidence investigating biomarker activity in lesions initially managed with a period of radiographic surveillance. In six localized and 12 metastatic ($n = 12$) tumors, Fujimoto et al. analyzed argyrophilic nucleolar organizer regions (AgNORs) and proliferating cell nuclear antigen (PCNA) activity, reporting that, in localized tumors, tumor doubling time was inversely proportional to, and significantly correlated with, AgNOR expression and PCNA activity [82]. In 18 patients with localized SRMs, Kato et al. measured cell proliferation and apoptosis using the marker Ki-67 and the transferase-mediated dUTP-biotin nick (TUNEL) assay. They reported that tumor growth rate was associated with a positive TUNEL ratio, but not with degree of Ki-67 immunostaining [83]. In an early series investigating growth kinetics of SRMs under observation, Oda et al. observed that the growth rate of incidentally found RCCs varied and that the initial clinical and pathological features did not predict subsequent tumor growth [84]. To further characterize these lesions, the authors examined cell proliferation, apoptosis, and angiogenesis in 16 incidentally found cases of RCC, using the Ki-67 labeling index (KI), apoptotic index (AI), and TUNEL technique. They found that while KI and AI were not associated with each other or tumor growth rates, the KI/AI ratio was strongly correlated with tumor growth rate ($r=0.71$; $p=0.01$) [85]. Unfortunately, the role of biomarkers in the selection and management of patients under AS is currently limited [54]. Until molecular markers specific for malignant or metastatic potential are identified and validated, alternative prognostic tools are required to help stratify risk in patients presenting with incidentally diagnosed SRMs.

Imaging Techniques

Currently, multiphase contrast-enhanced imaging (CT or MRI) scanning provides the best evaluation of a renal mass, namely enhancement characteristics, assessment of bilateral renal flow and function, and clinical (radiographic) staging data. Unfortunately, while contrast-based cross-sectional imaging can distinguish most renal cystic lesions from solid masses, it provides minimal biological information to predict a tumor's natural history. Existing imaging methods cannot definitively distinguish between benign and malignant solid tumors, RCC histologic subtypes, or indolent vs. aggressive tumor biology. Molecular imaging, such as positron emission tomography (PET), has the potential to characterize biologic processes at the cellular and subcellular level noninvasively in addition to providing the macroscopic detail obtained from CT or MRI. The use of 2-deoxy-2-[^{18}F] fluoro-D-glucose (^{18}F-FDG) to functionally image malignancies is based on the anticipated altered glycolytic pathway in malignant cells. When used in combination with standard CT, ^{18}F-FDG PET (PET-CT) provides both functional and anatomic tumor data thereby improving the diagnostic accuracy and tumor localization for a number of solid malignancies vs. either modality alone [86]. While there was initial enthusiasm for the utilization of ^{18}F-FDG-PET to diagnose, stage, or restage renal lesions, there are significant limitations to its clinical applicability. Summarized by Lawrentschuk et al., these series are comprised of a number of small reports (samples ranging from 4 to 66) with sensitivities for diagnosis ranging from 32% to 100% and for staging ranging from 47% to 75% [87]. While a majority of these studies were performed prior to combination scanning, reported false negative results are as high as 68%, severely limiting the utility of ^{18}F-FDG-PET for the initial assessment of primary renal masses.

Alternative molecular agents reflecting aberrant cellular pathways such as cellular oxidative metabolism, DNA synthesis, and tumor hypoxia tracers are currently under development and are in the early phases of investigation in RCC [88–90]. However, antibody-based molecular imaging, or immuno-PET, appears to offer a more clinically relevant strategy to improve molecular/biologic imaging in RCC. Immuno-PET offers the promise of highly selective binding to cancer-specific antigens to provide radiographically recognizable molecular targets, and enthusiasm for this imaging technique parallels recent progress in the development of small molecule targeted therapy for RCC. In an early phase I pilot study imaging 26 patients with renal masses prior to surgery, immuno-PET using a monoclonal antibody to CA IX labeled with ^{124}I (^{124}I-G250-PET) was able to discriminate between ccRCC and non-ccRCC with a high sensitivity (94%) and specificity (100%) and no serious drug-related adverse events [91]. This has led to considerable enthusiasm regarding the potential for the development of a first in class histologically specific imaging modality with the ability to offer relevant preoperative biological data. In a multi-institutional phase III study (REDECT trial) including 202 patients, ^{124}I-G250-PET/CT was able to discriminate ccRCC from non-ccRCC with a much higher sensitivity (86%) and specificity (87%) compared to conventional CT, with a 95% positive predictive value and no associated serious adverse events [92]. In comparison with previous efforts demonstrating only questionable or theoretical utility of molecular imaging to guide clinical decision making, results from the REDECT trial demonstrate that immuno-PET can be used to provide important preoperative diagnostic information that may help guide optimal therapy.

Preoperative Non-extirpative Assessment of Malignant Potential

Algorithms have been developed with the aim of predicting the biological potential of SRMs prior to intervention. Using a large institutional cohort, Lane et al. constructed a nomogram based on the findings that gender, tumor size, and smoking history were predictive of malignant vs. benign disease. However, the concordance index (CI) of this model was a modest 0.64. Furthermore, additional efforts to differentiate indolent from aggressive cancers yielded a CI of 0.56, accuracy that is only slightly better than a flip of a coin [56]. Utilizing a multi-institutional dataset, Jeldres et al. developed a tool with the aim of accurately predicting high-grade (Fuhrman grades 3–4) features at nephrectomy using four covariates (age at diagnosis, gender, tumor size, and symptom classification). Of these factors, only tumor size was significantly associated with high-grade disease on univariate analysis, and their most accurate multivariable model prediction of high-grade disease resulted in an accuracy similar to Lane's model (58.3%) [55]. Given the lower than acceptable accuracy of these early efforts to predict biology using demographic data, further evaluation of additional characteristics to more accurately predict pathologic features are necessary.

There is increasing evidence to suggest a relationship may exist between renal mass anatomy and pathology; however, only recently objective measures of renal mass anatomy have been described [93–95]. The R.E.N.A.L. Nephrometry Score is the first scoring system designed to assess reproducible and pertinent renal tumor anatomical attributes as they relate to surgical resectability [96], while alternative systems including P.A.D.U.A. [97] and the C-Index [98] have been published. Using a large prospectively maintained institutional cohort, Kutikov et al. evaluated the relationship between anatomical variables stratified by Nephrometry and malignant or high-grade pathologic features at the time of surgical resection. They found that total Nephrometry Score and all individual anatomic descriptor components significantly differed between tumor histology groups with the exception of the anterior/posterior (A) designation [99]. Papillary and chromophobe tumors had the lowest scores in each attribute indicating that they tended to be small, exophytic tumors with a polar distribution, resulting in low total Nephrometry Scores similar to benign lesions. Comparatively, clear cell carcinomas and uncommon yet more aggressive histologic subtypes (collecting duct, sarcomatoid) tended to be large, endophytic, interpolar lesions, thereby having higher total Nephrometry Scores. Based on these data, predictive nomograms integrating anatomic tumor attributes with patient's age and gender were constructed for preoperative prediction of tumor malignant histology (AUC 0.76) and high-grade features (AUC 0.73) [99]. This model represents the most accurate predictive model to date, with accuracy rates (particularly for tumor grade) that rival the results of contemporary percutaneous core biopsy series [56].

It is our hope that ultimately, the quantifiable probabilities of harboring malignant and high-grade pathology based on preoperative cross-sectional imaging can be objectively compared to competing risks of comorbid medical conditions and the morbidity of treatment itself. For example, using the Kutikov predictive model, an 80-year-old male with an enhancing renal mass with a Nephrometry Score of $1+3+1+a+2=7a$ has only a 26% chance of lesion malignancy. In turn, if the mass is indeed malignant, his chance of the cancer being high grade is approximately 30%. Overall, the patient has a 7.8% probability $(0.26 \times 0.30 = 0.078)$ of harboring high-grade malignancy. In contrast, an 80-year-old female with a Nephrometry Score $2+2+2+a+3h=9ah$ has a 92% chance of harboring a malignancy. If the tumor is malignant, the likelihood of high-grade disease is 59%. Unlike the 80-year-old male patient with "simple" tumor anatomy whose chance of having a high-grade malignancy is less than 10%, this female patient with a higher complexity renal mass which has a 54.2% chance $(0.92 \times 0.59 = 0.542)$ of harboring high-grade disease. With further refinement, these and other predictive models show significant potential for counseling patients newly diagnosed with SRMs, particularly elderly individuals with significant competing risks.

Indications for Observation and Contemporary Active Surveillance Protocols

When evaluating patients with newly diagnosed SRMs, it is helpful to stratify their risk status prior to choosing a treatment strategy. In our practice, each patient is categorized by absolute, relative, and elective indication for AS. Absolute indications include patients in whom surgery poses an immediate and unacceptable risk of mortality due to competing medical risks. Relative indications for observation include other concomitant disease states such as second malignancy, potential need for renal replacement therapy, and significant but not overriding medical comorbidities. Lastly, elective indications include patients who choose to pursue AS despite being low risk surgical candidates [100]. In our recent systematic review of all contemporary series of SRMs under AS, reason for AS was reported in eight studies ($N=312$ patients), consisting of elective (60.9%), relative (12.5%), and absolute (26.6%) indications [101].

When considering management options, it is the treating physician's responsibility to quantify factors affecting life expectancy, including performance status and operative risk, and compare these factors to the morbidity and mortality of untreated localized RCC. Often, this requires a team approach, including the patient's urologist, primary care provider, medical specialists (particularly cardiopulmonary and nephrology evaluation), and anesthesiologist. The potential need for postoperative renal replacement therapy must be strongly considered, particularly in elderly patients with diabetes, hypertension, and other systemic diseases that predispose to CKD. While the relationship between end-stage renal disease and adverse morbidity and mortality events is well recognized [102], recent large population-based cohort data have demonstrated that mild or moderate renal insufficiency determined by

reduced estimated glomerular filtration rates (GFRs) is associated with increased risks of death, cardiovascular events, and hospitalization [14]. As part of the initial evaluation, it is our practice to determine creatinine clearance and GFR to classify patient by CKD stage and refer patients to nephrology for further evaluation prior to pursuing definitive therapy. For patients considering AS who are adequate surgical candidates, an informed discussion must be held fully disclosing the current body of evidence as well as the limitations regarding known growth kinetics of SRMs under observation and risk of disease progression. Regardless of AS indication, when considering observation of an enhancing renal mass, both the patient and treating physician must understand that surveillance entails inherent calculated risk due to the heterogeneous and occasionally unpredictable behavior of RCC. In all cases, the primary goal of AS is to balance the risks of treatment vs. the risks of disease progression and development of metastasis.

To date there are no consistent surveillance protocols, and there have been no comparisons of the health care costs of active surveillance/delayed intervention with traditional surgical therapies or ablative techniques. Such comparisons are challenging, since patients must be matched not only by clinicopathological variables related to the renal mass, but also by associated comorbidities. Furthermore, costs of surgical morbidity and mortality must be captured in such datasets. In addition, surveillance of suspected malignant lesions carries implicit risks and effective surveillance protocols mandate a high degree of individual patient adherence. Current recommendations state that imaging should be performed with a consistent modality at defined intervals (3–6 months) [20]. The exact imaging interval is based on a qualitative decision by the treating physician, which is determined by clinicopathological risk factors specific to the renal mass and the patient's overall health status. In our practice, imaging is performed at 3- to 4-month intervals following initiation of AS to establish baseline SRM growth kinetics to guide the timing of additional imaging studies. In general, tumor size comparisons should be performed using consistent lesion characteristics [e.g., maximum tumor diameter (MTD) or estimated tumor volume (ETV)], while paying close attention to the cross-sectional cut from which the data is obtained across various radiographic studies [100]. Most importantly, patients must be appropriately counseled regarding management plans in the event that their tumor exhibits a rapid growth rate, a new lesion appears, or the onset of clinical symptoms occurs.

Natural History of Observed Renal Masses

Recent attention has been directed towards describing the natural history, or growth kinetics, of SRMs under observation in an effort to identify which lesions are safe to observe and which require early definitive intervention. Since surgical excision has historically been performed soon after diagnosis, there are limited existing data regarding the growth history of SRMS. The current body of evidence consists of small retrospective accounts of SRMs undergoing a delay prior to definitive treatment monitored with serial abdominal imaging at unspecified intervals [82–84, 103] and recent single institution series investigating outcomes in select patients intentionally managed with AS (all ≤level III evidence) [12, 100, 104–115].

Growth Kinetics

While there is considerable variation in the way tumor characteristics are reported across studies, the most reproducible method of reporting renal lesion growth is measurement of linear size (MTD), which assumes that the tumor is spherical and that growth occurs uniformly in all directions. The maximal cross-sectional diameter is measured with the growth rate expressed as the change in diameter per year (cm/year). When following a lesion with serial imaging it is essential at each study to perform lesion measurements at the same cross-sectional axial level for determination and comparison of interval growth. Despite

accurate and methodical measurements of tumor diameter, linear growth may not fully reflect the overall change in tumor volume. Indeed, calculation of volumetric growth, which may be easily determined on the basis of known cross-sectional dimensions, may better quantify biologic growth [116]. Tumor volume is calculated depending on the available dimensions reported on imaging data. If three dimensions are present, an ellipsoid volume formula ($0.5326xyz$) is utilized. If two dimensions are present, the formula $0.532xy(x+y/2)$ is used. If only one dimension is available, the formula for the volume of a sphere ($0.5326x^3$) is employed [113]. Such volume measurements may be more meaningful for solid lesions, as the growth rate in cystic lesions is confounded by the loss or accumulation of fluid that may not represent a true change in tumor mass. Using mass volume as a unit of measurement (mL or cm³), growth can then be expressed as change in ETV per year or tumor doubling time [117]. Relative proportional change in tumor diameter and volume can also be calculated and are expressed as percentage change in tumor size and volume per year [100].

Summary Data

In an attempt to consolidate these individual small experiences and identify growth trends in SRMs, Chawla et al. performed a meta-analysis of nine single institution retrospective series including 234 masses followed for a mean duration of 34 months. Initial MTD was 2.6 cm (range 1.73–4.08), mean growth rate was 0.28 cm/year, and pathologic confirmation was available in 46% (92% RCC or RCC variant) [118] (Fig. 10.4). We have recently updated these findings, performing a systematic literature review identifying 18 studies that included 880 patients with 936 SRMS (Table 10.1) [101]. Mean initial MTD was available in 14 studies ($N=586$), ranging from 1.73 to 7.2 cm at the time of diagnosis [82, 83, 100, 103, 104, 106–110, 112–114, 119]. Initial ETV was included in six studies ($N=284$), ranging from 6.0 to 83.5 cm³ at the time of diagnosis [100, 104, 107, 112, 113]. In comparison, MTD

Fig. 10.4 Tumor size vs. time in published series investigating small renal masses under a period of observation. Line slope and length represent mean growth rate and duration of follow-up, respectively. *N* represents the number of renal lesions followed in each individual series. (Reproduced with permission from "Chawla et al. The natural history of observed enhancing renal masses: Meta-analysis and review of the world literature. The Journal of Urology (2006); 175(2):427"; American Urological Association by Elsevier, Inc.)

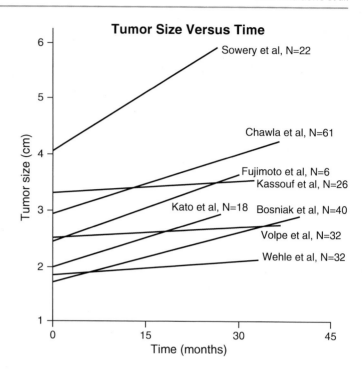

(range 2.4–3.78 cm) and ETV (range 18.2–116.4 cm³) at the conclusion of surveillance or time of intervention were available in seven (N=139) [82, 83, 103, 107, 110, 119] and two (N=45) [107, 113] studies, respectively. Imaging characteristic data was available in 14 studies (N=803) [82, 84, 100, 104–107, 109–113, 115, 119]; the majority (88.2%) of lesions were solid with 11.8% categorized as cystic. Multifocal disease was reported in 10.1% of patients. Mean change in maximal diameter per year was reported in 14 studies (N=586), ranging from 0.1 to 0.7 cm/year [82, 83, 100, 103, 104, 106–110, 112–114, 119]. Change in ETV per year was reported in seven studies (N=389), ranging from 2.7 to 26.8 cm³/year [100, 103, 104, 106, 107, 112, 113]. Pathologic data were available for 248 patients across 17 studies [82, 83, 100, 103–106, 108–115, 119] (Table 10.2), which revealed predominantly malignant disease (86.7%) of low-grade (81%) nature. However, specific use of percutaneous biopsy was rarely reported. Of available data from six studies (N=477) [105, 106, 110, 111, 119], only 85 patients (17.8%) had a biopsy performed as part of management planning. Of benign lesions, oncocytoma (12%) and

angiomyolipoma (1.6%) were most common. Of malignant lesions, predominant histologic subtypes included clear cell (67.2%) and papillary (14.5%) disease, while chromophobe (1.1%) and collecting duct carcinoma (0.5%) were uncommon. Eighteen patients (2.1%) developed metastatic disease over a mean period of observation of 40.2 months.

Representing perhaps the most robust data on the natural growth history of solid untreated tumors to date, Smaldone et al. performed a pooled analysis summarizing available individual level data from 275 patients (299 SRMs) meeting final inclusion criteria [101]. This analysis revealed a mean age of 66.9 ± 12.3 years (median 69; range 35–88) in 239 patients, while mean maximal tumor diameter (n=297) and ETV (n=297) at the time of diagnosis were 2.4 ± 1.4 cm (median 2; range 0.2–12) and 17.8 ± 63.9 cm³ (median 4.3; range 0.004–903.7), respectively. In comparison, mean maximal tumor diameter (n=263) and ETV (n=295) at the conclusion of observation were 3.2 ± 1.7 cm (median 2.8; range 0.9–15) and 34.3 ± 115.9 cm³ (median 11.5; range 0.27–1,765.1). With a mean duration of observation (n=298) of 33.6 ± 23.1 months (median 27.1;

Table 10.1 Clinical and cross-sectional imaging characteristics of small renal masses managed with active surveillance

Study	N (no. SRMs)	Mean age (years) (median; range)	Indication for AS No. (%)	Imaging characteristics No. (%)	Mean initial MTD (cm) (median; range)	Mean initial ETV (cm³) (median; range)	Mean final MTD (cm) (median; range)	Mean final ETV (cm³) (median; range)	Mean linear growth rate (cm/year) (median; range)	Mean volumetric growth rate (cm³/year) (median; range)	Mean follow-up (months) (median; range)	No. metastasis (%)
Fujimoto et al. [82]	6 (6)	59.7 (57; 47–70)	A—3 (50) R—0 E—3 (50)	Solid—6 (100)	2.47 (2.4, 1.7–3.4)		3.78 (3.8; 2.8–4.7)		0.57 (0.58; 0.39–0.74)		29 (20.3; 9.7–71)	0
Bosniak et al. [103]	37 (40)	65.1 (65.5; 42–84)		Multifocal—9 (24)	1.73 (1.8; 0.2–3.5)		3.11 (3; 1.2–7)		0.4 (0.36; 0–1.1)	5.26 (3.1; 0–42.1)	43.9 (39, 21–102)	0
Oda et al. [84]	16 (16)	54[a] (28–78)		Solid—16 (100)	2[a] (1–4.5)						25[a] (12–72)	0
Volpe et al. [113]	29 (32)	71[a] (27–84)		Solid—25 (78) Cystic—7 (22) Multifocal—N/A	2.48 (2.4; 0.9–3.9)	10.06 (7.01; 0.39–31.59)		18.2 (13.7; 0.3–63.7)	0.1	3.8 (1.2; 0–33.8)	35.3 (27.5; 5.3–143)	0
Wehle et al. [114]	29 (29)	70.5 (N/A; 51–88)			1.83 (N/A; 0.4–3.5)				0.12		32 (N/A; 10–89)	0
Kato et al. [83]	18 (18)	55.1 (56.5; 37–71)	E—18 (100)		1.98 (2; 0.8–3.4)		2.81 (2.8; 1.4–4.4)		0.42 (0.28; .08–1.6)		27 (22.5; 12–63)	0
Sowery et al. [112]	22 (22)	77[a] (60–92)	A—15 (68) E—7 (31.8)	Solid—15 (68) Cystic—7 (32)	4.08 (N/A; 2–8.8)	62.4 (N/A; 1.8–363)			0.86	24 (N/A)	26 (N/A)	1 (4.5)
Lamb et al. [109]	36 (36)	76.1 (77, 56–91)	A—14 (39) R—17 (47) E—5 (14)	Solid—36 (100)	7.2 (6; 3.5–20)				0.39 (0; 0–1.76)		27.7 (24; 3–136)	1 (2.8)
Kouba et al. [108]	43 (46)	67 (69, N/A)			2.92 (2.9; N/A)				0.7 (0.35; N/A)		35.8 (N/A)	0
Abou Youssif et al. [104]	35 (44)	71.8 (74, 29–90)		Solid—38 (86) Cystic—6 (14) Multifocal—N/A	2.2 (N/A; 0.5–4)	6.1 (4.4; 0.1–34.1)			0.21 (0.17; –0.3–1.9)	2.7 (0.83; –0.7–26.3)	47.6 (41; 6–160)	3 (8.6)
Fernando et al. [107]	13 (13)	80.4 (N/A, 66–88)	A—2 (15) R—1 (8) E—10 (77)	Solid—13 (100)	5.02 (N/A; 2–8.6)	83.5 (N/A; 4.2–338.8)	5.57 (N/A; 2–12.2)	116.4 (N/A; 4.2–618)	0.17	11.97 (N/A)	38.4 (N/A; 19–105)	1 (7.7)
Matsuzaki et al. [110]	15 (15)	67 (N/A; 44–87)	A—5 (33) E—10 (67)	Solid—15 (100)	2.2 (N/A; 1–3.9)		2.4 (N/A, 1–4.2)		0.06 (N/A; –0.09–0.28)		38 (N/A; 8–91)	0

(continued)

Table 10.1 (continued)

Study	N (no. SRMs)	Mean age (years) (median; range)	Indication for AS No. (%)	Imaging characteristics No. (%)	Mean initial MTD (cm) (median; range)	Mean initial ETV (cm³) (median; range)	Mean final MTD (cm) (median; range)	Mean final ETV (cm³) (median; range)	Mean linear growth rate (cm/year) (median; range)	Mean volumetric growth rate (cm³/year) (median; range)	Mean follow-up (months) (median; range)	No. metastasis (%)
Wong et al. [115][b]	1 (1)	78	A—1 (100)	Solid—1 (100)	2.5	6	5.9	96	2.7	71.9	15	1 (100)
Siu et al. [119]	41 (47)	68 (N/A, 34–84)	A—25 (53) E—22 (47)	Solid—47 (100) Multifocal—N/A	2 (N/A; 0.8–5)		2.6 (N/A; 0.8–6.9)		0.27 (N/A; −0.13–1.5)		29.5 (23.7; N/A)	1 (2.4)
Abouassaly et al. [105]	110	81[a] (76–95)		Solid—106 (96) Cystic—4 (4) Multifocal—N/A	2.5[a] (0.9–11.2)				0.26 (0.08; 0–3.3)		24 (N/A)	0
Beisland et al. [106]	63 (65)	76.6 (78.8; 56–89)		Solid—60 (92) Cystic—3 (5) Multifocal—N/A	4.3 (3.5; 1.3–11.1)				0.66 (0.31; −0.4–4.9)	26.8 (3.5; −4.8–277)	33 (37; 1–34)	2 (3.2)
Crispen et al. [100]	154 (173)	69 (71; 35–88)	A—18 (12) R—21 (13) E—115 (75)	Solid—147 (85) Cystic—26 (15) Multifocal—12 (8)	2.45 (2; 0.4–12)	20 (4.18; 0.3–904)			0.29 (0.15; −1.4–2.47)	17 (3; −20–431)	31 (24; 12–156)	3 (1.9)[c]
Rosales et al. [111]	212 (223)	71[a] (50–92)		Solid—183 (86) Cystic—40 (14)	2.8[a] (0.5–13.1)		3.7[a] (0.9–14.1)		0.34[a] (0.29–2.3)		35[a] (6–137)	4 (1.9)

SRM small renal mass, *AS* active surveillance, *MTD* mean linear tumor diameter, *ETV* estimated tumor, *A* absolute, *R* relative, *E* elective

[a]Median value

[b]Case report of a single small renal mass progressing to metastasis under observation, which was excluded from summary data

[c]Includes unpublished data

Table 10.2 Pathologic characteristics of small renal masses managed with a period of observation

Study No. (%)	No. with pathologic data	No. malignant	Pathologic grade		Histologic subtype—malignant					Histologic subtype—benign		
			High grade	Low grade	Clear cell	Papillary	Chromophobe	Collecting duct	Unable to characterize	AML	Oncocytoma	Cyst
Fujimoto et al. [82]	6	6 (100)	1 (17)	5 (83)	6 (100)							
Bosniak et al. [103]	26	22 (85)	0	22 (100)							4 (15)	
Oda et al. [84]	16	16 (100)	1 (6)	15 (94)								
Volpe et al. [113]	9	8 (89)	4 (50)	4 (50)	8 (89)						1 (11)	
Wehle et al. [114]	4	3 (75)	0	3 (100)							1 (25)	
Kato et al. [83]	18	18 (100)	3 (17)	15 (83)	15 (83)	3 (17)						
Sowery et al. [112]	2	2 (100)										
Lamb et al. [109]	24	23 (96)	1 (25)	3 (75)	18 (75)	1 (4)					1 (4)	
Kouba et al. [108]	14	12 (86)	2 (17)	10 (83)						1 (8)		1 (8)
Abou Youssif et al. [104]	8	6 (75)			4 (50)	2 (25)					2 (25)	
Matsuzaki et al. [110]	3	3 (100)	0	3 (100)	3 (100)							
Wong et al. [115]	1	1	0	1	1 (100)							
Siu et al. [119]	16	10 (63)			10 (63)						6 (37)	
Abouassaly et al. [105]	4	2	1 (50)	1 (50)	1 (25)	1 (25)			1 (25)		1 (25)	
Beisland et al. [106]	18	15 (83)	5 (50)	5 (50)	9 (60)	5 (33)			1 (7)		3 (17)	
Crispen et al. [100]	68	57 (84)	12 (23)	40 (77)	39 (68)	15 (26)	2 (4)	1 (2)	4 (17)	2 (3)	7 (10)	
Rosales et al. [111]	11	11 (100)			11 (100)							
Total	248	215/248 (86.7)	30/157 (19)	127/157 (81)	125/186 (67.2)	27/186 (14.5)	2/186 (1.1)	1/186 (0.5)	6/186 (3.2)	3/186 (1.6)	26/216 (12)	1/186 (0.5)

AML angiomyolipoma

range 5.3–156), calculated mean change in maximal diameter (linear growth rate; $n=263$) and
ETV (volumetric growth rate; $n=295$) per year
were 0.33 ± 0.41 cm/year (median 0.26; range
−1.4 to 2.7) and 7.3 ± 27.9 cm^3/year (median 1.9;
range −20.0 to 430.7).

Radiographic Predictors of Tumor Growth Rate and Malignant Potential

These data confirm initial observations that a
majority of localized renal tumors exhibit slow

radiographic growth with low metastatic potential
while under an initial period of observation.
However, early efforts to identify radiographic
characteristics associated with rapid growth rate
or aggressive malignant potential have been elusive, as no correlation or conflicting data has been
documented between tumor growth and patient
age [100, 108], initial MTD [57, 104, 105, 108,
113], tumor size >4 cm [106, 112], development
of clinical symptoms vs. incidental detection
[112], multifocality [120], or solid/cystic appearance [112, 113] (Fig. 10.5a, b). In fact, while initially assumed that larger tumors at presentation

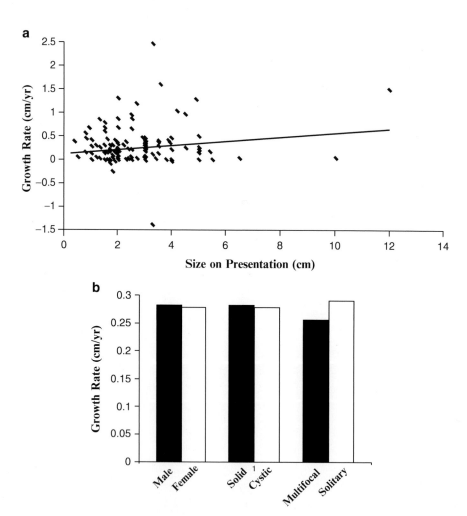

Fig. 10.5 (a) Observed tumor growth rate vs. tumor size
at presentation ($p>0.05$). (b) Observed tumor growth rate
comparing male vs. females, solid vs. cystic tumors, and
multifocal vs. solitary tumors ($p>0.05$ for all comparisons).

(Reproduced with permission from "Crispen et al.
Predicting growth of solid renal masses under active sur-
veillance. Urologic Oncology: Seminars and Original
Investigations (2008); 26(5):556–7"; Elsevier, Inc.)

may demonstrate faster growth rates, Crispen et al. demonstrated in a large single institutional series that when annual percent change in tumor size and volume is calculated, smaller tumors grow at proportionally faster rates compared to larger tumors [100]. This finding is suggestive of Gompertzian growth kinetics, which theorizes that a tumor's growth rate is initially exponential and then decreases with increasing size [121]. Although there are emerging anecdotal data suggesting that cT1b and even cT2 tumors may be judiciously observed for short periods in select patients with significant medical comorbidity [122], the biology of these lesions must be distinguished from the infrequent case of a localized mass with aggressive malignant potential that develops metachronous disease during a period of AS.

Additional efforts to characterize the malignant potential of SRMs have also yielded conflicting results and are severely limited by lack of compete pathologic assessment. In 18 patients who underwent surgical excision 12 or more months following diagnosis, Kato et al. reported that grade 3 lesions grew at significantly faster rates than grade 2 lesions (0.93 cm/year vs. 0.28 cm/year; $p=0.01$); however, these findings are limited by small sample size. In fact, in their dataset grade 1 lesions grew faster than grade 2 lesions (0.37 cm/year vs. 0.28 cm/year) although this did not reach statistical significance ($p=0.47$) [83]. From their retrospective series of 47 SRMs under surveillance, Siu et al. compared patients with proven RCC ($n=10$) vs. oncocytoma ($n=6$), reporting no differences in tumor growth rate (0.71 cm/year vs. 0.52 cm/year; $p=$NS) between groups [119]. In one of the largest single institution experiences to date (154 patients, 173 SRMs followed for a minimum of 12 months), Crispen et al. reported that SRMs stratified by Fuhrman grade and presence of benign histologic features exhibited no differences in growth rates [100]. In their original meta-analysis, when comparing pathologically confirmed RCCs with lesions managed with observation, Chawla et al. reported that initial MTD was similar between groups but the growth rate of proven malignant lesions was significantly greater (0.4 cm/year vs. 0.2 cm/year, $p=0.001$) compared to strictly observed lesions [118]. However, this does not account for selection bias and may reflect a trend towards earlier intervention in patients with rapid growth rates [68]. On further subanalysis of 76 SRMs (9 oncocytomas, 67 RCC variants) with available pathologic and growth kinetic data, the authors reported that both initial MTD (2.0 cm vs. 2.2 cm; $p=0.59$) and mean growth rate (0.1 cm/year vs. 0.4 cm/year; $p=0.15$) were comparable between groups [118]. These data, supported by positive growth rates documented in percutaneously biopsied oncocytomas managed subsequently with observation [123], suggest that a positive growth rate is not always indicative of malignant histology, and further assessment to identify characteristics predictive of aggressive malignant potential is necessary.

SRMs Undergoing Delayed Intervention

While consideration of preoperative indications for AS are important, it is equally important to review characteristics of lesions progressing to delayed intervention. In a large single institution review of 87 SRMs followed for more than 12 months, Crispen et al. reported that definitive treatment was delayed for ≥12 or 24 months in 69% and 33% of tumors, respectively. Of these, pathology assessment confirmed RCC in 84% of treated tumors, of which only 26% revealed aggressive histologic features. Importantly, despite delay in therapy, 76% of patients underwent nephron-sparing approaches and 60% were treated in a minimally invasive fashion. The authors concluded from these data that definitive therapy may be cautiously delayed in select patients without limiting available treatment options or incurring a high risk of disease progression [124].

From our systematic review (Table 10.3), 204 (23.2%) underwent delayed intervention after a mean period of observation [82–84, 100, 103–106, 108, 110–114, 119] ranging from 11.3 to 45.6 months ($N=151$) [83, 100, 103, 106, 108, 110, 113, 114]. Reason for progression to therapy was available in 11 series ($N=138$) [82, 100, 104–106, 110–114, 119] and consisted of patient preference (46.4%), improved medical condition

Table 10.3 Comparison of cross-sectional imaging characteristics and growth kinetics of small renal masses managed with observation alone and those who progressed to delayed intervention

Study	SRMs managed with observation alone					SRMs progressing to delayed intervention				
	No. SRMs	Mean initial MTD (cm)	Mean linear growth rate (cm/year)	Mean initial ETV (cm³)	Mean volumetric growth rate (cm³/year)	No. SRMs	Mean initial MTD (cm)	Mean linear growth rate (cm/year)	Mean final ETV (cm³)	Mean volumetric growth rate (cm³/year)
Fujimoto et al. [82]	1	1.8	0.55			5	2.6	0.58		
Bosniak et al. [103]	14	1.91	0.29		3.13	26	1.63	0.46		6.41
Volpe et al. [113]	23	2.3		8.34	3.5	9	2.93		14.5	4.54
Kato et al. [83]	0					18	1.98	0.42		
Kouba et al. [108][a]	32	3.07	0.61	6.5	1.17	14	2.59	0.9		
Abou Youssif et al. [104][a]	17	2.1	0.15			8	1.9	0.5	4	5.5
Matsuzaki et al. [110]	12	2.18	0.08			3	2.17	0		
Crispen et al. [100]	105	2.49	0.24	17.4	5.74	68	2.38	0.34	24	11.3
Rosales et al. [111][b]	197	2.61	0.34			15	3.56	1.75		
Total						Total				
Summary data (range)	204	1.8–3.07	0.08–0.61	6.5–17.4	1.17–5.74	151	1.63–3.56	0–1.75	4–24	4.54–11.3
Pooled analysis	155	2.4	0.25	15.7	5.6	129	2.2	0.39	22.9	9.7

SRM small renal mass, MTD maximum linear tumor diameter, ETV estimated tumor volume

[a]Individual data unavailable and was not utilized in pooled analysis evaluation of growth kinetics

[b]Only median values reported which were not included in final summary data

(6.3%), tumor growth (45.7%), or other (1.6%; retroperitoneal hematoma, concurrent surgical procedure). In our recent pooled analysis of individual level data, comparison of patients undergoing delayed intervention ($N = 129$) and those managed strictly with surveillance ($N = 155$) revealed similar initial MTD (2.4 cm vs. 2.2 cm; $p = 0.212$) and initial ETV (16.4 cm³ vs. 16.03 cm³; $p = 0.82$) at the time of diagnosis. However, significantly increased linear (0.26 cm/year vs. 0.39 cm/year; $p = 0.0001$) and volumetric (5.5 cm³/year vs. 8.8 cm³/year; $p = 0.001$) growth rates were observed in the patients undergoing active treatment [101]. While intuitive that lesions with faster growth kinetics would self-select for treatment, these data are confounded by lack of standardized criteria for intervention among contemporary surveillance protocols. Furthermore, similar to clinical experiences with AS in prostate cancer [25], a large proportion of patients (46% of those with available data) proceeded to intervention despite the absence of predetermined clinical or radiographic triggers.

SRMs Exhibiting "Zero Net Growth" While Under Surveillance

Observed linear growth rates range from 0.06 to 0.86 cm/year in contemporary individual series [82–84, 100, 103–114, 119], with summary data consistently reporting overall growth rates ranging from 0.28 to 0.32 cm/year [101, 118]. However, these data also reveal a subset of SRMs that demonstrate no interval growth on serial imaging while under observation. In single institution series of enhancing SRMs followed for more than 12 months (mean 29 months), Kunkle et al. compared radiographic characteristics in 35 (33%) lesions exhibiting zero net growth and 70 masses (67%) showing growth at 0.31 cm/year. No differences were seen with respect to patient age ($p = 0.96$), initial MTD ($p = 0.41$), solid/cystic appearance ($p = 1.0$), or incidental detection rate ($p = 0.38$) [125]. Not surprisingly, there was a significantly increased rate of intervention in lesions demonstrating positive growth rates (51% vs. 17%, $p = 0.001$). However, pathological

assessment revealed similar malignancy rates between groups (83% vs. 89%, $p = 0.56$), an observation which has been confirmed in other small series [103, 114]. Supporting this data, our recent systematic review reported that of 421 SRMs with available data, 29.5% exhibited zero net growth over time, and there was no difference in pathologic malignancy rate (84% vs. 93%, $p = 1.0$) between lesions exhibiting positive and zero growth [82, 83, 100, 103, 105, 107–110, 113–115, 119]. Pooled analysis of available individual level data (220 exhibiting growth vs. 65 patients exhibiting no growth) revealed no difference in initial MTD (2.3 cm vs. 2.5 cm; $p = 0.46$) between groups (Table 10.4) [101]. While these data confirm that lack of interval radiographic growth does not correlate with benign histology, an important observation is that no lesion demonstrating zero net growth while under surveillance has progressed to metastatic disease.

SRMs Progressing to Metastases While Under Surveillance

Progression to metastatic disease in patients with SRMs under AS is uncommon and poorly documented in the literature. Our recent systematic review identified 18 patients progressing to metastatic disease from a cohort of 880 patients with SRMs under AS (2.1%) [100, 104, 106, 107, 109, 111, 112, 115, 119, 126] (Table 10.5). Indications for active surveillance ($n = 13$) were absolute in 61.5% and elective in 38.5%. Pathologic confirmation of diagnosis was made in nine cases (50%); three with percutaneous biopsy [100, 111, 115], five at the time of surgical exploration [100, 104, 119], and one unknown [126]. Of the 11 patients with available information, three (72.7%) were diagnosed with distant visceral or bony disease with or without positive lymphadenopathy, and three patients were diagnosed with pathologic lymph node involvement only (27.3%). Histologic subtypes were predominantly clear cell (66.7%) [100, 104, 109, 115, 119, 126] and papillary (22.2%) [104, 111], with one lesion exhibiting mixed clear cell and papillary features (11.1%) [100]. Importantly, time to development

Table 10.4 Comparison of growth kinetics and pathologic characteristics in small renal masses exhibiting zero growth and positive growth during a period of observation

Study	SRMs with zero growth			SRMs with positive growth			
	No. with zero growth	Mean initial MTD (cm)	Pathologic characteristics	No. with positive growth	Mean initial MTD (cm)	Mean linear growth rate (cm/year)	Pathologic characteristics
Fujimoto et al. [82]	0			6	2.47	0.57	6—malignant (6—clear cell; 1 HG, 5 LG)
Bosniak et al. [103]	2	1.9	1—malignant (LG RCC)	38	1.72	0.42	4—benign (oncocytoma) 21—malignant (21 LG RCC)
Volpe et al. [113]	7	2.82		25	1.98		
Kato et al. [83]	0			18	1.98	0.42	18—malignant (15—clear cell, 3—papillary; 15—HG, 3—LG)
Matsuzaki et al. [110]	11	2.25	3—malignant (3 clear cell)	4	2	0.21	
Wong et al. [115][a]	0			1	2.5	2.7	1—LG clear cell RCC
Siu et al. [119][b]	21	1.9	2—malignant	26	2.1	0.5	8—malignant 6—benign (oncocytoma)
Abouassaly et al. [105][b]	38	2.49		51	2.87	0.56	2—malignant (1 clear cell, 1 papillary) 2—benign (1 oncocytoma, 1 atypical)
Crispen et al. [100]	45	2.5	8—malignant 1—benign (oncocytoma)	128	2.4	0.41	44—malignant 8—benign
Total				Total			
Summary data (range)	124	1.9–2.82	Malignant (93) Benign (7)	297	1.72–2.87	0.21–0.57	Malignant (84) Benign (16)
Pooled analysis	65	2.5		220	2.3	0.43	

SRM small renal mass, *MTD* maximum linear tumor diameter, *RCC* renal cell carcinoma, *HG* high grade, *LG* low grade

[a]Case report of a single small renal mass progressing to metastasis under observation, which was excluded from summary data

[b]Individual data unavailable and was not utilized in pooled analysis of growth kinetics

Table 10.5 Clinical and radiographic characteristics of documented small renal masses progressing to metastasis under a period of observation

Clinical series	Age (years); gender	Indication for AS	MTD at diagnosis (cm)	ETV at diagnosis (cm³)	MTD at metastasis (cm)	ETV at metastasis (cm³)	Time to metastasis (months)	Linear growth Rate (cm/year)	Volumetric growth rate (cm³/year)	Site of metastasis, pathologic data; outcome
Lamb et al. [109]	79	Elective[a]					132			Clear cell (FG 3) Alive at 136 months
Sowery et al. [112]	74; M	CHR	8.8	363	10.7	653	68	0.33	50.9	RPLAD, liver Managed with angioembolization, mortality at 70 months
Wong et al. [115]	78; F	CHR	2.5	6	5.9	95.8	15	2.7	71.8	RP LAD, pulmonary; clear cell (FG 2) Mortality at 20 months
Fernando et al. [107]	NA; F						20			Pulmonary Mortality at 22 months
Siu et al. [119]	NA; F	CHR	3	14.4	6	115	78	0.46	15.5	RP LAD; clear cell Attempted pNx which was aborted due to grossly positive lymphadenopathy. Patient ultimately died from locally advanced disease
Abou Youssif et al. [104]	NA	Elective[a]	2.7	10.5	5.8	103.9	40	0.94	28.3	Spine
	NA [104]	Elective	2.7	10.5	4.5	48.5	29	0.75	15.8	Pulmonary[b]; pT3aN0Mx; clear cell (FG 3) Nx at 26 months, mortality at 35 months
	NA [104]	Elective	4.5	33.5	4.8	46.6	37	0.1	4.8	Pancreas, RP LAD[b]; pT1bNxMx; papillary Nx at 13 months, developed metastasis at 37 months from diagnosis
Biesland et al. [106]	81	CHR	6.2	126.9						Mortality at 9 months from diagnosis
	82	CHR	6.7	160.2						
Crispen et al. [100]	84; M	CHR	3	11	8	102.1	54	1.1	20.2	Pulmonary Hospice, mortality
	70; F	CHR	3.2	16.6	4.8	51.1	63	0.3	6.6	RP LAD; pT1bN2Mx; mixed clear cell and papillary (FG 4) Partial Nx and lymph node dissection. No adjuvant therapy, deceased
	54; M [100]	CHR	2.7		6.5	80	38			RP LAD; pT3aN2Mx; clear cell (FG 2) Alive, no adjuvant therapy

(continued)

Table 10.5 (continued)

Clinical series	Age (years); gender	Indication for AS	MTD at diagnosis (cm)	ETV at diagnosis (cm³)	MTD at metastasis (cm)	ETV at metastasis (cm³)	Time to metastasis (months)	Linear growth Rate (cm/year)	Volumetric growth rate (cm³/year)	Site of metastasis, pathologic data; outcome
Rosales et al. [111]	NA		2	4.3	4.1	36.7	22[c]	1.2	18	papillary
	NA		3.1	15.9	3.8	29.2	22[c]	0.4	7.4	
	NA		5.1	70.7	6.1	120.9	22[c]	0.6	27.9	
	NA		7.2	198.8	8.7	350.7	22[c]	0.83	84.4	
Jewett et al. [126]	74; F	Elective	2.7	8.3	3.1	13.4	12	0.4	5.1	Pulmonary; clear cell (FG 2) Alive on tyrosine kinase inhibitors
Pooled analysis (n = 18)	75.1		4.3	70	5.9	132.1	40.2	0.77	27.4	

AS active surveillance, *MTD* maximum linear tumor diameter, *ETV* estimated tumor volume, *CHR* competing health risk, *LTF* lost to follow up, *Nx* nephrectomy, *pNx* partial nephrectomy, *RP LAD* retroperitoneal lymphadenopathy, *FG* Fuhrman grade

[a]Patient lost to follow up for prolonged period, metastasis documented at time patient represented

[b]Underwent nephrectomy prior to documentation of metastasis

[c]Mean time to metastasis in this cohort was 22 months, individual data per patient not available

of metastatic disease was a late event (mean 40.2, range 12–132 months).

Comparing patients who progressed to metastatic disease in our systematic review ($n=18$) with those who did not in our pooled cohort of patients with individual level data ($n=281$), the duration of observation was similar between groups (40.2 months vs. 33.3 months; $p=0.47$), but there were significant differences in mean patient age (75.1 years vs. 66.6 years; $p=0.03$). Trends in patients progressing to metastases included larger tumor size (4.1 cm vs. 2.3 cm; $p<0.0001$) and ETV (66.4 cm^3 vs. 15.1 cm^3; $p<0.0001$) at diagnosis as well as mean linear (0.80 cm/year vs. 0.30 cm/year; $p=0.0001$) and volumetric growth rates (27.1 cm^3/year vs. 6.2 cm^3/year; $p<0.0001$) [101].

When considering patient selection for AS protocols, the most important endpoint to consider is metastatic disease progression. While findings of our review suggest that the proportion of lesions that progressed was low (2.1%), these lesions demonstrated a rapid growth rate (0.8 cm/year) and were predominantly high-grade, clear cell histology, and $\geq$cT1b at the time of diagnosis (38% >4 cm), perhaps reflecting poor initial case selection or substantive competing risk [101]. Supporting this theory, elderly patients with absolute indications for surveillance were more common in the progression cohort, implying that they were not acceptable operative candidates at diagnosis despite concerning radiographic characteristics. Furthermore, because this group included some individuals who were lost to follow up it is conceivable that a proportion of these patients would have undergone definitive treatment if more closely followed.

There are significant limitations in the interpretation and application of existing AS data, including the quality of evidence (all $\leq$level III), significant selection bias, and lack of universal pathologic evaluation. These limitations are especially important to consider when evaluating the rate of progression to metastatic disease, as the inclusion of benign disease and exclusion of rapidly growing lesions might falsely lower the observed rate of disease progression [127]. However, despite these limitations, important

observations to consider are that metastasis was a late event (>3 years following diagnosis), all lesions that progressed were >3 cm at the time of metastasis, all demonstrated positive growth rates, and no lesion exhibiting zero net growth while under surveillance has developed metastases while under observation [101]. Of available characteristics, a positive growth rate may be the most accurate available predictor of potential for disease progression among readily available metrics and indicate the need for definitive intervention, while lesions demonstrating zero net growth may self-select for continued AS. There has been one reported case of a 73-year-old male with a 2.4 cm renal mass progressing to bony metastases at 5 months with no increase in tumor size [126]. It is unclear from available data whether this represents true clinical progression or occult undiagnosed systemic disease at the time of presentation and for this reason was excluded from our progression cohort. However, this example highlights the need for close scrutiny of contemporary surveillance protocols.

Conclusions

With the increased utilization of cross-sectional abdominal imaging, there has been a significant stage migration towards the incidental detection of small clinically localized renal masses <4 cm. The gold standard for the management of enhancing renal lesions remains surgical excision. However, despite a concurrent increase in surgical resection rates, cancer-specific mortality remains unchanged implying that a proportion of these SRMs may be indolent tumors that may not require surgical intervention. Although the contemporary body of literature on the natural history of untreated SRMs is limited, recent pooled data demonstrate that the vast majority demonstrate slow growth kinetics with a very low rate of progression to metastatic disease. Approximately 20–30% of SRMS exhibit zero net growth under observation, and while malignancy rates are equivalent when compared to lesions demonstrating positive growth, to date no zero growth lesion has progressed to metastatic disease nor has any

SRM been <3 cm at the time of progression. Analysis of lesions that have progressed to metastases under observation reveals that these tumors are more likely to be larger at diagnosis, high nuclear grade, with significantly more rapid growth kinetics. While improved methods of recognizing more aggressive phenotypes at the time of presentation are needed, metastatic progression in these patients still appears to be a late event. Of available characteristics, linear growth rate appears to be the most useful predictor of metastatic potential, and it seems reasonable that SRMs that demonstrate rapid growth kinetics should proceed to immediate definitive intervention while lesions exhibiting zero or minimal growth self-select for continued AS. We anticipate that as contemporary investigations progress, improved imaging techniques, utilization of percutaneous biopsy, and biomarker discovery will play more prominent roles in an effort to match treatment to individual tumor biology. In the interim, emphasis on preoperative nomograms stratifying SRM malignant potential and competing medical risks will continue to grow as more practitioners embrace AS as a viable treatment strategy. While prospective trials would be ideal, randomized comparisons with surgical excision and ablation are unlikely. In the absence of level I data, AS for localized solid renal masses should only be considered as an alternative to definitive surgical extirpation in select patients with limited life expectancy, competing health risks precluding surgery, or significant potential for requiring renal replacement therapy. When discussing observation of the incidentally diagnosed SRM, patients and clinicians must consider and accept the calculated risks of surveillance and consider all treatment trade-off decisions.

References

1. Jemal A, Siegel R, Xu J, et al. Cancer statistics, 2010. CA Cancer J Clin. 2010;60(5):277–300.
2. Chow WH, Devesa SS, Warren JL, et al. Rising incidence of renal cell cancer in the United States. JAMA. 1999;281(17):1628–31.
3. Hollingsworth JM, Miller DC, Daignault S, et al. Rising incidence of small renal masses: a need to reassess treatment effect. J Natl Cancer Inst. 2006;98(18):1331–4.
4. Cooperberg MR, Mallin K, Ritchey J, et al. Decreasing size at diagnosis of stage 1 renal cell carcinoma: analysis from the National Cancer Data Base, 1993 to 2004. J Urol. 2008;179(6):2131–5.
5. Kane CJ, Mallin K, Ritchey J, et al. Renal cell cancer stage migration: analysis of the National Cancer Data Base. Cancer. 2008;113(1):78–83.
6. Jayson M, Sanders H. Increased incidence of serendipitously discovered renal cell carcinoma. Urology. 1998;51(2):203–5.
7. Kutikov A, Fossett LK, Ramchandani P, et al. Incidence of benign pathologic findings at partial nephrectomy for solitary renal mass presumed to be renal cell carcinoma on preoperative imaging. Urology. 2006;68(4):737–40.
8. Crispen PL, Boorjian SA, Lohse CM, et al. Outcomes following partial nephrectomy by tumor size. J Urol. 2008;180(5):1912–7.
9. Remzi M, Ozsoy M, Klingler HC, et al. Are small renal tumors harmless? Analysis of histopathological features according to tumors 4 cm or less in diameter. J Urol. 2006;176(3):896–9.
10. Jemal A, Siegel R, Ward E, et al. Cancer statistics, 2008. CA Cancer J Clin. 2008;58(2):71–96.
11. Hollenbeck BK, Taub DA, Miller DC, et al. National utilization trends of partial nephrectomy for renal cell carcinoma: a case of underutilization? Urology. 2006;67(2):254–9.
12. Huang WC, Levey AS, Serio AM, et al. Chronic kidney disease after nephrectomy in patients with renal cortical tumours: a retrospective cohort study. Lancet Oncol. 2006;7(9):735–40.
13. McKiernan J, Simmons R, Katz J, et al. Natural history of chronic renal insufficiency after partial and radical nephrectomy. Urology. 2002;59(6):816–20.
14. Go AS, Chertow GM, Fan D, et al. Chronic kidney disease and the risks of death, cardiovascular events, and hospitalization. N Engl J Med. 2004;351(13):1296–305.
15. Huang WC, Elkin EB, Levey AS, et al. Partial nephrectomy versus radical nephrectomy in patients with small renal tumors – is there a difference in mortality and cardiovascular outcomes? J Urol. 2009;181(1):55–61 [discussion 2].
16. Thompson RH, Boorjian SA, Lohse CM, et al. Radical nephrectomy for pT1a renal masses may be associated with decreased overall survival compared with partial nephrectomy. J Urol. 2008;179(2):468–71 [discussion 72–3].
17. Gill IS, Kavoussi LR, Lane BR, et al. Comparison of 1,800 laparoscopic and open partial nephrectomies for single renal tumors. J Urol. 2007;178(1):41–6.
18. Lane BR, Gill IS. 7-Year oncological outcomes after laparoscopic and open partial nephrectomy. J Urol. 2010;183(2):473–9.
19. Scoll BJ, Uzzo RG, Chen DY, et al. Robot-assisted partial nephrectomy: a large single-institutional experience. Urology. 2010;75(6):1328–34.
20. Campbell SC, Novick AC, Belldegrun A, et al. Guideline for management of the clinical T1 renal mass. J Urol. 2009;182(4):1271–9.

21. Kutikov A, Kunkle DA, Uzzo RG. Focal therapy for kidney cancer: a systematic review. Curr Opin Urol. 2009;19(2):148–53.

22. Kunkle DA, Egleston BL, Uzzo RG. Excise, ablate or observe: the small renal mass dilemma – a meta-analysis and review. J Urol. 2008;179(4):1227–33 [discussion 33–4].

23. Kutikov A, Egleston BL, Wong YN, et al. Evaluating overall survival and competing risks of death in patients with localized renal cell carcinoma using a comprehensive nomogram. J Clin Oncol. 2010;28(2):311–7.

24. Welch HG, Black WC. Overdiagnosis in cancer. J Natl Cancer Inst. 2010;102(9):605–13.

25. Dall'Era MA, Cooperberg MR, Chan JM, et al. Active surveillance for early-stage prostate cancer: review of the current literature. Cancer. 2008;112(8):1650–9.

26. Klotz L, Zhang L, Lam A, et al. Clinical results of long-term follow-up of a large, active surveillance cohort with localized prostate cancer. J Clin Oncol. 2010;28(1):126–31.

27. Frank I, Blute ML, Cheville JC, et al. Solid renal tumors: an analysis of pathological features related to tumor size. J Urol. 2003;170(6 Pt 1):2217–20.

28. Thompson RH, Kurta JM, Kaag M, et al. Tumor size is associated with malignant potential in renal cell carcinoma cases. J Urol. 2009;181(5):2033–6.

29. Rothman J, Egleston B, Wong YN, et al. Histopathological characteristics of localized renal cell carcinoma correlate with tumor size: a SEER analysis. J Urol. 2009;181(1):29–33 [discussion 4].

30. Kunkle DA, Crispen PL, Li T, et al. Tumor size predicts synchronous metastatic renal cell carcinoma: implications for surveillance of small renal masses. J Urol. 2007;177(5):1692–6 [discussion 7].

31. Nguyen MM, Gill IS. Effect of renal cancer size on the prevalence of metastasis at diagnosis and mortality. J Urol. 2009;181(3):1020–7 [discussion 7].

32. Thompson RH, Hill JR, Babayev Y, et al. Metastatic renal cell carcinoma risk according to tumor size. J Urol. 2009;182(1):41–5.

33. Duffey BG, Choyke PL, Glenn G, et al. The relationship between renal tumor size and metastases in patients with von Hippel–Lindau disease. J Urol. 2004;172(1):63–5.

34. Frank I, Blute ML, Cheville JC, et al. An outcome prediction model for patients with clear cell renal cell carcinoma treated with radical nephrectomy based on tumor stage, size, grade and necrosis: the SSIGN score. J Urol. 2002;168(6):2395–400.

35. Karakiewicz PI, Briganti A, Chun FK, et al. Multi-institutional validation of a new renal cancer-specific survival nomogram. J Clin Oncol. 2007;25(11):1316–22.

36. Kattan MW, Reuter V, Motzer RJ, et al. A postoperative prognostic nomogram for renal cell carcinoma. J Urol. 2001;166(1):63–7.

37. Kim HL, Seligson D, Liu X, et al. Using tumor markers to predict the survival of patients with metastatic renal cell carcinoma. J Urol. 2005;173(5):1496–501.

38. Kim HL, Seligson D, Liu X, et al. Using protein expressions to predict survival in clear cell renal carcinoma. Clin Cancer Res. 2004;10(16):5464–71.

39. Patard JJ, Leray E, Rioux-Leclercq N, et al. Prognostic value of histologic subtypes in renal cell carcinoma: a multicenter experience. J Clin Oncol. 2005;23(12):2763–71.

40. Thompson RH, Leibovich BC, Lohse CM, et al. Dynamic outcome prediction in patients with clear cell renal cell carcinoma treated with radical nephrectomy: the D-SSIGN score. J Urol. 2007;177(2):477–80.

41. Zisman A, Pantuck AJ, Dorey F, et al. Mathematical model to predict individual survival for patients with renal cell carcinoma. J Clin Oncol. 2002;20(5):1368–74.

42. Zisman A, Pantuck AJ, Dorey F, et al. Improved prognostication of renal cell carcinoma using an integrated staging system. J Clin Oncol. 2001;19(6):1649–57.

43. Zisman A, Pantuck AJ, Wieder J, et al. Risk group assessment and clinical outcome algorithm to predict the natural history of patients with surgically resected renal cell carcinoma. J Clin Oncol. 2002;20(23):4559–66.

44. Cindolo L, Patard JJ, Chiodini P, et al. Comparison of predictive accuracy of four prognostic models for nonmetastatic renal cell carcinoma after nephrectomy: a multicenter European study. Cancer. 2005;104(7):1362–71.

45. Cindolo L, de la Taille A, Messina G, et al. A preoperative clinical prognostic model for non-metastatic renal cell carcinoma. BJU Int. 2003;92(9):901–5.

46. Raj GV, Thompson RH, Leibovich BC, et al. Preoperative nomogram predicting 12-year probability of metastatic renal cancer. J Urol. 2008;179(6):2146–51 [discussion 51].

47. Yaycioglu O, Roberts WW, Chan T, et al. Prognostic assessment of nonmetastatic renal cell carcinoma: a clinically based model. Urology. 2001;58(2):141–5.

48. Van Poppel H, Da Pozzo L, Albrecht W, et al. A Prospective, randomised EORTC intergroup phase 3 study comparing the oncologic outcome of elective nephron-sparing surgery and radical nephrectomy for low-stage renal cell carcinoma. Eur Urol. 2011;59:543–52.

49. Lane BR, Abouassaly R, Gao T, et al. Active treatment of localized renal tumors may not impact overall survival in patients aged 75 years or older. Cancer. 2010;116(13):3119–26.

50. Santos Arrontes D, Fernandez Acenero MJ, Garcia Gonzalez JI, et al. Survival analysis of clear cell renal carcinoma according to the Charlson comorbidity index. J Urol. 2008;179(3):857–61.

51. Hollingsworth JM, Miller DC, Daignault S, et al. Five-year survival after surgical treatment for kidney cancer: a population-based competing risk analysis. Cancer. 2007;109(9):1763–8.

52. Lughezzani G, Sun M, Budaus L, et al. Population-based external validation of a competing-risks nomogram for patients with localized renal cell carcinoma. J Clin Oncol. 2010;28(18):e299–300 [author reply e1].

53. Kutikov A, Egleston BL, Smaldone MC, et al. Quantification of competing risks of death with localized renal cell carcinoma (RCC): a comprehensive nomogram incorporating co-morbidities. In: Podium presentation; American Urologic Association meeting, Washington; 2011.

54. Uzzo RG. Renal masses – to treat or not to treat? If that is the question are contemporary biomarkers the answer? J Urol. 2008;180(2):433–4.

55. Jeldres C, Sun M, Liberman D, et al. Can renal mass biopsy assessment of tumor grade be safely substituted for by a predictive model? J Urol. 2009;182(6):2585–9.

56. Lane BR, Babineau D, Kattan MW, et al. A preoperative prognostic nomogram for solid enhancing renal tumors 7 cm or less amenable to partial nephrectomy. J Urol. 2007;178(2):429–34.

57. Crispen PL, Blute ML. Do percutaneous renal tumor biopsies at initial presentation affect treatment strategies? Eur Urol. 2009;55(2):307–9.

58. Lane BR, Samplaski MK, Herts BR, et al. Renal mass biopsy – a renaissance? J Urol. 2008;179(1):20–7.

59. Wang R, Wolf Jr JS, Wood Jr DP, et al. Accuracy of percutaneous core biopsy in management of small renal masses. Urology. 2009;73(3):586–90 [discussion 90–1].

60. Neuzillet Y, Lechevallier E, Andre M, et al. Accuracy and clinical role of fine needle percutaneous biopsy with computerized tomography guidance of small (less than 4.0 cm) renal masses. J Urol. 2004;171(5): 1802–5.

61. Lechevallier E, Andre M, Barriol D, et al. Fine-needle percutaneous biopsy of renal masses with helical CT guidance. Radiology. 2000;216(2):506–10.

62. Tsui KH, Shvarts O, Smith RB, et al. Prognostic indicators for renal cell carcinoma: a multivariate analysis of 643 patients using the revised 1997 TNM staging criteria. J Urol. 2000;163(4):1090–5 [quiz 295].

63. Leveridge M, Shiff D, Chung H, et al. Small renal mass needle core biopsy: outcomes of non-diagnostic percutaneous biopsy and role of repeat biopsy (abstract 821). J Urol. 2010;183(4):e321.

64. Blumenfeld AJ, Guru K, Fuchs GJ, et al. Percutaneous biopsy of renal cell carcinoma underestimates nuclear grade. Urology. 2010;76(3):610–3.

65. Khan AA, Shergill IS, Quereshi S, et al. Percutaneous needle biopsy for indeterminate renal masses: a national survey of UK consultant urologists. BMC Urol. 2007;7:10.

66. Wood BJ, Khan MA, McGovern F, et al. Imaging guided biopsy of renal masses: indications, accuracy and impact on clinical management. J Urol. 1999;161(5):1470–4.

67. Maturen KE, Nghiem HV, Caoili EM, et al. Renal mass core biopsy: accuracy and impact on clinical management. AJR Am J Roentgenol. 2007;188(2): 563–70.

68. Jewett MA, Zuniga A. Renal tumor natural history: the rationale and role for active surveillance. Urol Clin North Am. 2008;35(4):627–34. vii.

69. Rothman J, Crispen PL, Wong YN, et al. Pathologic concordance of sporadic synchronous bilateral renal masses. Urology. 2008;72(1):138–42.

70. Visapaa H, Bui M, Huang Y, et al. Correlation of Ki-67 and gelsolin expression to clinical outcome in renal clear cell carcinoma. Urology. 2003;61(4):845–50.

71. Delahunt B, Bethwaite PB, Thornton A, et al. Proliferation of renal cell carcinoma assessed by fixation-resistant polyclonal Ki-67 antibody labeling. Correlation with clinical outcome. Cancer. 1995;75(11):2714–9.

72. Shiina H, Igawa M, Urakami S, et al. Clinical significance of immunohistochemically detectable p53 protein in renal cell carcinoma. Eur Urol. 1997;31(1):73–80.

73. Shvarts O, Seligson D, Lam J, et al. p53 is an independent predictor of tumor recurrence and progression after nephrectomy in patients with localized renal cell carcinoma. J Urol. 2005;173(3):725–8.

74. Zhang X, Takenaka I. Cell proliferation and apoptosis with BCL-2 expression in renal cell carcinoma. Urology. 2000;56(3):510–5.

75. Tomisawa M, Tokunaga T, Oshika Y, et al. Expression pattern of vascular endothelial growth factor isoform is closely correlated with tumour stage and vascularisation in renal cell carcinoma. Eur J Cancer. 1999;35(1):133–7.

76. Bilim V, Yuuki K, Itoi T, et al. Double inhibition of XIAP and Bcl-2 axis is beneficial for retrieving sensitivity of renal cell cancer to apoptosis. Br J Cancer. 2008;98(5):941–9.

77. Hedberg Y, Davoodi E, Roos G, et al. Cyclin-D1 expression in human renal-cell carcinoma. Int J Cancer. 1999;84(3):268–72.

78. Sabo E, Miselevich I, Bejar J, et al. The role of vimentin expression in predicting the long-term outcome of patients with localized renal cell carcinoma. Br J Urol. 1997;80(6):864–8.

79. Tatokoro M, Saito K, Iimura Y, et al. Prognostic impact of postoperative C-reactive protein level in patients with metastatic renal cell carcinoma undergoing cytoreductive nephrectomy. J Urol. 2008;180(2): 515–9.

80. Bui MH, Seligson D, Han KR, et al. Carbonic anhydrase IX is an independent predictor of survival in advanced renal clear cell carcinoma: implications for prognosis and therapy. Clin Cancer Res. 2003;9(2):802–11.

81. Crispen PL, Boorjian SA, Lohse CM, et al. Predicting disease progression after nephrectomy for localized renal cell carcinoma: the utility of prognostic models and molecular biomarkers. Cancer. 2008;113(3): 450–60.

82. Fujimoto N, Sugita A, Terasawa Y, et al. Observations on the growth rate of renal cell carcinoma. Int J Urol. 1995;2(2):71–6.

83. Kato M, Suzuki T, Suzuki Y, et al. Natural history of small renal cell carcinoma: evaluation of growth rate,

histological grade, cell proliferation and apoptosis. J Urol. 2004;172(3):863–6.

84. Oda T, Miyao N, Takahashi A, et al. Growth rates of primary and metastatic lesions of renal cell carcinoma. Int J Urol. 2001;8(9):473–7.

85. Oda T, Takahashi A, Miyao N, et al. Cell proliferation, apoptosis, angiogenesis and growth rate of incidentally found renal cell carcinoma. Int J Urol. 2003;10(1):13–8.

86. Hicks RJ, Ware RE, Lau EW. PET/CT: will it change the way that we use CT in cancer imaging? Cancer Imaging. 2006;6:S52–62.

87. Lawrentschuk N, Davis ID, Bolton DM, et al. Functional imaging of renal cell carcinoma. Nat Rev Urol. 2010;7(5):258–66.

88. Lawrentschuk N, Poon AM, Foo SS, et al. Assessing regional hypoxia in human renal tumours using 18 F-fluoromisonidazole positron emission tomography. BJU Int. 2005;96(4):540–6.

89. Lawrentschuk N, Poon AM, Scott AM. Fluorine-18 fluorothymidine: a new positron emission radioisotope for renal tumors. Clin Nucl Med. 2006;31(12):788–9.

90. Oyama N, Okazawa H, Kusukawa N, et al. 11 C-Acetate PET imaging for renal cell carcinoma. Eur J Nucl Med Mol Imaging. 2009;36(3):422–7.

91. Divgi CR, Pandit-Taskar N, Jungbluth AA, et al. Preoperative characterisation of clear-cell renal carcinoma using iodine-124-labelled antibody chimeric G250 (124I-cG250) and PET in patients with renal masses: a phase I trial. Lancet Oncol. 2007;8(4):304–10.

92. Uzzo RG, Russo P, Chen D, et al. The multicenter phase III redect trial: a comparative study of 124 I-girentuximab-PET/CT versus diagnostic CT for the pre-operative diagnosis of clear cell renal cell carcinoma (ccRCC) (late breaking abstract; AUA, San Francisco); 2010.

93. Schachter LR, Bach AM, Snyder ME, et al. The impact of tumour location on the histological subtype of renal cortical tumours. BJU Int. 2006;98(1):63–6.

94. Venkatesh R, Weld K, Ames CD, et al. Laparoscopic partial nephrectomy for renal masses: effect of tumor location. Urology. 2006;67(6):1169–74 [discussion 74].

95. Weizer AZ, Gilbert SM, Roberts WW, et al. Tailoring technique of laparoscopic partial nephrectomy to tumor characteristics. J Urol. 2008;180(4):1273–8.

96. Kutikov A, Uzzo RG. The R.E.N.A.L. nephrometry score: a comprehensive standardized system for quantitating renal tumor size, location and depth. J Urol. 2009;182(3):844–53.

97. Ficarra V, Novara G, Secco S, et al. Preoperative aspects and dimensions used for an anatomical (PADUA) classification of renal tumours in patients who are candidates for nephron-sparing surgery. Eur Urol. 2009;56(5):786–93.

98. Simmons MN, Ching CB, Samplaski MK, et al. Kidney tumor location measurement using the C index method. J Urol. 2010;183(5):1708–13.

99. Kutikov A, Manley BJ, Canter DJ, et al. Anatomical features of enhancing renal masses predict histology and grade – an analysis using nephrometry (AUA abstract no. 1238). J Urol. 2010;183(4):e479.

100. Crispen PL, Viterbo R, Boorjian SA, et al. Natural history, growth kinetics, and outcomes of untreated clinically localized renal tumors under active surveillance. Cancer. 2009;115(13):2844–52.

101. Smaldone MC, Kutikov A, Canter DJ, et al. A critical analysis of active surveillance with delayed curative intent for the treatment of small renal masses. Podium presentation (#11); presented at the Society of Urologic Oncology; 2010.

102. Letourneau I, Ouimet D, Dumont M, et al. Renal replacement in end-stage renal disease patients over 75 years old. Am J Nephrol. 2003;23(2):71–7.

103. Bosniak MA, Birnbaum BA, Krinsky GA, et al. Small renal parenchymal neoplasms: further observations on growth. Radiology. 1995;197(3):589–97.

104. Abou Youssif T, Kassouf W, Steinberg J, et al. Active surveillance for selected patients with renal masses: updated results with long-term follow-up. Cancer. 2007;110(5):1010–4.

105. Abouassaly R, Lane BR, Novick AC. Active surveillance of renal masses in elderly patients. J Urol. 2008;180(2):505–8 [discussion 8–9].

106. Beisland C, Hjelle KM, Reisaeter LA, et al. Observation should be considered as an alternative in management of renal masses in older and comorbid patients. Eur Urol. 2009;55(6):1419–27.

107. Fernando HS, Duvuru S, Hawkyard SJ. Conservative management of renal masses in the elderly: our experience. Int Urol Nephrol. 2007;39(1):203–7.

108. Kouba E, Smith A, McRackan D, et al. Watchful waiting for solid renal masses: insight into the natural history and results of delayed intervention. J Urol. 2007;177(2):466–70 [discussion 70].

109. Lamb GW, Bromwich EJ, Vasey P, et al. Management of renal masses in patients medically unsuitable for nephrectomy – natural history, complications, and outcome. Urology. 2004;64(5):909–13.

110. Matsuzaki M, Kawano Y, Morikawa H, et al. Conservative management of small renal tumors. Hinyokika Kiyo. 2007;53(4):207–11.

111. Rosales JC, Haramis G, Moreno J, et al. Active surveillance for renal cortical neoplasms. J Urol. 2010;183(5):1698–702.

112. Sowery RD, Siemens DR. Growth characteristics of renal cortical tumors in patients managed by watchful waiting. Can J Urol. 2004;11(5):2407–10.

113. Volpe A, Panzarella T, Rendon RA, et al. The natural history of incidentally detected small renal masses. Cancer. 2004;100(4):738–45.

114. Wehle MJ, Thiel DD, Petrou SP, et al. Conservative management of incidental contrast-enhancing renal masses as safe alternative to invasive therapy. Urology. 2004;64(1):49–52.

115. Wong JA, Rendon RA. Progression to metastatic disease from a small renal cell carcinoma prospectively

followed with an active surveillance protocol. Can Urol Assoc J. 2007;1(2):120–2.

116. Mues AC, Landman J. Small renal masses: current concepts regarding the natural history and reflections on the American Urological Association guidelines. Curr Opin Urol. 2010;20(2):105–10.

117. Ozono S, Miyao N, Igarashi T, et al. Tumor doubling time of renal cell carcinoma measured by CT: collaboration of Japanese Society of Renal Cancer. Jpn J Clin Oncol. 2004;34(2):82–5.

118. Chawla SN, Crispen PL, Hanlon AL, et al. The natural history of observed enhancing renal masses: meta-analysis and review of the world literature. J Urol. 2006;175(2):425–31.

119. Siu W, Hafez KS, Johnston 3rd WK, et al. Growth rates of renal cell carcinoma and oncocytoma under surveillance are similar. Urol Oncol. 2007;25(2):115–9.

120. Crispen PL, Wong YN, Greenberg RE, et al. Predicting growth of solid renal masses under active surveillance. Urol Oncol. 2008;26(5):555–9.

121. Norton L. A Gompertzian model of human breast cancer growth. Cancer Res. 1988;48(24 Pt 1):7067–71.

122. Mues AC, Haramis G, Badani K, et al. Active surveillance for larger (cT1bN0M0 and cT2N0M0) renal cortical neoplasms. Urology. 2010;76(3):620–3.

123. Neuzillet Y, Lechevallier E, Andre M, et al. Follow-up of renal oncocytoma diagnosed by percutaneous tumor biopsy. Urology. 2005;66(6):1181–5.

124. Crispen PL, Viterbo R, Fox EB, et al. Delayed intervention of sporadic renal masses undergoing active surveillance. Cancer. 2008;112(5):1051–7.

125. Kunkle DA, Crispen PL, Chen DY, et al. Enhancing renal masses with zero net growth during active surveillance. J Urol. 2007;177(3):849–53 [discussion 53–4].

126. Jewett MA, Finelli A, Morash C, et al. Active surveillance of small renal masses: a prospective multicenter Canadian uro-oncology group trial: abstract no. 896. J Urol. 2009;181(4 supplement):320.

127. Crispen PL, Uzzo RG. The natural history of untreated renal masses. BJU Int. 2007;99(5 Pt B):1203–7.

Part III

Locally Advanced Disease

Locally Advanced Renal Cell Carcinoma

11

Stephen H. Culp and Christopher G. Wood

Introduction

Renal cell carcinoma (RCC) accounts for 3% of all adult malignancies and is the most lethal of the common genitourinary cancers. Surgery remains the standard of care for patients with localized disease. Independent predictors of both progression-free and overall survival in patients with non-metastatic RCC include tumor stage, grade, and regional lymph node involvement [1, 2]. Although patients with low-stage, low-grade tumors tend to do well, patients with locally advanced RCC demonstrate a high risk for both recurrence and progression of disease despite surgical therapy. In this chapter, we review locally advanced RCC, including venous involvement, extracapsular extension, and involvement of adjacent lymph nodes or organs.

Surgery is the mainstay of treatment for patients with locally advanced and non-metastatic disease, providing improved cancer-specific survival (CSS) that cannot be achieved with other modalities. In their study of patients with locally advanced disease (T3/T4, N0–2) but no evidence of distant disease using the surveillance epidemiology and end result (SEER) database, Zini et al. found that the 1-, 2-, 5-, and 10-year disease-specific survival for patients undergoing nephrectomy for locally advanced disease ($n = 6,575$) was 88.9%, 88.1%, 68.6%, and 57.5%, respectively [3]. For patients undergoing nonsurgical therapy (e.g., observation, systemic therapy, etc.) ($n = 282$), the corresponding numbers were 44.8%, 30.6%, 14.5%, and 10.6%. Nonsurgical therapy was associated with a 5.8-fold increased risk of death in patients with locally advanced but non-metastatic RCC. In patients with locally advanced disease, staging modalities should include a dedicated MRI or multiphase CT scan of the abdomen and chest. For patients with bone pain or an elevated alkaline phosphatase, a bone scan should also be obtained. For those with symptoms attributed to central nervous system involvement, appropriate imaging of the brain and/or spine should also be obtained [4].

Lymph Node Disease

Historically, lymph node involvement was seen in 23–35% of RCC cases [5]. More recently, however, isolated lymph node involvement is observed in only 3–5% of patients without clinical evidence of visceral metastatic disease. Obviously, the incidence of positive lymph nodes depends on the extent of lymph node dissection (LND) [6]. When only hilar and regional lymph nodes are resected, the incidence of lymph node

S.H. Culp
Department of Urology, University of Virginia Health System, Box 800422, Charlottesville, VA 22908, USA
e-mail: shc5e@virginia.edu

C.G. Wood (✉)
Department of Urology, The University of Texas MD Anderson Cancer Center, 1515 Holcombe Boulevard, Unit 1373, Houston, TX 77030, USA
e-mail: cgwood@mdanderson.org

Table 11.1 2010[a] and 2002[b] AJCC classification of renal cell carcinoma based on TNM staging

Stage	Primary tumor (T)	Lymph node (N)	Metastasis (M)
I	T1	N0	M0
II	T2	N0	M0
III	T1/T2	N1	M0
	T3	N0/N1	M0
IV	T4	Any N	M0
	Any T	N1[a] or N2[b]	M0
	Any T	Any N	M1

positive disease is 5–8%. However, the incidence of lymph node positivity can be as high as 38% when an extensive LND is performed [6]. Regardless, most patients with lymph node involvement will also have concurrent distant metastatic disease.

Table 11.1 details the staging of RCC pertinent to locally advanced disease, staged 3 and 4. According to the historic Robson staging system, lymph node positive disease was stage IIIb because the prognosis of patients with lymph node involvement was significantly worse than those classified Robson stages I–IIIa [7]. In the 2002 TMN AJCC staging criteria, a single node corresponds to stage IIIb or IIIc in the absence of metastatic disease and whether the primary tumor (T) stage was I/II or III, respectively. Two or more positive nodes correspond to stage IV in the 2002 TMN AJCC staging. However, in the most recent 2010 TMN AJCC staging criteria, only N0 or N1 (not N2) is used to determine stage III or IV disease in conjunction with T stage and metastatic status.

Preoperative evaluation of lymph node involvement has evolved over the past few decades with the advancement of imaging. CT imaging is the standard modality, with a sensitivity greater than 90% [8]. Sensitivity is decreased when only hilar lymph nodes are involved, with accuracies ranging from 43% to 83% [9, 10]. The risk of a false positive reading is increased in the presence of tumor thrombus or necrosis, because, when the latter is present, lymph nodes as large as 2 cm may be reactive rather than involved by tumor.

The risk of lymph node disease involvement increases with tumor stage. In their study of 104 consecutive patients undergoing an extended LND, Giuliani et al. found that when tumors were confined to the kidney, only 6% of patients had lymph node involvement. However, the incidence of lymph node disease increased to 46.4% with locally advanced disease and 61.0% when distant metastases were present. When vascular infiltration and distant metastases were both present, the incidence of lymph node disease was 66.6% [11]. In a later study, Zisman et al. examined 661 patients without metastatic disease and found that in patients with stage T2 or less disease (based on 1997 UICC TNM scheme), 3% had lymph node positive disease whereas 20% of patients with stage III/IV disease had lymph node positivity [12].

Lymph node involvement is also correlated with Fuhrman nuclear grade. In patients with lymph node negative disease, Pantuck et al. found that 67% had low-grade disease (Fuhrman grade I or II). However, 68% of patients with node positive disease had high grade disease (Fuhrman grade III or IV) [13]. In addition, Guiliani et al. found that 81% of grade III patients but only 25% of grade 1 tumors were node positive or metastatic [14].

RCC tumor histology is another potential predictor of regional lymph node involvement. In their study of 245 patients with non-metastatic papillary RCC undergoing nephrectomy at MDACC, Margulis et al. found that 13% harbored lymph node metastasis, compared to 8% in patients with clear cell histology ($p < 0.02$) [15]. Of interest, lymph node metastases in patients with papillary RCC seemed to demonstrate a more indolent course in that these patients had a 65% disease-specific survival compared to 19% for patients with regional lymph node disease and clear cell histology. In addition, in a subsequent study by Delacroix et al. examining 68 patients with RCC and pathological nodal involvement but no distant metastasis, papillary histology was an independent predictor of overall survival (HR 0.26; 95% CI 0.08, 0.85; $p = 0.026$) and patients with papillary RCC demonstrated a delayed time to recurrence (37.2 months) compared to patients with clear cell RCC (4.4 months) [16].

Multiple studies have shown that lymph node involvement is associated with decreased

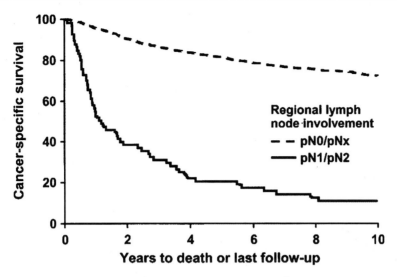

Fig. 11.1 Cancer-specific survival of patients with clear cell renal cell carcinoma treated with nephrectomy based on regional lymph node involvement (pN0/pNx vs. pN1/pN2). Reprinted with permission from Blute ML, Leibovich BC, Cheville JC, Lohse CM, Zincke H.

A protocol for performing extended lymph node dissection using primary tumor pathological features for patients treated with radical nephrectomy for clear cell renal cell carcinoma. The Journal of Urology 2004;172(2): 465–9

survival. In their study of 1,652 patients undergoing radical nephrectomy for unilateral non-metastatic sporadic clear cell RCC between 1970 and 2000, Blute et al. found that the 1-, 5-, and 10-year disease-specific survival of patients with pN0/pNx disease was 95.5%, 82.1%, and 72.5%, respectively. However, patients with pN1/pN2 disease demonstrated a much decreased 1-, 5-, and 10-year disease-specific survival of 52.2%, 20.9%, and 11.4% (Fig. 11.1) [17]. In addition, Margulis et al. found that 5-year CSS for patients with clear cell RCC and lymph node involvement was only 19% [15].

Potential predictors of survival in patients with lymph node disease and no evidence of metastasis include numbers of lymph nodes involved, lymph node density, and the presence of extranodal extension. In their study of 40 patients with clinical regional node-positive non-metastatic disease who underwent an extended LND, Canfield et al. found that survival was dependent on pathological node stage. Patients having pN1 disease (30%) had a median survival of 37.5 months whereas in patients with pN2 disease (70%), median survival was 14.5 months. In addition, on multivariate analysis, two or more

positive lymph nodes was an independent predictor of both decreased recurrence-free survival (HR 2.83; 95% CI 1.06, 7.61, p=0.039) and overall survival (HR 9.33; 95% CI 1.85, 47.09, p<0.01) [18]. The ratio of positive to total lymph nodes removed is also important in survival. In their study of 618 patients undergoing LND between 1983 and 1999, Terrone et al. found that 14.2% of patients had positive lymph nodes with a 5-year disease-specific survival of 18%. There was no difference in survival based on pN1 and pN2 or, as important, the number of lymph nodes removed. However, on multivariate analysis, poor prognostic factors included greater than four lymph nodes removed (p=0.02) and a lymph node density greater than 60% (p=0.01) [19]. Importantly, this study reported that the number of lymph nodes influenced the detection rate of metastasis. These authors reported that the incidence of lymph node metastasis was 3.4% when 12 or fewer nodes were removed at the time of nephrectomy; however, this increased to 10.5% when 13 or more lymph nodes were removed [19]. For patients with localized disease, lymph node positivity increased to 19.7% and 32.2% when <13 or ≥13 lymph nodes were removed at the time of surgery, respectively. These results were corroborated by Joslyn et al., examining data on 4,000 patients from the SEER registry, demonstrating that the incidence of lymph node detection significantly correlated with the number of lymph nodes removed at the time of nephrectomy [20]. Based on these studies, the sixth edition of the AJCC states that removal of eight or more nodes at the time of LND is required for adequate nodal staging in RCC [21].

The presence of extranodal extension of lymph node disease is also important in patient survival. Dimashkieh et al., in their review of 2,076 patients without metastatic disease, found that, although there was no difference in survival in patients based on pN1 vs. pN2 disease, patients with extranodal extension were twice as likely to die from their disease (5-year disease-specific survival of 18% vs. 35%) [21].

Lymph Node Dissection

Based on multiple studies, it is apparent that not only are there differences in patient survival based on lymph node involvement but also there is variability in survival based on extent of lymph node disease. The question then becomes when to perform an LND and how extensive does the dissection need to be? Studies to date are plagued by major limitations. Most have been retrospective, have included a small number of patients, and ultimately have shown a selection bias with respect to the performance of an LND. In addition, there is a lack of a standardized LND template as well as a standardized pathologic examination and defined postsurgical systemic treatment.

The benefits of LND undoubtedly include more accurate staging of the patient's disease and evaluation of prognosis. However, the therapeutic benefit remains controversial. Over the past two decades, there have been significant developments in other malignancies (breast, colon, and head and neck) demonstrating that removal of potentially diseased lymph nodes at the time of primary tumor surgery not only prolongs survival but also results in cure in a select number of

patients. In addition, lymph node removal in other GU malignancies (e.g., prostate, bladder, penile, and testicular germ cell tumors), initially only done for staging purposes, has been shown to demonstrate therapeutic benefit [9, 22, 23]. Therefore, in RCC, some could argue that it could mean possible cure in patients with disease limited to the retroperitoneum and that an LND would ultimately decrease the risk of local recurrence of disease. In addition, in the era of targeted systemic therapy, a LND would allow for sufficient cytoreduction in patients with systemic disease in order for them to respond better to adjuvant therapy. Nonetheless, there are potential risks of LND including bleeding, bowel injury, chylous ascites, and prolonged postoperative recovery.

Types of LND

Initial studies of renal lymphatic drainage by Alice Parker in 1939 on stillborn fetuses with Prussian blue dye demonstrated that the normal flow of renal lymphatics follows the arterial system to eventually coalesce in the renal sinus prior to draining into the regional lymphatics. Unfortunately, lymph node drainage in renal cancer is not always predictable [14, 24, 25]. Extensive neovascularization and collateral circulation induced by the primary kidney tumor may alter lymph node drainage [26]. Furthermore, lymphatic drainage of perinephric fat is not the same as the kidney, and therefore higher stage tumors will show additional drainage patterns not seen in the "normal" kidney [27].

According to Robson four decades ago, at a time when adequate preoperative imaging did not exist and up to 22.7% of patients undergoing radical nephrectomy had positive lymph nodes, the standard treatment of RCC should include a radical nephrectomy as well as removal of "the para-aortic and para-caval lymph nodes from the bifurcation of the aorta to the crus of the diaphragm" (Fig. 11.2) [28]. Traditionally, a *hilar* LND would include resection of all lymph nodes from the involved kidney to the inferior vena cava or the aorta for a right or left-sided tumor,

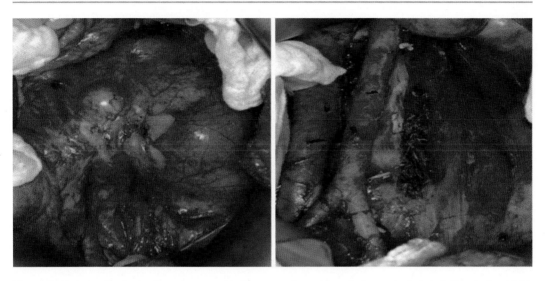

Fig. 11.2 Patient with renal cell carcinoma and bulky retroperitoneal lymphadenopathy before (*left*) and after (*right*) radical nephrectomy and complete lymph node dissection

respectively (Fig. 11.3). A *regional* LND would include resection of all hilar nodes as well as additional lymph nodes along the inferior vena cava or aorta for a right or left-sided tumor, respectively (Fig. 11.3). An *extended* LND for a left-sided tumor would include all para-aortic and interaortocaval lymph nodes from the aortic bifurcation to the crus of the diaphragm. For a right-sided tumor, an *extended* LND would include all paracaval as well as interaortocaval lymph nodes, the latter because 50% of positive lymph nodes in right-sided tumors will be within the interaortocaval region (Fig. 11.4) [29].

Multiple retrospective studies have shown a potential therapeutic benefit for performing an LND at the time of nephrectomy. Peters and Brown, in 1980, found that in patients undergoing an extended LND, both 1-year and 5-year survival were better (87.5% and 43.8%) compared to patients who did not undergo an LND (56.5% and 25.7%). The authors found an 18% improvement in 5-year survival in patients with stage C disease who underwent an LND [30]. However, this study lacked information regarding the number and extent of lymph node involvement. Furthermore, improved imaging over the following decades would likely make these results irrelevant. More recent and larger studies

include those by Herrlinger et al. in 1991 who prospectively examined 511 patients with non-metastatic disease and compared survival based on extended ($n=320$) vs. facultative (nodes resected for staging purposes only) ($n=191$) LND. The authors found that there was a 26% improvement in 5-year survival in patients with Stage I–II disease undergoing LND. Specifically, patients undergoing an extended LND had a 5- and 10-year survival of 66% and 56.1%, respectively. Patients undergoing a facultative LND had a 5- and 10-year survival of 58% and 40.9%, respectively. In interpreting these results, one must consider stage migration to account for the discrepancy between improvement in survival (26%) and incidence of positive lymph nodes (8%) [6]. In their review of 200 consecutive patients undergoing extended LND, of which 25% had metastatic disease at the time of surgery, Giuliani et al. found that patients with node-positive, non-metastatic disease undergoing LND had a survival statistically similar to those with pT3N0M0 disease and better than patients with M1 disease (47.9% 5-year and 31.9% 10-year) [14]. In the largest retrospective study to date examining 900 patients, Pantuck et al. found that there was a 5-month increase in median survival in patients undergoing any type of LND compared

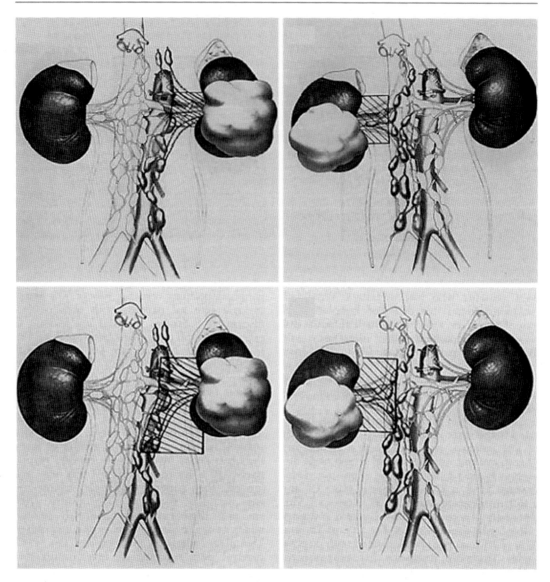

Fig. 11.3 Area of resection for hilar (*top*) and regional (*bottom*) lymph node dissection in renal cell carcinoma based on side of primary tumor. Reprinted with permis-sion from Wood DP, Jr. Role of lymphadenectomy in renal cell carcinoma. The Urologic Clinics of North America 1991;18(3):421–6

to those patients with clinically positive lymph nodes left in situ. In addition, performing an LND was an independent predictor of survival on mul-tivariate analysis in patients with clinical evi-dence of lymph node disease. Importantly, there was no measurable benefit in survival (overall or progression-free) in patients with clinically nega-tive lymph nodes undergoing LND [31].

Multiple studies have also demonstrated no clear benefit for performing an LND in patients with RCC, and this remains a very controversial topic. In their review of 554 patients diagnosed with RCC at autopsy between 1958 and 1982, Johnsen and Hellsten found that only five (<1%) patients had no metastatic disease and positive nodes limited to the retroperitoneum and therefore were amenable to potential cure with nephrectomy and LND alone [32]. In addition, Minervini and colleagues examined 167 patients without meta-static disease from 1990 to 1997 [33]. Fifty-nine

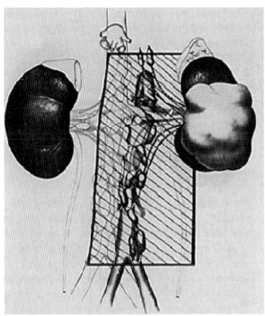 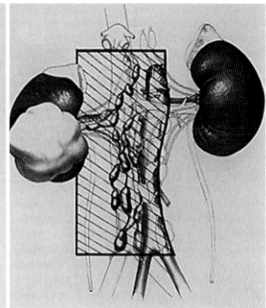

Fig. 11.4 Area of resection for extended lymph node dissection in renal cell carcinoma based on side of primary tumor. Reprinted with permission from Wood DP, Jr. Role of lymphadenectomy in renal cell carcinoma. The Urologic Clinics of North America 1991;18(3):421–6

of these patients underwent radical nephrectomy with regional LND, of which 49 of these had no clinical evidence of lymph node involvement. The LND consisted of dissection limited to the anterior, posterior, and lateral sides of the ipsilateral great vessel from the level of the renal vessels down to the IMA. Only one (2%) patient had a positive node on final pathology. Five-year survival was 79% and 78% for patients undergoing nephrectomy or nephrectomy with LND, respectively. In a larger study, Schafhauser et al. examined 1,035 patients and estimated that only 4% benefited from an extensive LND [34]. These studies suggest that LND do not provide a survival advantage in patients with RCC, especially those without clinical evidence of lymph node disease.

The only randomized trial examining the influence of LND on survival of patients with RCC was the EORTC 30881 trial [35, 36]. Seven hundred and seventy-two patients were randomized to undergo radical nephrectomy alone or radical nephrectomy with LND. The results showed that there was no discernable difference in CSS between the two groups. However, this was an underpowered study in that only 3.3% of

patients had node-positive disease. Most patients had low-stage and low-grade disease and therefore, based on previous studies, had a low risk for lymph node involvement. Furthermore, only 17% of patients progressed or died of RCC. Importantly, though, this study did demonstrate that morbidity from a standardized LND was low with few complications.

Various nomograms have been developed in order to help identify factors that are important for predicting lymph node disease and therefore provide better guidance on when to perform an LND. These nomograms can provide better preoperative surgical planning as well as counseling to the patient. In addition, nomograms can potentially identify those patients who may be best served with enrollment in neoadjuvant or adjuvant therapy trials. Blute et al. examined their results from 955 patients with non-metastatic clear cell RCC who underwent radical nephrectomy and LND from 1970 to 2000 [17]. Sixty-eight (7.1%) patients had pN1 or pN2 disease. On multivariate analysis, significant independent predictors of lymph node involvement were tumor size greater than 10 cm, pT3 or pT4

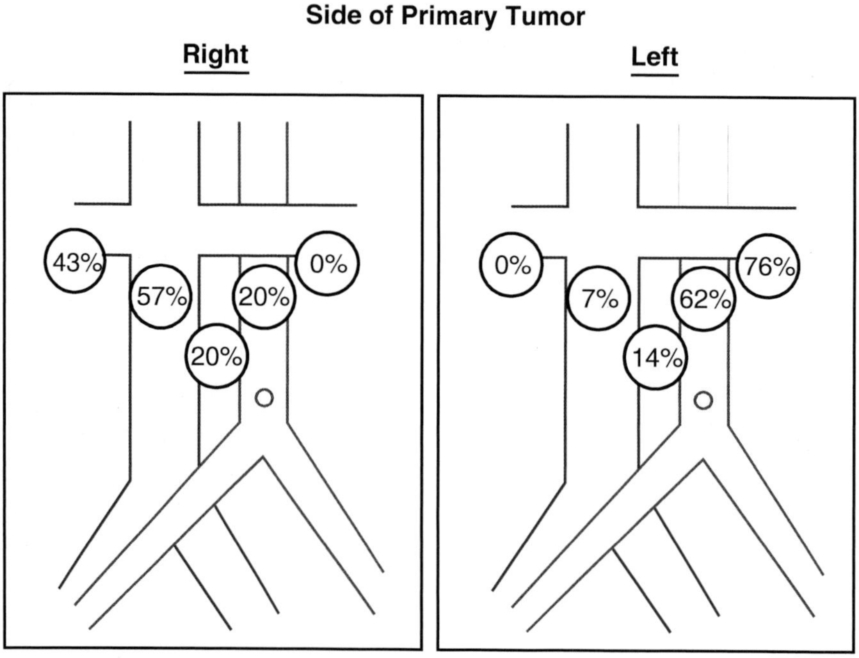

Side of Primary Tumor

Right   Left

Fig. 11.5 Location of pathological positive lymph nodes based on side of primary tumor. Percentage represents frequency of involved location in patients with lymph node positive disease. Reprinted with permission from Crispen PL, Breau RH, Allmer C, et al. Lymph node dissection at the time of radical nephrectomy for high-risk clear cell renal cell carcinoma: indications and recommendations for surgical templates. European Urology 59(1):18–23

disease, Fuhrman grade III or IV, and sarcomatoid de-differentiation. In addition, the presence of necrosis on pathology, although not significant, was included in their nomogram to identify patients who would benefit from an LND at the time of nephrectomy. Only six of 1,031 patients (0.6%) with 0 or 1 of the above features had positive lymph nodes. However, 62 (10%) patients with two or more features had lymph node disease. Overall, there was a fourfold increased risk with two or more features and a 50% increase if all five features were present. Therefore, the authors recommend an intraoperative risk assessment whereby the primary tumor would be sent for frozen pathologic analysis. An LND should be performed if two or more of the above features are present in the primary tumor. Of course, some could argue that an LND could be performed in the time needed to wait for the results from the frozen analysis. A more recent study by Crispen et al. validated these risk factors in patients with high-risk clear cell RCC and demonstrated the percentage of positive lymph nodes based on anatomic location (Fig. 11.5) [37].

A similar but more complex nomogram was developed based on results from 4,844 patients at MSKCC and the Mayo Clinic. Of these, 139 (2.9%) had lymph node positive disease. The accuracy of this nomogram for predicting pathologic node-positive disease was 76.1%. Factors involved in this nomogram included symptoms at presentation, history of hematuria, gender, ECOG performance status, comorbidity index, tumor location, preoperative hemoglobin level, tumor size, lymph nodes on imaging, and necrosis.

In an effort to develop a nomogram based on fewer factors, Hutterer et al. looked at 4,658 patients from seven centers [38]. Of these, 2,522 (54.1%) patients, of which 4.2% had positive lymph nodes, were used for development of a nomogram and 2,136 (45.9%) patients, of which 4.7% had lymph node disease, were used for validation of the nomogram. Prediction of lymph node involvement is based on tumor size, symptom classification (no symptoms, local, or systemic), and age. Based on their results, the AUC was 78.4% for the nomogram.

Summary of Lymph Node Management

Lymph node involvement in RCC is associated with a higher grade and stage of disease and compromised patient prognosis. Undoubtedly, LND at the time of surgery does provide improved staging and better ascertainment of patient prognosis. However, there is controversy as to whether an LND provides a therapeutic benefit. Patients with low-stage, organ-confined tumors are at a low risk to have lymph node disease and therefore an LND is not necessary in these patients. However, based on studies that demonstrate that an LND can be performed safely and with low morbidity, we would recommend that an LND be performed in patients with clinical or intraoperative evidence of nodal disease or locally invasive disease with associated risk factors. Further studies are needed to better define the role of LND in RCC, which will likely evolve with the new therapeutic strategies used to treat metastatic disease.

Tumor Thrombus

Inferior vena caval involvement by tumor thrombus occurs in 4–10% of patients with RCC [39, 40], with thrombus reaching the atrium in 1% of patients [41]. One-third of patients with tumor thrombus will have distant metastatic disease [42]. Tumor thrombus may be detected incidentally as with the primary tumor but if present, symptoms may include lower extremity edema, right-sided varicocele, pulmonary embolus, and caput medusa [43]. Additional findings may include proteinuria, right atrial mass, or a non-functioning renal unit.

Staging

According to the AJCC TMN 2009 staging system, renal thrombus located within the renal vein is pT3a, in the IVC below the hepatic veins is pT3b,

and above the diaphragm is pT3c. This most recent change in staging of tumor thrombus was supported by a large multi-institutional study of 1,215 patients reported by Martinez-Salamanca et al. [44]. Traditionally, the Mayo Classification of Tumor Thrombus [45] is as follows: level 0—thrombus in the renal vein only (detected clinically or during pathologic evaluation), level I—thrombus either at entry to renal vein or within the IVC less than 2 cm from the confluence of the renal vein and IVC, level II—thrombus within IVC greater than 2 cm distal to renal vein but below the hepatic veins, level III—thrombus involving the intrahepatic IVC, and IV—thrombus extends above the diaphragm or into the right atrium of the heart (Fig. 11.6).

Imaging

Various imaging modalities may be used to identify and evaluate thrombus associated with RCC. MRI has traditionally been used for this purpose; however, newer CT modalities, specifically multiplanar CT, can be as accurate as MRI, and CT is now the most commonly utilized modality for imaging IVC thrombi. Nonetheless, MRI is still preferred at many centers related to its accuracy for determining the true extent of tumor thrombus, the degree of IVC occlusion, and the existence of bland thrombus in the infrarenal IVC and any venous anomalies [46, 47]. During surgical resection, transesophageal echocardiography is frequently used to provide real-time imaging of the thrombus [48].

Surgical Resection

The first RCC thrombus ever resected was done in 1919. Once considered a death sentence, the thrombus was usually left in situ. The majority of patients undergoing removal of the kidney alone survived less than a year [49]. Currently, the surgical mortality from nephrectomy and high level IVC thrombectomy is 5–10% [50]. However, mortality can be as high as 40% if the thrombus extends above the diaphragm [51–53]. Fortunately,

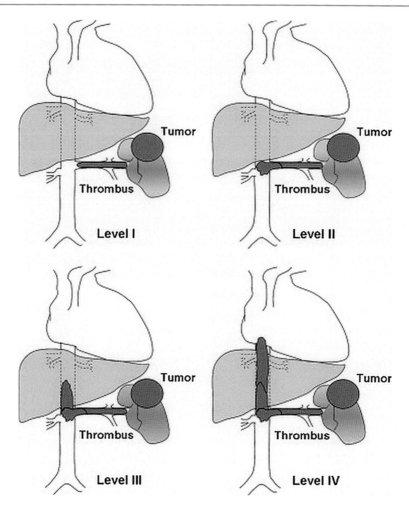

Fig. 11.6 Mayo classification of tumor thrombus based on level of inferior vena caval involvement in renal cell carcinoma. Reprinted with permission from Kirkali Z, Van Poppel H. A critical analysis of surgery for kidney cancer with vena cava invasion. European Urology 2007;52(3):658–62

45–70% of patients with non-metastatic disease can be cured with complete surgical resection [54, 55]. Five-year survival of patients with IVC thrombus ranges from 60% to 82% and 18% to 55% for patients without or with metastatic disease, respectively, who undergo surgical resection [56, 57] (Table 11.2).

Careful surgical planning prior to resection is paramount and may require a multidisciplinary approach. Radical nephrectomy with IVC thrombectomy is a complex procedure with potential for high morbidity [58] and a mortality rate of 10% [51–53]. Surgical management depends on the size of the tumor, the cranial extent of the thrombus, baseline surgical risk factors, and

Table 11.2 Five-year survival of patients with renal cell carcinoma and inferior vena cava tumor thrombus and no evidence of metastatic disease undergoing surgical resection

Study	Study year	Patient number	%Survival
Swierzewski	1994	100	64
Quek	2001	99	59
Zisman	2003	100	72
Blute	2004	191	59
Skinner	1989	43	57
Glazer	1996	18	57
Lubahn	2006	44	56

whether the thrombus is infiltrating the wall of the IVC [59]. Depending on the size of tumor and thrombus, there is potential for significant surgical blood loss as well as pulmonary embolism during thrombectomy.

The choice of incision depends on the size and location of tumor as well as thrombus extent but may involve a midline, Chevron, subcostal, or thoracoabdominal approach. For thrombi isolated to the renal vein or within 5 cm of the IVC/renal vein ostium, a flank incision may also be appropriate. Although we do not routinely perform it, preoperative embolization of the kidney may be done in order to decrease blood loss and to facilitate more direct access to the renal hilum and vessels. In addition, embolization may result in partial regression of the tumor thrombus and may decrease venous congestion in the primary tumor and thrombus [58, 60, 61].

Resection of a level I or II thrombus requires early control of the renal artery, ligation of any lumbar veins, and venous control both proximal and distal to the thrombus as well as the contralateral renal vein. If possible, the goal is to remove the diseased kidney and thrombus en bloc [62]. After proper mobilization of the kidney, ligation of the renal artery and lumbar veins, and clamping of the IVC and contralateral renal vein, the renal ostium is opened allowing removal of the diseased kidney and simultaneous extraction of the IVC thrombus. The IVC is oversewn being careful to avoid significant narrowing of the vessel (Fig. 11.7). For a level III thrombus, mobilization of the hepatic caudate lobe is required [63]. This allows access to IVC above the tumor thrombus and the ability to clamp below the intrahepatic veins. Tumor thrombus above the hepatic veins may require complete liver mobilization [64], veno-venous bypass, Pringle maneuver, and occlusion of select hepatic veins [65, 66]. Level IV thrombi may require circulatory arrest with [67, 68] or without hypothermia [69, 70]. There is an increased risk for coagulopathy, cerebral vascular incident, and myocardial infarction [67, 68, 70]. For patients with a level III or IV non-adherent thrombus, it may be possible to "milk" the thrombus back below the hepatic veins therefore avoiding the need for clamping the suprahepatic IVC.

It is not uncommon to find complete thrombosis of the IVC inferior to the tumor thrombus.

If possible, this bland thrombus may be removed at the time of removal of the tumor thrombus. If not possible, then it may be necessary to ligate the infrarenal IVC to avoid postoperative embolization of clot [71].

Boorjian et al. examined the Mayo Clinic experience in more than 400 patients in terms of complications from tumor thrombus resection [72]. They found that the incidence of both early (<30 days) and late (≥30 days) complications correlated with the level of tumor thrombus. If the IVC thrombus is small or there is incomplete obstruction of the IVC with minimal collateral, then vena caval clamping can result in profound hypotension and the need for a venous–venous bypass in order to augment venous return. With a left-sided renal tumor and venous/IVC occlusion, there are multiple methods of venous return (adrenal, inferior diaphragmatic, gonadal, ureteral, and lumbar) [73].

Clinicopathological Features

Multiple studies have examined the association of clinicopathologic features with the presence and level of tumor thrombus. The majority of renal tumors with associated thrombus are of clear cell histology with 5–28% of them having sarcomatoid de-differentiation [74–76]. In their study of 1,082 patients, Rabbani et al. reported that renal vein and IVC extension of tumor thrombus were present in 5.4% and 2.8% of patients, respectively [77]. Clear cell histology was significantly associated with an increased risk for thrombus while histologies such as oncocytoma and papillary RCC were significantly associated with a decreased risk [77]. Larger tumor thrombi are associated with higher Fuhrman nuclear grade and more advanced stage [45]. In examining markers associated with tumor thrombi, vascular endothelial growth factor expression was found not to be significantly associated with the level of tumor thrombus [78]. However, Ki67 expression was positively associated with the presence and level of tumor thrombus [79]. Higher level of thrombus is also associated with decreased response to immunotherapy and increased perioperative morbidity and mortality [80].

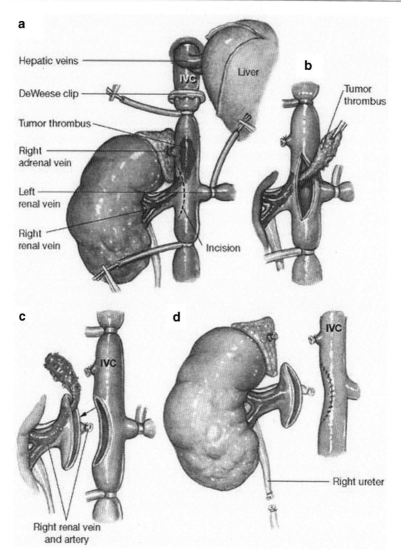

Fig. 11.7 Illustration of surgical resection of infrahepatic tumor thrombus from renal cell thrombus. Control of inferior vena cava (IVC) both proximal and distal to thrombus as well as contralateral renal vein is performed (**a**). The IVC is then opened to allow for mobilization of the tumor thrombus (**b**). The renal vein and tumor thrombus are then separated from the IVC (**c**) and the IVC is oversewn (**d**). Reprinted with permission from Wszolek MF, Wotkowicz C, Libertino JA. Surgical management of large renal tumors. Nature Clinical Practice 2008;5(1):35–46

Patient Survival

Complete resection of tumor thrombus in patients with non-metastatic disease can result in a survival greater than 50%. However, survival is dependent on level of tumor thrombus with an IVC thrombus extending above the diaphragm predicting a worse survival even after controlling for Fuhrman nuclear grade and ECOG performance status [81].

In addition, tumor thrombus level is associated with likelihood of metastatic disease. In a study of 56 patients, Ciancio et al. found that 10 of 49 patients with levels I–III thrombus and four of seven patients with level IV thrombus had distant metastasis [82].

In a study of 118 patients with pT3b or pT3c RCC from 1989 to 2006, Lambert et al. found that the 5-year CSS was 60.3% and 10% for patients without or with distant metastasis, respectively [83]. Importantly, the level of tumor thrombus was not an independent predictor of survival, only positive lymph node disease and tumor diameter greater than 7 cm. Another retrospective study of 1,192 patients with pT3b or pT3c disease from 13 European institutions (1982–2003) found no difference in survival based on IVC level of tumor thrombus. However, there was a significant difference in median survival of patients based on renal vein vs. IVC thrombus below or above the diaphragm (52 vs. 25.8 and 18 months, respectively) [84]. Unfortunately, based on the multi-institutional nature of the study, there was no ability to control for difference in surgical techniques or the use of adjuvant therapy. In a study of 153 patients, Moinzadeh and Libertino found that 5-year survival was similar between renal vein only and IVC tumor thrombus; however, 10-year overall survival was significantly different (66% vs. 29%, respectively) [85].

The impact of tumor thrombus level on survival depends on whether or not the patient has distant disease. In a study of 101 patients with pT3b disease between 1990 and 2006, Klaver et al. found that Mayo Clinic level of tumor thrombus was an independent predictor of CSS in patients with non-nodal, non-metastatic disease on multivariate analysis (median survival of 69, 26, and 21 months for levels I, II, and III tumor thrombus, respectively) [86]. However, in patients with either nodal or distant disease, tumor size and histologic subtype (but not level of tumor thrombus) were independent predictors of CSS.

Venous Wall Involvement

It is rare for a tumor thrombus to invade the wall of the IVC. However, when extensive invasion or caval adherence is present, partial or complete resection of the IVC may be required. When the IVC is chronically obstructed, resection of the cava with no replacement can be well tolerated with few sequelae [39, 87]. In the absence of adequate collateral circulation, however, resection can result in significant IVC narrowing and/or

lower extremity edema and a patch or interposition graft should be considered, either a PTFE, pericardial [88], or autologous venous graft [89]. Grafting techniques may be technically challenging and may therefore require the expertise of vascular surgery. Depending on which type of graft used and location, there may be an increased risk for infection [90], renal and/or hepatic failure, ascites, and lower extremity edema. Invasion of the wall of the inferior vena cava is a poor prognostic sign and is staged pT3c independent of the cephalad extent of the thrombus.

Zini et al. evaluated 32 patients undergoing nephrectomy from 2000 to 2006 with IVC involvement and found that renal vein ostium wall invasion was present in 13 (40.6%) patients [91]. RV ostium wall invasion was significantly associated with a higher recurrence rate, lower CSS, and higher level of tumor thrombus. From this study, CT imaging with cutoffs of 1.8 cm of IVC AP diameter and 1.4 cm of renal vein ostium diameter had a sensitivity of 90% for predicting invasion.

Budd–Chiari Syndrome

Although rare, some patients with RCC and IVC thrombus may have tumor involving the orifices of the hepatic veins. This results in Budd–Chiari syndrome (BCS) with occlusion of hepatic venous outflow, hepatic congestion, and potential progression to liver failure. Symptoms may include abdominal pain, hepatomegaly, ascites, jaundice, lower extremity edema, bleeding, and encephalopathy. Aggressive surgical management is required to prevent liver failure and death. Based on the anatomy and complexity of the surgery, dedicated transplant and thoracic surgeons should be involved.

In their review of 12 cases of BCS caused by RCC thrombus, Kume et al. divided patients into two groups, mild/silent and severe, based on the absence or presence of liver failure, respectively [92]. Patients with mild/silent disease had minimal hepatic dysfunction likely secondary to gradual or incomplete occlusion resulting in sufficient time to develop collateral outflow. Patients with severe disease, however, had sudden and complete occlusion resulting in significant liver failure and disseminated intravascular coagulation. Based on their experience, patients who underwent immediate thrombectomy for mild/silent disease avoided fulminant hepatic failure and their prognosis was similar to patients with IVC thrombus only. Although there is increased risk in patients with severe disease based on the presence of liver failure and consequent poor condition, management should be made on a case-by-case basis as a successful thrombectomy may lead to resolution of liver dysfunction. In the MDACC experience, five of six patients with BCS due to RCC thrombus have undergone complete thrombectomy and two are alive with no evidence of disease at 37 months (MDACC, unpublished data).

Extracapsular Extension

Perinephric Fat Invasion

Perinephric fat invasion has been shown by multiple studies to be a poor prognostic indicator in patients with RCC. There is controversy regarding the significance of focal vs. extensive perinephric fat invasion. Roberts et al. evaluated 186 patients with clinical T1 disease and found that 57 (31%) were upgraded to pT3a disease based on focal perinephric fat invasion [93]. Five-year CSS was not different between the two groups of patients (90.6% for pT1 and 97.5% for pT3a). Jung et al. retrospectively reviewed 198 patients to determine the impact of focal vs. extensive perinephric fat invasion [94]. All patients were free of nodal and distant metastasis. Of these patients, 57 and 61 had minimal (≤5mm) or extensive (>5 mm) perinephric fat invasion with 5-year survival rates of 85% and 76%, respectively. Therefore, based on this study, the prognosis of perinephric fat invasion did not depend on extent of involvement.

The presence of perinephric fat invasion in combination with other factors also results in a poorer outcome. In their review of 96 patients with pT3b RCC, Sweeney et al. found that the concomitant presence of perinephric fat invasion

resulted in a significant reduction in the median survival from 33 to 10 months [58]. Similar findings were found by Fujita et al. in their retrospective review of 43 patients with pT3b disease [95]. Patients with tumor thrombus only (tumor otherwise confined to the kidney) had a median CSS of 70.9 months, while patients with concomitant perinephric fat invasion had a median CSS of 25 months. Based on similar findings showing that perinephric fat invasion was not only an independent prognostic factor for patients with tumor thrombus but also seemed to have a greater impact on survival when present by itself, both Ficarra [96] and Thompson [97] and their associated colleagues proposed separate reclassification schemes in the TMN staging to include perinephric fat invasion as a prognostic factor and in an effort to more accurately stratify patients with pT3 RCC with respect to risk of disease recurrence. The scheme proposed by Ficarra and associates stratifies perinephric fat invasion or thrombus below the diaphragm as pT3a, perinephric fat invasion and tumor thrombus below diaphragm as pT3b, and adrenal gland involvement or tumor outside Gerota's fascia, or tumor thrombus above the diaphragm as pT4 disease [96]. The scheme proposed by Thompson and colleagues includes level 0 thrombus with no perinephric fat invasion as pT3a, perinephric invasion only as pT3b, level 0 thrombus with perinephric fat invasion or levels I–III thrombus with no fat invasion as pT3c, levels I–III thrombus with fat invasion or level IV thrombus as pT3d, and extension beyond Gerota's fascia as pT4 [97]. These proposals highlight the importance of capturing all adverse features when staging patients with locally advanced renal cancer, because they allow for more refined risk stratification.

Renal Sinus Invasion

The renal sinus is a fatty compartment located within the central aspect of the kidney, adjacent to the collecting system, and is composed of an abundance of lymphatics and small veins [98]. This potentially lends it to be an ideal location for propagation of tumor otherwise located within the renal capsule. Although, historically, renal sinus involvement was not routinely evaluated, the 2002 AJCC TMN staging placed renal sinus invasion as pT3a. The prognostic significance of renal sinus involvement remains somewhat controversial. Bonsib et al. demonstrated in a prospective study of 31 patients that tumors with renal sinus involvement were more often larger, displayed higher Fuhrman nuclear grades, and more frequently involved the renal vein and capsule, all of which would increase the metastatic potential of the tumor [99]. Thompson et al., in their evaluation of 205 patients with pT3a RCC, found that tumors with clear cell histology involving the renal sinus displayed higher aggressiveness compared to tumors invading the perinephric fat lateral to the kidney, demonstrating a higher propensity for metastasis to lymph nodes, a higher Fuhrman nuclear grade, and a greater proportion of sarcomatoid de-differentiation [100]. In addition, on multivariate analysis, renal sinus invasion remained an independent predictor of poor survival in patients with pT3a disease. However, in contrast to the above findings, other authors have found similar patient survival rates between those with renal sinus involvement and those with perinephric fat invasion [101]. Specifically, Margulis et al., in their review of patients at MDACC, did not find a significant difference in disease-specific survival between perinephric fat and renal sinus invasion (54.1% and 50.8%, respectively, $p = 0.782$). These differences in findings may reflect the higher number of patients and increased incidence of renal sinus invasion (56% vs. 21%) in the series by Margulis et al. [102].

Collecting System Invasion

Renal tumor involvement of the urinary collecting system has not been extensively studied and its implications remain unclear. Terrone et al., in their study of 671 patients at two institutions, found that involvement of the collecting system by tumor was low (8.8%) and was not an independent prognostic factor [103]. In contrast,

Klatte et al., in evaluation of 519 patients with intracapsular RCC, found that renal capsule and collecting system involvement occurred in 21.6% and 7.5% of patients, respectively [103]. There was a significant association of collecting system involvement and microvascular invasion, and collecting system invasion was an independent predictor of progression-free survival (RR 3.78). Further studies are undoubtedly needed to better elucidate the impact of collecting system invasion on disease recurrence and patient survival.

Adjacent Organ Involvement (T4 Disease)

The incidence of adjacent organ involvement in RCC ranges from 5% to 15% [104]. Renal tumors are more likely to compress rather than invade adjacent structures. Additionally, large renal masses can frequently induce a significant degree of reactive changes which may obliterate surgical tissue planes and therefore mimic T4 disease [105]. The poor prognosis in patients with T4 disease is compounded by the fact that a majority of these patients also have nodal or distant metastases, high-grade tumors, or sarcomatoid de-differentiation [97]. However, only 1% of patients without distant disease undergoing nephrectomy have pT4 disease [106]. Organs at risk for tumor invasion include the ipsilateral adrenal gland, posterior abdominal wall, paraspinous muscles, diaphragm, liver, spleen, duodenum, pancreas, and colon (Fig. 11.8). Patients may experience significant pain when the tumor involves the paraspinous muscles and nerve roots. T4 disease is associated with a poor prognosis with a 5-year survival of 5–18% [96, 97]. Unfortunately, complete surgical excision of tumor and any involved organs represents the only chance for cure. Incomplete resection of the primary tumor results in a dismal prognosis with greater than 90% of patients dying within 1 year from disease progression [107].

In one of the larger series of locally invasive disease, Karellas et al. evaluated 38 patients with pT3 or pT4 disease undergoing radical nephrectomy with adjacent organ/structure resection [108].

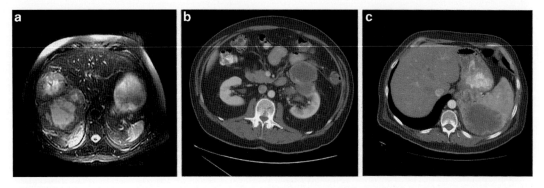

Fig. 11.8 Preoperative imaging of renal cell carcinoma with adjacent organ involvement (pT4 disease): right primary renal tumor invading liver (**a**), left primary renal tumor involving descending colon (**b**), and left primary renal tumor invading spleen (**c**)

The liver was the most common organ involved (ten cases), 68% of patients were pT4, clear cell was the most common histology (95% of cases), and 14 (37%) patients had a positive surgical margin. Median survival of patients was 11.7 months after surgical resection and surgical margin status was the only significant factor predicting disease recurrence and death. In a separate study at MDACC, Margulis et al. evaluated 30 patients with suspected T4 disease without distant metastasis [109]. The colon, pancreas, and diaphragm were the most common adjacent organs involved. Compared to patients with pT3 or lower RCC, pT4 disease was an independent predictor on multivariate analysis of decreased recurrence-free survival (10 months vs. 28 months) and decreased CSS (22 months vs. 65 months). Importantly, a significant number of these patients (60%) were downstaged on final pathology and no tumor characteristic was predictive of pT4 disease. Therefore, the authors concluded that prediction of pT4 disease cannot be adequately done by pre- or intra-operative findings.

Preoperative planning is vitally important for patients with locally advanced RCC. This requires careful imaging to define organs at risk, and patients should be counseled about the probable need for en bloc resection of adjacent organs. A formal bowel preparation should be instituted if hemicolectomy is planned, and vaccination protocols should be considered if sple-

nectomy is likely. The surgical approach can be tailored to fit the challenges of the situation on an individual basis. Preoperative embolization can be considered selectively, particularly for tumor encasing the hilum, in an effort to facilitate dissection in this area.

Ipsilateral adrenal invasion occurs in approximately 6% of advanced RCC tumors [110, 111] and is found in 2.5% of nephrectomy specimens [112]. When adrenal invasion is present, the 5-year CSS is 42%. Preoperative CT imaging has a sensitivity and specificity of 90% and 99%, respectively, for detecting adrenal involvement by the renal tumor [104]. Ito et al. evaluated 30 patients with ipsilateral adrenal involvement and compared them to 926 control patients without adrenal involvement [113]. Independent predictors for ipsilateral adrenal involvement on multivariate analysis were tumor size greater than 5.5 cm, distant disease separate from the adrenal gland, retroperitoneal lymph node involvement, and clinical stage T3 or higher. Based on their results, the authors conclude that the adrenal may be spared if the tumor size is less than 5.5 cm, there is no evidence of distant or lymph node disease, clinical stage remains less than T3, and there is no evidence of adrenal involvement on CT imaging. Surprisingly, upper pole involvement by the renal tumor was not predictive of adrenal gland involvement. In a separate study examining when the adrenal gland can be spared, Paul et al.

examined 866 consecutive patients from 1983 to 1999 [114]. Of these, 27 (3.1%) had ipsilateral adrenal gland involvement. Based on their study, the authors concluded that the adrenal gland can be spared if the primary tumor size is less than 8 cm, and there is no evidence of lymph node or distant metastasis.

Another study by Tsui et al. evaluating 511 patients from 1986 to 1998 found that 29 (5.7%) patients had adrenal involvement, 58.6% of which were local extension of disease [115]. CT imaging had a 99.4% negative predictive value for predicting adrenal gland involvement. There was no correlation between tumor size and adrenal gland involvement. In contrast to other studies, an upper pole tumor was prognostic for adrenal gland involvement.

There has been controversy regarding correct staging of ipsilateral adrenal gland involvement. Before 1987, infiltration of the adrenal gland was not considered as a prognostic factor. The 2002 AJCC TMN staging listed adrenal gland involvement as pT3a disease. However, multiple studies have shown that patients with direct invasion of the ipsilateral adrenal gland have a worse prognosis compared to patients with perinephric fat invasion (also pT3a). Because of this, the 2009 AJCC TMN staging now lists direct involvement of the ipsilateral adrenal gland as pT4 disease.

In a retrospective study of 1,087 patients, Han et al. found that 187 had perinephric fat involvement and 27 (2.5%) had direct adrenal invasion [112]. The latter group was twice as likely to present with gross hematuria (59% vs. 33%) and more likely to have lymph node involvement (52% vs. 26%, $p < 0.001$). Median survival was compromised in patients with adrenal gland invasion (12.5 months) compared to those with perinephric fat invasion (36 months). In addition, whereas 5-year survival of those with perinephric invasion alone was 36%, 5-year survival of those with adrenal gland invasion was 0%.

The multi-institutional European study by Ficarra et al. demonstrated that patients with adrenal gland invasion should be classified into two subgroups based on venous involvement by tumor thrombus [96]. Median survival of patients was much worse in those with venous involvement (12 months) compared to those without (24 months).

Postoperative Surveillance

After surgical treatment, predictors of tumor recurrence include tumor histology, Fuhrman nuclear grade, stage of tumor, margin status, and the presence of lymph node involvement [114]. Therefore, patients with locally advanced RCC (≥pT3 stage and/or LN+disease) have a higher risk of disease recurrence and progression despite definitive surgical therapy. In their series examining patients with pT3N0/Nx RCC undergoing nephrectomy with curative intent, Levy et al. found that 39% of patients developed metastases with a median time to progression of 17 months (range 2, 88) [117]. Likewise, Stephenson et al., in their study of 495 patients with pT1–T3 RCC, 5-year disease-free survival and time to progression were 67% and 14 months for patients with pT3a tumors, respectively, and 57% and 9 months for patients with pT3b tumors [118]. Based on these results as well as other studies [119, 120], recommended surveillance for patients with pT3N0 RCC after surgery includes physical exam, laboratory studies (chemistry, liver function tests, alkaline phosphatase), and chest X-ray every 6 months for 3 years and then annually thereafter. An abdominal CT scan should be performed every 6 months for the first 2 years then at year 3 and 5 unless an abnormality is discovered. For patients with lymph node disease at the time of surgery regardless of stage, Canfield et al. reported a 70% progression rate with a median time to progression of 4.9 months [18]. In their study of 45 patients with pTanyN+M0 RCC, Saidi et al. found that the progression rate was 64% with a median time to progression of 9 months [121]. Most disease will progress within a year with >90% having progressed within 3 years of surgery. Common sites of progression include the retroperitoneal lymph nodes, lung, liver, bone, kidney fossa, and brain. Based on these results and other studies [122], the surveillance recommended for patients with lymph node positive disease includes physical exam, laboratory studies (including liver function tests), chest X-ray, and CT of the abdomen and pelvis at months 3 and 6 and then every 6 months for 3 years and then annual thereafter.

The UCLA group developed an evidence-based surveillance system based on stratifying groups based on risk after surgery for localized or locally advanced disease [123]. Based on their results, most patients with locally advanced RCC would be classified as high-risk, having the highest recurrence rate of disease (58.1%) at 5 years and the shortest median time to disease recurrence (9.5 months). For patients without evidence of lymph node positive disease, these authors recommend physical examination, laboratory studies, and chest CT every 6 months for the first 3 years and then annually thereafter except for the chest CT which can be alternated with a chest X-ray. CT imaging of the abdomen should be performed every 6 months for the first 2 years and then yearly thereafter. Due to the low incidence of brain or bone metastasis in the absence of associated symptoms, the authors do not recommend routine radionucleotide bone scans or brain imaging in the asymptomatic patient. Secondary to the higher risk of disease recurrence, the authors recommend a more stringent follow-up for patients with lymph node positive disease. These patients should undergo physical examination, laboratory studies, and CT chest/abdomen at 3, 6, 12, 18, 24, 36 months and annually thereafter [123].

Conclusion

Patients with locally advanced RCC demonstrate a high risk for both recurrence and progression of disease and decreased survival compared to patients with localized RCC. Aggressive surgical resection, when feasible, remains the best treatment for locally advanced RCC. Although management of locally advanced disease can be a challenge, excellent outcomes can be achieved through careful preoperative planning and meticulous surgical technique. Postoperative surveillance protocols are intensive, and these patients should be considered for adjuvant trials of systemic therapy.

References

1. Zisman A, Pantuck AJ, Wieder J, et al. Risk group assessment and clinical outcome algorithm to predict the natural history of patients with surgically resected renal cell carcinoma. J Clin Oncol. 2002;20(23):4559–66.
2. Leibovich BC, Blute ML, Cheville JC, et al. Prediction of progression after radical nephrectomy for patients with clear cell renal cell carcinoma: a stratification tool for prospective clinical trials. Cancer. 2003;97(7):1663–71.
3. Zini L, Perrotte P, Jeldres C, et al. Nephrectomy improves the survival of patients with locally advanced renal cell carcinoma. BJU Int. 2008;102(11):1610–4.
4. Motzer RJ, Agarwal N, Beard C, et al. NCCN clinical practice guidelines in oncology: kidney cancer. J Natl Compr Canc Netw. 2009;7(6):618–30.
5. Marshall FF. Lymphadenectomy for renal cell carcinoma. BJU Int. 2005;95 Suppl 2:34.
6. Herrlinger A, Schrott KM, Schott G, Sigel A. What are the benefits of extended dissection of the regional renal lymph nodes in the therapy of renal cell carcinoma. J Urol. 1991;146(5):1224–7.
7. Motzer RJ, Bander NH, Nanus DM. Renal-cell carcinoma. N Engl J Med. 1996;335(12):865–75.
8. Hilton S. Imaging of renal cell carcinoma. Semin Oncol. 2000;27(2):150–9.
9. Studer UE, Scherz S, Scheidegger J, et al. Enlargement of regional lymph nodes in renal cell carcinoma is often not due to metastases. J Urol. 1990;144(2 Pt 1):243–5.
10. Johnson CD, Dunnick NR, Cohan RH, Illescas FF. Renal adenocarcinoma: CT staging of 100 tumors. Am J Roentgenol. 1987;148(1):59–63.
11. Giuliani L, Martorana G, Giberti C, Pescatore D, Magnani G. Results of radical nephrectomy with extensive lymphadenectomy for renal cell carcinoma. J Urol. 1983;130(4):664–8.
12. Zisman A, Pantuck AJ, Dorey F, et al. Improved prognostication of renal cell carcinoma using an integrated staging system. J Clin Oncol. 2001;19(6):1649–57.
13. Pantuck AJ, Zisman A, Dorey F, et al. Renal cell carcinoma with retroperitoneal lymph nodes. Impact on survival and benefits of immunotherapy. Cancer. 2003;97(12):2995–3002.
14. Giuliani L, Giberti C, Martorana G, Rovida S. Radical extensive surgery for renal cell carcinoma: long-term results and prognostic factors. J Urol. 1990;143(3):468–73 [discussion 73–4].
15. Margulis V, Tamboli P, Matin SF, Swanson DA, Wood CG. Analysis of clinicopathologic predictors of oncologic outcome provides insight into the natural history of surgically managed papillary renal cell carcinoma. Cancer. 2008;112(7):1480–8.
16. Delacroix SE, Jr., Chapin BF, Chen JJ, Nogueras-Gonzalez GM, Tamboli P, Matin SF, et al. Can a

durable disease-free survival be achieved with surgical resection in patients with pathological node positive renal cell carcinoma? The Journal of urology. 2011;186(4):1236–41. Epub 2011/08/19.

17. Blute ML, Leibovich BC, Cheville JC, Lohse CM, Zincke H. A protocol for performing extended lymph node dissection using primary tumor pathological features for patients treated with radical nephrectomy for clear cell renal cell carcinoma. J Urol. 2004;172(2):465–9.

18. Canfield SE, Kamat AM, Sanchez-Ortiz RF, Detry M, Swanson DA, Wood CG. Renal cell carcinoma with nodal metastases in the absence of distant metastatic disease (clinical stage TxN1-2M0): the impact of aggressive surgical resection on patient outcome. J Urol. 2006;175(3 Pt 1):864–9.

19. Terrone C, Guercio S, De Luca S, et al. The number of lymph nodes examined and staging accuracy in renal cell carcinoma. BJU Int. 2003;91(1):37–40.

20. Joslyn SA, Sirintrapun SJ, Konety BR. Impact of lymphadenectomy and nodal burden in renal cell carcinoma: retrospective analysis of the National Surveillance, Epidemiology, and End Results database. Urology. 2005;65(4):675–80.

21. Dimashkieh HH, Lohse CM, Blute ML, Kwon ED, Leibovich BC, Cheville JC. Extranodal extension in regional lymph nodes is associated with outcome in patients with renal cell carcinoma. J Urol. 2006;176(5):1978–82 [discussion 82–3].

22. Raj GV, Bochner BH. Radical cystectomy and lymphadenectomy for invasive bladder cancer: towards the evolution of an optimal surgical standard. Semin Oncol. 2007;34(2):110–21.

23. Stephenson AJ, Bosl GJ, Motzer RJ, Bajorin DF, Stasi JP, Sheinfeld J. Nonrandomized comparison of primary chemotherapy and retroperitoneal lymph node dissection for clinical stage IIA and IIB nonseminomatous germ cell testicular cancer. J Clin Oncol. 2007;25(35):5597–602.

24. Hulten L, Rosencrantz M, Seeman T, Wahlqvist L, Ahren C. Occurrence and localization of lymph node metastases in renal carcinoma. A lymphographic and histopathological investigation in connection with nephrectomy. Scand J Urol Nephrol. 1969;3(2):129–33.

25. Saitoh H, Hida M, Nakamura K, Satoh T. Distant metastasis of urothelial tumors of the renal pelvis and ureter. Tokai J Exp Clin Med. 1982;7(3):355–64.

26. Freedland SJ, Dekernion JB. Role of lymphadenectomy for patients undergoing radical nephrectomy for renal cell carcinoma. Rev Urol. 2003;5(3):191–5.

27. DeKernion JB. Lymphadenectomy for renal cell carcinoma. Therapeutic implications. Urolog Clin North Am. 1980;7(3):697–703.

28. Robson CJ, Churchill BM, Anderson W. The results of radical nephrectomy for renal cell carcinoma. J Urol. 1969;101(3):297–301.

29. Wood Jr DP. Role of lymphadenectomy in renal cell carcinoma. Urol Clin North Am. 1991;18(3):421–6.

30. Peters PC, Brown GL. The role of lymphadenectomy in the management of renal cell carcinoma. Urol Clin North Am. 1980;7(3):705–9.

31. Pantuck AJ, Zisman A, Dorey F, et al. Renal cell carcinoma with retroperitoneal lymph nodes: role of lymph node dissection. J Urol. 2003;169(6):2076–83.

32. Johnsen JA, Hellsten S. Lymphatogenous spread of renal cell carcinoma: an autopsy study. J Urol. 1997;157(2):450–3.

33. Minervini A, Lilas L, Morelli G, et al. Regional lymph node dissection in the treatment of renal cell carcinoma: is it useful in patients with no suspected adenopathy before or during surgery? BJU Int. 2001;88(3):169–72.

34. Schafhauser W, Ebert A, Brod J, Petsch S, Schrott KM. Lymph node involvement in renal cell carcinoma and survival chance by systematic lymphadenectomy. Anticancer Res. 1999;19(2C):1573–8.

35. Blom JH, van Poppel H, Marechal JM, et al. Radical nephrectomy with and without lymph-node dissection: final results of European Organization for Research and Treatment of Cancer (EORTC) randomized phase 3 trial 30881. Eur Urol. 2009;55(1):28–34.

36. Blom JH, van Poppel H, Marechal JM, et al. Radical nephrectomy with and without lymph node dissection: preliminary results of the EORTC randomized phase III protocol 30881. EORTC Genitourinary Group. Eur Urol. 1999;36(6):570–5.

37. Crispen PL, Breau RH, Allmer C, et al. Lymph node dissection at the time of radical nephrectomy for high-risk clear cell renal cell carcinoma: indications and recommendations for surgical templates. Eur Urol. 2011;59(1):18–23.

38. Hutterer GC, Patard JJ, Perrotte P, et al. Patients with renal cell carcinoma nodal metastases can be accurately identified: external validation of a new nomogram. Int J Cancer. 2007;121(11):2556–61.

39. Kearney GP, Waters WB, Klein LA, Richie JP, Gittes RF. Results of inferior vena cava resection for renal cell carcinoma. J Urol. 1981;125(6):769–73.

40. Hatcher PA, Anderson EE, Paulson DF, Carson CC, Robertson JE. Surgical management and prognosis of renal cell carcinoma invading the vena cava. J Urol. 1991;145(1):20–3 [discussion 3–4].

41. Marshall FF. Renal cell carcinoma: surgical management of regional lymph nodes and inferior vena-caval tumor thrombus. Semin Surg Oncol. 1988;4(2):129–32.

42. Skinner DG, Pfister RF, Colvin R. Extension of renal cell carcinoma into the vena cava: the rationale for aggressive surgical management. J Urol. 1972;107(5):711–6.

43. Wszolek MF, Wotkowicz C, Libertino JA. Surgical management of large renal tumors. Nat Clin Pract. 2008;5(1):35–46.

44. Martinez-Salamanca JI, Huang WC, Millan I, et al. Prognostic impact of the 2009 UICC/AJCC TNM staging system for renal cell carcinoma with venous extension. Eur Urol. 2011;59(1):120–7.

45. Kirkali Z, Van Poppel H. A critical analysis of surgery for kidney cancer with vena cava invasion. Eur Urol. 2007;52(3):658–62.

46. Oto A, Herts BR, Remer EM, Novick AC. Inferior vena cava tumor thrombus in renal cell carcinoma: staging by MR imaging and impact on surgical treatment. Am J Roentgenol. 1998;171(6):1619–24.

47. Goldfarb DA, Lorig R, Zelch M, Patrone P, Bukowski RM, Pontes JE. Right renal mass with vena caval thrombus. J Urol. 1990;143(3):574–7.

48. Mizoguchi T, Koide Y, Ohara M, Okumura F. Multiplane transesophageal echocardiographic guidance during resection of renal cell carcinoma extending into the inferior vena cava. Anesth Analg. 1995;81(5):1102–5.

49. Mootha RK, Butler R, Laucirica R, Scardino PT, Lerner SP. Renal cell carcinoma with an infrarenal vena caval tumor thrombus. Urology. 1999;54(3):561.

50. Otaibi MA, Tanguay S. Locally advanced renal cell carcinoma. Can Urol Assoc J. 2007;1(2 Suppl):S55–61.

51. Staehler G, Brkovic D. The role of radical surgery for renal cell carcinoma with extension into the vena cava. J Urol. 2000;163(6):1671–5.

52. Blute ML, Leibovich BC, Lohse CM, Cheville JC, Zincke H. The Mayo Clinic experience with surgical management, complications and outcome for patients with renal cell carcinoma and venous tumour thrombus. BJU Int. 2004;94(1):33–41.

53. Gettman MT, Boelter CW, Cheville JC, Zincke H, Bryant SC, Blute ML. Charlson co-morbidity index as a predictor of outcome after surgery for renal cell carcinoma with renal vein, vena cava or right atrium extension. J Urol. 2003;169(4):1282–6.

54. Glazer AA, Novick AC. Long-term followup after surgical treatment for renal cell carcinoma extending into the right atrium. J Urol. 1996;155(2):448–50.

55. Zisman A, Wieder JA, Pantuck AJ, et al. Renal cell carcinoma with tumor thrombus extension: biology, role of nephrectomy and response to immunotherapy. J Urol. 2003;169(3):909–16.

56. Skinner DG, Pritchett TR, Lieskovsky G, Boyd SD, Stiles QR. Vena caval involvement by renal cell carcinoma. Surgical resection provides meaningful long-term survival. Ann Surg. 1989;210(3):387–92 [discussion 92–4].

57. Swierzewski DJ, Swierzewski MJ, Libertino JA. Radical nephrectomy in patients with renal cell carcinoma with venous, vena caval, and atrial extension. Am J Surg. 1994;168(2):205–9.

58. Sweeney P, Wood CG, Pisters LL, et al. Surgical management of renal cell carcinoma associated with complex inferior vena caval thrombi. Urol Oncol. 2003;21(5):327–33.

59. Zini L, Haulon S, Decoene C, et al. Renal cell carcinoma associated with tumor thrombus in the inferior vena cava: surgical strategies. Ann Vasc Surg. 2005;19(4):522–8.

60. Schwartz MJ, Smith EB, Trost DW, Vaughan Jr ED. Renal artery embolization: clinical indications and experience from over 100 cases. BJU Int. 2007;99(4): 881–6.

61. Novick AC, Kaye MC, Cosgrove DM, et al. Experience with cardiopulmonary bypass and deep hypothermic circulatory arrest in the management of retroperitoneal tumors with large vena caval thrombi. Ann Surg. 1990;212(4):472–6 [discussion 6–7].

62. Wotkowicz C, Wszolek MF, Libertino JA. Resection of renal tumors invading the vena cava. Urol Clin North Am. 2008;35(4):657–71. vii.

63. Gallucci M, Borzomati D, Flammia G, et al. Liver harvesting surgical technique for the treatment of retro-hepatic caval thrombosis concomitant to renal cell carcinoma: perioperative and long-term results in 15 patients without mortality. Eur Urol. 2004;45(2):194–202.

64. Ciancio G, Hawke C, Soloway M. The use of liver transplant techniques to aid in the surgical management of urological tumors. J Urol. 2000; 164(3 Pt 1):665–72.

65. Ciancio G, Soloway M. Renal cell carcinoma invading the hepatic veins. Cancer. 2001;92(7): 1836–42.

66. Burt JD, Bowsher WG, Joyce G, et al. The management of renal cell carcinoma with inferior vena-caval involvement. Aust N Z J Surg. 1993;63(1):25–9.

67. Marshall FF, Reitz BA, Diamond DA. A new technique for management of renal cell carcinoma involving the right atrium: hypothermia and cardiac arrest. J Urol. 1984;131(1):103–7.

68. Vaislic CD, Puel P, Grondin P, et al. Cancer of the kidney invading the vena cava and heart. Results after 11 years of treatment. J Thorac Cardiovasc Surg. 1986;91(4):604–9.

69. Marshall VF, Middleton RG, Holswade GR, Goldsmith EI. Surgery for renal cell carcinoma in the vena cava. J Urol. 1970;103(4):414–20.

70. Stewart JR, Carey JA, McDougal WS, Merrill WH, Koch MO, Bender Jr HW. Cavoatrial tumor thrombectomy using cardiopulmonary bypass without circulatory arrest. Ann Thorac Surg. 1991;51(5):717–21 [discussion 21–2].

71. Al Otaibi M, Abou Youssif T, Alkhaldi A, et al. Renal cell carcinoma with inferior vena caval extention: impact of tumour extent on surgical outcome. BJU Int. 2009;104(10):1467–70.

72. Boorjian SA, Sengupta S, Blute ML. Renal cell carcinoma: vena caval involvement. BJU Int. 2007;99 (5 Pt B):1239–44.

73. Karnes RJ, Blute ML. Surgery insight: management of renal cell carcinoma with associated inferior vena cava thrombus. Nat Clin Pract. 2008;5(6): 329–39.

74. Rigaud J, Hetet JF, Braud G, et al. Surgical care, morbidity, mortality and follow-up after nephrectomy for renal cancer with extension of tumor thrombus into the inferior vena cava: retrospective study since 1990s. Eur Urol. 2006;50(2):302–10.

75. Goetzl MA, Goluboff ET, Murphy AM, et al. A contemporary evaluation of cytoreductive nephrectomy

with tumor thrombus: morbidity and long-term survival. Urol Oncol. 2004;22(3):182–7.

76. Parekh DJ, Cookson MS, Chapman W, et al. Renal cell carcinoma with renal vein and inferior vena caval involvement: clinicopathological features, surgical techniques and outcomes. J Urol. 2005;173(6):1897–902.

77. Rabbani F, Hakimian P, Reuter VE, Simmons R, Russo P. Renal vein or inferior vena caval extension in patients with renal cortical tumors: impact of tumor histology. J Urol. 2004;171(3):1057–61.

78. Bensalah K, Rioux-Leclercq N, Vincendeau S, Guille F, Patard JJ. Is tumour expression of VEGF associated with venous invasion and survival in pT3 renal cell carcinoma? Prog Urol. 2007;17(2):189–93.

79. Rey D, Pfister C, Gobet F, Martinez S, Staerman F, Grise P. Study of the prognostic value of DNA ploidy and proliferation index (Ki-67) in renal cell carcinoma with venous thrombus. Prog Urol. 2003;13(6):1300–6.

80. Klatte T, Pantuck AJ, Riggs SB, et al. Prognostic factors for renal cell carcinoma with tumor thrombus extension. J Urol. 2007;178(4 Pt 1):1189–95 [discussion 95].

81. Kim HL, Zisman A, Han KR, Figlin RA, Belldegrun AS. Prognostic significance of venous thrombus in renal cell carcinoma. Are renal vein and inferior vena cava involvement different? J Urol. 2004;171 (2 Pt 1):588–91.

82. Ciancio G, Livingstone AS, Soloway M. Surgical management of renal cell carcinoma with tumor thrombus in the renal and inferior vena cava: the University of Miami experience in using liver transplantation techniques. Eur Urol. 2007;51(4):988–94 [discussion 94–5].

83. Lambert EH, Pierorazio PM, Shabsigh A, Olsson CA, Benson MC, McKiernan JM. Prognostic risk stratification and clinical outcomes in patients undergoing surgical treatment for renal cell carcinoma with vascular tumor thrombus. Urology. 2007;69(6):1054–8.

84. Wagner B, Patard JJ, Mejean A, et al. Prognostic value of renal vein and inferior vena cava involvement in renal cell carcinoma. Eur Urol. 2009;55(2):452–9.

85. Moinzadeh A, Libertino JA. Prognostic significance of tumor thrombus level in patients with renal cell carcinoma and venous tumor thrombus extension. Is all T3b the same? J Urol. 2004;171(2 Pt 1):598–601.

86. Klaver S, Joniau S, Suy R, Oyen R, Van Poppel H. Analysis of renal cell carcinoma with subdiaphragmatic macroscopic venous invasion (T3b). BJU Int. 2008;101(4):444–9.

87. Ciancio G, Soloway M. Resection of the abdominal inferior vena cava for complicated renal cell carcinoma with tumour thrombus. BJU Int. 2005;96(6):815–8.

88. Marshall FF, Reitz BA. Supradiaphragmatic renal cell carcinoma tumor thrombus: indications for vena caval reconstruction with pericardium. J Urol. 1985;133(2):266–8.

89. Caldarelli G, Minervini A, Guerra M, Bonari G, Caldarelli C, Minervini R. Prosthetic replacement of the inferior vena cava and the iliofemoral vein for urologically related malignancies. BJU Int. 2002;90(4):368–74.

90. Hardwigsen J, Baque P, Crespy B, Moutardier V, Delpero JR, Le Treut YP. Resection of the inferior vena cava for neoplasms with or without prosthetic replacement: a 14-patient series. Ann Surg. 2001; 233(2):242–9.

91. Zini L, Destrieux-Garnier L, Leroy X, et al. Renal vein ostium wall invasion of renal cell carcinoma with an inferior vena cava tumor thrombus: prediction by renal and vena caval vein diameters and prognostic significance. J Urol. 2008;179(2):450–4 [discussion 4].

92. Kume H, Kameyama S, Kasuya Y, Tajima A, Kawabe K. Surgical treatment of renal cell carcinoma associated with Budd-Chiari syndrome: report of four cases and review of the literature. Eur J Surg Oncol. 1999;25(1):71–5.

93. Roberts WW, Bhayani SB, Allaf ME, Chan TY, Kavoussi LR, Jarrett TW. Pathological stage does not alter the prognosis for renal lesions determined to be stage T1 by computerized tomography. J Urol. 2005;173(3):713–5.

94. Jung SJ, Ro JY, Truong LD, Ayala AG, Shen SS. Reappraisal of T3N0/NxM0 renal cell carcinoma: significance of extent of fat invasion, renal vein invasion, and adrenal invasion. Hum Pathol. 2008;39(11):1689–94.

95. Fujita T, Iwamura M, Yanagisawa N, et al. Prognostic impact of perirenal fat or adrenal gland involvement in patients with pT3b renal cell carcinoma. Urology. 2007;69(5):839–42.

96. Ficarra V, Galfano A, Guille F, et al. A new staging system for locally advanced (pT3-4) renal cell carcinoma: a multicenter European study including 2,000 patients. J Urol. 2007;178(2):418–24 [discussion 23–4].

97. Thompson RH, Cheville JC, Lohse CM, et al. Reclassification of patients with pT3 and pT4 renal cell carcinoma improves prognostic accuracy. Cancer. 2005;104(1):53–60.

98. Satyapal KS. Classification of the drainage patterns of the renal veins. J Anat. 1995;186(Pt 2):329–33.

99. Bonsib SM, Gibson D, Mhoon M, Greene GF. Renal sinus involvement in renal cell carcinomas. Am J Surg Pathol. 2000;24(3):451–8.

100. Thompson RH, Leibovich BC, Cheville JC, et al. Is renal sinus fat invasion the same as perinephric fat invasion for pT3a renal cell carcinoma? J Urol. 2005;174(4 Pt 1):1218–21.

101. Margulis V, Tamboli P, Matin SF, Meisner M, Swanson DA, Wood CG. Location of extrarenal tumor extension does not impact survival of patients with pT3a renal cell carcinoma. J Urol. 2007;178(5):1878–82.

102. Terrone C, Cracco C, Guercio S, et al. Prognostic value of the involvement of the urinary collecting system in renal cell carcinoma. Eur Urol. 2004;46(4):472–6.

103. Klatte T, Chung J, Leppert JT, et al. Prognostic relevance of capsular involvement and collecting system invasion in stage I and II renal cell carcinoma. BJU Int. 2007;99(4):821–4.

104. Lam JS, Breda A, Belldegrun AS, Figlin RA. Evolving principles of surgical management and prognostic factors for outcome in renal cell carcinoma. J Clin Oncol. 2006;24(35):5565–75.

105. Connolly J, Eisner D, Goldman S, Stutzman R, Steiner M. Benign retroperitoneal fibrosis and renal cell carcinoma. J Urol. 1993;149(6):1535–7.

106. Margulis V, Wood CG. Update on staging controversies for locally advanced renal cell carcinoma. Expert Rev Anticancer Ther. 2007;7(7):909–14.

107. Dekernion JB, Ramming KP, Smith RB. The natural history of metastatic renal cell carcinoma: a computer analysis. J Urol. 1978;120(2):148–52.

108. Karellas ME, Jang TL, Kagiwada MA, Kinnaman MD, Jarnagin WR, Russo P. Advanced-stage renal cell carcinoma treated by radical nephrectomy and adjacent organ or structure resection. BJU Int. 2009;103(2):160–4.

109. Margulis V, Sanchez-Ortiz RF, Tamboli P, Cohen DD, Swanson DA, Wood CG. Renal cell carcinoma clinically involving adjacent organs: experience with aggressive surgical management. Cancer. 2007;109(10):2025–30.

110. Tsui KH, Shvarts O, Smith RB, Figlin RA, deKernion JB, Belldegrun A. Prognostic indicators for renal cell carcinoma: a multivariate analysis of 643 patients using the revised 1997 TNM staging criteria. J Urol. 2000;163(4):1090–5. quiz 295.

111. Antonelli A, Cozzoli A, Simeone C, et al. Surgical treatment of adrenal metastasis from renal cell carcinoma: a single-centre experience of 45 patients. BJU Int. 2006;97(3):505–8.

112. Han KR, Bui MH, Pantuck AJ, et al. TNM T3a renal cell carcinoma: adrenal gland involvement is not the same as renal fat invasion. J Urol. 2003;169(3):899–903 [discussion 4].

113. Ito K, Nakazawa H, Marumo K, et al. Risk factors for ipsilateral adrenal involvement in renal cell carcinoma. Urology. 2008;72(2):354–8.

114. Paul R, Mordhorst J, Busch R, Leyh H, Hartung R. Adrenal sparing surgery during radical nephrectomy in patients with renal cell cancer: a new algorithm. J Urol. 2001;166(1):59–62.

115. Tsui KH, Shvarts O, Barbaric Z, Figlin R, de Kernion JB, Belldegrun A. Is adrenalectomy a necessary component of radical nephrectomy? UCLA experience with 511 radical nephrectomies. J Urol. 2000;163(2):437–41.

116. Lam JS, Shvarts O, Leppert JT, Figlin RA, Belldegrun AS. Renal cell carcinoma 2005: new frontiers in staging, prognostication and targeted molecular therapy. J Urol. 2005;173(6):1853–62.

117. Levy DA, Slaton JW, Swanson DA, Dinney CP. Stage specific guidelines for surveillance after radical nephrectomy for local renal cell carcinoma. J Urol. 1998;159(4):1163–7.

118. Stephenson AJ, Chetner MP, Rourke K, et al. Guidelines for the surveillance of localized renal cell carcinoma based on the patterns of relapse after nephrectomy. J Urol. 2004;172(1):58–62.

119. Sandock DS, Seftel AD, Resnick MI. A new protocol for the followup of renal cell carcinoma based on pathological stage. J Urol. 1995;154(1):28–31.

120. Ljungberg B, Hanbury DC, Kuczyk MA, et al. Renal cell carcinoma guideline. Eur Urol. 2007;51(6):1502–10.

121. Saidi JA, Newhouse JH, Sawczuk IS. Radiologic follow-up of patients with T1–3a, b, c or T4N+M0 renal cell carcinoma after radical nephrectomy. Urology. 1998;52(6):1000–3.

122. Han KR, Pantuck AJ, Bui MH, et al. Number of metastatic sites rather than location dictates overall survival of patients with node-negative metastatic renal cell carcinoma. Urology. 2003;61(2):314–9.

123. Lam JS, Shvarts O, Leppert JT, Pantuck AJ, Figlin RA, Belldegrun AS. Postoperative surveillance protocol for patients with localized and locally advanced renal cell carcinoma based on a validated prognostic nomogram and risk group stratification system. J Urol. 2005;174(2):466–72 [discussion 72; quiz 801].

Neoadjuvant Targeted Therapy and Consolidative Surgery

12

Sean P. Stroup and Ithaar H. Derweesh

Introduction

Although great strides have been made in the diagnosis and treatment of renal cell carcinoma, approximately 30–40% of patients continue to present with locally advanced or metastatic disease at initial diagnosis [1]. With improved response rates and tolerability of targeted agents [2–4], the concept of primary targeted therapy followed by consolidative surgery has emerged as a novel paradigm for the management of select patients with locally advanced RCC. Herein we discuss patient selection criteria for this strategy, including the concept of response to therapy and consolidative nephrectomy, and assess the quality of emerging data using primary systemic therapy in the treatment of patients with locally advanced RCC. We will also highlight perioperative patient safety concerns and the arguments for and against utilization of primary systemic targeted therapy. Finally, we discuss current and future directions for investigation regarding this topic.

Rationale and Potential Limitations of Primary Targeted Therapy for Management of Locally Advanced Renal Cell Carcinoma

Background

Important advances in the understanding of the molecular and genetic components of RCC have ushered in a new era of targeted molecular therapy. These treatments have primarily focused on blocking signaling pathways associated with the von Hippel–Lindau tumor suppressor gene. Inactivation of this gene leads to elevated levels of hypoxia-inducible factor alpha (HIF-a) and overexpression of vascular endothelial growth factor (VEGF) [4]. Small molecule inhibitors of this pathway targeting the VEGF receptor tyrosine kinase and mammalian target of rapamycin (mTOR) pathways have proven efficacy. Landmark studies in the past decade helped pave the way for approval of sorafenib, sunitinib, temsirolimus, everolimus, and recently pazopanib and axinitib. Other studies identified a role for bevacizumab in combination with interferon-alfa for mRCC. These agents have demonstrated improved survival outcomes over traditional immunotherapeutic regimens with better tolerability [3, 4].

Rationale for Primary Targeted Therapy

Using these agents in the neoadjuvant setting for locally advanced renal cell carcinoma represents

S.P. Stroup • I.H. Derweesh (✉)
Division of Urology, Department of Surgery,
Moores UCSD Cancer Center, University of California
San Diego School of Medicine, 3855 Health Sciences
Drive, Mail Code 0987, La Jolla, CA 92093-0987, USA
e-mail: sstroup@ucsd.edu; iderweesh@gmail.com;
iderweesh@ucsd.edu

S.C. Campbell and B.I. Rini (eds.), *Renal Cell Carcinoma: Clinical Management*, Current Clinical Urology,
DOI 10.1007/978-1-62703-062-5_12, © Springer Science+Business Media New York 2013

a new and promising treatment paradigm. Neoadjuvant targeted therapy offers the potential advantage of tumor downstaging which may make surgical interventions possible in some patients who would not otherwise be surgical candidates. Reduction of the primary tumor and metastatic disease may also make any surgical intervention less morbid, provided sufficient washout time is given to limit wound complications. Furthermore, as the biological understanding of RCC advances, tissue provided from initial biopsy may provide a genetic tumor fingerprint that would allow more individualized targeted therapy with a chance for better patient selection and efficacy.

Potential Limitations of Primary Systemic Targeted Therapy

Counterarguments to upfront TKI therapy identify treatment-related presurgical morbidity and a lack of high level evidence supporting the approach as concerns. Neoadjuvant TKI strategies may also complicate the surgical procedure, unnecessarily delay surgery, and/or increase the risk of perioperative morbidity. Despite being oral agents, these agents are associated with a significant degree of toxicity. Postoperative wound healing, infection, spontaneous bowel perforation, and cardiovascular morbidity with hypertension and declines in left ventricular ejection fraction are among the most feared complications in surgical patients. Theoretical concerns also exist about the risk of starting, stopping, and restarting TKIs. Selection of tumors resistant to targeted therapy is a potential adverse outcome of this strategy.

Primary Targeted Therapy Followed by Planned Surgical Consolidation

Patient Selection

A number of factors are important in determining whether a patient is suitable for initial targeted molecular therapy followed by consolidative surgery

as part of a multimodal approach for management of mRCC. Neoadjuvant targeted therapy strategies may be primarily considered for patients with locally advanced disease with direct invasion into surrounding organs and in those with large, bulky tumors for whom resection might be particularly challenging [5, 6]. In these cases, initial targeted therapy may reduce surgical morbidity by shrinking the tumor and minimizing resection of neighboring organs or structures, although the degree of this response is variable and usually limited (see Fig. 12.1) [2, 7]. Patients with renal vein or inferior vena cava thrombi have also been selected for treatment with upfront targeted therapy as a means to reduce the tumor thrombus level, although the data supporting this is largely anecdotal [8]. Patients with bulky central or hilar tumors in the setting of locally advanced disease with imperative indication for nephron-sparing surgery may also benefit from primary targeted therapy prior to planned nephron-sparing surgery (see Fig. 12.1). Level III evidence exists in the form of several small series examining neoadjuvant (presurgical) targeted therapy before cytoreductive surgery which suggest the approach appears safe [9–11].

Renal Mass Biopsy

In recent years the accuracy and safety of renal mass biopsy have improved substantially due to refinements in CT- and MRI-guided techniques. Pretreatment tumor biopsies to confirm histology should be performed before embarking on neoadjuvant therapy. The diagnostic accuracy of renal mass biopsy for clinically confined renal tumors has improved from about 82% before 2001 to more than 95% currently. Noninformative biopsies continue to be seen in 10–15% of cases, while false negative rates now approach 1% and the incidence of symptomatic complications is low with <2% requiring some form of intervention. Needle tract seeding also appears to be exceptionally low. The addition of fine needle aspiration may complement the standard core biopsy and is particularly helpful when assessing extrarenal metastatic lesions. Biopsy of locally

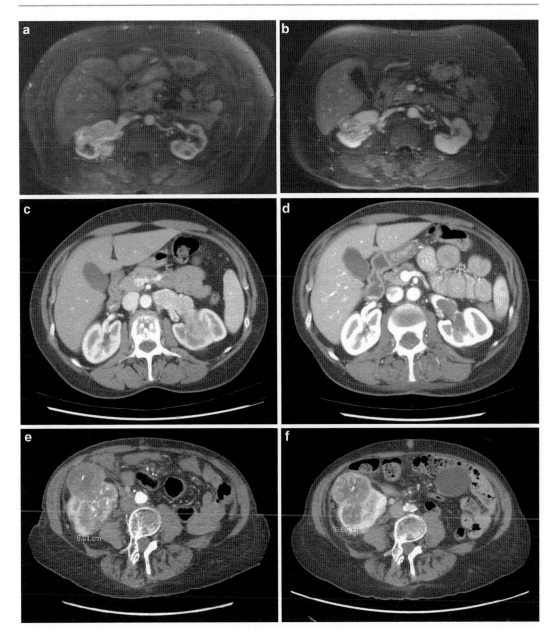

Fig. 12.1 Representative neoadjuvant targeted treatment scenarios. (**a**, **b**) A 68-year-old female with stage III CKD presented with a 6.30 cm right renal mass and a high R.E.N.A.L. score. The patient underwent biopsy which confirmed CC-RCC, followed by two cycles of primary sunitinib resulting in reduction of the mass to 3.25 cm, thus facilitating nephron-sparing surgery. (**c**, **d**) A 51-year-old female presented with bone and lung mets and a 9.1 cm left renal mass with a renal vein thrombus. After confirming mCC-RCC, the patient underwent two cycles of sunitinib and radiation therapy to her clavicular and spinal mets, resulting in reduction of her thrombus and tumor to 7.4 cm, thereby enabling laparo-endoscopic single site left radical nephrectomy and renal vein thrombectomy. (**e**, **f**) A 56-year-old female with CKD and a solitary kidney presented with an 8 cm renal mass and pancreatic metastases. After confirmatory biopsy for CC-RCC, the patient underwent two cycles of sunitinib, resulting in reduction of the primary tumor to 6.7 cm and facilitating cytoreductive nephron-sparing surgery

advanced RCC is more challenging, because these tumors have a more broad differential diagnosis, potentially including adrenal neoplasms, urothelial-based tumors, lymphoma, and a variety of other malignancies. Tumor necrosis is also more common in this population, and multiple cores including peripherally based ones should be considered. Most studies suggest that clear cell tumors tend to respond best to targeted therapies in any setting, and biopsy may play a role in patient selection and for guiding choice of therapy.

Although precise Fuhrman grading and tumor subtype histology are not always accurately determined, the addition of histopathologic and molecular imaging techniques to renal mass biopsy represents an important potential advance. Interphase fluorescence in situ hybridization (FISH) has been used to identify abnormalities in chromosomes 3, 7, 10, 13, 17, and 21 and the locus 3p25–26 [12]. The technique improved the diagnostic accuracy in subtyping RCC from 87% to 94%. Polymerase chain reaction has also been used to amplify CA-IX from FNA specimens and results in enhanced sensitivity and specificity [12, 13]. Finally, newer techniques of molecular profiling, gene expression, and proteomic analysis applied to renal mass biopsy may further refine the role of neoadjuvant systemic therapy prior to debulking nephrectomy by refinement of risk and outcome stratification. Such strategies may eventually further decrease patient morbidity and improve outcomes, but remain investigational at present [14].

Selection of Targeted Molecular Therapy and Duration of Therapy

A variety of agents have been used in the neoadjuvant setting before debulking nephrectomy. Most experience has been gained using sunitinib, as this agent has been associated with better response rates and more impressive downsizing. Alternative therapies may include interferon-alfa with bevacizumab in patients who can tolerate this regimen or temsirolimus in those with non-clear cell histology. Pazopanib is also a promising agent for tumor downsizing, given its impressive

response rates that have approximated those of sunitinib [15].

In most cases, the clinical response to therapy is assessed after two or three cycles. With this strategy, clinicians can determine tumor progression and offer alternative therapy. After two or three cycles of sunitinib before planned nephrectomy most studies have reached a maximum clinical benefit, and prolonging therapy beyond this point is likely to be counterproductive. In the multinational study from the UK and the Netherlands, after two or three cycles, 73% had clinical benefit with a partial response in 6%. Ultimately 71% of this group went on to consolidative nephrectomy [16].

Radiographic Response to Therapy

Tumor response to therapy is generally assessed by CT/MRI every two to three cycles of treatment and defined according to the response evaluation criteria in solid tumors (RECISTs) v.1.1 [17]. The clinical response of the primary tumor is classified as complete response, partial response, stable disease, or progressive disease. Progressive disease is defined as a greater than 20% increase in sum of longest diameters from nadir or the appearance of new lesions. Partial responders are identified with greater than 30% reduction in the sum of target lesion diameters, while stable disease is within these limits.

Level III evidence exists demonstrating a moderate response to primary targeted therapy in the setting of the primary tumor. Important work by van der Velt and colleagues helped to establish tumor response parameters for neoadjuvant treatment. They evaluated the effects of sunitinib on the primary tumor in 17 patients with initially unresectable advanced RCC [2]. Partial response or stable disease was seen in 16 of 17 (94.1%) patients by RECIST, while 13 (76.5%) had a volume reduction of the primary tumor between 18% and 64%. They also noted that the 31% median reduction in tumor volume was associated with increased areas of central necrosis. Three (18%) patients eventually underwent nephrectomy with good perioperative outcomes.

Utilization of Primary Targeted Therapy Prior to Debulking Radical Nephrectomy

Robert et al. reported on the first case of complete remission after neoadjuvant sunitinib. In a 78-year-old woman with locally advanced RCC with vena cava thrombus extension, 6 months of neoadjuvant therapy led to sufficient downstaging and a complete tumor response [18]. This and other case reports contributed to the initial excitement about the possibility of dramatic tumor downstaging with targeted therapy. Larger studies have helped to better quantify expected tumor shrinkage.

The experience of Thomas and colleagues from the Cleveland Clinic is informative, as they reported the response of advanced primary renal tumors to treatment with neoadjuvant sunitinib [19]. In their series, 19 patients with advanced renal cell carcinoma deemed unsuitable for initial nephrectomy due to locally advanced disease or extensive metastatic burden were treated with standard dosing sunitinib (50 mg daily for 4 weeks followed by 2 weeks off therapy). No patients experienced complete response. Primary tumor partial responses were noted in three patients (16%), stable disease in seven (37%), and nine (47%) had disease progression in the primary tumor. With a median of two cycles of TKI therapy, primary tumor shrinkage was observed in eight patients (42%) with an average decrease in primary tumor size of 24% (range

2–46%). At median follow-up of 6 months (range 1–15), four patients (21%) had undergone nephrectomy and five died of disease progression. No unexpected surgical morbidity was encountered. Viable tumor was present in all four specimens.

Sorafenib has been evaluated in the presurgical setting by Cowey and colleagues from the University of North Carolina Group. In a prospective nonrandomized study, the authors examined a histologically heterogeneous RCC population (17 localized, 13 metastatic), noting a primary reduction in 77% of patients with a mean diameter reduction of 9.6% in the primary tumor [20].

These and other similar studies (Table 12.1) demonstrate that most tumors may experience a modest decrease in size, which can potentially facilitate tumor resection in the setting of metastatic and locally advanced disease. However, further investigation is necessary to provide more detailed outcomes data and to refine selection criteria.

Development of central necrosis has also been noted as a unique tumor response to TKIs, but it is rare to see complete eradication of malignant elements, and resection of residual masses is strongly advocated if possible. In the van der Velt study, treatment with sunitinib led to decreases in the median density of the solid component of the renal tumors suggesting an increase in the degree of central necrosis, with an average reduction of 16 HU (82–66). A multinational group from the UK and the Netherlands also noted that necrosis was a prominent feature at nephrectomy in 49%

Table 12.1 Primary targeted therapy for renal cell carcinoma

Agent/type of study	Patient population	No. of patients with primary tumor shrinkage	Amount of primary tumor shrinkage
Sunitinib (retrospective) [19]	"Unresectable" RCC ($n=19$)	42%	24% (range 2–46%)
Sunitinib (retrospective) [2]	M+ patients with primary tumor in place ($n=17$)	76%	12% (range 2–33%)
Sunitinib (prospective, phase II) [21]	M+ patients with primary tumor in place ($n=52$)	Not stated	12% (range 8–35%)
Sorafenib (prospective) [20]	≥T2 RCC; 17 localized; 13 M+ ($n=30$)	77%	9.6% (range 1–40%)
Bevacizumab (±erlotinib) (prospective) [22]	M+ patients with primary tumor in place ($n=50$)	52%	(range 1–≤30%)
Sunitinib (retrospective) [11]	Localized ($n=7$) and M+ ($n=5$); imperative NSS ($n=12$)	100%	21% (range 4.7–46%)

of patients [21]; however, a pT0 response has only rarely been reported [18].

Utilization of Primary Targeted Therapy in the Setting of Tumor Thrombus

Neoadjuvant targeted therapy has been investigated in the setting of tumor thrombus to see whether this approach could improve operative characteristics and decrease perioperative morbidity and mortality. Karakiewicz et al. reported on a 75-year-old woman who presented with an 11-cm left renal mass, ECOG status 0, and extension of tumor thrombus into the right atrium [23]. After two cycles of sunitinib therapy, the tumor regressed into the IVC below the hepatic veins. This significantly reduced the extent of the surgery. At this point, only Level III and IV evidence has been reported to examine the outcomes in this setting.

In one of the largest retrospective series, Cost et al. evaluated the cytoreductive effects of targeted molecular therapies on in situ level II or higher inferior vena cava tumor thrombi [8]. The main outcome measured was a change in the clinical level of tumor thrombus following TMT. They also measured radiographic responses in thrombus size and location before and after TMT. Before targeted therapy, thrombus level was II in 18 patients (72%), III in five patients (20%), and IV in two patients (8%). Sunitinib was initial therapy for 12 cases, while alternative targeted molecular treatments (TMTs) were administered in 13. Following TMT, seven patients (28%) had a measurable increase in thrombus height, 7 (28%) had no change, and 11 (44%) had a decrease. One patient (4%) had an increase in thrombus-level classification, 21 (84%) had stable thrombi level, and in three (12%) the thrombus level decreased. There was only one case (4%) where the surgical approach was potentially affected by tumor thrombus regression (levels IV–III). Statistically significant predictors of tumor thrombus response to targeted therapy could not be identified. The authors concluded that TMT had a minimal clinical effect on RCC tumor thrombi.

The retrospective design of these data and lack of prospective, protocol-driven criteria for patient selection limit our ability to extrapolate this experience to all patients with locally advanced RCC. While Cost et al. represents the largest reported experience with in situ caval tumor thrombi treated with targeted therapy, there is insufficient statistical power to assess the usefulness of TMTs for tumor thrombus cytoreduction on a larger scale. A prospective study with more formalized inclusion criteria may better answer these questions.

Utilization of Primary Targeted Therapy Prior to Nephron Sparing Surgery

Presurgical targeted therapy has been reported in an attempt to downsize tumors in patients with imperative indications for partial nephrectomy, and in patients with tumors potentially amenable to staged nephron-sparing approaches. In one case report, 15 months after undergoing a left radical nephrectomy for a pT3bN0M0 high-grade clear cell RCC, a 62-year-old woman was found to have two enhancing renal masses in her remaining right kidney without evidence of other metastatic disease [24]. Her performance status was excellent. Neoadjuvant targeted therapy led to a 20% reduction in tumor size and stable disease over six cycles. The authors contended that the course of treatment allowed the lesions that were not previously amenable to nephron sparing surgery, to be resected successfully with negative margins while avoiding the need for renal replacement therapy.

Our group reported on the efficacy of neoadjuvant TKI therapy prior nephron-sparing surgery in 12 patients with 14 tumors in the setting of locally advanced and/or metastatic disease and with imperative indication for nephron-sparing surgery; all patients had bulky local disease or central lesions [11]. We observed a mean tumor size reduction of 21.1%, and noted a partial response in 4 of 14 (28.6%) tumors and stable disease in the remaining ten (71.4%) tumors. All attempted partial nephrectomies were successful with negative margins, and at a mean follow-up of 24 months, 10 of 12 patients are alive, with one dying from metastatic RCC. Three of the 14 renal units developed delayed urinary leaks, which only occurred in those given postoperative sunitinib. These data demonstrate that in well selected patients with imperative indications for nephron-sparing surgery in the setting of locally advanced disease, primary TKI therapy results in tumor response and may facilitate or enable challenging partial nephrectomy. While all planned renal units were successfully salvaged, patients who subsequently underwent further systemic therapy were at high risk for developing a delayed urine leak, which is likely due to the potent anti-angiogenic and antiproliferative effects of sunitinib, and is analogous to wound healing data reported in other studies.

Further study is requisite to determine the utility of nephron-sparing surgery in this setting, particularly in assessing the benefits of cancer control weighed against the risk of chronic kidney disease and cardiovascular death [22, 25].

Safety, Toxicity, and Side Effects of Primary Targeted Therapy

Perioperative Safety of Neoadjuvant Therapy

Tyrosine kinase inhibitors and mTOR inhibitors can have notable toxicities based upon their unique and novel mechanisms action. Proangiogenic pathways have important roles in tissue healing and integrity. Hence, disturbance of these pathways may lead to increased incidence of delayed wound healing, fascial disruption, and incisional hernia [26, 27]. These agents will also block the natural regeneration of the microvasculature and might thus predispose the patient to postoperative bleeding or thrombotic events [28–30].

Fatigue, nausea, diarrhea, hepatotoxicity, and myelosuppression are fairly common in patients taking these agents and could impact quality of life prior to surgery or delay consolidative surgery [27]. TKI-associated hand–foot syndrome may also be a factor at higher toxicity grades. Most toxicities are reversible and manageable if a sufficient washout period is allowed before surgery. Most series of primary TKI therapy before debulking nephrectomy have provided reassuring

safety profiles and encouraging results [5, 30]. Thomas et al. reported perioperative complications in 16% of patients with fatigue (74%), abnormal taste (43%), diarrhea (31%), and hand–foot syndrome (32%) being most common [19, 31]. Margulis et al. found that patients treated with preoperative targeted therapy experienced marginally increased rates of wound related complications, although this did not reach statistical significance. In multivariate analysis, the type of preoperative systemic therapy and its duration and interval from discontinuation of systemic therapy to surgery were not associated with the development of perioperative morbidity. In addition, none of the surgical parameters such as EBL, rate of blood transfusion or operative time were different between the studied patient cohorts treated with or without TMT, suggesting that the procedural difficulty was not affected by preoperative administration of TMT. However, most of these consolidative surgical experiences for RCC have been rather limited and further data will be required.

Silberstein and colleagues described complications of targeted therapy in the setting of partial nephrectomy [11]. They found delayed urine leaks in 3 of 14 renal units undergoing nephron-sparing surgery after neoadjuvant sunitinib. It is important to note that all had a bulky tumor burden that required extensive collecting-system reconstruction. All patients resumed sunitinib 4 weeks after surgery. Conservative measures that included temporary discontinuation of sunitinib and placement of ureteral and perirenal drains led to resolution of fistulae in all patients. Satisfactory healing after partial nephrectomy, as observed in the majority of patients this series, represents a strong indication that consolidative surgery can be performed safely given appropriate surgical expertise and a meticulous approach.

Wound Healing

Concerns remain about perioperative morbidity, wound healing and long-term outcomes. Targeted agents have a variety of half-lives; with temsirolimus at 17 h, sorafenib at 1–2 days, sunitinib at 4 days, and the bevacizumab infusion at 17 days is the longest. To minimize the effect on wound healing, most series have advocated at least a 2-week washout period for most oral TKIs and at least 4 weeks for bevacizumab. Despite these recommendations, some have reported good outcomes in patients who did not suspend therapy before surgery. In a paper by Margulis and colleagues, there appeared to be no difference in perioperative complications between those stopping TKIs 1 day or 14 days before surgery [29]. In the Jonasch study, presurgical treatment of patients with bevacizumab before surgery resulted in a 20.9% rate of delayed wound healing, vs. 2% for non-treated patients [26]. Further, these complications range from superficial to deep fascial and may significantly delay restarting targeted therapy. Bowel perforation is also a known, but rare complication of treatment with TKIs and should be considered in the postoperative setting in patients with extensive lysis of adhesions, bowel manipulation, or resections [32, 33].

Cardiovascular Toxicity

Cardiovascular toxicity, hypertension, and venous thrombosis are also concerning side effects of sunitinib and sorafenib that may complicate the perioperative course [34]. VEGF inhibitors block the natural regeneration of the microvessels and could potentially affect vascular and coronary integrity. Sunitinib has the greater potential for inducing cardiac toxicity with up to a 21% of patients experiencing a decline in left ventricular ejection fraction below the lower limit of normal. Sunitinib has also been shown to increase the QTc interval and care should be used when prescribing this regimen to patients with any history of ventricular arrhythmias, or co-administering medications that also prolong the OT interval [32]. Close measurement of electrolytes to prevent hypokalemia and hypomagnesemia is also warranted.

Thromboembolic Complications

Tyrosine kinase inhibitors may increase risk of developing arterial and venous thromboembolic events and consideration should be given to using low-dose aspirin or unfractionated or low-molecular-weight heparin during the perioperative period to reduce the risk of these events. Pooled data from five randomized controlled trials that included a total of 1,745 patients with metastatic colorectal, breast, or non-small-cell lung carcinoma treated with bevacizumab supports a concern in this area, particularly when targeted agents are used along with chemotherapy [30]. Using Cox proportional hazards regression, treatment with bevacizumab and chemotherapy, compared with chemotherapy alone, was associated with increased risk for an arterial thromboembolic event (HR = 2.0, 95% CI = 1.05–3.75; $p = 0.031$) but not for a venous thromboembolic event (HR = 0.89, 95% CI = 0.66–1.20; $p = 0.44$). The absolute rate of developing an arterial thromboembolism was 5.5 events per 100 person-years for those receiving combination therapy and 3.1 events per 100 person-years for those receiving chemotherapy alone (ratio = 1.8, 95% CI = 0.94–3.33; $P = 0.076$). Therefore combination treatment with bevacizumab and chemotherapy, compared with chemotherapy alone, was associated with an increased risk of arterial thromboembolism but not venous thromboembolism. Whether this will apply to patients with RCC who do not received conventional cytotoxic chemotherapy or to TKIs that have a different mechanism of action when compared to bevacizumab, is not known.

Future Directions

Based on the limited data currently available, neoadjuvant TKI therapy followed by consolidative surgery appears to be a promising approach for select patients with locally advanced tumors or to facilitate or enable challenging partial nephrectomies, but it is important to emphasize that this approach is still experimental, and further work is required.

While several randomized studies are aimed at answering the question of utility and timing of cytoreductive nephrectomy in the setting of mRCC [34], currently no prospective randomized studies exist to evaluate utility of primary targeted therapy in the setting of locally advanced disease. Indeed, these studies are necessary from several different standpoints independent of work on mRCC for the following reasons: (a) The primary question being asked is not the utility or desirability of the operation, but of the pre-surgical pharmacologic intervention, (b) as nephron-sparing surgery is increasingly applied to larger tumors in the setting of imperative indications more information is necessary on the efficacy and desirability of neoadjuvant targeted therapy, and (c) tissue obtained prior to and after primary pharmacological intervention should be utilized in translational investigation to gain further insight into risk stratification, tumor response, and outcomes which may better select appropriate patients for this approach in the future.

Conclusion

Initial TKI therapy in the setting of locally advanced disease represents a paradigm shift that is promising but still very much investigational. This strategy may help to facilitate less morbid resection of high risk surgical disease and improve the outcomes of nephron-sparing surgery for bulky or locally extensive tumors, in addition to providing tissue for translational applications. Retrospective studies have provided important preliminary insights into the feasibility of primary targeted therapy for locally extensive disease and the natural course and outcomes of a neoadjuvant TKI approach. While clinical trials are underway to evaluate the utility and timing of cytoreductive nephrectomy in the setting of mRCC, further investigation from prospective randomized clinical trials is also required to assess the role of targeted therapy in the treatment of locally advanced RCC. Morbidity after consolidative surgery in this setting appears to be relatively low but the current experience remains limited, and meticulous surgical technique and withholding of TKI for a least a few half lives prior to and after surgery should be strongly considered.

References

1. Hollingsworth JM, Miller DC, Daignault S, Hollenbeck BK. Rising incidence of small renal masses: a need to reassess treatment effect. J Natl Cancer Inst. 2006;98:1331–4.
2. van der Veldt AA, Meijerink MR, van den Eertwegh AJ, et al. Sunitinib for treatment of advanced renal cell cancer: primary tumor response. Clin Cancer Res. 2008;14:2431–6.
3. Motzer RJ, Hutson TE, Tomczak P, et al. Sunitinib versus interferon alfa in metastatic renal-cell carcinoma. N Engl J Med. 2007;356:115–24.
4. Motzer RJ, Bukowski RM. Targeted therapy for metastatic renal cell carcinoma. J Clin Oncol. 2006;24:5601–8.
5. Wood CG, Margulis V. Neoadjuvant (presurgical) therapy for renal cell carcinoma: a new treatment paradigm for locally advanced and metastatic disease. Cancer. 2009;115 Suppl 10:2355–60.
6. Margulis V, Wood CG. Pre-surgical targeted molecular therapy in renal cell carcinoma. BJU Int. 2009;103:150–3.
7. Bex A, van der Veldt AA, Blank C, et al. Neoadjuvant sunitinib for surgically complex advanced renal cell cancer of doubtful resectability: initial experience with downsizing to reconsider cytoreductive surgery. World J Urol. 2009;27:533–9.
8. Cost NG, Delacroix Jr, SE, Sleeper JP, et al. The impact of targeted molecular therapies on the level of renal cell carcinoma vena caval tumor thrombus. Eur Urol. 2011;59:912–8.
9. Wood CG. Multimodal approaches in the management of locally advanced and metastatic renal cell carcinoma: combining surgery and systemic therapies to improve patient outcome. Clin Cancer Res. 2007;13:697s–702.
10. Shuch B, Riggs SB, LaRochelle JC, et al. Neoadjuvant targeted therapy and advanced kidney cancer: observations and implications for a new treatment paradigm. BJU Int. 2008;102(6):692–6.
11. Silberstein JL, Millard F, Mehrazin R, et al. Feasibility and efficacy of neoadjuvant sunitinib before nephron-sparing surgery. BJU Int. 2010;106:1270–6.
12. Samplaski MK, Zhou M, Lane BR, Herts B, Campbell SC. Renal mass sampling: an enlightened perspective. Int J Urol. 2011;18:5–19.
13. Li G, Cuilleron M, Cottier M, et al. The use of MN/CA9 gene expression in identifying malignant solid renal tumors. Eur Urol. 2006;49:401–5.
14. Valera VA, Li-Ning TE, Walter BA, Roberts DD, Linehan WM, Merino MJ. Protein expression profiling in the spectrum of renal cell carcinomas. J Cancer. 2010;1:184–96.
15. Bukowski RM. Critical appraisal of pazopanib as treatment for patients with advanced metastatic renal cell carcinoma. Cancer Manag Res. 2011;3:273–85.
16. van der Veldt AA, Boven E, Helgason HH, et al. Predictive factors for severe toxicity of sunitinib in

unselected patients with advanced renal cell cancer. Br J Cancer. 2008;99:259–65.

17. Eisenhauer EA, Therasse P, Bogaerts J, et al. New response evaluation criteria in solid tumours: revised RECIST guideline (version 1.1). Eur J Cancer. 2009;45:228–47.

18. Robert G, Gabbay G, Bram R, et al. Case study of the month. Complete histologic remission after sunitinib neoadjuvant therapy in T3b renal cell carcinoma. Eur Urol. 2009;55:1477–80.

19. Thomas AA, Rini BI, Lane BR, et al. Response of the primary tumor to neoadjuvant sunitinib in patients with advanced renal cell carcinoma. J Urol. 2009;181:518–23.

20. Cowey CL, Amin C, Pruthi RS, et al. Neoadjuvant clinical trial with sorafenib for patients with stage II or higher renal cell carcinoma. J Clin Oncol. 2010;28:1502–7.

21. Powles T, Kayani I, Blank C, et al. The safety and efficacy of sunitinib before planned nephrectomy in metastatic clear cell renal cancer. Ann Oncol. 2011;22:1041–7.

22. Go AS, Chertow GM, Fan D, McCulloch CE, Hsu CY. Chronic kidney disease and the risks of death, cardiovascular events, and hospitalization. N Engl J Med. 2004;351:1296–305.

23. Karakiewicz PI, Suardi N, Jeldres C, et al. Neoadjuvant sutent induction therapy may effectively down-stage renal cell carcinoma atrial thrombi. Eur Urol. 2008;53:845–8.

24. Ansari J, Doherty A, McCafferty I, Wallace M, Deshmukh N, Porfiri E. Neoadjuvant sunitinib facilitates nephron-sparing surgery and avoids long-term dialysis in a patient with metachronous contralateral renal cell carcinoma. Clin Genitourin Cancer. 2009;7:E39–41.

25. Weight CJ, Larson BT, Fergany AF, et al. Nephrectomy induced chronic renal insufficiency is associated with increased risk of cardiovascular death and death from any cause in patients with localized cT1b renal masses. J Urol. 2010;183:1317–23.

26. Jonasch E, Wood CG, Matin SF, et al. Phase II presurgical feasibility study of bevacizumab in untreated patients with metastatic renal cell carcinoma. J Clin Oncol. 2009;27:4076–81.

27. Scappaticci FA, Fehrenbacher L, Cartwright T, et al. Surgical wound healing complications in metastatic colorectal cancer patients treated with bevacizumab. J Surg Oncol. 2005;91(3):173–80.

28. Hong MH, Kim HS, Kim C, et al. Treatment outcomes of sunitinib treatment in advanced renal cell carcinoma patients: a single cancer center experience in Korea. Cancer Res Treat. 2009;41:67–72.

29. Margulis V, Matin SF, Tannir N, et al. Surgical morbidity associated with administration of targeted molecular therapies before cytoreductive nephrectomy or resection of locally recurrent renal cell carcinoma. J Urol. 2008;180:94–8.

30. Scappaticci FA, Skillings JR, Holden SN, et al. Arterial thromboembolic events in patients with metastatic carcinoma treated with chemotherapy and bevacizumab. J Natl Cancer Inst. 2007;99:1232–9.

31. Eisen T, Ahmad T, Flaherty KT, et al. Sorafenib in advanced melanoma: a Phase II randomised discontinuation trial analysis. Br J Cancer. 2006;95:581–6.

32. Pfizer. Highlights of prescribing information. New York; 2006. http://www.pfizer.com/files/products/uspi_sutent.pdf. Accessed 6 Feb 2011.

33. Pfizer. Temsirolimus [prescribing information]. Madison, NJ; 2008. http://www.pfizerpro.com/content/showlabeling.asp?id=490. Accessed 6 Feb 2011

34. Biswas S, Kelly J, Eisen T. Cytoreductive nephrectomy in metastatic clear-cell renal cell carcinoma: perspectives in the tyrosine kinase inhibitor era. Oncologist. 2009;14:52–9.

Part IV

Advanced Disease

Biology of Renal Cell Carcinoma (Vascular Endothelial Growth Factor, Mammalian Target of Rapamycin, Immune Aspects)

Alexandra Arreola and W. Kimryn Rathmell

Introduction

Considering for a moment only clear cell renal cell carcinoma (ccRCC), we can focus on the unique biology of this renal tumor subtype, which accounts for the majority (>70%) of all cases of renal cell carcinoma (RCC). Although familial RCC occurs in fewer than 5% of cases of kidney cancer, there is much that has been learned from genetic studies from families with ccRCC. The majority of familial ccRCC occurs in association with the familial von Hippel–Lindau (VHL) family cancer syndrome, which is characterized by multifocal bilateral ccRCC in addition to pheochromocytoma/peripheral neuroendocrine tumor (PNET) and hemangioblastomas of the retina, cerebellum, and spine [1]. In 1994, it was recognized that the majority of sporadic ccRCC cases were also associated with inactivation of the *VHL* gene as the primary genetic perturbation, thus providing a valuable resource for understanding this pivotal genetic event driving the development of RCC [1].

Molecules Mediating RCC Pathophysiology

von Hippel–Lindau

Lessons from VHL Disease

To understand the pathways currently targeted for therapy of RCC, we must first explore the lessons that we have learned from the study of VHL disease. As alluded to above, the tumor suppressor gene *VHL* has been associated with a familial predisposition for various cancers including, hemangioblastomas (central nervous tumors that originate in the vascular system), pheochromocytomas (adrenal gland tumors), as well as clear cell renal carcinoma. Specifically, some families bear increased risk for one or more of these classic three tumor manifestations. VHL disease has, therefore, been classified according to these clinical manifestations as Type 1, 2A, 2B, and 2C [2]. In this classification, VHL Type 1 disease is highly associated with ccRCC and hemangioblastoma, but poses no risk for the development of the pheochromocytoma, whereas Types 2A, 2B, and 2C all present this risk. Within Type 2 disease, however, Type 2A presents some risk for ccRCC, Type 2B presents high risk for ccRCC, and Type 2C patients *exclusively* develop

A. Arreola
Department of Genetics, Lineberger Comprehensive
Cancer Center, University of North Carolina,
450 West Drive, CB 7295, Chapel Hill, NC 27599, USA

W.K. Rathmell (✉)
Department of Medicine, Lineberger Comprehensive
Cancer Center, University of North Carolina,
450 West Drive, CB 7295, Chapel Hill, NC 27599, USA

Department of Genetics, Lineberger Comprehensive
Cancer Center, University of North Carolina,
450 West Drive, CB 7295, Chapel Hill, NC 27599, USA
e-mail: Rathmell@med.unc.edu

pheochromocytoma, this subtype having no association with ccRCC [3].

The identification of these RCC-associated subtypes within the VHL disease spectrum gave way to a better understanding of the function of *VHL* gene and its role in RCC [4]. A variety of *VHL* mutations occur, including several higher frequency hot spots, spread over virtually the entirety of the gene. All of the major structural mutations are associated with ccRCC, but not risk for pheochromocytoma. Therefore, when a subset of families were found to carry structurally intact missense mutations of *VHL*, which also shared association with ccRCC risk, it provided new insight into the specific tumor suppressive action of the protein. Among the missense mutations, those associated with greater penetrance for RCC largely affected the portions of the *VHL* gene that encode for domains that either disrupt the participation of pVHL with its known partners in the E3-ubiquitin ligase complex in which pVHL plays the role of the key substrate recognition component or prevents binding to a key family of substrates of that complex, the hypoxia-inducible factors (HIFs), which we will discuss below [5]. This classification and the identification of genotype/phenotype-linked *VHL* mutations provide an interesting starting point for defining domains and functions of the pVHL protein that are integral to the development of ccRCC. These relationships have given way to a genetic and molecular understanding of *VHL* gene target regulation, primarily the regulation of the HIF pathway [6], which, as we shall see, has altered the paradigm for understanding and treating ccRCC.

VHL Mutation in Sporadic RCC

While patients with sporadic RCC commonly have a deletion of a portion of chromosome 3p that encompasses the *VHL* gene, most of the *VHL* mutations also associated with sporadic RCC are missense mutations that result in inactivation of the VHL protein (pVHL) either completely or partially. *VHL* functions as a classical tumor suppressor gene, such that disruption of VHL tumor suppressor activity requires biallelic inactivation in accordance with Knudson's two-hit hypothesis [7–9].

The chromosomal deletions that are encountered are therefore thought to primarily represent loss of heterozygosity (LOH) events.

pVHL partners with Elongin C, Elongin B, Ring Box Protein 1 (Rbx1/Roc1), and Cullin 2 to form an E3 ubiquitin ligase complex known as VBC [10–14]. This E3-ubiquitin ligase complex resembles the canonical complex SCF in its structure and function, with pVHL performing the function of the F-box protein [15]. Its role, therefore, is to provide the complex's target specificity. Several target proteins have been identified, but the most notable to date are the hypoxia-inducible factors HIF-1α and HIF-2α [16]. Representative hotspot missense mutations identified in *VHL* occur in residues that produce mutant proteins affecting the ability of pVHL to properly bind the VBC complex or reduce its affinity for detecting HIF-1α and HIF-2α subunits. This work gave way to the investigation of differential affinity and thereby, regulation, of HIF-α subunits by pVHL and the VBC complex [17].

VHL: Regulation of HIF and the Cellular Hypoxic Response

As the substrate recognition molecule in the E3-ubiquitin ligase complex VBC, under normal oxygen conditions pVHL is responsible for recognizing and recruiting the HIF-α subunits to the VBC complex where they will undergo polyubiquitination, targeting them for subsequent proteosomal degradation [18, 19]. Under conditions of oxygen deprivation (<4% Oxygen), pVHL fails to recognize HIF-α, and the proteins are stabilized as a result of avoiding degradation. Because the HIF proteins are translated at a high basal rate, stabilization of these proteins means they can accumulate to high levels very rapidly, in a matter of minutes.

The essence of this oxygen dependency comes from a post-translational modification that occurs in the presence of molecular oxygen. HIF-α factors contain an oxygen-dependent domain which hosts proline residues that are hydroxylated by an iron and oxygen-dependent family of enzymes called the HIF prolyl hydroxylases (PHD). pVHL specifically targets the prolyl hydroxylated forms of HIF-α. Thus, under low-oxygen conditions,

HIF PHD are unable to hydroxylate HIF-α subunits, and unhydroxylated HIF-α escape recognition by the VBC complex. The HIF-αfactors translocate to the nucleus, by way of heterodimerizing with the nuclear transporter HIF-1β, and promote the transcription of various target genes involved in the cellular response to limiting oxygen supply. Some notable target genes, which facilitate the hypoxic response, include platelet-derived growth factor (PDGF), vascular endothelial growth factor (VEGF), and carbonic anhydrase IX (CAIX), all of which are current or emerging targets of therapy.

VHL as a Tumor Suppressor

In ccRCC, as a result of *VHL* mutation, HIF factor stabilization is a constant feature of the cancer cells. The role pVHL plays in the prevention of cancer is a fascinating intersection of a normal physiological response to environmental stimuli derailed in the extreme. These cells, therefore, have constitutive stabilization of HIF factors, constitutive target gene activation, and little dynamic regulation of these factors. The condition of tonic activation of the hypoxia response pathway *in the presence of oxygen* has been termed pseudohypoxia. This condition sets the stage for a unique targeted therapy paradigm in RCC.

HIF Biology

HIF-1, HIF-2, and HIF-3: A Family of Transcription Factors Deregulated in Cancer

HIFs-1, -2, and -3 form a family of basic helix–loop–helix transcription factors that each heterodimerize in the cytoplasm with a stably expressed nuclear transport protein, HIF-1β also known as aryl hydrocarbon receptor nuclear translocator (ARNT). HIF-1α and HIF-2α subunits are most similar in structure and DNA-binding domains; although they are known to regulate some of the same gene targets there is increasing evidence of their differential regulation of hypoxia-inducible genes [20]. Difference in the balance of HIF-1α and HIF-2α produces stable variation in the downstream target genes, which we will discuss further in this chapter. HIF-3α exists in at least four splice variants whose functions are still largely uncharacterized, but are known to have additional DNA-binding elements that lack homology with HIF-1α or HIF-2α. Future work with HIF-3α will likely lend further insight into the influences on an individual tumor's transcriptional profile, but a full understanding of this factor's participation in ccRCC remains to be developed.

HIF Regulation and Function

HIF-α subunits that have averted proteosomal degradation, as a result of hypoxia or inactive pVHL as previously described, accumulate and are able to bind HIF-β partners which are then referred to as HIF-1 or HIF-2, according to the α subunit component of the complex. These newly formed HIF transcription factors translocate to the nucleus, bind hypoxia response elements (HREs) in gene promoter or enhancer regions and thereby regulate transcription of various target genes involved in numerous cellular functions. HIFs regulate a variety of cellular processes including: apoptosis, erythropoiesis, angiogenesis, energy metabolism, and cell proliferation. The most commonly dysregulated and explored target genes are VEGF [21], PDGF, CAIX, GLUT1/SLC2A1, and genes involved in glycolysis. We will discuss the implications of these deregulated target genes for supporting tumor cell growth later in this chapter.

Although HIF-1α and HIF-2α deregulation in ccRCC is primarily associated with *VHL* mutation or loss, there are other cellular processes that can influence the basal levels of each HIF factor. At the transcriptional level there are factors which bind in the promoter region of either *HIF-1α* or *HIF-2α*. One notable feature of *HIF-2α* transcriptional regulation is the participation of iron regulatory protein (IRP1) in regulating *HIF-2α* gene expression. This iron-dependent process involves IRP1 binding to a stem-loop structure in the *HIF-2α* 5′ untranslated region, effectively blocking transcription [22]. Similar mechanisms may be involved in *HIF-1α* regulation and may present unique opportunities for therapeutic targeting.

Perhaps most intriguing to the present discussion, it has been observed that HIF is also regulated at a translational level by mTOR complex 1 (mTORC1) mediated cap-dependent translation. HIF-1α is one of a panel of proteins specifically produced in response to mTOR-related signaling, and this effect on translation feeds the high basal rate of protein production, such that HIF-1α can accumulate very rapidly under hypoxic conditions. This also provides a valuable strategy to limit the extent of HIF-1α protein that can achieve stabilization, by blocking this important pathway with mTOR inhibitors. However, HIF-2 does not appear to be affected by mTORC1, but rather its production occurs downstream of the alternate complex mTORC2. We will review mTORC1 signaling mechanisms below, but new strategies with inhibitors which block activation of both complexes are under development.

HIF Role in RCC Tumorigenesis and Progression by Transcriptional Regulation of HIF Target Genes: Focus on VEGF

A very large repertoire of hypoxia response genes are regulated by the HIF family of transcription factors. We will focus on one of these targets, VEGF, that has made major strides in the road toward the development of effective therapeutic options for advanced RCC. Initiation and progression of RCC is dependent on the recruitment of endothelial cells to the tumor cells for the formation of new vasculature, the ability of cancer cells to overcome a hypoxic environment and thrive, as well as to manage an increased metabolic state of the cells. The survival of renal cancer cells requires direct transcriptional regulation of these pathways by HIF family members [23]. The development and maintenance of the dense vascular network associated with RCC is largely driven by HIF's transcriptional regulation of pro-angiogenic factors such as VEGF.

VEGF is itself a soluble growth factor that is secreted from cells to promote pro-angiogenic signals to the local environment. It therefore presents an interesting and tractable target for inhibition as a strategy to intercept this signal emanating from tumor cells. Such growth factor ligands mediate their effects by binding and activating cognate receptors, which in the case of VEGF are present on the surface of endothelial cells. VEGF receptors (VEGFRs) are a part of a family of receptor tyrosine kinases (RTKs) that are activated by extracellular growth factors to initiate a signaling cascade and promote cell mitogenesis. In addition to promoting angiogenesis, VEGF has other activities detailed below that also enable this factor to have potent effects on the general health of the tumor. As such, this factor among the many transcriptionally activated genes associated with HIF provides an ideal target to select for therapeutic development.

HIF1 Vs. HIF2: Convergent and Divergent Activities in RCC

Based on the differential regulation activity via pVHL and the VBC complex on the two major HIF-α family members and the other means of modulating HIF expression, it is no surprise that the spectrum of HIF-1α and HIF-2 expression is variable. However, adding to this source of tumor variability, HIF-1α and HIF-2 appear to not only maintain many similar gene targets, but also have sets of gene targets that are more commonly or specifically regulated by either HIF-1α or HIF-2α [20, 24]. As such, varying levels of HIF-1α and HIF-2α expression in renal carcinoma are associated with upregulation of certain pathways. Tumors expressing both factors (H1H2) were found to promote glucose consumption over HIF-2α expressing tumors (H2) [25]. Similarly, pVHL-deficient H1H2 clear cell renal carcinomas display upregulated mTOR and MAPK signaling pathways, while those H2 carcinomas have upregulated c-Myc activity and showed increased proliferative capacity [26]. Both groupings displayed increased angiogenesis and deregulation of VEGF transcript. Differential regulation of HIFs and their target genes can therefore provide valuable information as to what genetic and molecular perturbations influence tumor biology and may give clues as to the potential for response to therapies targeting the mTOR or VEGF signaling pathways [27]. This chapter will focus on two commonly targeted pathways

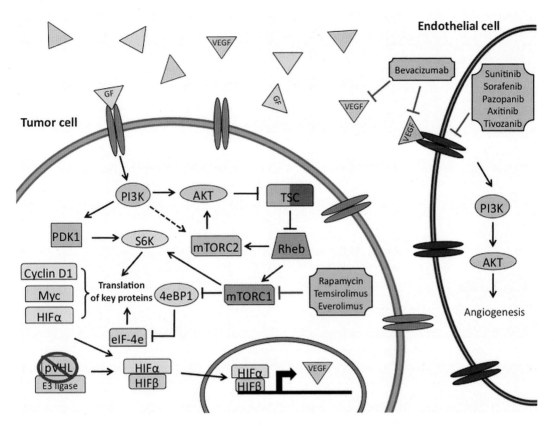

Fig. 13.1 Signaling pathways and current therapies for advanced RCC. (*1*) The effects of VHL loss and HIF stabilization on transcriptional activity provides the chief mode of induction of VEGF, a secreted growth factor that stimulates the expansion and maturation of endothelial cells by engaging VEGF receptors on the endothelial cell surface. One targeted antibody therapy, bevacizumab, directly inhibits VEGF ligands from activating receptor tyrosine kinases. Tyrosine kinase inhibitors are indicated which are currently in use targeting the intracellular kinase domain to prevent activation of VEGF receptor-mediated signaling pathways in endothelial cells. (2) Endothelial cells responding to VEGF and tumor cells responding to other growth factor stimuli activate transmembrane receptor tyrosine kinases and subsequently the PI3K/Akt/mTOR signal transduction cascade, intersecting with HIF regulation at the level of protein translation. Various targeted therapies against mTORC1 are indicated

for therapy in RCC: VEGF, a HIF target and potent regulator of tumor vascularity, and mTOR, a regulator of HIF expression and global cell maintenance (Fig. 13.1).

Vascular Endothelial Growth Factor

The Family of VEGF Ligands and VEGF Receptors

VEGF, a Historical Perspective

VEGF was first identified in 1948, known then as soluble "angiogenic factor X" which could promote the growth of vessels [28]. Even in the early studies it was recognized that regional tissues liberated a substance that promoted the expansion of existing blood vessel networks, termed angiogenesis, and supported the formation of new vessels, termed neovascularization. This process was also noted to occur along a substrate gradient to reach a region of tissue in need of vascular supply. For the next half-century these principles have formed the foundation of investigations into normal and tumor angiogenesis, and VEGF has remained as the single most potent and ubiquitous angiogenic growth factor in cell biology.

VEGF, also known as vascular permeability factor (VPF), functions as both a mitogen and an important regulator of endothelial vessel physiology. VEGF was formally identified in 1989 as a secreted mitogen specific to endothelial cells [29, 30]. In tumors, VEGF exerts its mitogenic growth effect on the vascular endothelial cells, promoting both proliferation and new vessel formation, as well as directing forward extension along a growth factor gradient. In many cancer situations, oxygen diffusion is unable to penetrate into the deeper regions of the tumor. This triggers a hypoxic response as we have described above, resulting in HIF stabilization and resultant transcriptional activation of VEGF. For the case of ccRCC, and other tumors that have acquired constitutive HIF deregulation, it is important to consider that the driving transcriptional force for VEGF expression is not regulated by physiological gradients of oxygen. In these conditions, VEGF is being transcriptionally induced independently of tumor oxygen status, and therefore may achieve much higher levels and also promote an even more vigorously disorganized assortment of endothelium as a result of unrestrained endothelial mitogenic and neovascularization processes.

Because of the importance of VEGF in this critical process of tumor angiogenesis, it has become a central player in the arena of targeted drug development for many tumors, including RCC. For years, the influence of angiogenesis and the impact on oxygen and nutrient delivery to rapidly growing tumors has been a basic factor of tumor biology as it impacts such key clinically relevant factors as drug delivery, surgical resection strategies, and sensitivity to radiation therapy. This chapter will provide an overview of the biology of VEGF and relevant pro-angiogenic cofactors, as well as the current status of therapeutics specifically targeting this key molecule in the treatment of RCC.

VEGF Protein Structure and Isoforms

VEGF actually refers to a family of related peptides, each with restricted tissue expression and receptor specificity. VEGFA is the primary factor targeted in the treatment of cancer. The protein is structurally related to the PDGF family, sharing homology with both PDGF-α and PDGF-β. The

original VEGFA was identified as a secreted peptide of 45 kDa, although the apparent molecular mass is approximately 20 kDa under reducing conditions, confirming substantial modification of the protein [31].

The active portion of the protein is a 26 amino acid signal sequence at the N terminus of the multiple isoforms of the protein. At least nine isoforms arise due to the alternative splicing of a single gene [32]. The primary protein of this family is a 165 amino acid member (VEGF165) [29]. In addition to VEGF165, there are also two common 121 amino acid (VEGF121) and 189 amino acid (VEGF189) forms. Finally, a 145 amino acid isoform (VEGF145) has been identified in association with tumor angiogenesis. The various isoforms all arise from one 8 exon gene and arise through alternative splicing [33]. VEGF189 represents the complete 8 exon transcript. VEGF165 lacks exon 6, VEGF145 lacks exon 7, and VEGF 121 lacks both exons 6 and 7. VEGF165 is the predominant isoform with basic charge and moderate affinity for heparin, making it locally sequestered in the extracellular matrix following secretion with slow diffusion, setting up the gradient along which physiologic endothelial responses occur [31]. By contrast VEGF121 has little affinity for heparin and is liberated freely from the cell, but VEGF189, as a result of additional basic residues, binds heparin strongly and is fully sequestered in the extracellular matrix [34].

The activity of the various isoforms continues to be an area of active investigation, but is beyond the scope of this chapter. The important message is that all VEGFA isoforms are liberated in response to HIF-mediated transcriptional induction, providing local and distant effects on the tumor environment. It stands to reason, however, that currently available neutralizing antibody preparations target common portions of VEGFA, and thus restrict VEGFA signaling from most if not all of the isoforms. This assessment requires further validation, and failure to fully neutralize isoforms due to exon selection or local environment restrictions could be potentially a major source of drug resistance.

Related family members, VEGFB, VEGFC, and VEGFD are also regulated by HIF transcriptional activation and expressed in a host of tumor environments. These distinct genes interact with a separate group of related receptors, some involved in endothelial cell growth and others involved in lymphatic vessel development [35, 36]. In particular, VEGFB targets the endothelial receptor VEGFR1 (Flt1), whereas VEGFA isoforms engage the VEGF receptor 2 (VEGFR2, Flk1, KDR) to induce endothelial cell growth. However, both VEGFA isoforms and VEGFB can bind to soluble VEGFR1. Although investigations continue to examine potential activities of these proteins in tumor biology, a definitive role for these related proteins in tumor development or maintenance has not been conclusively demonstrated. Therefore, although targeting these pathways may eventually be developed in cancer therapy, there is no current role in RCC, and the focus of this chapter will be exclusively on VEGFA.

Regulation of VEGF: Management at Many Levels

Much of what we understand about VEGF regulation does come from investigations of the expression in tumors or tumor-related tissues. Major advances have been made in the quantitative assessment of parameters or factors directly associated with tumor angiogenesis. Histologically, quantitation of intra-tumoral microvessel density (MVD) correlates well with the measurement of pro-angiogenic factors, primarily VEGF, in the serum of cancer patients. Most of the attention has been directed to VEGF and its cognate receptors in tumor angiogenesis.

Gene expression of VEGF is regulated by a variety of factors including growth factors, p53 mutation, estrogen receptor activation, thyroid-stimulating hormone, nitric oxide, and hypoxia. Inappropriate activation of the hypoxia response pathway, as discussed above, and elsewhere in this text, is a major mechanism of VEGF transcriptional regulation in RCC [37, 38]. In RCC, HIF complex binds to a conserved hypoxia response element (HRE) proximal to a CREB element (cAMP response element) located in the VEGF 5′ promoter region. The C-terminal transactivation domain of HIF-α interacts with the p300/CBP (CREB binding protein) coactivator to induce transcription at the VEGF locus [39–41]. This transcriptional regulation via HIF appears to be the dominant regulatory mechanism for major VEGFA stimulation, and inhibition of binding at the consensus HRE promoter sequence suppresses transcriptional activation of VEGF [42]. Based on nuclear runoff transcriptional assays the transcriptional rate for VEGF is increased at least two- to threefold by hypoxia [43].

VEGF is also regulated in response to hypoxia at the level of mRNA stability. Both the 5′ and 3′ untranslated regions of VEGF confer increased mRNA stability. In particular the increase in VEGF level in response to hypoxia is at least partly contributed by post-transcriptional mechanisms [44]. Under normoxic conditions VEGF mRNA is extremely labile, with a very short half-life [45–47], and experiments have demonstrated an increase in half-life by as much as eightfold under hypoxic conditions. The specific mechanisms of maintaining VEGF stability remain to be determined, but likely involve compensatory regulation by hypoxia or HIF-regulated tumor microRNAs [48].

The effect of hypoxia on VEGF translation has been understudied, and much less is known about the mechanisms and significance of these translational controls. Hypoxia appears to play opposite roles on cap-dependent translation and internal ribosomal entry (IRE) translation. Global protein translation that involves the traditional 5′-m7-GTP capping processing is inhibited by hypoxic signals, whereas induction by IRE preserves the translation of a small number of factors critical for the physiological response to oxygen deprivation, including VEGF as well as HIF-1α [49]. Much more is likely to be learned about this dynamic and potentially important mechanism of VEGF regulation in cancer as well as normal physiology.

VEGF Function

VEGF protein is a potent mitogen of both capillary and vascular endothelial cells [29, 31]. It is perhaps the only chemokine with direct activity to stimulate proliferation and migration of endothelial cells, promoted through binding and dimerization of cell surface transmembrane

VEGF receptors which also impacts the vascular physiology, causing vessel dilation and vascular permeability. The receptors FLT1 (VEGFR1) and KDR/FLK1 (VEGFR2), mentioned above as receptors for VEGFB and VEGFA, respectively, comprise the major classifications of endothelial receptors that bind VEGF. These receptors are only present on endothelial cells and data suggests that the multiple isoforms of VEGF compete for binding on the receptor. Specifically, it is important to note that VEGF145, the major tumor-associated isoform, will inhibit the binding of VEGF165 to the KDR/FLK1/VEGFR2 receptor, although binding by either results in receptor activation and downstream signaling.

Both VEGF145 and VEGF189 have highly basic residues that permit them to reside stably in the extracellular matrix. This structural organization of VEGFA species residing in the extracellular matrix surrounding the secreting cell spatially fixes them as chemokines to direct vessel growth [50]. In addition, the VEGF family regulates the permeability of both mature and developing vessels in a dose-dependent manner [51–56]. Even these seemingly distant activities, however, occur through interactions with the FLT1 and KDR/FLK1 receptor family. Finally, VEGF has been implicated in maintaining the blood–brain barrier, and facilitating glucose transport across this essential barrier during periods of physiological crisis.

VEGF and Cancer

It was not until 1995 that the importance of VEGF and its receptor system in tumor angiogenesis was fully recognized as a feature not only promoting cancer growth, but essential for tumor maintenance as well. This suggested a potential therapeutic option specifically targeting this aspect of tumor biology [57]. Since then, a revolution in targeted therapy has evolved multiple strategies to achieve the inhibition of tumor angiogenesis. Because of the unique molecular characteristics of constitutive, non-hypoxia-dependent HIF activation and VEGF expression in RCC, this cancer is an ideal system in which to examine these emerging therapeutics specifically targeting VEGF signaling and provide important proof of concept work.

As alluded to above, the vascularization of tumors provides a provocative target for therapy for several reasons. First, in adults, the formation of new vessels is an event essentially relegated to pathologic conditions, with the exception of wound healing. The pathological event that demonstrates the efficiency of this process most elegantly is the growth of solid tumors. By promoting VEGF signaling, cancer cells co-opt host vessels, sprout new vessels from existing ones, and/or recruit endothelial cells from the bone marrow. Second, the resulting vasculature is structurally and functionally abnormal, lacking vascular tone or proper pericyte support structures and is highly permeable with global disorganization. Therefore, this unique tumor vasculature provides a distinctive target for inhibitory therapy [37].

A large amount of data has supported the importance of VEGF and its cognate receptors in tumor angiogenesis given that VEGF is measurably increased in tumors and the surrounding extracellular matrix. VEGF has also been shown to be elevated in the serum of patients with non-small-cell lung cancer, colorectal, breast, ovarian, uterine, and RCC [58–63]. As detailed above, a variety of mechanisms account for the increase in VEGF, with activation of the hypoxic response pathway via the transcription factors HIF-1α and HIF-2α as the most classic mechanism of induction. Despite the consistency with which VEGF is elevated in the tumor phenotype, it remains an unpredictable tumor marker [64]. Many other pathologic or inflammatory states can cause serum elevations of VEGF and VEGF levels themselves vary somewhat widely in intrapatient measurement, limiting its use as an independent biomarker. One potential problem with serum measurement of VEGF is the high concentration of VEGF in platelets, which release their contents during the collection of serum samples [65, 66]. It is also interesting to note that disruption in VEGF signaling with VEGF RTK inhibitors leads to an increase in serum VEGF, presumably as a result of feedback mechanisms or reduced turnover of the receptor/ligand pairs.

RCC presents a unique clinical setting in which a tumor type nearly universally usurps a pro-angiogenic cellular homeostatic mechanism. Cell culture model systems of RCC have demonstrated a direct link between *VHL* mutation and upregulation of VEGF. RCC cells in which *VHL* is mutant express abundant levels of VEGF mRNA and protein, and reconstitution of these cells with a wild-type *VHL* cDNA restores predicted patterns of VEGF hypoxia responsive regulation [21]. Thus, increased expression of VEGF and the consequences of that increased expression are expected and predictable events in the development of most RCC.

Targeting VEGF and VEGF Receptors

The notion of targeting tumor angiogenesis is not unique to RCC. Certainly, the requirement of increased vascularity, or recruitment of vasculature by solid tumors, is a well-established hallmark of cancer [67]. VEGFA can be targeted by a humanized neutralizing antibody, bevacizumab, which was previously approved as an adjunct to chemotherapy for other cancers [68]. Although bevacizumab has shown limited activity as a single agent in many other tumors, the drug provides an important addition to chemotherapy, as the reduction in tumor-produced VEGF results in normalization of the vasculature for more effective penetration of the chemotherapy.

In advanced RCC the situation is somewhat different, as the tumor cells produce abundant levels of VEGF in a manner unregulated by normal control mechanisms. The result is a notoriously abundant and disorganized vasculature. What was speculated, but was unknown, was whether as a result these tumors would be *more dependent* on tumor endothelium to support continued growth. In fact, phase II data suggested that these tumors were, in fact, highly dependent on the supporting vasculature, and reductions in tumor volume followed treatment targeting VEGF ligand [69]. As will be discussed elsewhere in this volume, bevacizumab is now approved for RCC in combination with interferon-alpha [69].

Of course, as a secreted ligand, VEGF-mediated mitogen activity is dependent upon engagement of its receptor. As discussed above, there are multiple VEGF receptors expressed on tumor endothelial cells and possibly other components of the tumor stroma. It is important to note that functional VEGF receptors have not yet been identified on renal carcinoma cells. Thus, the effect of inhibiting VEGF receptor signaling rests primarily in preventing tumor angiogenesis; additionally, withdrawal of the VEGF signal to endothelial cells induces their regression. In elegant work by Bhatt et al., the tumor vasculature is virtually absent from the tumor shortly after treatment with VEGF RTK inhibitors [70, 71]. Indeed, RCC tumors treated with VEGF receptor TKIs display marked central necrosis, consistent with cell death as a result of removing the vascular supply [72, 73].

Later chapters in this volume will detail the development of VEGF RTK inhibitors, but the success of this therapeutic strategy is owed to the unique dependency of RCC on the disordered vasculature. It is important to recognize that as with most tyrosine kinase inhibitors, those used for the treatment of RCC are not exclusively inhibitory to VEGF receptors. However, as more is learned about the VEGF receptor inhibitors that have been developed the theme that emerges is of inhibition of VEGF receptor 2, as the critical mediator of RCC tumor angiogenesis. The first two tyrosine kinase inhibitors developed for advanced RCC are sunitinib [74] and sorafenib [75]. Pazopanib is another tyrosine kinase inhibitor (TKI) recently approved for use in RCC therapy targeting all VEGF receptors as well as PDGFR-α and β, and c-Kit to inhibit endothelial cell proliferation [76] (Table 13.1). Finally, additional VEGF RTK inhibitors currently emerging are tivozanib [80] and axitinib, both of which inhibit VEGF receptors 1–3 as well as PDGFR-β [81]. These therapeutics will be discussed in depth in the following chapters.

Mammalian Target of Rapamycin

PI3Kinase, Akt, and mTOR, a Common Pathway in Cancer Biology

The mammalian target of rapamycin (mTOR) is an intracellular serine-threonine kinase that can be regulated by upstream growth factor signals and acts as a master regulator of cell functions by influencing multiple downstream pathways.

Table 13.1 Targeted receptors and tyrosine kinase inhibitor therapies [75–79]

Receptor	Ligand	Primary receptor role	High affinity target therapy
VEGFR-1 (Flt-1)	VEGF-A VEGF-B	Angiogenesis, vasculogenesis	Sunitinib, pazopanib, axitinib, tivozanib
VEGFR-2 (Flk1/KDR)	VEGF-A VEGF-C VEGF-D VEFG-E	Angiogenesis, vasculogenesis	Sorafenib, sunitinib, pazopanib, axitinib, tivozanib
VEGFR-3 (Flt4)	VEGF-C VEGF-D	Lymphangiogenesis	Sorafenib, sunitinib, pazopanib, axitinib, tivozanib
PDGFR-α	PDGF	Angiogenesis	Sunitinib, pazopanib, axitinib
PDGFR-β	PDGF	Angiogenesis	Sorafenib, sunitinib, pazopanib, axitinib, tivozanib
c-Kit	SCF	Mast cell growth	Sunitinib

SCF cytokine stem cell factor, *PDGFR* platelet-derived growth factor receptor, *VEGFR* vascular endothelial growth factor receptor

Evolutionarily conserved TOR is required for mouse embryonic development as is seen by embryonic lethality of mTOR−/− mice [82]. mTOR is also a gatekeeper of many cellular regulatory roles including cell growth, metabolism, proliferation, and cell signaling. The pathway of signal transduction implicating mTOR complex signaling will be discussed below, as well as the effects of mTOR pathway inhibition on tumor and normal cells (Fig. 13.1).

Engagement of ligands to their cognate RTKs on tumor or supporting cells initiates a classical signaling cascade, which activates phosphoinositide 3-kinase (PI3K) resulting in the generation of phosphatidylinositol-3,4,5-triphosphate (PIP3) from PIP2. PI3K activity is regulated by its heterodimer subunits, p85 regulatory subunit and the catalytic subunit p110 that together tightly regulate cell growth and proliferation once stimulated by growth factor RTKs activated by ligand engagement, overexpression, or oncogenic mutation [83]. This enzyme is negatively regulated by the gatekeeper protein phosphatase and tensin homolog (PTEN), which acts as a major tumor suppressor protein in many cancers.

In a step highly dependent on intracellular localization, PIP2 propagates the PI3K signal by recruiting cytoplasmic protein kinase B (Akt/PKB) to the cell membrane where it can be activated by polycystin-1 (PDK1) [84, 85]. It is important to note that Akt exists in three isoforms, Akt1, Akt2, and Akt3, which for the purposes of this chapter will be considered together, but which have variations in activity that can impact the degrees or direction of signaling through these pathways [86]. This signaling pathway is one of the many simultaneous levels of regulation, as well as feedback loops, such that straightforward interpretation of the pathway is often difficult. As an example, mTOR complex 2 (mTOR2), which we will discuss below, also participates in Akt activation at the cell membrane.

One downstream target of Akt is the tuberous sclerosis complex (TSC, a heterodimeric complex TSC1/TSC2), which normally functions to inhibit the highly active Ras-related GTPase Rheb (Ras homolog enriched in brain), by converting it to its inactive GDP-bound state. Thus, activation of Akt leads to the inactivation of downstream TSC resulting in Rheb activation and an increase of cell growth, proliferation, and cell survival. The most significant function of Rheb-GTP is its activation of mTOR. mTOR is a highly conserved ser/thr kinase, first identified as the ultimate target of inhibition of the immune suppressant rapamycin. The activation of these targets results in cell growth and survival and is a potent promoter of tumorigenesis.

Understanding the Role of mTORC1/2 Subunits

mTOR is comprised of two signaling complexes mTORC1 and mTORC2 (mentioned above as a feedback activator of Akt) which differentially regulate HIF-1α and HIF-2α protein translation, respectively, and therefore have roles in different cellular processes with regards to RCC biology [87]. mTORC1 is composed of mTOR, regulatory-associated protein of mTOR (raptor), and G protein β-subunit-like (GβL) and is largely regulated through the PI3K/Akt pathway as discussed above [88]. mTORC2 is composed of mTOR, rapamycin-insensitive companion of target of rapamycin (Rictor) and GβL [89]. Rictor is necessary for a feedback phosphorylation of the serine-threonine protein kinase Akt, reactivating this pathway [90].

In an interesting twist on the VHL/HIF pathway discussed above, the production of HIF factors has been linked to mTORC1-mediated cap-dependent translation. In particular, HIF-1α protein translation appears to be dependent on active mTORC1, and this mechanism of disrupting HIF signaling in RCC has been exploited in the therapeutic arena as discussed elsewhere. What remains less certain is the influence of mTOR signaling on HIF-2α translation. Recent evidence suggests that HIF-1α abundance can be influenced by both mTORC1 and mTORC2, but that HIF-2α translation is specifically regulated within the mTOR signaling pathway via mTORC2 [86, 91].

mTOR Targets Dysregulated in Advanced RCC

S6 Kinase-1 and Eukaryote Initiation Factor 4E

Activation of mTOR leads to phosphorylation of ribosomal S6 kinase-1 (S6K) and eukaryote translation initiation factor 4E-binding protein (4EBP), two translation-regulating factors to promote cell proliferation and survival. 4EBP directly binds eukaryote initiation factor 4E (eIF-4E) and prevents it from binding to the other translation initiation factor complex subunits, and this repression is released upon mTOR-mediated phosphorylation [92]. When 4EBP is inactivated by phosphorylation, eIF-4E binds to its other partners as well as the 5′cap of mRNA transcripts [93]. Activated S6K results in a downstream effect of increased translation of mRNA encoding ribosomal proteins as well as increased

translation of mRNAs that encode for HIFs, c-Myc, and cyclin D1 [94].

HIF Factors

As alluded to above, mTORC1 is a known positive regulator of HIF-1α. This upregulation of HIF protein translation is required by cancerous cells in times of hypoxic stress for the continued transcriptional activation of angiogenic factors such as VEGF, as a way to maintain blood supply for sustained cell proliferation [94]. HIF-1α protein levels are reduced upon treatment of renal carcinoma cells by the current mTOR inhibitors [95]. However, issues remain with targeted effects of these drugs in in situ tumors, and the degree to which HIF is downregulated in the continued face of absent *VHL* regulation. Reducing overall HIF levels is likely one component of mTOR inhibitor activity in renal carcinomas, but other features of the pathway that promote global cell proliferation are also likely integral to its activity.

mTOR Pathway as a Target for Treating RCC

Rapamycin was the first mTOR inhibitor isolated from *Streptomyces hygroscopicus* that showed antiproliferative activity in human cancer cells [96]. Rapamycin binds an immunophilin receptor, FKBP12, to inhibit mTOR activation. Temsirolimus and everolimus inhibit mTORC1 by a similar mechanism and have both been shown to reduce in vitro levels of HIF-1α and further have been shown to have disease activity. Temsirolimus has been approved for use as first-line therapy of advanced RCC for patients with a poor prognosis [97–99]. Everolimus also binds FKBP12 to inhibit downstream mTOR signaling [100]. It is approved for patients with advanced RCC that have failed treatment with a VEGF RTK inhibitor such as sorafenib or sunitinib [101]. These compounds are functional by disengaging a terminal step in a highly complex and intertwined signaling pathway, the understanding of which may help guide the most appropriate use of these agents, or the directions for developing next generation inhibitors of this signaling pathway. Finally, the discussion in this chapter has focused on biological aspects of ccRCC, but it is important to note that mTOR signaling pathways can be important, and have indeed been implicated very strongly in non-clear cell histologies, suggesting that this pathway may be more universally applicable to renal tumor biology.

Immunology in RCC

The Intersection of Immune System Physiology and Renal Tumor Biology

Prior to the advent of targeted therapies taking aim at VEGF and mTOR signaling, most therapeutic attention in ccRCC was directed toward immunotherapy. RCC remains one of the most immune-responsive solid tumors, for reasons that remain incompletely understood. Despite the promising moves forward with targeted therapy, immunotherapy remains the only treatment which has been shown to induce prolonged and durable complete responses, such that treatment with high-dose interleukin 2 (IL-2) remains a mainstay of therapy at many specialty centers, and intensive efforts remain focused on the development of new less toxic and more broadly effective therapies in this arena [102].

Infiltration of immune cells is a frequently encountered feature of RCC. This infiltrate is highly heterogeneous, and can include T cells (CD4 and CD8), regulatory T cells, dendritic cells, natural killer (NK) cells, macrophages, and B cells of various stages of differentiation [103]. The impact of these various components on tumor behavior or response to either immunotherapy or targeted therapies is not known at this time. This infiltrate commonly locates itself along the plethora of vessels integrated in the tumor, but can also be found within the tumor stroma itself. While the specific contributions of these immune infiltrates are not well understood, these factors can produce a state of profound immunosuppression of the tumor. This is seen not only in the patients who elicit dramatic responses to immunotherapy, but also in the patients who reside with dormant tumors for prolonged periods of time, only to develop explosive disease at a later time point, suggesting a break in tolerance that could potentially be rectified with therapeutic immune modulation. The next section will discuss what is known about T cell tolerance and RCC.

Immunosurveillance in RCC

Immunosurveillance describes the process of innate and adaptive immunity processes identifying and eliminating host-derived cells that have been altered chemically or genetically [104]. The concept of immunosurveillance has been recently amended to put forward a proposal that host–tumor relationships depend on a process termed immunoediting. According to this hypothesis, initially the immune system recognizes and eliminates the majority of immunogenic tumor cells, leading to a state of equilibrium in which the immune system holds the tumor cells in a steady state, where tumor growth is equal to the immune system's capability to control it. Finally, the tumor escapes immune regulatory mechanisms by downregulating immunogenic epitopes, developing local or systemic immune suppressor mechanisms, or by increasing the rate of tumor growth leading to the immune response being overrun [105].

The tumor promotes this local immunosuppression often as a result of tumor-secreted cytokines such as IL-10 and TGF-β. In an interesting intersection of immunology and angiogenesis, VEGF secretion by tumors and stroma has also been implicated in local immunosuppression. VEGFA can also act as a chemoattractant for macrophages via VEGF receptor Flt-1, recruiting these potent immune mediators to the tumor where they might produce local responses or alternatively become reprogrammed to recognize tumor cells as self [106]. These cytokines inhibit cytotoxic immunity and may also promote the differentiation and recruitment of regulatory cells. These cells include regulatory T cells (Treg) and myeloid-derived suppressor cells (MDSCs) [107]. These immune system subsets provide an interesting opportunity to target the balance of immunologic sensors and mediators shift the immune system in favor of increased tumor immunosurveillance.

Summary and a Look Forward

Conclusions

RCC is a tumor type that has established the paradigm that understanding the biology of the cancer will lead to fruitful innovations in treatment of patients. As a result of the discoveries relating frequent *VHL* loss or mutation to HIF family stabilization, the major source of VEGF elevation has been revealed. In addition to the canonical pathway, there are influences on VEGF expression from within the pathway (mutation effects of *VHL*, patterns of HIF deregulation) as well as extrinsic influences on VEGF expression (including transcriptional and translational regulatory mechanisms). A robust understanding of these influences has enabled us to better understand how to target VEGF and angiogenic signaling and provides clues for combating drug resistance.

mTOR signaling is similarly complex. This important pathway provides the growth control signals from numerous cellular pathways, and it is regulated at many levels, including feedback loops. Current strategies specifically target the mTORC1 complex, which provides a unique tactic to reduce HIF-1α levels, but scrutiny of the pathway suggests that targeting further upstream or dual targeting of mTORC1 and mTORC2 may hold even more promise. Those initiatives are anxiously awaited as we work to understand how best to select among the currently available agents for our patients.

Finally, the immune system in RCC is clearly a uniquely balanced arrangement. The features of individual host or tumor environments that provide for competent tumor immunosurveillance continue to undergo investigation. The potential to harness the immune system for strategic management of RCC continues to be an important goal.

Future Directions

The future of targeted and immune-based therapies will rely on the expanded exploration and understanding of these highly regulated pathways. New strategies to more effectively or more precisely target the specific mediators of tumor growth will emerge from the more sophisticated understanding of these pathways in RCC. We see the signs of these new therapies already on the horizon: multifaceted targeting of the mTOR signaling pathway at the levels of PI3K, PDK, Akt, and mTORC2 as well as mTORC1; new strategies to target VEGF and alternate pro-angiogenic pathways, as well as strategies to target HIF family members directly, immune-modulating strategies that address issues of co-stimulation, T cell subset activation, and the restoration of immunosurveillance. The biology of this cancer continues to provide an elegant roadmap for therapeutic strategy development, which in turn will direct us toward increasingly effective and less toxic therapies.

References

1. Ong KR, Woodward ER, Killick P, Lim C, Macdonald F, Maher ER. Genotype–phenotype correlations in von Hippel Lindau disease. Hum Mutat. 2007;28(2):143–9.
2. Zbar B. Von Hippel–Lindau disease and sporadic renal cell carcinoma. Cancer Surv. 1995;25:219.
3. Zbar B, Kishida T, Chen F, et al. Germline mutations in the Von Hippel–Lindau disease (VHL) gene in families from North America, Europe, and Japan. Hum Mutat. 1996;8(4):348–57.
4. Crossey PA, Richards FM, Foster K, et al. Identification of intragenic mutations in the Von Hippel–Lindau disease tumour suppressor gene and correlation with disease phenotype. Hum Mol Genet. 1994;3(8):1303.
5. Latif F, Tory K, Gnarra J, et al. Identification of the von Hippel–Lindau disease tumor suppressor gene. Science. 1993;260(5112):1317.
6. Clifford SC, Cockman ME, Smallwood AC, et al. Contrasting effects on HIF-1 regulation by disease-causing pVHL mutations correlate with patterns of tumourigenesis in von Hippel–Lindau disease. Hum Mol Genet. 2001;10(10):1029.
7. Linehan W, Lerman M, Zbar B. Identification of the VHL gene: its role in renal carcinoma. JAMA. 1995;273(7):564–70.
8. Knudson AG. Mutation and cancer: statistical study of retinoblastoma. Proc Natl Acad Sci USA. 1971;68(4):820.
9. Hamano K, Esumi M, Igarashi H, et al. Biallelic inactivation of the von Hippel–Lindau tumor suppressor gene in sporadic renal cell carcinoma. J Urol. 2002;167(2):713–7.
10. Duan DR, Pause A, Burgess WH, et al. Inhibition of transcription elongation by the VHL tumor suppressor protein. Science. 1995;269(5229):1402.

11. Kibel A, Iliopoulos O, DeCaprio JA, Kaelin Jr WG. Binding of the von Hippel–Lindau tumor suppressor protein to elongin B and C. Science. 1995;269(5229):1444.

12. Kamura T, Koepp D, Conrad M, et al. Rbx1, a component of the VHL tumor suppressor complex and SCF ubiquitin ligase. Science. 1999;284(5414):657.

13. Pause A, Lee S, Worrell RA, et al. The von Hippel–Lindau tumor-suppressor gene product forms a stable complex with human CUL-2, a member of the Cdc53 family of proteins. Proc Natl Acad Sci USA. 1997;94(6):2156.

14. Lonergan KM, Iliopoulos O, Ohh M, et al. Regulation of hypoxia-inducible mRNAs by the von Hippel–Lindau tumor suppressor protein requires binding to complexes containing elongins B/C and Cul2. Mol Cell Biol. 1998;18(2):732.

15. Clifford SC, Astuti D, Hooper L, Maxwell PH, Ratcliffe PJ, Maher ER. The pVHL-associated SCF ubiquitin ligase complex: molecular genetic analysis of elongin B and C, Rbx1 and HIF-1alpha in renal cell carcinoma. Oncogene. 2001;20(36):5067.

16. Maxwell PH, Wiesener MS, Chang GW, et al. The tumor suppressor protein VHL targets hypoxia inducible factores for oxygen-dependent proteolysis. Development. 1995;121:4005–16.

17. Knauth K, Bex C, Jemth P, Buchberger A. Renal cell carcinoma risk in type 2 von Hippel–Lindau disease correlates with defects in pVHL stability and HIF-1 interactions. Oncogene. 2005;25(3):370–7.

18. Maxwell P, Wiesener M, Chang G, et al. The tumour suppressor protein VHL targets hypoxia inducible factors for oxygen-dependent proteolysis. Nature. 1999;399:271–5.

19. Cockman ME, Masson N, Mole DR, et al. Hypoxia inducible factor- binding and ubiquitylation by the von Hippel–Lindau tumor suppressor protein. J Biol Chem. 2000;275(33):25733.

20. Hu CJ, Wang LY, Chodosh LA, Keith B, Simon MC. Differential roles of hypoxia-inducible factor 1 alpha}(HIF-1 {alpha}) and HIF-2 {alpha in hypoxic gene regulation. Mol Cell Biol. 2003;23(24):9361.

21. Iliopoulos O, Levy AP, Jiang C, Kaelin WG, Goldberg MA. Negative regulation of hypoxia-inducible genes by the von Hippel–Lindau protein. Proc Natl Acad Sci USA. 1996;93(20):10595.

22. Zimmer M, Doucette D, Siddiqui N, Iliopoulos O. Inhibition of hypoxia-inducible factor is sufficient for growth suppression of VHL–/–tumors. Mol Cancer Res. 2004;2(2):89–95.

23. Kondo K, Kim WY, Lechpammer M, Kaelin Jr WG. Inhibition of HIF2alpha is sufficient to suppress pVHL-defective tumor growth. PLoS Biol. 2003;1(3):E83.

24. Raval RR, Lau KW, Tran MGB, et al. Contrasting properties of hypoxia-inducible factor 1 (HIF-1) and HIF-2 in von Hippel–Lindau-associated renal cell carcinoma. Mol Cell Biol. 2005;25(13):5675.

25. Ferrara N. Role of vascular endothelial growth factor in the regulation of angiogenesis. Kidney Int. 1999;56(3):794–814.

26. Gordan JD, Lal P, Dondeti VR, et al. HIF-[alpha] effects on c-Myc distinguish two subtypes of sporadic VHL-deficient clear cell renal carcinoma. Cancer Cell. 2008;14(6):435–46.

27. Gordan JD, Bertout JA, Hu CJ, Diehl JA, Simon MC. HIF-2 [alpha] promotes hypoxic cell proliferation by enhancing c-myc transcriptional activity. Cancer Cell. 2007;11(4):335–47.

28. Michaelson I. The mode of development of the vascular system of the retina, with some observations on its significance for certain retinal diseases. Trans Ophthalmol Soc UK. 1948;68:137–80.

29. Leung DW, Cachianes G, Kuang WJ, Goeddel DV, Ferrara N. Vascular endothelial growth factor is a secretedangiogenicmitogen.Science.1989;246(4935):1306.

30. Keck PJ, Hauser SD, Krivi G, et al. Vascular permeability factor, an endothelial cell mitogen related to PDGF. Science. 1989;246(4935):1309.

31. Ferrara N, Henzel WJ. Pituitary follicular cells secrete a novel heparin-binding growth factor specific for vascular endothelial cells. Biochem Biophys Res Commun. 1989;161(2):851–8.

32. Takahashi H, Shibuya M. The vascular endothelial growth factor (VEGF)/VEGF receptor system and its role under physiological and pathological conditions. Clin Sci. 2005;109:227–41.

33. Tischer E, Mitchell R, Hartman T, et al. The human gene for vascular endothelial growth factor. Multiple protein forms are encoded through alternative exon splicing. J Biol Chem. 1991;266(18):11947.

34. Ferrara N, Davis-Smyth T. The biology of vascular endothelial growth factor. Endocr Rev. 1997;18(1):4–25.

35. Paavonen K, Mandelin J, Partanen T, et al. Vascular endothelial growth factors C and D and their VEGFR-2 and 3 receptors in blood and lymphatic vessels in healthy and arthritic synovium. J Rheumatol. 2002;29(1):39.

36. Kukk E, Lymboussaki A, Taira S, et al. VEGF-C receptor binding and pattern of expression with VEGFR-3 suggests a role in lymphatic vascular development. Development. 1996;122(12):3829.

37. Tsuzuki Y, Fukumura D, Oosthuyse B, Koike C, Carmeliet P, Jain RK. Vascular endothelial growth factor (VEGF) modulation by targeting hypoxia-inducible factor-1 hypoxia response element VEGF cascade differentially regulates vascular response and growth rate in tumors. Cancer Res. 2000;60(22):6248.

38. Shweiki D, Itin A, Soffer D, Keshet E. Vascular endothelial growth factor induced by hypoxia may mediate hypoxia-initiated angiogenesis. Nature. 1992;359(6398):843–5.

39. Lando D, Peet DJ, Whelan DA, Gorman JJ, Whitelaw ML. Asparagine hydroxylation of the HIF transactivation domain: a hypoxic switch. Science. 2002;295(5556):858.

40. Dames SA, Martinez-Yamout M, De Guzman RN, Dyson HJ, Wright PE. Structural basis for Hif-1/

CBP recognition in the cellular hypoxic response. Proc Natl Acad Sci USA. 2002;99(8):5271.

41. Kobayashi A, Numayama-Tsuruta K, Sogawa K, Fujii-Kuriyama Y. CBP/p300 functions as a possible transcriptional coactivator of Ah receptor nuclear translocator (Arnt). J Biochem. 1997;122(4):703.

42. Olenyuk BZ, Zhang GJ, Klco JM, Nickols NG, Kaelin Jr WG, Dervan PB. Inhibition of vascular endothelial growth factor with a sequence-specific hypoxia response element antagonist. Proc Natl Acad Sci USA. 2004;101(48):16768.

43. Levy AP, Levy NS, Wegner S, Goldberg MA. Transcriptional regulation of the rat vascular endothelial growth factor gene by hypoxia. J Biol Chem. 1995;270(22):13333.

44. Damert A, Machein M, Breier G, et al. Up-regulation of vascular endothelial growth factor expression in a rat glioma is conferred by two distinct hypoxia-driven mechanisms. Cancer Res. 1997;57(17):3860.

45. Levy AP, Levy NS, Goldberg MA. Hypoxia-inducible protein binding to vascular endothelial growth factor mRNA and its modulation by the von Hippel–Lindau protein. J Biol Chem. 1996;271(41): 25492.

46. Stein I, Neeman M, Shweiki D, Itin A, Keshet E. Stabilization of vascular endothelial growth factor mRNA by hypoxia and hypoglycemia and coregulation with other ischemia-induced genes. Mol Cell Biol. 1995;15(10):5363.

47. Levy AP, Levy NS, Goldberg MA. Post-transcriptional regulation of vascular endothelial growth factor by hypoxia. J Biol Chem. 1996;271(5): 2746.

48. Liu H, Brannon AR, Reddy AR, et al. Identifying mRNA targets of microRNA dysregulated in cancer: with application to clear cell renal cell carcinoma. BMC Syst Biol. 2010;4(1):51.

49. Liu L, Simon MC. Regulation of transcription and translation by hypoxia. Cancer Biol Ther. 2004;3(6):492.

50. Poltorak Z, Cohen T, Sivan R, et al. VEGF145, a secreted vascular endothelial growth factor isoform that binds to extracellular matrix. J Biol Chem. 1997;272(11):7151.

51. Senger DR, Perruzzi CA, Feder J, Dvorak HF. A highly conserved vascular permeability factor secreted by a variety of human and rodent tumor cell lines. Cancer Res. 1986;46(11):5629.

52. Collins P, Connolly D, Williams T. Characterization of the increase in vascular permeability induced by vascular permeability factor in vivo. Br J Pharmacol. 1993;109(1):195.

53. Roberts W, Palade G. Increased microvascular permeability and endothelial fenestration induced by vascular endothelial growth factor. J Cell Sci. 1995;108:2369.

54. Dvorak HF, Brown LF, Detmar M, Dvorak AM. Vascular permeability factor/vascular endothelial growth factor, microvascular hyperpermeability, and angiogenesis. Am J Pathol. 1995;146(5):1029.

55. Wu H, Huang Q, Yuan Y, Granger HJ. VEGF induces NO-dependent hyperpermeability in coronary venules. Am J Physiol. 1996;271(6):H2735.

56. Hippenstiel S, Krull M, Ikemann A, Risau W, Clauss M, Suttorp N. VEGF induces hyperpermeability by a direct action on endothelial cells. Am J Physiol. 1998;274(5):L678.

57. Folkman J. Clinical applications of research on angiogenesis. N Engl J Med. 1995;333(26):1757.

58. Brattström D, Bergqvist M, Larsson A, et al. Basic fibroblast growth factor and vascular endothelial growth factor in sera from non-small cell lung cancer patients. Anticancer Res. 1998;18(2A):1123–7.

59. Guidi A. Vascular permeability factor (vascular endothelial growth factor) expression and angiogenesis in cervical neoplasia. J Natl Cancer Inst. 1995;87(16):1237.

60. Gasparini G, Bonoldi E, Gatti C, et al. Prognostic significance of vascular endothelial growth factor protein in node-negative breast carcinoma. J Natl Cancer Inst. 1997;89(2):139.

61. Yamamoto Y, Toi M, Kondo S, et al. Concentrations of vascular endothelial growth factor in the sera of normal controls and cancer patients. Clin Cancer Res. 1996;2(5):821.

62. Li XF, Gregory J, Ahmed A. Immunolocalisation of vascular endothelial growth factor in human endometrium. Growth Factors. 1994;11(4):277–82.

63. Salven P, Ruotsalainen T, Mattson K, Joensuu H. High pre-treatment serum level of vascular endothelial growth factor (VEGF) is associated with poor outcome in small-cell lung cancer. Int J Cancer. 1998;79(2):144–6.

64. Fuhrmann Benzakein E, Ma MN, Rubbia Brandt L, et al. Elevated levels of angiogenic cytokines in the plasma of cancer patients. Int J Cancer. 2000; 85(1):40–5.

65. Mhle R, Green D, Moore MAS, Nachman RL, Rafii S. Constitutive production and thrombin-induced release of vascular endothelial growth factor by human megakaryocytes and platelets. Proc Natl Acad Sci USA. 1997;94(2):663.

66. Webb NJA, Myers CR, Watson CJ, Bottomley MJ, Brenchley PEC. Activated human neutrophils express vascular endothelial growth factor (VEGF). Cytokine. 1998;10(4):254–7.

67. Hanahan D, Weinberg RA. The hallmarks of cancer. Cell. 2000;100(1):57–70.

68. Hurwitz H, Fehrenbacher L, Novotny W, et al. Bevacizumab plus irinotecan, fluorouracil, and leucovorin for metastatic colorectal cancer. N Engl J Med. 2004;350(23):2335.

69. Yang JC, Haworth L, Sherry RM, et al. A randomized trial of bevacizumab, an anti-vascular endothelial growth factor antibody, for metastatic renal cancer. N Engl J Med. 2003;349(5):427.

70. Bhatt RS, Wang X, Zhang L, et al. Renal cancer resistance to antiangiogenic therapy is delayed by restoration of angiostatic signaling. Mol Cancer Ther. 2010;9:2793–802.

71. Atkins MB, Choueiri TK, Cho D, Regan M, Signoretti S. Treatment selection for patients with metastatic renal cell carcinoma. Cancer. 2009; 115(S10):2327–33.

72. Cowey CL, Fielding JR, Kimryn Rathmell W. The loss of radiographic enhancement in primary renal cell carcinoma tumors following multitargeted receptor tyrosine kinase therapy is an additional indicator of response. Urology. 2010;75(5): 1108–13.

73. Cowey CL, Amin C, Pruthi RS, et al. Neoadjuvant clinical trial with sorafenib for patients with stage II or higher renal cell carcinoma. J Clin Oncol. 2010;28(9):1502.

74. Motzer RJ, Rini BI, Bukowski RM, et al. Sunitinib in patients with metastatic renal cell carcinoma. JAMA. 2006;295(21):2516.

75. Escudier B, Eisen T, Stadler WM, et al. Sorafenib in advanced clear-cell renal-cell carcinoma. N Engl J Med. 2007;356(2):125.

76. Ward JE, Stadler WM. Pazopanib in renal cell carcinoma. Clin Cancer Res. 2010;16(24):5923.

77. Cowey CL, Hutson TE, Figlin R. Pazopanib in the treatment of renal cell carcinoma. Clin Investig. 2011;1(1):75–85.

78. Motzer RJ, Hutson TE, Tomczak P, et al. Sunitinib versus interferon alfa in metastatic renal-cell carcinoma. N Engl J Med. 2007;356(2):115.

79. Bhargava P, Esteves B, Al-Adhami M, et al. Activity of tivozanib (AV-951) in patients with renal cell carcinoma (RCC): subgroup analysis from a phase II randomized discontinuation trial (RDT). Proc Am Soc Clin Onc. 2010;28:4599.

80. Bhargava P, Esteves B, Nosov D, et al. Updated activity and safety results of a phase II randomized discontinuation trial (RDT) of AV-951, a potent and selective VEGFR1, 2, and 3 kinase inhibitor, in patients with renal cell carcinoma (RCC). Proc Am Soc Clin Onc. 2009;27:5032.

81. Rini BI, Wilding G, Hudes G, et al. Phase II study of axitinib in sorafenib-refractory metastatic renal cell carcinoma. J Clin Oncol. 2009;27(27):4462.

82. Murakami M, Ichisaka T, Maeda M, et al. mTOR is essential for growth and proliferation in early mouse embryos and embryonic stem cells. Mol Cell Biol. 2004;24(15):6710.

83. Engelman JA, Luo J, Cantley LC. The evolution of phosphatidylinositol 3-kinases as regulators of growth and metabolism. Nat Rev Genet. 2006;7(8):606–19.

84. Wullschleger S, Loewith R, Hall MN. TOR signaling in growth and metabolism. Cell. 2006; 124(3):471–84.

85. Hay N, Sonenberg N. Upstream and downstream of mTOR. Genes Dev. 2004;18(16):1926.

86. Toschi A, Lee E, Gadir N, Ohh M, Foster DA. Differential dependence of hypoxia-inducible factors 1 and 2 on mTORC1 and mTORC2. J Biol Chem. 2008;283(50):34495.

87. Zheng XF, Fiorentino D, Chen J, Crabtree GR, Schreiber SL. TOR kinase domains are required for two distinct functions, only one of which is inhibited by rapamycin. Cell. 1995;82(1):121–30.

88. Kim DH, Sarbassov DD, Ali SM, et al. mTOR interacts with raptor to form a nutrient-sensitive complex that signals to the cell growth machinery. Cell. 2002;110(2):163–75.

89. Jacinto E, Loewith R, Schmidt A, et al. Mammalian TOR complex 2 controls the actin cytoskeleton and is rapamycin insensitive. Nat Cell Biol. 2004;6(11): 1122–8.

90. Guertin DA, Sabatini DM. Defining the role of mTOR in cancer. Cancer Cell. 2007;12(1):9–22.

91. Linehan WM, Srinivasan R, Schmidt LS. The genetic basis of kidney cancer: a metabolic disease. Nat Rev Urol. 2010;7(5):277–85.

92. Hara K, Maruki Y, Long X, et al. Raptor, a binding partner of target of rapamycin (TOR), mediates TOR action. Cell. 2002;110(2):177–89.

93. Sonenberg N, Gingras AC. The mRNA 5′cap-binding protein eIF4E and control of cell growth. Curr Opin Cell Biol. 1998;10(2):268–75.

94. Hudson CC, Liu M, Chiang GG, et al. Regulation of hypoxia-inducible factor 1 alpha expression and function by the mammalian target of rapamycin. Mol Cell Biol. 2002;22(20):7004.

95. Thomas GV, Tran C, Mellinghoff IK, et al. Hypoxia-inducible factor determines sensitivity to inhibitors of mTOR in kidney cancer. Nat Med. 2005; 12(1):122–7.

96. Vezine C, Kudelski A, Sehgal S. Rapamycin (AY-22.989), a new antifungal antibiotic. I. Taxonomy of the producing streptomycete ans isolation of the active principle. J Antibiot (Tokyo). 1975;28:721–6.

97. Hudes G, Carducci M, Tomczak P, et al. Temsirolimus, interferon alfa, or both for advanced renal-cell carcinoma. N Engl J Med. 2007;356(22):2271.

98. Wang Y, Wang X, Subjeck J, Shrikant P, Kim H. Temsirolimus, an mTOR inhibitor, enhances antitumour effects of heat shock protein cancer vaccines. Br J Cancer. 2011;104:643–52.

99. Dutcher J, de Souza P, McDermott D, et al. Effect of temsirolimus versus interferon-α on outcome of patients with advanced renal cell carcinoma of different tumor histologies. Med Oncol. 2009; 26(2):202–9.

100. Kirova YM, Servois V, Chargari C, Amessis M, Zerbib M, Beuzeboc P. Further developments for improving response and tolerance to irradiation for advanced renal cancer: concurrent (mTOR) inhibitor RAD001 and helical tomotherapy. Invest New Drugs. 2012;30:1241–3.

101. Motzer RJ, Escudier B, Oudard S, et al. Efficacy of everolimus in advanced renal cell carcinoma: a double-blind, randomised, placebo-controlled phase III trial. Lancet. 2008;372(9637):449–56.

102. Bedke J, Stenzl A. Immunologic mechanisms in RCC and allogeneic renal transplant rejection. Nat Rev Urol. 2010;7(6):339–47.

103. Gouttefangeas C, Stenzl A, Stevanovi S, Rammensee HG. Immunotherapy of renal cell carcinoma. Cancer Immunol Immunother. 2007;56(1):117–28.
104. Schreiber T, Podack E. A critical analysis of the tumour immunosurveillance controversy for 3-MCA-induced sarcomas. Br J Cancer. 2009; 101(3):381–6.
105. Dunn GP, Bruce AT, Ikeda H, Old LJ, Schreiber RD. Cancer immunoediting: from immunosur-veillance to tumor escape. Nat Immunol. 2002;3(11): 991–8.
106. Barleon B, Sozzani S, Zhou D, Weich HA, Mantovani A, Marme D. Migration of human monocytes in response to vascular endothelial growth factor (VEGF) is mediated via the VEGF receptor flt-1. Blood. 1996;87(8):3336.
107. Curiel TJ. Tregs and rethinking cancer immunother-apy. J Clin Invest. 2007;117(5):1167–74.

Prognostic Factors in Advanced Renal Cell Carcinoma

14

Michael M. Vickers and Daniel Y.C. Heng

Introduction

The management of metastatic renal cell carcinoma (mRCC) has undergone dramatic changes over the past 5 years with the median progression-free survival (PFS) of patients with mRCC improving significantly due to the introduction of agents targeting the vascular endothelial growth factor (VEGF) and mammalian target of rapamycin (mTOR) pathways [1–8]. The heterogeneity of mRCC has long been recognized and as such, factors associated with clinical outcomes have been explored and identified.

A prognostic factor can be defined as a situation, condition, or patient characteristic that can be used to estimate the chance of recovery from a disease or the chance of disease recurrence [9]. Early prognostic models for mRCC focused on the anatomic extent of tumors [10], whereas more modern models focus on patient, laboratory, and tumor- and treatment-related factors. This stratification of patients into different risk groups is important for patient counseling, risk-directed therapy, clinical trial design, and also for interpretation of study results.

We will review the most common prognostic models (see Table 14.1) that have incorporated combinations of these variables for the stratification of mRCC patients treated with immunotherapy, agents targeting the VEGF pathway and agents targeting the mTOR pathway.

Previously studied prognostic factors for advanced renal cell carcinoma can broadly be grouped into four categories (Fig. 14.1). Patient-related factors such as performance status are a large driver of prognosis. Tumor burden is intuitively obvious as a larger tumor burden should lead to a poorer prognosis. Proinflammatory markers are elevated in mRCC because of the immune response elicited by the primary tumor. Finally, treatment-related factors such as the time from initial diagnosis to treatment are important because a short interval suggests more aggressive disease while a longer interval suggests more indolent disease.

Most recently, hyponatremia has been identified as an independent clinical prognostic factor. In an assessment of prognostic factors in 120 consecutive patients and validated in another 120 patients treated with subcutaneous, low-dose interleukin-2 or interferon-alpha, Jeppensen et al. [17] demonstrated that hyponatremia (serum sodium less than the lower limit of normal) was an independent prognostic factor for worse survival and was also predictive of lack of response to cytokine therapy. Further, using retrospective data from 885 patients who received VEGF targeted therapies, hyponatremia (sodium < 135 mmol/L) remained a significant predictor for poorer overall

M.M. Vickers • D.Y.C. Heng (✉)
Department of Oncology, Tom Baker Cancer Centre,
University of Calgary, 1331 29th Street, NW, Calgary,
AB T2N 4N2, Canada
e-mail: Michael.vickers@albertahealthservices.ca;
    daniel.heng@albertahealthservices.ca

S.C. Campbell and B.I. Rini (eds.), *Renal Cell Carcinoma: Clinical Management*, Current Clinical Urology, 249
DOI 10.1007/978-1-62703-062-5_14, © Springer Science+Business Media New York 2013

Table 14.1 Summary table of variables included in prognostic models

Variable	Immunotherapy era			VEGF era		
	MSKCC [11] (1° endpoint OS)	Groupe Française d'Immunothérapie [12] (1° endpoint OS)	IKCWG [13] (1° endpoint OS)	CCF [14] (1° endpoint PFS)	International mRCC Consortium [15] (1° endpoint OS)	Sunitinib phase III [16] (1° endpoint OS)
Performance status	√	√	√	√	√	√
Interval to treatment	√		√	√	√	√
Number of metastases		√	√			
Bone metastases						√
Disease-free interval		√				
Signs of inflammation		√				
Immunotherapy treatment			√			
Hemoglobin	√	√	√		√	√
Corrected calcium	√		√	√	√	√
LDH	√		√			√
Neutrophils				√	√	
Alkaline phosphatase			√			
White blood cell count			√			
Thrombocytosis				√	√	

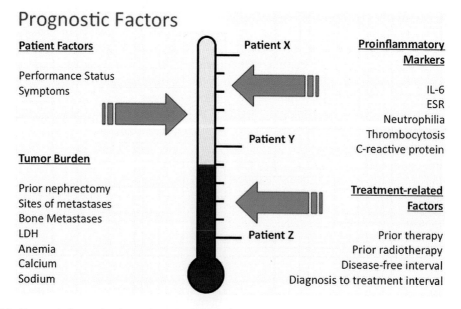

Fig. 14.1 Prognostic factors in advanced renal cell carcinoma

survival (OS) and time to treatment failure (TTF) on multivariate analysis even after adjustment for other known poor prognostic factors [18]. The underlying mechanism is unknown but may be related to higher tumor burden causing SIADH in patients with more extensive pulmonary or brain metastases.

Prognostic Factor Models in the Immunotherapy Era

Memorial Sloan Kettering Cancer Center

The incorporation of clinical and laboratory variables into a prognostic model for patients with mRCC was first accomplished by Motzer et al. [19] from the Memorial Sloan Kettering Cancer Center (MSKCC) and validated by the Cleveland Clinic group [20]. A retrospective analysis was performed on data from 670 patients enrolled on 24 consecutive MSKCC clinical trials (immunotherapy and chemotherapy) from 1975 to 1996. Patients were included if they had stage IV disease, measurable lesions, adequate Karnofsky performance status (KPS), adequate organ function, and nonsignificant comorbidities. Multivariate analysis revealed that low hemoglobin (< lower limit of normal), high lactate dehydrogenase (LDH) (>1.5 upper limit of normal), elevated corrected serum calcium (>10 mg/dL), absence of nephrectomy, and low KPS (<80%) were independent predictors of poor survival. Using these variables, patients were then placed into three risk groups: favorable (0 risk factors), intermediate (1–2 risk factors), and poor risk (3–5 risk factors). The median survival was significantly different with survivals of 19.9, 10.3, and 3.9 months for favorable, intermediate, and poor risk groups, respectively. Subsequent exploration of prognostic factors in patients treated on clinical trials with interferon-α (IFN-α) revealed lactate dehydrogenase, hemoglobin, corrected calcium, KPS and interval from RCC diagnosis to IFN-α treatment remained significant in multivariate analysis [11]. Consequently, cytoreductive nephrectomy did not remain significant in this analysis and was replaced by interval from RCC diagnosis to IFN-α. During

the time frame between these analyses, cytoreductive nephrectomy was shown to improve survival prior to IFN-α therapy, and, as IFN-α was standard therapy at the time, time to IFN-α therapy was a more appropriate risk factor. With these updated MSKCC risk groups, median survival was 29.6, 13.8, and 4.9 months for favorable, intermediate, and poor risk groups. This prognostic model subsequently became the standard for risk stratification for clinical trials.

Groupe Française d'Immunothérapie

To further assess prognostic factors in the immunotherapy era, Negrier et al. [12] evaluated clinical and biochemical variables in 1,563 enrolled on five clinical trials of IFN or IL-2, or both. Nine parameters were independent poor prognostic factors and included signs of inflammation, time interval from renal tumor to metastases (<12 months), ECOG performance status (PS) ($\geq$1), number of circulating neutrophils (>7.5 $\times$ 10^3/L), presence of liver metastases, presence of bone metastases, number of metastatic sites (>1), elevated alkaline phosphatase (>100 UI/L), and low hemoglobin level (<115 (female) and <130 (male) g/L). Five of these factors (PS, number of metastatic sites, time interval from renal tumor to metastases, signs of inflammation and hemoglobin level) were selected (based on literature survey) and integrated into two risk models for overall survival: one with five risk groups and the other with three risk groups. In addition, four factors were significant for predicting rapid progression (within 3 months of cytokine initiation) and included: presence of hepatic metastases, elevated neutrophil count, <1 year from renal tumor to metastases, and two or more metastatic sites.

International Kidney Cancer Working Group Prognostic Model

In an incredible collaborative effort, researchers from Europe and the USA developed a large database of 3,748 patients entered into clinical trials between 1975 and 2002 [13]. The majority of patients had received IFN-α or IL-2 therapy (72%), while the remainder received chemotherapy/hormonal therapy (25%) only or other treatments (3%). Multivariable analysis revealed that treatment, PS, number of metastatic sites, interval from diagnosis to treatment, pretreatment hemoglobin, white blood cell count, LDH, alkaline phosphatase, and calcium were independent prognostic factors. Integration of these factors into three risk groups revealed survivals of 27.8 months (favorable) 11.4 months (intermediate) and 4.1 months (poor).

Prognostic Factors in VEGF Era

As the therapeutic options for the treatment of mRCC have changed over the past decade, treatment with cytokine therapy has lost favor as more effective therapies have emerged. Agents targeting VEGF and the mTOR have revolutionized the treatment landscape. Consequently, the prognostic factors outlined above required reevaluation in the setting of newer therapies. These prognostic factors may still be applicable as relevant patient, tumor, or laboratory factors.

Cleveland Clinic Foundation Criteria

With the development of multiple agents targeting the VEGF pathway, reassessment of prognostic factors in mRCC was necessary. Choueiri et al. [14] were the first to report the Cleveland Clinic experience of prognostic factors for patients with mRCC treated with VEGF inhibiting agents. Retrospective data was collected from 120 clinical trial patients who had histologically proven clear cell mRCC and were treated with anti-VEGF therapies. MSKCC risk groups, CCF risk groups and a number of other clinical, biochemical/hematologic, and histologic factors were assessed for their prognostic value. Five factors proved to be prognostic for PFS in multivariate analysis. ECOG PS (≥1 vs. 0), time from diagnosis to current treatment (<2 years vs. ≥2 years), abnormal baseline

corrected serum calcium (<8.5 or >10 vs. 8.5–10 mg/dL), high platelet count (>300 vs. ≤300 K/μL), and higher absolute neutrophil count (ANC) (>4.5 vs. ≤4.5 K/μL) (lymphocyte count was dropped from the original model as it did not remain significant on bootstrap validation). In calculation of risk, one point was given for each variable except for corrected serum calcium which received two points. The median PFS was 20.1, 13, and 3.9 months for favorable (0–1 prognostic factors), intermediate (two prognostic factors), and poor (>2 prognostic factors) risk groups, respectively. This was the first report of prognostic factors for PFS in the targeted therapy era.

International mRCC Consortium Database

To further explore and validate prognostic factors in the anti-angiogenic era, Heng et al. [15] performed a retrospective, multicenter study of patients with mRCC treated with VEGF-targeted therapy (sunitinib, sorafenib and bevacizumab). Using consecutive patient data from seven cancer centers across North America, 645 patients were identified and demographic, clinical and laboratory variables were correlated with overall survival. Multivariable analysis revealed that like the MSKCC criteria, low hemoglobin (<lower limit of normal), elevated corrected serum calcium (>upper limit of normal), low KPS (<80%), and time from initial diagnosis to initiation therapy of <1 year, were independent predictors of survival. In addition to these, absolute neutrophil count and thrombocytosis (both > upper limit of normal) were also found to be independent predictors of survival. The biologic rationale behind the use of platelet and neutrophil counts has not been clearly characterized. Platelets are acute phase reactants and contain VEGF, platelet-derived growth factor, and transforming growth factor beta which are important in angiogenesis and tumor progression [21, 22]. Neutrophilia may be representative of the inflammatory process which has been implicated in the prognosis of patients [23].

Patients with, zero adverse factors (favorable risk) had a median OS which was not reached, one to two adverse factors (intermediate risk) had a median OS of 27 months, and three to six adverse factors (poor risk) had a median OS of 8.8 months. The strength of this study was that it was multicentered and included patients that were treated on or off clinical trials with a variety of VEGF-targeted agents which improved its generalizability. The model was tested in sunitinib and sorafenib-treated patients separately which revealed similar results. This model was internally validated using the bootstrap method and studies are underway for external validation.

Prognostic Factors from the Sunitinib Phase III Trial

As the standard treatment of mRCC moved away from cytokine therapy and into the targeted era, validation of MSKCC prognostic criteria was required. Using individual patient data (375 patients with clear cell RCC) from the sunitinib arm of a phase III randomized clinical trial of sunitinib versus IFN-α [2], the following variables were assessed for their prognostic significance: corrected calcium levels, the number of metastatic sites, hemoglobin levels, prior nephrectomy, presence of lung and liver metastases, Eastern Cooperative Oncology Group (ECOG) performance status, thrombocytosis, time from diagnosis to treatment, and alkaline phosphatase and lactate dehydrogenase levels [24]. Corrected serum calcium levels, the number of metastatic sites, the presence of hepatic metastases, thrombocytosis, serum lactate dehydrogenase levels, and the time from diagnosis to treatment were identified as important independent predictors of PFS and were incorporated into a predictive nomogram for 12 months PFS.

Patil et al. [16] reported prognostic factors of PFS and OS in 750 patients treated in both the sunitinib and IFN-α arms of the trial outlined above. Multivariate analysis showed that ECOG PS >0, absence of nephrectomy, LDH levels, platelet count, and ≥2 metastatic sites were significantly associated with PFS in patients

treated with sunitinib. For OS, ECOG PS >0, time from diagnosis to treatment <1 year, LDH, corrected calcium levels, hemoglobin levels, and bone metastasis were found to be significant prognostic factors. Consequently, of the six prognostic factors for OS, five were described in the original MSKCC model.

The strengths of this study include that the model was derived from prospectively followed clinical trials patients. This revealed that the MSKCC model can be used in the era of targeted therapy and the presence of bone metastases could be added. Evaluation of this new model will need to be performed on a larger set of patients and prospectively evaluated.

Prognostic Factors in mTOR-Treated Patients

In the phase III trial that established the efficacy of temsirolimus in poor prognosis mRCC, eligible patients required at least three of the following features: LDH > 1.5 times the upper limit of normal, hemoglobin below the lower limit of normal, a corrected serum calcium >10 mg/dL (2.5 mmol/L), time from initial diagnosis to randomization of less than a year, KPS of 60–70, and metastasis in multiple organs [7]. In an exploratory analysis, patients younger than age 65 and those with a serum LDH greater >1.5 times the upper limit of normal had a greater overall survival when treated with temsirolimus. It was unclear why an elevated LDH would be associated with longer overall survival as other models have suggested this to be a poor prognostic feature. It is possible that of the six poor prognostic eligibility criteria, an elevated LDH may select out a population that may benefit from temsirolimus. This finding will require external validation to confirm its prognostic potential in this population of patients.

Similarly, pretreatment prognostic profiles were assessed in the RECORD-1 trial which evaluated everolimus versus best supportive care after progression during or within 6 months of sunitinib and/or sorafenib [8]. The MSKCC risk criteria was shown to influence OS with 12-month probabilities of survival of 70% (favorable risk), 56% (intermediate risk), and 26% (poor risk). Multivariable analysis revealed that the risk of death was significantly higher in those with intermediate or poor risk compared with favorable risk patients. Additional factors associated with decreased PFS and OS included liver or bone metastases, elevated neutrophils, and prior treatment with sunitinib.

Limitations and How We Can Improve Prognostication

There are limitations to our current prognostic models. All of these models are retrospective and have not been prospectively validated or compared against each other. There are also limits to their generalizability as some are from single institutions which may involve homogenous populations. Others involve only patients enrolled in clinical trials only which may have differing eligibility criteria and have a tendency to select for healthier populations. There are also issues of missing data in these studies. For example, markers of inflammation such as C-reactive protein are not routinely ordered and therefore are not often collected in retrospective analyses. Finally, models developed from the immunotherapy era may not be relevant in VEGF era and require validation in this new treatment paradigm.

A good prognostic model should be easy to use, be generalizable, and have good discriminatory accuracy to be able to correctly place a patient in the correct prognostic group. The maximum concordance (c-index), which is an indicator of how well the prognostic model can correctly differentiate between a good risk patient and a poor risk patient, ranges around 0.74 [15]. We have probably reached our maximum prognostic accuracy and discrimination with clinical factors alone.

This could perhaps be increased if we are able to add biomarkers to these prognostic models. For example, Xu et al. [25] recently reported the effect of angiogenic and exposure-related genes (*IL8*, *FGFR2*, *VEGFA*, *FLT4*, and *NR1I2*) on survival in patients treated with pazopanib in a phase II and phase III trials. Specific germline single

nucleotide polymorphisms (SNPs) of these genes were significantly associated with overall survival. These findings require prospective validation and could potentially be added to the current clinical prognostic models to increase their predictive ability.

Conclusions

With the changing treatment paradigm of mRCC, evaluation of preexisting and possible new prognostic factors are required. The most commonly used prognostic model is the MSKCC risk criteria which integrates two clinical and three laboratory values and has been validated in clinical trial patients treated with immunotherapy. The mRCC database Consortium model is similar and was derived in the era of contemporary VEGF-targeted therapies. All of these models have stratified patients into favorable, intermediate, and poor risk groups and includes information which is easily available.

The integration of biomarkers and clinical variables into nomograms has the potential to provide more meaningful information on prognosis than either alone. Attempts at improving prognostication through molecular profiling has revealed some promising results [26]; however, much work remains before biomarkers enter into clinical decision making for mRCC.

References

1. Motzer RJ, Bander NH, Nanus DM. Renal-cell carcinoma. N Engl J Med. 1996;335(12):865–75.
2. Motzer RJ, Hutson TE, Tomczak P, et al. Overall survival and updated results for sunitinib compared with interferon alfa in patients with metastatic renal cell carcinoma. J Clin Oncol. 2009;27(22):3584–90.
3. Escudier B, Eisen T, Stadler WM, et al. Sorafenib for treatment of renal cell carcinoma: final efficacy and safety results of the phase III treatment approaches in renal cancer global evaluation trial. J Clin Oncol. 2009;27(20):3312–8.
4. Sternberg CN, Davis ID, Mardiak J, et al. Pazopanib in locally advanced or metastatic renal cell carcinoma: results of a randomized phase III trial. J Clin Oncol. 2010;28(6):1061–8.
5. Escudier B, Bellmunt J, Negrier S, et al. Phase III trial of bevacizumab plus interferon alfa-2a in patients

with metastatic renal cell carcinoma (AVOREN): final analysis of overall survival. J Clin Oncol. 2010;28(13):2144–50.

6. Rini BI, Halabi S, Rosenberg JE, et al. Phase III trial of bevacizumab plus interferon alfa versus interferon alfa monotherapy in patients with metastatic renal cell carcinoma: final results of CALGB 90206. J Clin Oncol. 2010;28(13):2137–43.

7. Hudes G, Carducci M, Tomczak P, et al. Temsirolimus, interferon alfa, or both for advanced renal-cell carcinoma. N Engl J Med. 2007;356(22):2271–81.

8. Motzer RJ, Escudier B, Oudard S, et al. Phase 3 trial of everolimus for metastatic renal cell carcinoma: final results and analysis of prognostic factors. Cancer. 2010;116(18):4256–65.

9. National Cancer Institute Dictionary of Cancer Terms; 2011. http://www.cancer.gov/dictionary/. Accessed on March 3, 2011.

10. Guinan P, Sobin LH, Algaba F, et al. TNM staging of renal cell carcinoma: workgroup no. 3. Union International Contre le Cancer (UICC) and the American Joint Committee on Cancer (AJCC). Cancer. 1997;80(5):992–3.

11. Motzer RJ, Bacik J, Murphy BA, Russo P, Mazumdar M. Interferon-alfa as a comparative treatment for clinical trials of new therapies against advanced renal cell carcinoma. J Clin Oncol. 2002;20(1):289–96.

12. Negrier S, Escudier B, Gomez F, et al. Prognostic factors of survival and rapid progression in 782 patients with metastatic renal carcinomas treated by cytokines: a report from the Groupe Francais d'Immunotherapie. Ann Oncol. 2002;13(9):1460–8.

13. Royston P, Bacik J, Elson P, Manola J, Mazumdar M. A consensus prognostic factor model for survival in patients with metastatic renal cell carcinoma: a Kidney Cancer Association's International Kidney Cancer Working Group (IKCWG) study. J Clin Oncol. 2007;25(Suppl 18) [Abstr 5109].

14. Choueiri TK, Rini B, Garcia JA, et al. Prognostic factors associated with long-term survival in previously untreated metastatic renal cell carcinoma. Ann Oncol. 2007;18(2):249–55.

15. Heng DY, Xie W, Regan MM, et al. Prognostic factors for overall survival in patients with metastatic renal cell carcinoma treated with vascular endothelial growth factor-targeted agents: results from a large, multicenter study. J Clin Oncol. 2009;27(34):5794–9.

16. Patil S, Figlin RA, Hutson TE, et al. Prognostic factors for progression-free and overall survival with sunitinib targeted therapy and with cytokine as first-line therapy in patients with metastatic renal cell carcinoma. Ann Oncol. 2011;22(2):295–300.

17. Jeppesen AN, Jensen HK, Donskov F, Marcussen N, von der Maase H. Hyponatremia as a prognostic and predictive factor in metastatic renal cell carcinoma. Br J Cancer. 2010;102(5):867–72.

18. Schutz FA, Xie W, Heng DY, et al. The effect of low serum sodium on treatment outcome to vascular endothelial growth factor (VEGF)-targeted therapy in metastatic renal cell carcinoma: results from a large international collaboration. J Clin Oncol. 2011;29(Suppl 7) [Abstr 322].

19. Motzer RJ, Mazumdar M, Bacik J, Berg W, Amsterdam A, Ferrara J. Survival and prognostic stratification of 670 patients with advanced renal cell carcinoma. J Clin Oncol. 1999;17(8):2530–40.

20. Mekhail TM, Abou-Jawde RM, Boumerhi G, et al. Validation and extension of the Memorial Sloan-Kettering prognostic factors model for survival in patients with previously untreated metastatic renal cell carcinoma. J Clin Oncol. 2005;23(4):832–41.

21. Mohle R, Green D, Moore MA, Nachman RL, Rafii S. Constitutive production and thrombin-induced release of vascular endothelial growth factor by human mega-karyocytes and platelets. Proc Natl Acad Sci USA. 1997;94(2):663–8.

22. O'Byrne KJ, Dobbs N, Propper D, Smith K, Harris AL. Vascular endothelial growth factor platelet counts, and prognosis in renal cancer. Lancet. 1999;353(9163): 1494–5.

23. Donskov F, von der Maase H. Impact of immune parameters on long-term survival in metastatic renal cell carcinoma. J Clin Oncol. 2006;24(13): 1997–2005.

24. Motzer RJ, Bukowski RM, Figlin RA, et al. Prognostic nomogram for sunitinib in patients with metastatic renal cell carcinoma. Cancer. 2008;113(7):1552–8.

25. Xu C, Ball HA, Bing CN, et al. Association of genetic markers in angiogenesis- or exposure-related genes with overall survival in pazopanib (P) treated patients (Pts) with advanced renal cell carcinoma. J Clin Oncol. 2011;29:7s (suppl 7; abstr 303).

26. Vickers MM, Heng DY. Prognostic and predictive biomarkers in renal cell carcinoma. Target Oncol. 2010;5(2):85–94.

Integration of Surgery in Metastatic Renal Cancer

Tom Powles and Axel Bex

Role of Nephrectomy in Metastatic Disease

Historical Considerations

Historically, the incidence of spontaneous regression, and the occasional indolent course of pulmonary metastases, had prompted the concept of removal of asymptomatic primary tumours in metastatic renal cell carcinoma (mRCC) [1–4]. However, while most urologists agreed that palliative nephrectomy for symptomatic primary lesions in systemic disease is justified, removing asymptomatic tumours without effective systemic treatment was highly controversial. Freed [5] suggested in 1977 that nephrectomy may be beneficial for patients with primary metastatic disease. He speculated that nephrectomy may halt the disease progress via up-regulation of the host immune mechanisms and that the immune-rich environment of the lung may explain sponta-

T. Powles (✉)
Department of Medical Oncology,
Barts Cancer Institute, St Bartholomew's Hospital London,
Queen Mary University of London,
West Smithfield, London EC1A 7BE, UK
e-mail: Thomas.powles@bartsandlondon.nhs.uk

A. Bex
Division of Surgical Oncology, Department of Urology,
The Netherlands Cancer Institute, Amsterdam,
The Netherlands

neous regression of lung-only metastases after nephrectomy. Before the advent of systemic immunotherapy, spontaneous regression of single pulmonary lesions had been reported in up to approximately 5% of patients after cytoreductive nephrectomy (CN). However, solitary metastasis occurs in under 5% of patients making this approach an exception to the rule [6, 7]. Barney et al. reported on a patient who survived 23 years after nephrectomy and lobectomy for pulmonary metastases [8]. Since then many authors reported similar results with metastasectomy of solitary or multiple lesions after CN. Skinner et al. reported a 29% 5-year survival in a series of 41 patients in whom one or two metastases were excised in addition to nephrectomy [9], and Tolia et al. reported a 35% 5-year survival in a similar series [6]. In a retrospective study on the natural history of untreated metastatic renal cell carcinoma (mRCC), deKernion et al. [1] noted that CN was associated with a 6% mortality rate but overall these patients had a better outcome than those who did not have surgery. In the absence of effective systemic therapy and randomized data in this arena, the consensus was that nephrectomy may be beneficial when a limited number of metastases were present and aggressive treatment of these metastases may be warranted [10]. This data was potentially influenced by selection bias; therefore, two large randomized trials investigating the role of nephrectomy were planned and completed.

S.C. Campbell and B.I. Rini (eds.), *Renal Cell Carcinoma: Clinical Management*, Current Clinical Urology,
DOI 10.1007/978-1-62703-062-5_15, © Springer Science+Business Media New York 2013

Randomized Prospective Trials of Nephrectomy Followed by Immunotherapy Vs. Immunotherapy Alone

The emergence of immunotherapy for patients with metastatic renal cell cancer provided the basis for further investigation of the role of CN in metastases [11].

In 2001 data from two randomized phase III trials comparing nephrectomy followed by immunotherapy vs. immunotherapy alone became available. These prospective trials of the SWOG and EORTC groups both demonstrated a prolonged survival for the nephrectomy plus interferon-α arms as opposed to the interferon alone arms [12, 13]. In 2004 a combined analysis of these two trials showed a median survival of 13.6 months for nephrectomy plus interferon vs. 7.8 months for interferon alone [14]. The survival was strongly influenced by performance status. These trials had a number of concerns. Importantly, 25% of the patients in each arm of the SWOG study died within the first 4 months of treatment regardless of the study arm, suggesting patient selection may be suboptimal. Additionally, the responses in the metastatic sites to IFN-α in both arms were low and did not differ significantly from each other (3.6% vs. 3.3%). These results question the hypothesis that nephrectomy makes interferon therapy more responsive by enhancing the immune repertoire. Despite the improvement in survival following CN in combination with IFN-a, the mechanism is still not fully understood and several factors have been proposed. The often large primary tumour may attract and trap circulating antibodies and immune cells and secrete co-stimulatory molecules that down-regulate immune responses. Alternatively, tumour cells may secrete pro-angiogenic growth factors, such as vascular endothelial growth factor (VEGF), platelet-derived growth factor, fibroblast growth factor and transforming growth factor-β1 [15–17]. Removal of a large tumour bulk may result in reduced expression of the oncogenic factors. This is especially true as immune therapy has at best only modest effects on tumour growth.

IL-2 (sc or IV) was widely given as an alternative to interferon. Indeed high-dose IL-2 is still given to highly selected patients with curative intent [18]. No randomized trial has been performed to investigated the role of IL-2 with or without CN, which is in part due to the conclusive findings of the randomised trials with interferon [12, 13]. In a letter to the New England Journal of Medicine, Pantuck et al. published a retrospective analysis of 89 selected patients who underwent nephrectomy followed by sc IL-2 [19]. These patients had similar inclusion criteria for the SWOG trial and the median survival was 16.7 months. The authors plotted the Kaplan–Meyer survival curves over the data from the SWOG interferon trial and argued that, despite the retrospective nature of the data, nephrectomy followed by interleukin-2-based immunotherapy may be preferable. This was highly controversial and disputable. Nevertheless subcutaneous IL-2 was routinely used instead of interferon in North America.

The results of these prospective SWOG and EORTC-GU randomized phase III trials with interferon established the role of CN in the era of cytokine therapy [12, 13]. Subset analysis showed that performance status and the Memorial Sloan Kettering Cancer Center (MSKCC) risk score were both important in predicting benefit with CN [20]. Other subgroups which appeared to benefit from CN included patients with a significant tumour burden of the primary tumour, absence of significant co-morbidity, absence of central nervous system metastasis and low risk of surgical morbidity [21]. Culp and co-workers more recently identified a number of prognostic factors predicting benefit from CN. These added a number of factors to the MSKCC prognostic score. These factors included raised plasma lactate dehydrogenase, low serum albumin, symptoms caused by metastatic sites, sites of disease (liver metastasis and specific lymphadenopathy) and clinical ≥T3 for the primary tumour stage [22].

Overall the data from the pre-targeted therapy era showed that CN had a clear role in mRCC. Although it did not increase the response to cytokine therapy, it had a remarkable effect on overall survival (a median of 6.3-month OS advantage [14]). Subgroups of patients were identified which appeared to glean most benefit from this surgery, including those with a good performance status and favourable MSKCC risk score. Therefore, the combination of surgery and cytokine therapy was given as part of a multimodality management for patients with systemic disease.

Role of Nephrectomy in the Era of Targeted Therapy

The introduction of novel drugs targeting angiogenesis has resulted in a substantial improvement in outcome for mRCC. Currently approved agents include receptor tyrosine kinase inhibitors (TKIs), VEGF antibodies and mammalian target of rapamycin inhibitors (mTORs) [23–27]. Details on the efficacy of these agents are summarized in previous chapters. The vast majority of the data investigating CN and targeted therapy together focus on the VEGF TKIs such as sunitinib [28–34], there is very little data on mTORs and VEGF antibodies and CN [24, 35].

Sunitinib is, at present, the most commonly used first-line treatment in mRCC. It is associated with an objective response rate of 39% (vs. 8% with IFN-a) and median progression-free survival (PFS) was significantly prolonged at 11 months (vs. 5 months for interferon) [36]. The median overall survival is over 2 years. Based on this pivotal trial, sunitinib was registered in the USA and Europe in 2007. More recently pazopanib has been approved by both the FDA and EMEA in the first-line setting. It also shows a PFS in the first-line setting of approximately 11 months with impressive response rates and is therefore an alternative to sunitinib [27]. While there is phase II data and enrolling phase III studies investigating CN with sunitinib and other agents, there is currently a lack of data with CN and pazopanib.

The majority of patients (~90%) in the pivotal sunitinib and pazopanib registration studies had nephrectomy prior to entry. However, no information is provided how many of these patients had a previous nephrectomy for locally confined disease and developed systemic metastasis subsequently or had an upfront nephrectomy for synchronous mRCC. Because patients

with metachronous mRCC have a more latent progression, this may influence the results. In addition, little is known of the response rate of the primary tumours as most had been previously removed. There is subgroup analysis comparing the PFS of patients who did and did not undergo initial CN. The results are hampered by patient selection and sample size. However the results showed a numerical advantage for prior CN [11 months (range, 11–13 months) vs. 6 months (range, 4–11 months), respectively; $p = 0.0889$] [37]. Comparisons of responses in the metastatic sites and primary renal tumour show that the primary tumour response rates are lower (<10%) [33].

Other retrospective series have reported a similar advantage for patients undergoing CN. Choueiri et al. reported on 314 patients with mRCC of whom 201 underwent CN [38]. Using univariable analysis, they showed that CN was associated with a median OS of 19.8 months, compared with 9.4 months for patients who did not undergo CN ($p < 0.0001$). However, the benefit was absent in the poor prognostic risk group. Similarly, a retrospective population-based study from Canada suggested that prior CN in patients treated with TKIs is associated with improved OS in mRCC, independent of other prognostic variables [39]. A very recent Dutch population-based study concluded that even after accounting for prognostic profile patients with mRCC still benefited from CN with a 50% reduction in mortality [40]. However, the inherent bias of retrospective analysis does not allow to definitely conclude that patients derive a benefit from CN. In addition, patients who received targeted therapy without CN, while CN was considered as the standard of care, are obviously different from those who had CN and subsequently received TKIs.

The assumption that CN has a role in the era of targeted therapy, based on the randomized data with interferon, is flawed. It is argued by those in favour of medical therapy alone that, unlike cytokine therapy, targeted therapy controls the disease in the majority of the patients and CN does not change clinical outcome. Indeed the delay in starting targeted therapy during

CARMENA

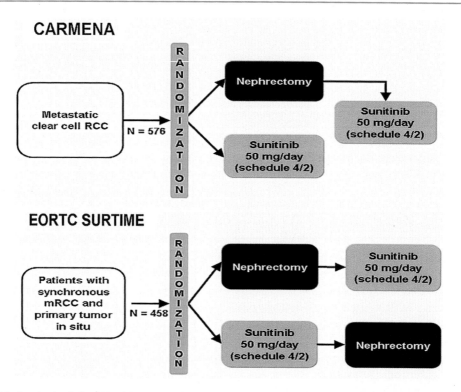

EORTC SURTIME

Fig. 15.1 Randomized phase III trials to investigate role and sequence of cytoreductive nephrectomy (CN) in primary metastatic renal cell carcinoma. The primary endpoint is overall survival in the CARMENA trial and progression-free survival in the EORTC SURTIME trial

the preoperative period for nephrectomy may be counterproductive. Others feel that there is no reason why the data from the cytokine era should not apply in the targeted therapy era, especially in those patients where primary renal tumour accounts for the vast majority of the volume of the disease [41, 42]. In addition over 90% of patients in the pivotal studies in the era of targeted had nephrectomies. Therefore it is argued that it should continue as standard of care until proven otherwise.

To answer this important question two distinct randomized phase III trials, investigating CN, have been developed and are now recruiting patients with untreated primary mRCC. The CARMENA trial investigates the role of CN by comparing sunitinib alone with nephrectomy followed by sunitinib [43]. This design is identical to the positive trials performed in the cytokine era. The second study addresses the sequencing of nephrectomy and sunitinib by comparing initial CN followed by sunitinib with presurgical

sunitinib follows by CN (the EORTC 30073 SURTIME trial) [44] (Fig. 15.1).

CARMENA (NCT00930033), which has been recruiting patients in France and the United Kingdom since 2009, is the pivotal trial to investigate the impact of CN on outcome in the era of targeted therapy. Patients with mRCC (with clear cell histology on biopsy) (ECOG PS 0 or 1), without prior systemic therapy or surgical interventions, are randomized to either nephrectomy followed by sunitinib or sunitinib alone [43]. The primary endpoint of this non-inferiority trial is overall survival and will include over 1,000 patients. The estimated completion date is 2016. In this study patients in the systemic therapy only arm can have palliative nephrectomy later in the disease process if deemed necessary for symptomatic control (Fig. 15.1).

It may be that as in the cytokine era, only specific subgroups of patients benefit from CN. One area of interest is whether the fractional volume of the primary renal cancer removed compared to the metastatic sites is relevant. It is intuitive that the higher the proportion of tumour burden removed the better. This theory is supported by a retrospective series which shows if the fractional percentage of tumour volume removed at nephrectomy is greater than 95%, patients have a better outcome [45]. Recent data supports this association in the era of targeted therapy [46].

How this theoretical and clinical benefit from CN applies to targeted therapies is currently unresolved and the CARMENA trial is designed to answer this important scientific question.

Nephrectomy for Symptomatic Primary Tumours

Patients with primary mRCC rarely present with debilitating symptoms related to the primary tumour, such as flank pain, gross haematuria or paraneoplastic syndromes. In the pre-targeted therapy era the overall survival of these patients was short [47]. As expected, CN alone was unable to reliably elevate symptoms from paraneoplastic syndromes [48]. In the era of targeted therapy symptomatic primary tumours should be removed where possible. Starting with upfront systemic therapy should only be considered where the tumour is inoperable, or the disease is particularly aggressive (MSKCC poor risk disease).

Angioinfarction of the primary renal tumour may be considered as a less invasive alternative to surgery. Data in the era of targeted therapy is lacking. The authors would consider angioinfarction in a small minority of patients. These include patients with metastatic disease and who are deemed inoperable but have persistent symptoms from the primary tumours despite systemic therapy.

Upfront Systemic Treatment Prior to Nephrectomy in Metastatic Disease

The History of Initial Systemic Therapy Followed by Nephrectomy

To date, only few retrospective studies specifically addressed the combination of initial immunotherapy followed by CN in patients with primary

mRCC [49]. Some authors recognized that initial immunotherapy followed by nephrectomy may have the advantage of circumventing the reported morbidity of initial nephrectomy, without compromising the concept of immunotherapy and cytoreduction. The potential advantages of systemic therapy followed by nephrectomy were that those individuals with cytokine refractory disease could be easily identified and selected out, sparing them nephrectomy. On the other hand if, as was speculated, nephrectomy was required to achieve a response to cytokine therapy, this approach of initial cytokine therapy could potentially miss responders.

The published series in the cytokine era are small. They focus on retrospective series of highly selected patients, or subset analysis from larger series which is open to selection bias, or small prospective series which are difficult to interpret [50–53] (Table 15.1).

Others reported selectively on those patients who responded to initial immunotherapy followed by complete surgical remissions by nephrectomy or resection of residual lesions [54–56] (Table 15.2).

In summary all these retrospective series noted the feasibility of immunotherapy with the primary in situ and remarked on the significant disease-free survival that could be achieved in selected patients. Efficacy data is very difficult to interpret from this data. It is noteworthy that some authors reported an effect of immunotherapy with IL-2 even on the primary tumour, which was generally believed not to occur from the prospective data [55, 57]. It should be remembered that high-dose IL-2 is still given to selected patients with curative intent in the era of targeted therapy. A number of prognostic factors exist which are used to identify these patients, one of which is prior nephrectomy. Therefore upfront high-dose IL-2 prior to nephrectomy cannot be recommended.

While randomized prospective trials comparing nephrectomy followed by IFN-α vs. IFN-α alone reported in favour of surgery and immunotherapy [14], no randomized trial was performed addressing upfront cytokine therapy. This may in part be due to the lack of robust data and the low response rate seen in the primary tumour. As a

Table 15.1 Retrospective series of initial immunotherapy (IMT) followed by cytoreductive nephrectomy

Source	No. of patients receiving IMT	IMT	No. of patients with cytoreduction	Response MS[a]		Median survival entire group (range	Survival after cytoreduction
				CR	PR		
Fleischmann et al. [50]	10	IL-2/LAK	2	3		5 months (2–18)	4, 9, 18 months
Spencer et al. [51]	12	IL-2/IFN-A	11	1	3	Not published	Not published
Rackley et al. [52]	25	IL-2 based	3	2	1	14 months (1–48)	18, 42, 48 months
Wagner et al. [53]	51	IL-2 based	3	1	2	13 months (1–86)	4, 11, 88 months

CR complete response, *PR* partial response, *IL-2* interleukin 2, *IFN-A* interferon-alpha, *LAK* lymphokine-activated killer cells
[a]*MS* metastatic sites

Table 15.2 Retrospective series of selected patients with objective response to initial immunotherapy (IMT) followed by nephrectomy or resection of metastases to no evidence of disease

Source	No. of patients	IMT	sNED	Median survival (range)
Sherry et al. [54]	16	IL-2	16	11 months (4–44)
Sella et al. [55]	17	IFN-A	17	26 months (6–34)
Krishnamurti et al. [56]	14	IL-2 based	14	44 months (4–97)

sNED surgically resected to no evidence of disease, *IL-2* interleukin-2, *IFN-A* interferon-alpha

consequence the timing of nephrectomy and immunotherapy in multimodality treatment of primary mRCC remains controversial. This controversy continues in the era of targeted therapy.

Presurgical Targeted Therapy Prior to Planned Nephrectomy

The randomized data supporting the role of nephrectomy in metastatic disease in the era of cytokine therapy has resulted in it being adopted as standard of care in the targeted therapy era as well [21, 58]. However there are concerns that the delay associated with planning, performing and recovering from nephrectomy may result in systemic progression of disease. Indeed it is reported that a high percentage of patients do not receive systemic therapy after CN due to surgical morbidity/mortality or disease progression. In a multi-institutional experience, Kutikov et al. described that 43 of 141 patients undergoing CN never received systemic therapy due to rapid disease progression in 30%, patient refusal in 23% and perioperative death in 19% [59]. CARMENA will address this important issue. It may be that nephrectomy prior to systemic therapy in patients with aggressive disease is counterproductive as it denies to some patients the opportunity to receive systemic therapy. This issue was not such a major concern in the cytokine era when treatment was largely ineffective, but in the modern era, where control of systemic disease is the norm, the delay associated with nephrectomy may be harmful in some individuals. A potential way around this problem is to perform a finite period of upfront systemic therapy prior to nephrectomy, resulting in a theoretically benefit from both immediate systemic therapy and nephrectomy.

Another potential advantage of this upfront targeted therapy approach may be the downsizing of the primary renal tumour facilitating surgery. It was hoped that this reduction in the primary tumour would be in the region of 30% (as seen in the metastatic sites), and even make inoperable patients operable [60]. Two prospective studies recently addressed this issue with sunitinib [33]. A fixed period of sunitinib (12–18 weeks) was given prior to nephrectomy and showed the median response rate of the primary tumour to be only 14%. This series did include some patients with T4 disease (10%) who had a reduction in tumour size and subsequent surgery. Nevertheless the overall effects on the primary tumour in terms of size was modest and lower than those responses seen in the metastatic sites. Moreover, fibrosis was reposted as being prominent at the surgery, potentially making the operation more complex. Therefore the conclusion that sunitinib facilitates surgery is questionable. However this work with other series has shown that surgery can be performed safely after targeted therapy [32, 33].

Perhaps the most attractive aspect of upfront targeted therapy is that patients with primary refractory disease, and a short life expectancy, can be spared nephrectomy. Again this is controversial as it could be argued that the nephrectomy itself increased the response rate and therefore a lower proportion of patients with primary refractory disease. A recent phase II study reported on the PFS and OS of 66 patients treated with upfront sunitinib prior to planned nephrectomy in primary metastatic disease [34]. This series included patients with MSKCC intermediate and poor risk disease. Although numbers were small and the study was not randomized, the proportion of patients with primary refractory disease was in line with expectations (17%). The study also identified a subgroup of patients with a favourable outcome. These patients, with MSKCC intermediate risk disease and clinical benefit (stable disease by RECIST) prior to surgery, had a median overall survival of over 2 years. One of the notable features of this work was the frequent occurrence of disease progression (36% by RECIST v1.1) during the surgery-related treatment break (median 29 days). Surgery requires treatment to be stopped for at least 1 day before and 14 days after surgery to avoid complications such as delayed wound healing. The consequences of the progression during this treatment break remain unknown. However over 70% of patients achieve subsequent disease stabilization when sunitinib was recommenced after surgery. While

the principle of disease progression on treatment is concerning, rebound of the tumour during the 2-week treatment-free interval is well described on sunitinib and may be less worrying.

Another area of concern is the potential for primary tumour growth during the period of upfront targeted therapy making operable tumours inoperable. Initial reports from a retrospective study of 19 patients with advanced renal cell carcinoma (RCC) and the primary tumour in situ showed nine (47%) had progressive disease (PD) in the primary tumour [61]. Others have observed progression of caval thrombi [62]. This may indicate that in a proportion of patients upfront therapy may result in progression of the primary tumour. More recent larger series countered this argument showing that no patients became inoperable after a period of sunitinib (Table 15.3). This work was supported by other studies with bevacizumab, where again no patients became inoperable.

While the reduction in the size of the primary tumour is modest, one of the more intriguing aspects of this is that the response itself may be prognostic. Recent data suggest a reduction in the longest diameter of 10–13% or more (median) is prognostic in multivariate analysis [34, 63]. This may turn out to be useful information in a setting where identifying patients who are benefiting from therapy has proved elusive. Another factor which required further consideration is that the median reported necrosis rate is over 50% in pretreated tumours. Therefore while the tumours may not be reducing in size dramatically there are extensive changes at a molecular level. These are nicely illustrated with functional imaging before and after therapy (Figs. 15.2, 15.3, and 15.4).

Another area of the major concern surrounding upfront targeted therapy prior to nephrectomy is that a large proportion of patients (approximately 30%) do not go on to have the planned nephrectomy. The most common reasons for this include primary progression of disease and patients choice [34]. Some argue that selecting out patients with TKI refractory disease is constructive as they can potentially switch to an alternative therapy, while others argue that this may be detrimental to outcome.

Table 15.3 Summary of studies investigating upfront targeted therapy prior to nephrectomy in metastatic disease

Study	Cowey et al. [67]	Powles et al. [33, 34]	Jonasch et al. [35]
Number of patients	30	66	50
Duration of upfront therapy	1–8 weeks	12–16 weeks	8 weeks
Agent used	Sorafenib	Sunitinib	Bevacizumab ± erlotinib
% Reduction of the renal tumour during upfront therapy	9.6%	14.5%	Approximately 5%
Duration in hospital (median)	Laparoscopic = 3.7 days Open = 7.5 days	7 days	5 days
Median blood loss (median)	Laparoscopic = 150 ml Open = 950 ml	725 ml	400 ml
Surgery-related deaths	0	1 2%	2 (4%)
Duration of surgery (median)	Laparoscopic = 135 min Open = 185 min	189 min	165 min
Delayed wound healing	1 (3%)	6 (13%)	9 (20%)
Serious complications (Clavien–Dindo classification III–V)	NA	4 (11%)	NA

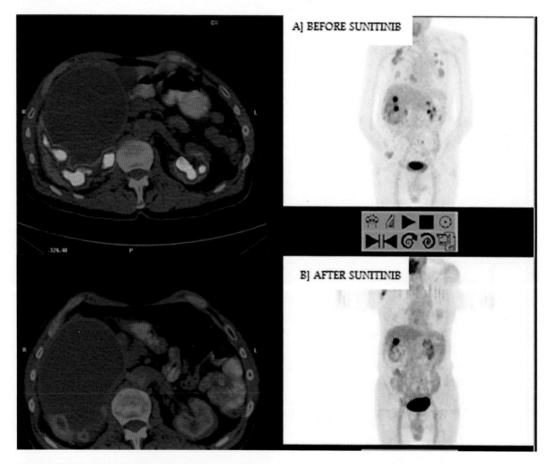

Fig. 15.2 FDG PET CT before (**a**) and after (**b**) sunitinib (18 weeks) in a large cystic renal tumour. This FDGPET CT shows no change in the size of the renal tumour after 18 weeks of sunitinib. However the tumour does show a metabolic response (63% reduction in SUV) to sunitinib. This demonstrates the dynamic changes occurring at a molecular level

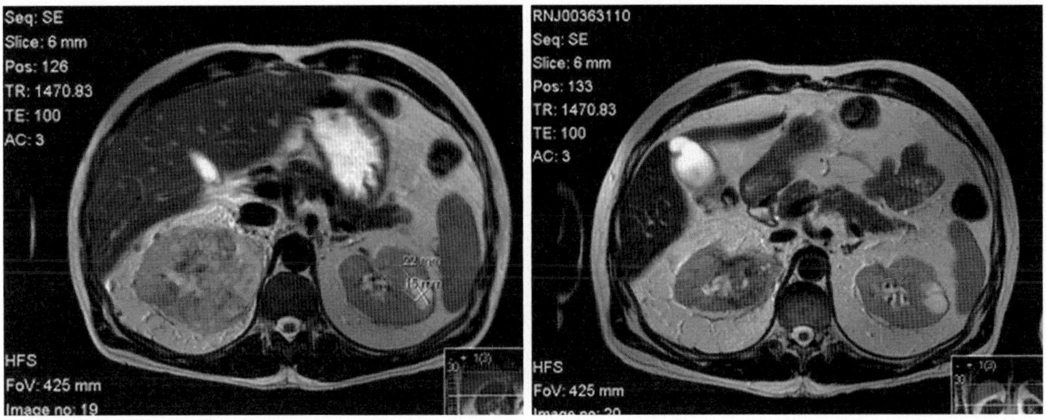

Fig. 15.3 This pair of CT scans before and after sunitinib therapy shows how a dramatic response to sunitinib therapy. (**a**) CT scan showing a large renal tumour prior to sunitinib therapy. (**b**) CT scan showing a large renal tumour responding to sunitinib therapy (72% reduction in largest diameter)

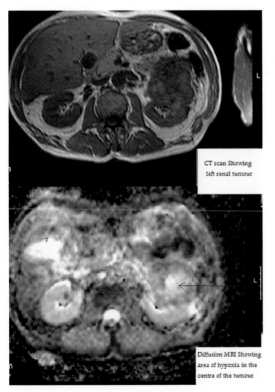

Fig. 15.4 CT scan and diffusion MRI of a left-sided renal tumour. These pair of scans shows a primary renal tumour with CT and diffusion MRI. At the centre of the left renal tumour (*red arrow*) is a bright area which represents necrosis, which is associated with a poor prognosis. This diffusion MRI scan demonstrates the heterogeneous nature of the renal cancer

A further consideration for this approach is the potential advantage of collection of sequential tissue during systemic therapy. Initial reports suggest that tissue taken at baseline does not predict outcome. However dynamic changes to molecular markers during therapy, which could potentially be identified from the tissue taken after a period of systemic therapy, may unlock the key to systemic resistance [64]. This drive towards personalized therapy is desirable in renal cancer, as there are a number of systemic treatment options without any truly predictive markers. These changes are being investigated by a number of consortiums and results are expected over the next 2 years. Areas of concern focus on tumour heterogeneity, unstandardized methods of tissue collection, differing methods of analysis and reproducibility of results.

Therefore, the principle of upfront targeted therapy prior to nephrectomy has both advantages and disadvantages and may even identify mechanisms of acquired resistance. It requires robust evaluation before it is incorporated into treatment algorithms.

A consistent feature of recent studies is a proportion of patients opt out of CN as they are reluctant to stop effective systemic treatment. This may result in the need for delayed nephrectomy later in the disease process, when the patient may be less well or the tumours become unresectable. Therefore with the current data available the authors feel that nephrectomy should be encouraged where possible in patients opting for a period of upfront targeted therapy prior to planned nephrectomy. Indeed the combination of sunitinib and surgery (CN and metastasectomy) has resulted in complete remissions in some selected individuals [65]. In a recent series 33% of these patients were taken off treatment for a median of 7 months (range 1–31 months) after achieving complete remission [66]. This approach, with a treatment-free interval, is attractive. While it is outside the remit of standard guidelines it is worthy of further investigation as targeted therapy is associated with significant short- and long-term side effects.

Other phase II studies have evaluated the role of upfront bevacizumab and sorafenib in this setting [35, 67]. Results appear similar to those seen with sunitinib, although direct comparisons are not possible (Table 15.2). One notable feature is the gap between targeted therapy and surgery with bevacizumab is longer than that seen with the TKIs (4 weeks vs. 24 h) due to its longer half-life [35]. Surgical-related complications in these studies were similar with 2% surgical-related mortality, 400–500 ml of blood loss during surgery and a postoperative stay between 5 and 7 days. Targeted therapy was restarted 2–4 weeks postoperatively. The commonest postoperative complication was delayed would healing, which occurred in 14–20%. It is speculated that restarting systemic therapy too early (before 3 weeks) may increase this proportion. Therefore, it appears that sunitinib can be safely discontinued 24 h prior to surgery [33]. However restarting targeted therapy is more controversial and waiting until full healing of the surgical scar has occurred is important.

A retrospective analysis attempted to identify whether upfront targeted therapy was associated with increased surgical morbidity or perioperative complications by comparing results with a matched cohort of 58 patients who underwent upfront surgery [32]. Results showed no difference between the two groups, and while this analysis is not robust, the above data is unable to identify particular concerns with the upfront approach at this stage.

There is debate about the optimal duration of targeted therapy prior to surgery in this population. The effect of downsizing the primary tumour is most prominent in the first 3–5 months [63, 68]. An underpowered exploratory analysis compared two and three cycles of sunitinib prior to surgery and could find no difference between these two regimens [33]. However only a few days of targeted therapy can induce maximal inhibition of cell proliferation [69], but these changes are unlikely to be clinically meaningful.

To formally test this paradigm of presurgical therapy prior to nephrectomy, a phase III trial was designed to investigate the sequence of CN and systemic therapy. This prospective, randomized EORTC trial has now opened in the Netherlands, Belgium, Italy, the United Kingdom and Canada comparing immediate vs. deferred CN in patients with synchronous mRCC (EORTC 30073, SURTIME) [44]. The principal objective of this trial is to investigate whether the sequence of nephrectomy in patients who receive sunitinib has an effect on patient outcome. The primary endpoint is PFS. Secondary endpoints include OS, safety, overall response to treatment in the deferred nephrectomy arm (including the proportion of patients who become unresectable) and the effect of nephrectomy on early progression in both arms. The investigators plan to enroll 458 patients over a 36-month period, with the final analysis performed after observation of 380 progressions or deaths and a minimum follow-up of 1.5 years for all patients. In addition, tissue and serum will be collected to identify genetic- and protein-profiles predictive of response. Together CARMENA and SURTIME will address the role of CN in the targeted therapy era.

The Role of the MSKCC Prognostic Score in Selecting Patients for CN

Patients with metastatic renal cancer can be stratified for outcome by the MSKCC risk score [20]. All three groups benefit from targeted therapy, although temsirolimus rather than VEGF

TKIs is considered standard of therapy in patients with poor risk disease [24, 70]. There are few data on the role of CN in these risk groups. This is particularly relevant to the MSKCC poor risk group which have a short overall survival, and where progression of disease may be rapid. These patients are often symptomatic from systemic disease at baseline and commencing targeted therapy immediately appears wise. Retrospective data questions the role of nephrectomy in this population and data on patients treated with upfront sunitinib followed by interval CN in this group showed no patients survived over 2 years [34]. Therefore the role of surgery in this group appears very questionable irrespective of its timing.

The role of CN in intermediate risk disease is also unclear and controversial. The delay associated with surgery may result in disease progression while, on the other hand, removing large bulky tumours accounting for the majority of the disease burden appears beneficial in retrospective series. Both initial nephrectomy and upfront TKI therapy followed by nephrectomy appear attractive in this population. Provocative data from 42 patients with intermediate risk disease showed impressive OS results with the "upfront" approach (over 70% 2-year survival in selected patients with clinical benefit) [34]. Finally patients with good risk disease should usually be considered for nephrectomy, at least until CARMENA reports, as delaying targeted therapy does not seem to have a detrimental effect on outcome and may allow consideration of other approaches such as high-dose IL-2 or metastasectomy in this population.

Metastasectomy in Metastatic Renal Cancer

Metastasis from RCC may be present at diagnosis or develop after nephrectomy. In the modern era, the vast majority of patients with systemic disease should be treated with targeted therapy. This is of proven benefit in randomized trials [71, 72]. The decision to surgically remove metastases rather than treating with targeted therapy is complex and controversial. There is retrospective data showing impressive outcomes associated with metastasectomy, especially in those patients with isolated metastasis to the lung or loco-regional lymph nodes [73–75]. This data is generated from a number of single institutional studies in the pre-targeted therapy era and is open to patient selection bias. Moreover these patients have an excellent outcome with targeted therapy, high-dose IL-2 or even initial observation. Therefore the applicability of the metastasectomy data, generated from the cytokine era, is unclear. Targeted therapy seldom results in a complete remission; therefore, the continued investigation of metastasectomy appears justified in selected individuals. Its role in conjunction with targeted therapy is exciting [76]. Down-staging limited metastatic disease with systemic therapy followed by surgical resection appears attractive and is the focus of clinical trials [77]. Also surgery may be justified in isolated progression in a single metastasis after a period of targeted therapy. The benefit of removing this focus of resistance is unclear. Surgery is not uncommon in this setting, especially to brain metastasis.

There is a select group of patients with metastatic clear cell renal cancer who have prolonged survival. These patients are likely to have distinct biological and clinical characteristics. Long-term remission or even spontaneous regression of metastasis can occur in this population. This same group tends to be the group offered metastasectomy. Therefore it is almost impossible to tell whether the surgery is altering the biology of the disease. Other potently curative treatments such as high-dose IL-2 are also offered to patients with clear cell histology, isolated metastatic disease and a good performance status. Therefore in this distinct group, four potential competing treatment options are available including surveillance, targeted therapy, metastasectomy or high-dose IL-2. Careful consideration of the pros and cons of each option is required. This section will deal with the selection of patients for metastasectomy in the era of targeted therapy. This may be used alone or in combination with one of the other treatment options.

The first report of metastasectomy goes back to 1939 [8]. One of the first series reporting on metastasectomy described surgery in 41 selected patients with solitary lesions in the lungs, pleura, central nervous system or abdomen and dates back to 1978. The disease-specific survival was 27 months with a 3-year survival of 59% [1]. These data supported by other similar results at the time [9] led to partial acceptance of metastasectomy in selected individuals.

While it was acknowledged that an isolated relapse, for example in the lung, after previous nephrectomy may be treated with metastasectomy it was less clear about patients who presented with a synchronous unresected renal tumour and metastatic disease. This was addressed in a study of 179 patients, in which the 5-year survival rate after resection of solitary lesions at various sites was 22% for synchronous vs. 39% for metachronous metastases [78]. This data also supports the hypothesis that patients with isolated relapse run a less aggressive course than those who present with synchronous unresected disease.

This leads to the issue surrounding the number of metastatic lesions which can successfully be removed. Recent retrospective reports suggest that the surgical resection of over three lesions is of benefit compared to unmatched controls who did not have surgery [74]. A further retrospective series examined this issue in more detail and showed that the outcome of removal of 1–6 lung lesions was associated with a better outcome compared to seven or more lung lesions removed [79].

One of the consistent features of this retrospective data is that surgical complete resection is associated with a good outcome [79, 80]. Negative surgical margins after resection of lung metastasis were associated with a 46.6 months median overall survival in one series [81]. There are two possible explanations for this. Firstly, patients who achieve a complete resection have a lower tumour burden than those where complete resection is not possible, which will influence outcome. Alternatively the surgery is genuinely altering the behavioural pattern of the disease.

Removal of a Single Metastasis in the Pre-TKI Era

The largest series to report on removal of a single metastatic site originates from the MD Anderson [78]. One hundred and seventy-nine patients (8.5%) of 2,100 patients who were known to have metastatic renal cancer between 1984 and 1997 underwent resection for a solitary metastatic lesion. While the overall survival for the cohort was impressive (29% at 5 years), perhaps the most important factor to affect outcome was the anatomical site of surgical removal. Patients with lung and loco-regional metastasis fared better than those with brain, bone or liver metastasis. Five-year survival rates for solitary metastases were over 50% for lungs/local regional disease. This dropped to 20% for visceral organs, approximately 15% for bone and 13% for brain. Other studies have supported these findings [74, 82]. Therefore surgical removals of lesions outside of the lungs and loco-regional area as initial treatment for metastatic disease required careful consideration in the era of targeted therapy. The one exception to this is the brain which required particular consideration and will be discussed later in this section.

Further attempts have been made to identify patients with solitary metastases who benefit from metastasectomy [73, 74, 83]. The most consistent findings are that those patients who have complete surgical removal of isolated lung or loco-regional disease at first relapse have an excellent outcome. This is perhaps the clearest indication for metastasectomy, especially those patients with lung or loco-regional disease and should be considered an accepted treatment option despite the absence of randomized data.

Surgical Removal of Multiple Metastasis in the Pre-TKI Era

The removal of multiple metastasis is more controversial. Logic dictates that as the number of lesions increases, the chances of unidentified lesions being missed which are too small to characterize with cross sectional.

Nevertheless, prior to the development of targeted therapy these were few treatment options and metastasectomy was widely employed in some institutions. The limited data available suggests that removal of up to six lung metastases is warranted (5-year survival of 32% vs. 0% [81]).

However removal of multiple metastases from multiple sites consistently shows poor outcome results [10, 84]. Systemic targeted therapy is more attractive in these patients.

Perhaps the most comprehensive and convincing data supporting metastasectomy in multiple sites of metastatic disease comes from the Mayo Clinic (1976–2006) [80]. Overall 125 (14%) underwent complete surgical resection of all metastases. These patients were compared to the remaining population with metastatic disease ($n = 762$). Complete surgical resection was associated with a significant prolongation of cancer-specific survival (median = 4.8 years vs. 1.3 years; $p < 0.001$). This benefit was not isolated to patients with disease isolated to the lungs. Patients with a complete resection of non-pulmonary metastasis had a 5-year cancer-specific survival rate of 32.5% vs. 12.4% for those without complete resection ($p < 0.001$). Complete resection remained predictive of improved survival for patients who had ≥3 metastatic lesions ($p < 0.001$). The authors of this work conclude that surgical resection should be considered where complete resection is possible irrespective of anatomical locations and number of sites of metastatic disease. Due to patient selection bias and in the absence of randomized data this approach cannot be recommended. However when this data is considered within the context of other series, multiple resections may be considered with caution where complete resection is easily achievable, especially in those patients with a limited number of lung metastasis.

Repeated surgical resection for metastatic disease has been described [85, 86]. It almost certainly reflects a subgroup with a more benign course of the disease and can result in exceptionally long survival lasting more than 10 years in these selected individuals. In a series of 141 patients with complete resection of solitary metastases 5-year survival rates after complete resection of second and third metastases were not different compared with initial metastasectomy (46 and 44%, respectively, vs. 43% 5-year OS rates; $p \geq 0.05$) [84]. This data needs to be interpreted with caution due to selection bias.

MSKCC Prognosis Score for Metastatic Disease and Metastasectomy

One of the most commonly used prognostic models is the MSKCC risk score which stratifies patients into three risk groups (good, intermediate and poor). Retrospective data comparing those patients who had metastasectomy with those who did not suggest surgery is associated with the survival advantage in both the good and intermediate risk groups with conflicting data in the poor risk group [87, 88]. It is unclear how much of this benefit is due to patient selection rather than the surgery itself. These data are derived from the pre-targeted therapy era, initial treatment with metastasectomy in the intermediate and poor risk group seems counterintuitive and should usually be avoided in the authors' opinion.

Site-Specific Metastasectomy

Resection of Pulmonary Metastases

Metastasis in the lungs occurs in 74% of patients in autopsy studies making them the most common metastatic sites [89] [90]. There are a number of small retrospective studies focusing on the role of metastasectomy in the cytokine era [84, 91–95]. These studies show the outcome is good (5-year survival rate of 37–54%) in this highly selected population [79, 80, 84, 96–104]. Also, a number of prognostic factors were consistently identified in multivariate analyses (Table 15.1), the most important of which were incomplete resection and number of metastasis removed (>6) [79–81, 84, 100, 103, 104]. The occurrence of simultaneous lymph node metastases and pulmonary metastasis has a detrimental effect on the outcome (median survival decreased from 102 to 19 months [104]). These less impressive results associated with tumour resection from multiple organs are not consistent throughout the literature however [80], but it does underline the caution required before embarking on major surgery to multiple sites, especially in the era of targeted therapy. Other significant factors associated with a poor outcome include a short disease-free interval from nephrectomy to relapse and the presence of synchronous metastasis [79, 81, 84, 99, 100, 103, 105]. Interestingly, the type of resection was not associated with a survival advantage and modern ablation techniques may be an alternative to surgical resection in select patients [106].

Resection of Liver Metastases

Liver metastases occur in 8–30% of patients with RCC [20]. They rarely occur in isolation and are often associated with a poor outcome [74, 78, 82]. Therefore there are few retrospective series focusing on liver metastasectomy [107–112]. The 5-year survival rates range between 8 and 38.9% in these series. The largest retrospective study analysed the outcome of 88 patients with liver metastasis as the only site [110]. Sixty-eight patients underwent resection and were compared to 20 who refused. The median 5-year overall survival rate after resection was 62.2% vs. 29.3% in the retrospective control. In both cohorts 79% received systemic therapy (immune-based therapy). These results appear impressive, although they contradict some of the smaller series where outcome is much less good. More importantly, hepatic metastasectomy is associated with significant morbidity (20%) and mortality (30%) [110, 111]. Therefore some recommend ablative techniques in this population based on very small numbers [113]. Overall the data on resection of liver metastasis is limited, surgical-related morbidity is high and the remaining patients invariably die from metastatic disease despite surgery. Resection of isolated liver metastasis as the only site of relapse may be warranted. These patients should always be discussed in a multidisciplinary setting.

Surgery for Bone Metastases

Bone metastases are observed in up to a quarter of patients with metastatic renal cancer and are frequently symptomatic [20]. The true prevalence of solitary bone metastasis is not known but they rarely occur in isolation (5.3%) [84].

Randomized prospective data in patients with bone metastasis from various malignancies demonstrated that direct decompressive surgery plus postoperative radiotherapy is superior to treatment with radiotherapy alone for patients with spinal cord compression caused by metastatic cancer [114]. In this study only a minority had renal cancer. Nevertheless this surgical approach is justified in this population for palliative reasons. In view of this randomized data, this is probably the strongest indication for surgery to a metastatic site. Surgery can also be performed to alleviate pain and for pathological fractures or strengthening a long bone which is prone to fracture due to a lesion [115]. While this surgery is often performed there is limited data regarding outcome or fracture rate. These procedures are often given in conjunction with radiotherapy [114].

In terms of the effect of surgery on outcome, only small series in a select group have reported. The results are conflicting. In a series of 38 cases with bone metastasis from RCC 13 evaluable patients had solitary lesions removed with a 5-year survival rate of approximately 50% for the entire cohort [116]. Conversely, two further reports show the 5-year survival results for surgical resection of a single bone metastasis at only 8–13% [80, 117]. A retrospective review of the literature showed a long disease-free interval, appendicular skeletal location and solitary metastases were correlated with longer survival [116].

The largest series addressing a variety of surgery for bone metastasis includes over 300 patients [115]. While symptomatic benefit can occur in the majority of patients, the median 5-year survival was 11 and 5% died in the postoperative period. This highlights the caution required for these patients prior to embarking on a surgical procedure. Wider resection may lessen the risk of recurrence at the same location [118]. Radiotherapy is clearly attractive and established alternative to surgery and these decisions should be made in the context of a multidisciplinary setting. Surgery seems most justified in those patients with bone disease threatening cord compression, where there is randomized data to support its use.

Metastasectomy of Brain Metastasis

Brain metastasis occurs in 2–17% of patients with renal cancer [119–121]. It is symptomatic in approximately 80% of cases. If left untreated, median survival is less than 4 months [122]. The selection of patients for metastasectomy is crucial in this population as the majority of patients have aggressive disease. There is also uncertainty about the effectiveness of targeted therapy in the CNS. For patients who present with brain disease the performance status, number of metastasis, MSKCC prognostic score and extracranial tumour burden should be considered [123–125]. A combination of whole brain radiotherapy (WBRT) and targeted therapy would be the standard treatment options for the majority of these patients.

A retrospective series of WBRT alone survival of patients with single brain metastases from RCC was only 4.4 months, while different small surgical series suggested a median survival of over 12 months [123, 126, 127]. These are clearly not comparable and were performed prior to the development of targeted therapy. However surgical excision of isolated metastasis in patients with a good performance status may be justified and associated with modest outcomes.

Stereotactic radiosurgery (SRS) can provide effective local control and is comparable to surgery even for multiple lesions and recurrent metastases [128]. Data from two series are available and the median overall survival was 11–13 months, with the majority of patients dying from systemic disease [125, 129]. Overall both SRS and surgery are being widely used in the era of targeted therapy, despite the lack of data. This is especially true in patients on systemic targeted therapy who have isolated relapse in the brain. Further data is urgently required.

Surgery for Locally Recurrent Disease and Lymph Node Metastases

Renal cancer-related nodal metastasis is an independent predictor of prognosis in patients who do not have metastatic disease [130]. The outcome of these patients is poor with post-surgical recurrence occurs in 70% and median overall survival of 20 months. Retrospective analysis suggests that removal of suspicious lymph nodes at the time of nephrectomy is associated with improved outcome [131]. Indeed a portion of patients with local lymph node involvement are cured with surgery

[132]. However, more widespread involvement is more sinister [133, 134]. Surgical management of local recurrence has been reported by the MD Anderson group [135]. Results show median survival of over 5 years and this approach should be considered in conjunction with subsequent systemic therapy. Factors associated with a poor outcome included positive surgical margin after resection, size of tumour recurrence, sarcomatoid features of the tumour, raised serum alkaline phosphatase and increased lactate dehydrogenase.

Small series also exist on the adrenalectomy in renal cancer. Isolated adrenal metastasis should be considered for surgery because it is associated with excellent long-term survival in individual patients [136–138].

There is a lack of comprehensive data reporting on the management of isolated lymph node relapse. Case reports detailing good outcomes are available [139, 140]. Overall, as with other organ involvement surgical resection of isolated metastasis needs to be considered in the context of the renal cancer disease pattern.

Perhaps the most useful data for lymph node surgery comes from a retrospective series of 101 patients who underwent resection of pulmonary metastases. In this work the prognostic value of concurrent hilar and mediastinal lymph node involvement was evaluated [104]. Overall 35% of patients had lymph node involvement which was associated with a worse prognosis. Indeed this poor outcome suggests patients with concurrent lung and thoracic lymph node involvement should not be surgical candidates [104].

Overall surgical intervention of local recurrence appears attractive. The role of lymphadenectomy in metastatic disease is less certain and does not seem warranted. Isolated lymph node relapse is rare and data lacks on the role of surgery.

Metastasectomy Following Systemic Therapy

The introduction of targeted therapy had complicated the role of metastasectomy in renal cancer. The principle of down-staging a tumour with systemic treatment followed by surgery to remove residual disease is attractive . In addition removal of isolated areas of disease progression after targeted therapy, such as a brain metastasis is feasible. However there is a lack of prospective data or even robust retrospective data to support these approaches.

The concept of systemic treatment followed by complete surgical resection of metastasis has been investigated in the cytokine era [141]. Over 8 years 38 patients with responsive or stable potentially resectable mRCC after cytokine treatment were enrolled. The numbers were too small to derive any definitive conclusions. The median overall survival was 4.7 years (range 3.0–7.8 years) with a median time to progression of 1.8 years (0.8–3.1 years). Twenty-one percent of the patients remained disease free. This is a highly selected population, and the results need further quantification. Therefore a similar German trial investigating this approach in the era of targeted therapy is planned.

The hypothesis of TKI therapy followed by surgery is supported by several cases [77, 142–144]. The largest cohort investigating this approach includes 22 [76]. The metastatic sites removed varied but mainly included the retroperitoneum and lung. At a median follow-up of more than 2 years 21 of the 22 patients were alive. This approach appears attractive in these selected patients, but more robust randomized data is required before this can be considered a standard approach. Perhaps one of the main advantages of this combined approach is that it may allow selected patients a specific period off targeted therapy prior to relapse. This concept of intermittent therapy after surgically induced complete response is attractive and clinical trials are planned.

Summary

The role of metastasectomy is unproven in this setting. Virtually all of the studies reported have impressive results but they represent a highly selected population of patients. Robust studies in the era of targeted therapy are lacking and are required if this is to widely accepted in treatment algorithms.

References

1. deKernion JB, Ramming KP, Smith RB. The natural history of metastatic renal cell carcinoma: a computer analysis. J Urol. 1978;120:148–52.
2. Johnson DE, Kaesler KE, Samuels ML. Is nephrectomy justified in patients with metastatic renal carcinoma? J Urol. 1975;114(1):27–9.
3. Middleton RG. Surgery for metastatic renal cell carcinoma. J Urol. 1967;97(6):973–7.
4. Montie JE, Stewart BH, Straffon RA, Banowsky LH, Hewitt CB, Montague DK. The role of adjunctive nephrectomy in patients with metastatic renal cell carcinoma. J Urol. 1977;117(3):272–5.
5. Freed SZ, Halperin JP, Gordon M. Idiopathic regression of metastases from renal cell carcinoma. J Urol. 1977;118(4):538–42.
6. Tolia BM, Whitmore Jr WF. Solitary metastasis from renal cell carcinoma. J Urol. 1975;114(6):836–8.
7. Tongaonkar HB, Kulkarni JN, Kamat MR. Solitary metastases from renal cell carcinoma: a review. J Surg Oncol. 1992;49(1):45–8.
8. Barney JD, Churchill J. Adenocarcinoma of the kidney with metastasis to the lung. J Urol. 1939; 42(269):271.
9. Skinner DG, Colvin RB, Vermillion CD, Pfister RC, Leadbetter WF. Diagnosis and management of renal cell carcinoma. A clinical and pathologic study of 309 cases. Cancer. 1971;28(5):1165–77.
10. Neves RJ, Zincke H, Taylor WF. Metastatic renal cell cancer and radical nephrectomy: identification of prognostic factors and patient survival. J Urol. 1988;139(6):1173–6.
11. Bukowski RM. Immunotherapy in renal cell carcinoma. Oncology (Williston Park). 1999;13(6): 801–10.
12. Flanigan RC, Salmon SE, Blumenstein BA, et al. Nephrectomy followed by interferon alfa-2b compared with interferon alfa-2b alone for metastatic renal-cell cancer. N Engl J Med. 2001;345(23): 1655–9.
13. Mickisch GH, Garin A, Van Poppel H, de Prijck L, Sylvester R. Radical nephrectomy plus interferon-alfa-based immunotherapy compared with interferon alfa alone in metastatic renal-cell carcinoma: a randomised trial. Lancet. 2001;358(9286):966–70.
14. Flanigan RC, Mickisch G, Sylvester R, Tangen C, Van Poppel H, Crawford ED. Cytoreductive nephrectomy in patients with metastatic renal cancer: a combined analysis. J Urol. 2004;171(3): 1071–6.
15. Crispen PL, Sheinin Y, Roth TJ, et al. Tumor cell and tumor vasculature expression of B7-H3 predict survival in clear cell renal cell carcinoma. Clin Cancer Res. 2008;14(16):5150–7.
16. Jacobsen J, Rasmuson T, Grankvist K, Ljungberg B. Vascular endothelial growth factor as prognostic factor in renal cell carcinoma. J Urol. 2000;163(1): 343–7.

17. Tatsumi T, Herrem CJ, Olson WC, et al. Disease stage variation in CD4+ and CD8+ T-cell reactivity to the receptor tyrosine kinase EphA2 in patients with renal cell carcinoma. Cancer Res. 2003; 63(15):4481–9.

18. Shablak A, Sikand K, Shanks JH, Thistlethwaite F, Spencer-Shaw A, Hawkins RE. High-dose interleukin-2 can produce a high rate of response and durable remissions in appropriately selected patients with metastatic renal cancer. J Immunother. 2011;34(1): 107–12.

19. Pantuck AJ, Belldegrun AS, Figlin RA. Nephrectomy and interleukin-2 for metastatic renal-cell carcinoma. N Engl J Med. 2001;345(23):1711–2.

20. Motzer RJ, Mazumdar M, Bacik J, Berg W, Amsterdam A, Ferrara J. Survival and prognostic stratification of 670 patients with advanced renal cell carcinoma. J Clin Oncol. 1999;17(8): 2530–40.

21. Chowdhury S, Harper PG, Choueiri TK. The role of cytoreductive nephrectomy for renal cell carcinoma in the era of targeted therapy. Nature Clin Pract Oncol. 2008;5(12):698–9.

22. Culp SH, Tannir NM, Abel EJ, et al. Can we better select patients with metastatic renal cell carcinoma for cytoreductive nephrectomy? Cancer. 2010;116(14): 3378–88.

23. Escudier B, Szczylik C, Hutson TE, et al. Randomized phase II trial of first-line treatment with sorafenib versus interferon Alfa-2a in patients with metastatic renal cell carcinoma. J Clin Oncol. 2001;27(8):1280–9.

24. Hudes G, Carducci M, Tomczak P, et al. Temsirolimus, interferon alfa, or both for advanced renal-cell carcinoma. N Engl J Med. 2007;356(22):2271–81.

25. Motzer RJ, Hutson TE, Tomczak P, et al. Sunitinib versus interferon alfa in metastatic renal-cell carcinoma. N Engl J Med. 2007;356(2):115–24.

26. Rini BI, Halabi S, Rosenberg JE, et al. Phase III trial of bevacizumab plus interferon alfa versus interferon alfa monotherapy in patients with metastatic renal cell carcinoma: final results of CALGB 90206. J Clin Oncol. 2001;28(13):2137–43.

27. Sternberg CN, Davis ID, Mardiak J, et al. Pazopanib in locally advanced or metastatic renal cell carcinoma: results of a randomized phase III trial. J Clin Oncol. 2010;28(6):1061–8.

28. Abel EJ, Wood CG. Cytoreductive nephrectomy for metastatic RCC in the era of targeted therapy. Nat Rev Urol. 2001;6(7):375–83.

29. Bex A, Blank C, Meinhardt W, van Tinteren H, Horenblas S, Haanen J. A phase II study of presurgical sunitinib in patients with metastatic clear-cell renal carcinoma and the primary tumor in situ. Urology. 2011;78:832–7.

30. Choueiri TK, Xie W, Kollmannsberger C, et al. The impact of cytoreductive nephrectomy on survival of patients with metastatic renal cell carcinoma receiving vascular endothelial growth factor targeted therapy. J Urol. 2011;185(1):60–6.

31. Hellenthal NJ, Underwood W, Penetrante R, et al. Prospective clinical trial of preoperative sunitinib in patients with renal cell carcinoma. J Urol. 2010;184(3):859–64.

32. Margulis V, Matin SF, Tannir N, et al. Surgical morbidity associated with administration of targeted molecular therapies before cytoreductive nephrectomy or resection of locally recurrent renal cell carcinoma. J Urol. 2008;180:94–8.

33. Powles T, Kayani I, Blank C, et al. The safety and efficacy of sunitinib before planned nephrectomy in metastatic clear cell renal cancer. Ann Oncol. 2011;22:1041–7.

34. Powles T, Blank C, Chowdhury S, et al. The outcome of patients treated with sunitinib prior to planned nephrectomy in metastatic clear cell renal cancer. Eur Urol. 2011;60:448–54.

35. Jonasch E, Wood CG, Matin SF, et al. Phase II presurgical feasibility study of bevacizumab in untreated patients with metastatic renal cell carcinoma. J Clin Oncol. 2009;27(25):4076–81.

36. Motzer RJ, Hutson TE, Tomczak P, et al. Overall survival and updated results for sunitinib compared with interferon alfa in patients with metastatic renal cell carcinoma. J Clin Oncol. 2009;27(22):3584–90.

37. Motzer RJ, Figlin RA, Hutson TE, et al. Sunitinib versus interferon-alfa (IFN-α) as first-line treatment of metastatic renal cell carcinoma (mRCC): updated results and analysis of prognostic factors. J Clin Oncol. 2001;25 (18S) [Abstract].

38. Choueiri TK, Xie W, Kollmannsberger C, et al. The impact of cytoreductive nephrectomy on survival of patients with metastatic renal cell carcinoma receiving vascular endothelial growth factor targeted therapy. J Urol. 2011;185(1):60–6.

39. Warren M, Venner PM, North S, et al. A population-based study examining the effect of tyrosine kinase inhibitors on survival in metastatic renal cell carcinoma in Alberta and the role of nephrectomy prior to treatment. Can Urol Assoc J. 2001;3(4):281–9.

40. Aben KK, Heskamp S, Janssen-Heijnen ML, et al. Better survival in patients with metastasised kidney cancer after nephrectomy: a population-based study in the Netherlands. Eur J Cancer. 2011;47:2023–32.

41. Margulis V, Wood CG. Cytoreductive nephrectomy in the era of targeted molecular agents: is it time to consider presurgical therapy? Eur Urol. 2008;54(3): 480–92.

42. Wood CG. Multimodal approaches in the management of locally advanced and metastatic renal cell carcinoma: combining surgery and systemic therapies to improve patient outcome. Clin Cancer Res. 2007;13(2):697s–702.

43. US National Institutes of Health. Clinical trial to assess the importance of nephrectomy (CARMENA). ClinicalTrials gov; 2009. http://clinicaltrials.gov/ct2/show/NCT00930033. Accessed 28 Jul 2010)

44. US National Institutes of Health. Immediate surgery or surgery after sunitinib malate in treating patients with metastatic kidney cancer. ClinicalTrials gov; 2010.

http://clinicaltrials.gov/ct2/show/NCT01099423. Accessed 5 May 2010

45. Pierorazio PM, McKiernan JM, McCann TR, Mohile S, Petrylak D, Benson MC. Outcome after cytoreductive nephrectomy for metastatic renal cell carcinoma is predicted by fractional percentage of tumour volume removed. BJU Int. 2007;100(4):755–9.

46. Barbastefano J, Garcia JA, Elson P, et al. Association of percentage of tumour burden removed with debulking nephrectomy and progression-free survival in patients with metastatic renal cell carcinoma treated with vascular endothelial growth factor-targeted therapy. BJU Int. 2010;106(9):1266–9.

47. Flanigan RC, Yonover PM. The role of radical nephrectomy in metastatic renal cell carcinoma. Semin Urol Oncol. 2001;19(2):98–102.

48. Walther MM, Patel B, Choyke PL, et al. Hypercalcemia in patients with metastatic renal cell carcinoma: effect of nephrectomy and metabolic evaluation. J Urol. 1997;158(3 Pt 1):733–9.

49. Bex A, Horenblas S, Meinhardt W, Verra N, de Gast GC. The role of initial immunotherapy as selection for nephrectomy in patients with metastatic renal cell carcinoma and the primary tumor in situ. Eur Urol. 2002;42(6):570–4.

50. Fleischmann JD, Kim B. Interleukin-2 immunotherapy followed by resection of residual renal cell carcinoma. J Urol. 1991;145(5):938–41.

51. Spencer WF, Linehan WM, Walther MM, et al. Immunotherapy with interleukin-2 and alpha-interferon in patients with metastatic renal cell cancer with in situ primary cancers: a pilot study. J Urol. 1992;147(1):24–30.

52. Rackley R, Novick A, Klein E, Bukowski R, McLain D, Goldfarb D. The impact of adjuvant nephrectomy on multimodality treatment of metastatic renal cell carcinoma. J Urol. 1994;152(5 Pt 1):1399–403.

53. Wagner JR, Walther MM, Linehan WM, White DE, Rosenberg SA, Yang JC. Interleukin-2 based immunotherapy for metastatic renal cell carcinoma with the kidney in place. J Urol. 1999;162(1):43–5.

54. Sherry RM, Pass HI, Rosenberg SA, Yang JC. Surgical resection of metastatic renal cell carcinoma and melanoma after response to interleukin-2-based immunotherapy. Cancer. 1992;69(7):1850–5.

55. Sella A, Swanson DA, Ro JY, et al. Surgery following response to interferon-alpha-based therapy for residual renal cell carcinoma. J Urol. 1993;149(1):19–21.

56. Krishnamurthi V, Novick AC, Bukowski RM. Efficacy of multimodality therapy in advanced renal cell carcinoma. Urology. 1998;51(6):933–7.

57. Haas GP, Redman BG, Rao VK, Dybal E, Pontes JE, Hillman GG. Immunotherapy for metastatic renal cell cancer: effect on the primary tumor. J Immunother Emphasis Tumor Immunol. 1993;13(2):130–5.

58. Bex A, Jonasch E, Kirkali Z, et al. Integrating surgery with targeted therapies for renal cell carcinoma: current evidence and ongoing trials. Eur Urol. 2010;58(6):819–28.

59. Kutikov A, Uzzo RG, Caraway A, et al. Use of systemic therapy and factors affecting survival for patients undergoing cytoreductive nephrectomy. BJU Int. 2010;106(2):218–23.

60. Abel EJ, Culp SH, Tannir NM, Tamboli P, Matin SF, Wood CG. Early primary tumor size reduction is an independent predictor of improved overall survival in metastatic renal cell carcinoma patients treated with sunitinib. Eur Urol. 2011;60(6):1273–9.

61. Thomas AA, Rini BI, Lane BR, et al. Response of the primary tumor to neoadjuvant sunitininb in patients with advanced renal cell carcinoma. J Urol. 2009;181:518–23.

62. Bex A, van der Veldt AA, Blank C, Meijerink MR, Boven E, Haanen JB. Progression of a caval vein thrombus in two patients with primary renal cell carcinoma on pretreatment with sunitinib. Acta Oncol. 2010;49(4):520–3.

63. Abel EJ, Culp SH, Tannir NM, Tamboli P, Matin SF, Wood CG. Early primary tumor size reduction is an independent predictor of improved overall survival in metastatic renal cell carcinoma patients treated with sunitinib. Eur Urol. 2011;60:1273–9.

64. Signoretti S, Bratslavsky G, Waldman FM, et al. Tissue-based research in kidney cancer: current challenges and future directions. Clin Cancer Res. 2008;14(12):3699–705.

65. Johannsen M, Florcken A, Bex A, et al. Can tyrosine kinase inhibitors be discontinued in patients with metastatic renal cell carcinoma and a complete response to treatment? A multicentre, retrospective analysis. Eur Urol. 2009;55:1430–8.

66. Johannsen M, Staehler M, Ohlmann CH, et al. Outcome of treatment discontinuation in patients with metastatic renal cell carcinoma and no evidence of disease following targeted therapy with or without metastasectomy. Ann Oncol. 2010;22:657–63.

67. Cowey CL, Amin C, Pruthi RS, et al. Neoadjuvant clinical trial with sorafenib for patients with stage II or higher renal cell carcinoma. J Clin Oncol. 2010;28(9):1502–7.

68. van der Veldt AA, Meijerink MR, van den Eertwegh AJ, et al. Sunitinib for treatment of advanced renal cell cancer: primary tumor response. Clin Cancer Res. 2008;14(8):2431–6.

69. Guix M, Granja NM, Meszoely I, et al. Short preoperative treatment with elotinib inhibits tumor cell proliferation in hormone receptor-positive breast cancers. J Clin Oncol. 2008;26(6):897–906.

70. Patil S, Figlin RA, Hutson TE, et al. Prognostic factors for progression-free and overall survival with sunitinib targeted therapy and with cytokine as first-line therapy in patients with metastatic renal cell carcinoma. Ann Oncol. 2010;22:295–300.

71. Escudier B, Kataja V. Renal cell carcinoma: ESMO clinical recommendations for diagnosis, treatment and follow-up. Ann Oncol. 2001;20 Suppl 4:81–2.

72. Gore ME, Escudier B. Emerging efficacy endpoints for targeted therapies in advanced renal cell

carcinoma. Oncology (Williston Park). 2006;20(6 Suppl 5):19–24.

73. Antonelli A, Zani D, Cozzoli A, Cunico SC. Surgical treatment of metastases from renal cell carcinoma. Arch Ital Urol Androl. 2005;77(2):125–8.

74. Han KR, Pantuck AJ, Bui MH, et al. Number of metastatic sites rather than location dictates overall survival of patients with node-negative metastatic renal cell carcinoma. Urology. 2003;61(2):314–9.

75. Russo P, O'Brien MF. Surgical intervention in patients with metastatic renal cancer: metastasectomy and cytoreductive nephrectomy. Urol Clin N Am. 2008;35(4):679–86.

76. Karam JA, Rini BI, Varella L, et al. Metastasectomy after targeted therapy in patients with advanced renal cell carcinoma. J Urol. 2011;185(2):439–44.

77. Patard JJ, Thuret R, Raffi A, Laguerre B, Bensalah K, Culine S. Treatment with sunitinib enabled complete resection of massive lymphadenopathy not previously amenable to excision in a patient with renal cell carcinoma. Eur Urol. 2009;55:237–9.

78. Swanson DA. Surgery for metastases of renal cell carcinoma. Scand J Surg. 2004;93(2):150–5.

79. Pfannschmidt J, Hoffmann H, Muley T, Krysa S, Trainer C, Dienemann H. Prognostic factors for survival after pulmonary resection of metastatic renal cell carcinoma. Ann Thorac Surg. 2002;74(5): 1653–7.

80. Alt AL, Boorjian SA, Lohse CM, Costello BA, Leibovich BC, Blute ML. Survival after complete surgical resection of multiple metastases from renal cell carcinoma. Cancer. 2011;117:2873–82.

81. Hofmann HS, Neef H, Krohe K, Andreev P, Silber RE. Prognostic factors and survival after pulmonary resection of metastatic renal cell carcinoma. Eur Urol. 2005;48(1):77–81.

82. van der Poel HG, Roukema JA, Horenblas S, van Geel AN, Debruyne FM. Metastasectomy in renal cell carcinoma: a multicenter retrospective analysis. Eur Urol. 1999;35(3):197–203.

83. Russo P, Synder M, Vickers A, Kondagunta V, Motzer R. Cytoreductive nephrectomy and nephrectomy/complete metastasectomy for metastatic renal cancer. Sci World J. 2007;7:768–78.

84. Kavolius JP, Mastorakos DP, Pavlovich C, Russo P, Burt ME, Brady MS. Resection of metastatic renal cell carcinoma. J Clin Oncol. 1998;16(6):2261–6.

85. Szendroi A, Szendroi M, Szucs M, Szekely E, Romics I. 11-Year survival of a renal cell cancer patient following multiple metastasectomy. Can J Urol. 2010;17(6):5475–7.

86. Yamaguchi K, Kawata N, Nagane Y, et al. Metastasectomy for renal cell carcinoma as a strategy to obtain complete remission. Int J Clin Oncol. 2010;15(5):519–22.

87. Eggener SE, Yossepowitch O, Pettus JA, Snyder ME, Motzer RJ, Russo P. Renal cell carcinoma recurrence after nephrectomy for localized disease: predicting survival from time of recurrence. J Clin Oncol. 2006;24(19):3101–6.

88. Eggener SE, Yossepowitch O, Kundu S, Motzer RJ, Russo P. Risk score and metastasectomy independently impact prognosis of patients with recurrent renal cell carcinoma. J Urol. 2008;180(3):873–8.

89. Weiss L, Harlos JP, Torhorst J, et al. Metastatic patterns of renal carcinoma: an analysis of 687 necropsies. J Cancer Res Clin Oncol. 1988;114(6):605–12.

90. Saitoh H, Nakayama M, Nakamura K, Satoh T. Distant metastasis of renal adenocarcinoma in nephrectomized cases. J Urol. 1982;127:1092–5.

91. Katzenstein AL, Purvis Jr R, Gmelich J, Askin F. Pulmonary resection for metastatic renal adenocarcinoma: pathologic findings and therapeutic value. Cancer. 1978;41(2):712–23.

92. Dernevik L, Berggren H, Larsson S, Roberts D. Surgical removal of pulmonary metastases from renal cell carcinoma. Scand J Urol Nephrol. 1985;19(2): 133–7.

93. Fukuda M, Satomi Y, Senga Y, et al. [Results of pulmonary resection for metastatic renal cell carcinoma]. Hinyokika Kiyo. 1987;33(7):993–7.

94. Tanguay S, Swanson DA, Putnam Jr JB. Renal cell carcinoma metastatic to the lung: potential benefit in the combination of biological therapy and surgery. J Urol. 1996;156(5):1586–9.

95. Fourquier P, Regnard JF, Rea S, Levi JF, Levasseur P. Lung metastases of renal cell carcinoma: results of surgical resection. Eur J Cardiothorac Surg. 1997;11(1):17–21.

96. Assouad J, Petkova B, Berna P, Dujon A, Foucault C, Riquet M. Renal cell carcinoma lung metastases surgery: pathologic findings and prognostic factors. Ann Thorac Surg. 2007;84(4):1114–20.

97. Cerfolio RJ, Allen MS, Deschamps C, et al. Pulmonary resection of metastatic renal cell carcinoma. Ann Thorac Surg. 1994;57(2):339–44.

98. Friedel G, Hurtgen M, Penzenstadler M, Kyriss T, Toomes H. Resection of pulmonary metastases from renal cell carcinoma. Anticancer Res. 1999;19(2C): 1593–6.

99. Friedel G, Pastorino U, Buyse M, et al. [Resection of lung metastases: long-term results and prognostic analysis based on 5206 cases–the international registry of lung metastases]. Zentralbl Chir. 1999;124(2): 96–103.

100. Kanzaki R, Higashiyama M, Fujiwara A, et al. Long-term results of surgical resection for pulmonary metastasis from renal cell carcinoma: a 25-year single-institution experience. Eur J Cardiothorac Surg. 2011;39(2):167–72.

101. Marulli G, Sartori F, Bassi PF, dal Moro F, Gino Favaretto A, Rea F. Long-term results of surgical management of pulmonary metastases from renal cell carcinoma. Thorac Cardiovasc Surg. 2006; 54(8):544–7.

102. Mineo TC, Ambrogi V, Tonini G, Nofroni I. Pulmonary metastasectomy: might the type of resection affect survival? J Surg Oncol. 2001;76(1):47–52.

103. Piltz S, Meimarakis G, Wichmann MW, Hatz R, Schildberg FW, Fuerst H. Long-term results after

pulmonary resection of renal cell carcinoma metastases. Ann Thorac Surg. 2002;73(4):1082–7.

104. Winter H, Meimarakis G, Angele MK, et al. Tumor infiltrated hilar and mediastinal lymph nodes are an independent prognostic factor for decreased survival after pulmonary metastasectomy in patients with renal cell carcinoma. J Urol. 2010;184(5):1888–94.

105. Murthy SC, Kim K, Rice TW, et al. Can we predict long-term survival after pulmonary metastasectomy for renal cell carcinoma? Ann Thorac Surg. 2005;79(3):996–1003.

106. Shu Yan Huo A, Lawson Morris D, King J, Glenn D. Use of percutaneous radiofrequency ablation in pulmonary metastases from renal cell carcinoma. Ann Surg Oncol. 2009;16(11):3169–75.

107. Fujisaki S, Takayama T, Shimada K, et al. Hepatectomy for metastatic renal cell carcinoma. Hepatogastroenterology. 1997;44(15):817–9.

108. Alves A, Adam R, Majno P, et al. Hepatic resection for metastatic renal tumors: is it worthwhile? Ann Surg Oncol. 2003;10(6):705–10.

109. Lang H, Nussbaum KT, Weimann A, Raab R. [Liver resection for non-colorectal, non-neuroendocrine hepatic metastases]. Chirurg. 1999;70(4):439–46.

110. Staehler MD, Kruse J, Haseke N, et al. Liver resection for metastatic disease prolongs survival in renal cell carcinoma: 12-year results from a retrospective comparative analysis. World J Urol. 2010;28(4):543–7.

111. Stief CG, Jahne J, Hagemann JH, Kuczyk M, Jonas U. Surgery for metachronous solitary liver metastases of renal cell carcinoma. J Urol. 1997;158(2):375–7.

112. Thelen A, Jonas S, Benckert C, et al. Liver resection for metastases from renal cell carcinoma. World J Surg. 2007;31(4):802–7.

113. Goering JD, Mahvi DM, Niederhuber JE, Chicks D, Rikkers LF. Cryoablation and liver resection for noncolorectal liver metastases. Am J Surg. 2002; 183(4):384–9.

114. Patchell RA, Tibbs PA, Regine WF, et al. Direct decompressive surgical resection in the treatment of spinal cord compression caused by metastatic cancer: a randomised trial. Lancet. 2005;366(9486):643–8.

115. Lin PP, Mirza AN, Lewis VO, et al. Patient survival after surgery for osseous metastases from renal cell carcinoma. J Bone Joint Surg Am. 2007;89(8): 1794–801.

116. Althausen P, Althausen A, Jennings LC, Mankin HJ. Prognostic factors and surgical treatment of osseous metastases secondary to renal cell carcinoma. Cancer. 1997;80(6):1103–9.

117. Baloch KG, Grimer RJ, Carter SR, Tillman RM. Radical surgery for the solitary bony metastasis from renal-cell carcinoma. J Bone Joint Surg Br. 2000; 82(1):62–7.

118. Les KA, Nicholas RW, Rougraff B, et al. Local progression after operative treatment of metastatic kidney cancer. Clin Orthop Relat Res. 2001;390:206–11.

119. Levy DA, Slaton JW, Swanson DA, Dinney CP. Stage specific guidelines for surveillance after radi-

cal nephrectomy for local renal cell carcinoma. J Urol. 1998;159(4):1163–7.

120. Ljungberg B, Alamdari FI, Rasmuson T, Roos G. Follow-up guidelines for nonmetastatic renal cell carcinoma based on the occurrence of metastases after radical nephrectomy. BJU Int. 1999; 84(4):405–11.

121. Sandock DS, Seftel AD, Resnick MI. A new protocol for the followup of renal cell carcinoma based on pathological stage. J Urol. 1995;154(1):28–31.

122. Decker DA, Decker VL, Herskovic A, Cummings GD. Brain metastases in patients with renal cell carcinoma: prognosis and treatment. J Clin Oncol. 1984;2(3):169–73.

123. Sperduto PW, Chao ST, Sneed PK, et al. Diagnosis-specific prognostic factors, indexes, and treatment outcomes for patients with newly diagnosed brain metastases: a multi-institutional analysis of 4,259 patients. Int J Radiat Oncol Biol Phys. 2010; 77(3):655–61.

124. Cannady SB, Cavanaugh KA, Lee SY, et al. Results of whole brain radiotherapy and recursive partitioning analysis in patients with brain metastases from renal cell carcinoma: a retrospective study. Int J Radiat Oncol Biol Phys. 2004;58(1):253–8.

125. Muacevic A, Kreth FW, Mack A, Tonn JC, Wowra B. Stereotactic radiosurgery without radiation therapy providing high local tumor control of multiple brain metastases from renal cell carcinoma. Minim Invasive Neurosurg. 2004;47(4):203–8.

126. Wronski M, Maor MH, Davis BJ, Sawaya R, Levin VA. External radiation of brain metastases from renal carcinoma: a retrospective study of 119 patients from the M.D. Anderson Cancer Center. Int J Radiat Oncol Biol Phys. 1997;37(4):753–9.

127. Wronski M, Arbit E, Russo P, Galicich JH. Surgical resection of brain metastases from renal cell carcinoma in 50 patients. Urology. 1996; 47(2):187–93.

128. Marko NF, Angelov L, Toms SA, et al. Stereotactic radiosurgery as single-modality treatment of incidentally identified renal cell carcinoma brain metastases. World Neurosurg. 2010;73(3):186–93.

129. Sheehan JP, Sun MH, Kondziolka D, Flickinger J, Lunsford LD. Radiosurgery in patients with renal cell carcinoma metastasis to the brain: long-term outcomes and prognostic factors influencing survival and local tumor control. J Neurosurg. 2003;98(2): 342–9.

130. Canfield SE, Kamat AM, Sanchez-Ortiz RF, Detry M, Swanson DA, Wood CG. Renal cell carcinoma with nodal metastases in the absence of distant metastatic disease (clinical stage TxN1-2 M0): the impact of aggressive surgical resection on patient outcome. J Urol. 2006;175(3):864–9.

131. Pantuck AJ, Zisman A, Dorey F, et al. Renal cell carcinoma with retroperitoneal lymph nodes: role of lymph node dissection. J Urol. 2003;169(6): 2076–83.

132. Pantuck AJ, Zisman A, Dorey F, et al. Renal cell carcinoma with retroperitoneal lymph nodes. Impact on survival and benefits of immunotherapy. Cancer. 2003;97(12):2995–3002.

133. Freedland SJ, deKernion JB. Role of lymphadenectomy for patients undergoing radical nephrectomy for renal cell carcinoma. Rev Urol. 2003;5(3): 191–5.

134. Phillips CK, Taneja SS. The role of lymphadenectomy in the surgical management of renal cell carcinoma. Urol Oncol. 2004;22(3):214–23.

135. Margulis V, McDonald M, Tamboli P, Swanson DA, Wood CG. Predictors of oncological outcome after resection of locally recurrent renal cell carcinoma. J Urol. 2009;181(5):2044–51.

136. Dieckmann KP, Wullbrand A, Krolzig G. Contralateral adrenal metastasis in renal cell cancer. Scand J Urol Nephrol. 1996;30(2):139–43.

137. Kessler OJ, Mukamel E, Weinstein R, Gayer E, Konichezky M, Servadio C. Metachronous renal cell carcinoma metastasis to the contralateral adrenal gland. Urology. 1998;51(4):539–43.

138. Onishi T, Ohishi Y, Goto H, Suzuki H, Asano K. Metachronous solitary metastasis of renal cell carcinoma to the contralateral adrenal gland after nephrectomy. Int J Clin Oncol. 2000;5(1):36–40.

139. Assouad J, Riquet M, Berna P, Danel C. Intrapulmonary lymph node metastasis and renal cell carcinoma. Eur J Cardiothorac Surg. 2007;31(1):132–4.

140. Kanzaki R, Higashiyama M, Okami J, Kodama K. Surgical treatment for patients with solitary metastasis in the mediastinal lymph node from renal cell carcinoma. Interact Cardiovasc Thorac Surg. 2009; 8(4):485–7.

141. Daliani DD, Tannir NM, Papandreou CN, et al. Prospective assessment of systemic therapy followed by surgical removal of metastases in selected patients with renal cell carcinoma. BJU Int. 2009;104(4): 456–60.

142. Rini BI, Shaw V, Rosenberg JE, Kim ST, Chen I. Patients with metastatic renal cell carcinoma with long term disease-free survival after treatment with sunitinib and resection of residual metastases. Clin Genitourin Cancer. 2006;5(3):232–4.

143. Shuch B, Riggs SB, LaRochelle JC, et al. Neoadjuvant targeted therapy and advanced kidney cancer: observations and implications for a new treatment paradigm. BJU Int. 2008;102:692–6.

144. Thibault F, Rixe O, Meric JB, et al. Neoadjuvant therapy for renal cancer. Prog Urol. 2008;18(4): 256–8.

Immunotherapy for Renal Cell Carcinoma

16

Diwakar Davar, Moon Fenton, and
Leonard J. Appleman

Introduction

The first suggestion that renal cell carcinoma (RCC) could be a target of the immune system came from the occasional spontaneous regressions that have been documented in patients with metastatic RCC over the past century [1–3]. Spontaneous regressions are sometimes associated with cytoreductive nephrectomy, although the rate of regression is low and variable between series [4, 5]. In a randomized study of interferon-γ 1b, 6 patients out of 91 in the placebo arm had spontaneous tumor regression [6, 7]. These cases were subjected to blinded central radiology review, and there were three complete responses and three partial responses (defined as greater than 50% decrease in sum of tumor diameters). Conversely, recurrences of renal carcinoma after nephrectomy have been described as long as 33 years after presentation. One explanation for this observation is loss of immune control of a radiographically occult tumor population [8, 9].

D. Davar
Division of General Internal Medicine,
University of Pittsburgh Medical Center, 200 Lothrop
Street, Pittsburgh, PA 15213, USA
e-mail: davard@upmc.edu

M. Fenton • L.J. Appleman (✉)
Division of Hematology-Oncology, University
of Pittsburgh Medical Center, 5150 Centre Avenue,
Pittsburgh, PA 15232, USA
e-mail: fentonm@upmc.edu; applemanlj@upmc.edu

Cancer immunotherapy can generally be characterized as active (requiring the participation of antigen-specific host cells) or passive (dependent on exogenous antibodies or T lymphocytes). Cancer immunotherapy can also be specific to particular tumor antigens or components or nonspecific (stimulation of the immune system by cytokines or adjuvant without specific antigenic material). Active and passive, specific and nonspecific immunotherapeutic approaches to RCC have all been investigated in the clinic.

Cytokine Therapy

The use of cytokines represents an active, nonspecific cancer immunotherapy. The premise underlying cytokine therapy is that nonspecific activation of immune system in a patient with cancer will allow tumor-specific immune response to develop to the point that they acquire clinical antitumor activity.

Interleukin-2

Interleukin-2 (IL-2) was identified in 1976 as a soluble factor in the conditioned medium of phytohemagglutinin-stimulated human lymphocytes that selectively enabled the growth of T cells in culture [10]. Initial in vitro and clinical studies were performed using IL-2 purified from culture supernatants of the Jurkat T leukemia cell line [11]. Interleukin-2 was subsequently cloned and

S.C. Campbell and B.I. Rini (eds.), *Renal Cell Carcinoma: Clinical Management*, Current Clinical Urology,
DOI 10.1007/978-1-62703-062-5_16, © Springer Science+Business Media New York 2013

produced recombinantly from *Escherichia coli* [12, 13]. The availability of large quantities of recombinant IL-2 allowed the in vitro expansion of lymphokine-activated killer (LAK) cells for adoptive immunotherapy, as well as the direct administration of large doses of IL-2 to patients. IL-2 was tested as an anti-neoplastic agent and demonstrated antitumor activity in a range of murine tumor models [14, 15].

The first phase I study of interleukin-2 in humans was reported by Lotze, Rosenberg and colleagues at the National Cancer Institute in 1984 [11]. No responses were seen using the relatively small quantities of IL-2 available as the nonrecombinant product purified from Jurkat cells. Clinical responses in patients with melanoma were seen in subsequent studies in which larger quantities of interleukin-2 available from recombinant production in *E. coli* were used [16]. The NCI group subsequently showed that the combination of high-dose IL-2 (720,000 or 600,000 IU/kg) with a LAK cell infusion had activity in metastatic renal cell cancer [17]. Fyfe and colleagues subsequently reported the combined results of seven phase II studies of bolus high-dose IL-2 in patients with metastatic RCC [18]. In this report, patients with metastatic RCC were with recombinant IL-2 dosed at 720,000 or 600,000 IU/kg delivered by a 15 min intravenous (IV) infusion every 8 h over 5 days consecutively for up to 14 consecutive doses. A single course of therapy consisted of two cycles as described above. Patients who had radiographic responses or stable disease were retreated with a second course after 12 weeks, generally for up to three courses in total. Overall response rate (RR) was 14% (36/255) with a complete response (CR) and partial response (PR) rates of 5% (12/255) and 9% (24/255), respectively (see Table 16.1). This led to the United States Food and Drug Administration (FDA) approving high-dose (HD) bolus recombinant interleukin-2 (Aldesleukin, Proleukin) for the treatment of patients with metastatic RCC in 1992.

High-dose bolus IV IL-2 administration is associated with severe multisystem toxicity [27]. Adverse manifestations are directly related to lymphocyte infiltration in various organs and a cytokine release by immune cells activated by IL-2, which results in a capillary leak syndrome causing hypovolemia and fluid accumulation in the extravascular space. Systemic effects such as fever and a sepsis-like syndrome are thought to be related to the IL-2-mediated release of tumor necrosis factor (TNF) by mononuclear cells. Other effects include cardiac (arrhythmia), renal (renal dysfunction), hematologic (thrombocytopenia, anemia, leucopenia), gastrointestinal (diarrhea), and metabolic (metabolic acidosis). Earlier studies did report an approximately 20% incidence of catheter-related bacteremia but improved infection control measures and the use of removable peripherally inserted central catheters (PICCs) have reduced this considerably. IL-2-related toxicities generally resolve within 2–3 days of cessation of therapy.

IL-2 Therapy: Alternative Schedules

The associated toxicities (up to 4% treatment-related mortality) and high cost associated with IL-2 administration led some researchers to investigate regimens containing lower doses of IL-2 or combinations of other agents—including 5-fluorouracil and IFN-α—with low-dose IL-2 in an attempt to decrease toxicity whilst maintaining therapeutic efficacy.

A French multicenter phase III trial published in the New England Journal of Medicine in 1998 compared continuous infusion intermediate dose IL-2 (5-day continuous infusion at 18×10^6 IU/m^2 of body-surface area daily), subcutaneous IFN-α (18×10^6 IU/m^2 thrice weekly for 10 weeks), and combination of the two agents in 425 patients with metastatic RCC [22]. Response rates at 25 weeks were significantly greater in the combined therapy group—overall RR of 14% (19/140) in the combined IL-2/IFN-α arm compared to 1% (4/138) and 6% (9/147) in the IL-2-alone and IFN-alpha alone arms, respectively. Event-free survival was also significantly higher in the combination group (20% at 1 year) vs. the IL-2-receiving group (15%) or the interferon-alpha group (12%) ($p = 0.01$). However, none of the

Table 16.1 Selected studies of cytokine therapy in advanced renal cell cancer

Author	Design	Participants	Interventions	Results
Rosenberg [19]	Single-center phase III RCT stratified by tumour type	$N=97$; median age 41–50 years (all histol); PS(0) 77% (all histol); male 66%	1. IL-2 2.16 MU/kg/day[a] i.v. with LAK 2. IL-2 2.16 MU/kg/day[a] i.v. without, LAK	HD IL-2 with LAK (24/85 = 28%) vs. HD IL-2 w/out LAK (16/79 = 20%)
Yang [20]	Single-center phase III RCT, stratified by melanoma vs. RCC, nephrectomy	$N=56$; median age 41–50; PS(0) 73% (melanoma + RCC); M/F NA	1. IL-2 2.16 MU/kg/day[a] i.v. alternating with PEG-IL2 3(–6) MU/kg i.v. weekly 2. IL-2 2.16 MU/kg/day[a] i.v.	HD IL-2 (13/65 = 20%) vs. LD IL-2 (9/60 = 15%)
Yang [21]	Single-center phase III RCT	$N=305$; median age 41–50 years; PS(0) 81%; male 70%	1. IL-2 i.v. 2.16 MU/kg/day[a] 2. IL-2 i.v. 0.216 MU/kg/day[a]	HD IL-2 (33/155 = 21%) vs. LD IL-2 (19/149 = 13%)
Negrier [22]	Multicenter, phase III RCT	$N=425$; ECOG PS 0–2 (72–83% PS 0); post-nephrectomy 92–94%	1. HD IL-2 per protocol[a] 2. SC IFN-α 18 × 10^6 IU/m² 3 days/week × 10 weeks (induction) followed by 13 weeks (maintenance) 3. HD IL-2 per protocol with SC IFN-α 6 × 10^6 IU/m² during each IL-2 cycle	*Response (CR + PR + SD)* – At 10 weeks: 6.5% (group 1) vs. 7.5% (group 2) vs. 18.6% (group 3) – At 25 weeks: 2.9% (group 1) vs. 6.1% (group 2) vs. 13.6% (group 3) *Survival:* Event-free survival rates at 1 year: 15% (group 1) vs. 12% (group 2) vs. 20% (group 3)
Yang [23]	Three-arm single center phase III RCT	$N=283$; male 71%	As for Yang 2003a(i), 3rd arm added: IL-2 0.125–0.25 MU/kg s.c. d 1–5/week	HD IL-2 (20/96 = 21%) vs. LD IL-2 (10/92 = 11%) vs. SC IL-2 (9/93 = 10)
McDermott [24]	Multicenter phase III RCT; stratified for site (liver/bone Y/N), PS 0 vs. 1, nephrectomy status	$N=193$; median age 54 years; PS(0) 60%; male 68%; Nx 69% (note only pts with PD were enrolled)	1. IL-2 5–15 MU/m²/day[a] s.c. + IFN-α2b 5 MU/m² thrice weekly 2. IL-2 1.8 MU/kg/day[a] i.v.	HD IL-2 (22/95 = 23%) vs. LD IL-2 + IFN (9/91 = 10%)
Negrier [25]	Multicenter, phase III RCT	$N=492$; median age 61 years; clear cell histo 79%; post-nephrectomy 96%	1. MPA[b] 200 mg daily 2. SC IFN-α 9 × 10^6 IU/m² thrice weekly for 10 weeks 3. SC intermediate dose IL-2 (5-day continuous infusion at 9 × 10^6 IU/m² daily) 4. – (2) + (3)	*Response (CR + PR)* – At 12 weeks: 2% (group 1) vs. 4% (group 2) vs. 4% (group 3) vs. 10% (group 4) – At 6 months: 2% (group 1) vs. 8% (group 2) vs. 4% (group 3) vs.7% (group 4) *Survival:* – OS (months): 14.9 (group 1) vs. 15.2 (group 2) vs. 15.3 (group 3) vs. 16.8 (group 4) – PFS (months): 3.0 (group 1) vs. 3.4 (group 2) vs. 3.4 (group 3) vs. 3.8 (group 4)

(continued)

Table 16.1 (continued)

Author	Design	Participants	Interventions	Results
McDermott [26]	Multicenter, nonrandomized, prospective study	$N=120$; median age unknown; PS(0) 60%; MSKCC intermediate risk 71%; clear cell histo 96%; post-nephrectomy 99%	HD IL-2 per FDA approved-protocol[c]	*Response (CR + PR) at time of reporting (ASCO 2011):* – RR: 29% (35/120 with 7 CR, 28 PR and 20 ongoing responses) *Survival at time of reporting (ASCO 2011):* – PFS (months): median 4.4 (20 ongoing)

[a]HD IL-2 protocol—induction cycle consisting of 18×10^6 MU/m^2/day$\times$5 days for two courses separated by 6 days with 3 weeks rest between cycles and maintenance cycle consisting of 18×10^6 MU/m^2/day$\times$5 days followed by 3 weeks rest

[b]*MPA* medroxyprogesterone (Farlutal; Pfizer, Paris, France)

[c]FDA-approved HD IL-2 protocol—18×10^6 MU/m^2/day (6×10^5 MU/m^2/dose q8)$\times$5 days (maximum 14 doses) followed by 9 days rest, then repeated with each cycle=5 days of treatment

three regimens tested had any advantage in terms of overall survival (OS).

Multiple trials comparing various intermediate-dose and low-dose schedules of IL-2 have been published—these trials produced response and survival rates comparable to those reported for HD IL-2 with significantly less acute toxicity (see Table 16.1). Generally, objective response (OR) rates were 15% with a CR rate of 7% and PR rate of 8%, respectively.

A National Cancer Institute (NCI) phase III study compared HD IL-2 to two different low dose regimens—an inpatient intravenous bolus regimen using 10% of the standard dose (72,000 IU/kg/dose intravenously every 8 h for a maximum of 28 doses) and an outpatient regimen using SC IL-2 (250,000 U/kg/dose in week 1 and then 125,000 U/kg/dose during subsequent 5 weeks) [23]. After noting that HD IL-2 appeared to result in significantly more responses compared to either low dose IV IL-2 or SC IL-2, the authors concluded that LD IL-2 regimens had some biologic activity in metastatic RCC but that given the higher response rates associated with HD IL-2, this was to be recommended in suitable patients with the caveat that none of the tested regimens had demonstrated any survival benefit.

The Cytokine Working Group (CWG) conducted a randomized phase III trial to compare HD IL-2 (600,000 IU/kg/dose intravenously

every 8 h for a maximum of 28 doses) to combination low-dose IL-2 (5 MIU/m^2 subcutaneously every 8 h for three doses on day 1, then daily 5 days/week for 4 weeks) and IFN-α (5 MIU/m^2 subcutaneously three times per week for 4 weeks) in patients with metastatic RCC [24]. Three-year PFS was the primary endpoint. PFS in the HD IL-2 group was 10.5% at 3 years vs. 3.3% in the low-dose IL-2/IFN arm ($p=0.082$). HD IL-2 resulted in response rate of 22%, significantly better than the 10% for LD IL-2/IFN. There were more complete responses in the HD IL-2 arm (8.3% vs. 3.3% for the IL-2/IFN combination ($p=0.214$). Seven out of 95 subjects in the HD IL-2 arm maintained complete remission through the last analysis, and none in the IFN arm ($p=014$). In addition, HD IL-2 administration resulted in a median OS of 17.5 months (vs. 13 for IL-2/IFN-α; $p=0.211$). Based on the results of the NCI and CWG group studies described above, HD IL-2 is the preferred regimen for fit patients who are treated with the objective of long-term disease control.

IL-2 Therapy: Adjuvant Therapy

IL-2 has been evaluated in the adjuvant setting by several investigators in an attempt to extend the progression-free survival (PFS) benefit seen in the metastatic setting to patients at high risk of recurrence post-resection. A pilot trial conducted by investigators at the University of Minnesota published in 2006 studied the effects of adjuvant low-dose IL-2 given in a dose-escalating fashion to 41 patients with resected RCC at high risk for recurrent disease (TNM stages III and IV resected distant metastases) [28]. Patients received SC IL-2 twice daily at either 4 or 8 MIU/m^2 per day in two different schedules for each dosing level. No statistically significant difference between any of the treatment arms with respect to disease-free survival or 3-year survival was noted in this trial.

Clark et al. conducted a randomized trial of adjuvant high-dose therapy via the CWG. Sixty-nine patients who were at high risk of recurrence post-nephrectomy were enrolled [29]. One course of standard dose HD IL-2 was given vs. observation in a randomized 1:1 fashion to patients who were within 12 weeks status post-nephrectomy. At an interim analysis performed at 24 months, only 72% of expected events had occurred leading the investigators to terminate the trial early as it was thought that there was a <1% chance of observing the stated 30% actual improvement in 2-year DFS, should the trend of events continue. At the time of publication it was noted that DFS in the IL-2 treatment arm averaged 19.5 months vs. 36 months in the observation arm. The authors concluded that adjuvant HD IL-2 failed to demonstrate a clinically meaningful benefit when administered postoperatively to patients with resected high-risk RCC.

Italian investigators have investigated low-dose IL-2 in combination with IFN-α in resected high-risk RCC. Three hundred and ten patients have been randomized to control vs. immunotherapy consisting of a 4-week cycle of LD IL-2 (subcutaneously 1 million IU/m^2 twice daily on D1–2 followed by 1 million IU/m^2 once daily on D3–5) with IFN-α (subcutaneously 1.8 million IU/m^2 on days 3 and 5). Cycles were repeated every 4 months for the first 2 years and every 6 months for the remaining 3 years for a total of 12 cycles in 5 years. Whilst DFS was similar for the 5 years of observation, at 10 years it appeared that treatment reduced risk of relapse with an estimated hazard ratio (HR) for treatment of 0.84 (95% CI 0.54–1.33,

$p=0.47$). The reduction in risk was greatest for patients with lower tumor grade.

IL-2 Therapy: HD IL-2 Combinations

The toxicity profile of IL-2 has been previously detailed. In an effort to improve response rates and/or survival benefit without significantly adding to toxicity, several groups have attempted to pair HD IL-2 with additional agents.

A CWG trial in which bevacizumab, a monoclonal antibody-directed against the vascular endothelial growth factor (VEGF) receptor, was added to standard dose HD IL-2 in patients with histologically confirmed metastatic RCC with predominantly clear cell histology [30]. Overall RR was 29% with CR 8% and PR 20%. Median PFS was 9 months with a 2-year PFS of 15%. Toxicity was comparable to single agent HD IL-2.

IL-2 has also been tested in combination with the small molecule tyrosine kinase inhibitors (TKIs). In a multicenter Italian study, 128 treatment-naive patients with metastatic RCC were enrolled to sorafenib alone or combination daily sorafenib plus subcutaneous IL-2 administered five times per week for 6 of every 8 weeks [31]. The initial dose administered was 4.5 million international units (MIU), but after enrollment of 40 total subjects, the dose of IL-2 was reduced to 3 MIU due to asthenia. The primary endpoint of the study was PFS. The PFS of the combination group was 33 weeks vs. 30 weeks for sorafenib alone ($p=0.109$). Although there was a trend toward improved PFS with sorafenib plus IL-2 in the subjects with MSKCC low risk (47 weeks vs. 41 weeks), the PFS in the intermediate risk group was 21 weeks for sorafenib plus IL-2 vs. 29 weeks for sorafenib alone. The authors concluded that low-dose interleukin-2 failed to improve outcomes with first-line sorafenib therapy for mRCC.

IL-2 Therapy: Predictors of Response

Given the antecedent toxicities associated with IL-2 administration, there exists a clear and pressing need to identify reliable clinical predictors of response to limit therapy to those most likely to benefit. The consistent survival benefit in a minority of nonselected patient populations treated with IL-2 suggests that there exist tumor-specific and/or host-specific phenotypes that confer susceptibility to immunotherapy emphasizing the need to identify reliable predictors of response.

A clinical algorithm, the UCLA SANI score (survival after nephrectomy and immunotherapy), was developed based upon the outcomes in 173 patients who had nephrectomy followed by IL-2-based therapy. The factors that predicted survival and response to IL-2 were regional lymph node status (N0 vs. N1 vs. N2), symptoms, location of metastases (bone only or lung only vs. multiple sites or other sites), sarcomatoid histology, and TSH level (2 mIU/L vs. 2.0–4.8 mIU/L vs. >4.8 mIU/L) [32]. Median survival for the low risk group (0 risk factors) was 47 months after nephrectomy and immunotherapy. Median survival for the intermediate risk group (one to three risk factors) was 19 months, and median survival for the high risk group was only 5 months.

Investigators have long known that certain subtypes of RCC portend for especially poor outcomes. MSKCC researchers established that metastatic non-clear-cell RCC was associated with resistance to systemic therapy including IL-2 and poor outcomes [33]. After analyzing patients with respect to therapy received, Upton et al. noted that patients with non-clear-cell RCC or clear-cell RCC with papillary or >50% granular features tended to respond poorly to IL-2 [34].

Researchers analyzing tumor tissue to identify putative biomarkers to aid in prognostication and/ or prediction of response to therapy had previously identified several candidates of interest. By gene profiling tumor specimens, Pantuck et al. were able to identify a set of 73 genes whose expression appears to distinguish complete responders from non-responders [35]. Complete responders to IL-2 have a signature gene and protein expression pattern that includes carbonic anhydrase IX (CAIX), PTEN, and CXCR4. CAIX may function to help cells proliferate in hypoxic conditions and appears to be inductively increased in many tumor types as opposed to normal tissue.

In an analysis of 321 patients using a monoclonal antibody designed to detect CAIX expression, Bui et al. demonstrated CAIX expression in primary tumors was seen in 79% of all patients and was associated with improved survival and was independently associated with survival [36]. Patients in the series who were long-term responders to IL-2-based treatment also had high CAIX expression. A retrospective analysis performed by Atkins et al. further validated the utility of CAIX analysis and established that CAIX expression is correlated with response to IL-2, OS and better histopathologic risk subtype [37]. When the percentage of CAIX-positive tumor cells was used to dichotomize IL-2 treatment responders, 78% of the IL-2 treatment responders had high CAIX expression (>85%) compared with 51% of non-responders.

Genome-wide analyses are now being performed to identify alleles that are predictive of benefit from IL-2 and other systemic treatments. An array-based comparative genomic hybridization analysis identified loss of chromosome 4, 9, and 17p as possible predictors of non-response to IL-2 [38].

Prospective assessment of candidate predictors of IL-2 response was evaluated in the High-Dose Aldesleukin (IL-2) "Select" Trial [39, 40]. One hundred and twenty patients with metastatic or unresectable histologically confirmed RCC of any histologic type were enrolled and treated with standard bolus HD IL-2. The primary endpoint of the study was tumor response rate. The primary objective was to determine whether prospective selection of patients would result in a doubling of the response rate vs. historical series (from 14% to 28%). Surprisingly, the response rate for the entire study population was 28% (30% for the 115 subjects with clear cell carcinoma), whereas the median PFS was 4.2 months, close to the value seen historically. Surprisingly, the response rate in subjects in the prospectively assigned poor risk histology group was 33% ($n = 24$), and subjects with low CAIX expression (hypothesized to predict poor risk) had a response rate of 38%. Central review of histology and CAIX expression did not predict response to IL-2. No patients with a high risk UCLA SANI score responded to IL-2, and this group had inferior PFS. Analysis of additional biomarkers measured in blood and tumor tissues is ongoing. The high response rate seen in this study likely reflects the more stringent selection of patients for study entry in the modern era of alternative targeted therapies. It is likely that only those subjects felt most likely to benefit from IL-2 were identified for study screening. There is still much room to improve upon the response rate of 30% seen among the patients with clear cell RCC enrolled in the study. Given the toxicity of HD IL-2, the identification of biomarkers predictive of response remains an important unmet need.

IL-2 Therapy: Relapses

Although complete and partial responses with IL-2 therapy can be long-lasting, most patients eventually relapse. A series from the NCI reported on the pattern of relapse in 107 patients with metastatic RCC who had previously responded to IL-2-based therapy. Overall, 70% of all treated patients relapsed with most (55/64, 86%) occurring in patients with prior PRs as opposed to less than half as often (20/43, 43%) in patients with prior CRs. Interestingly, relapses tended to occur in previously identified sites of disease in patients with PRs whilst patients relapsing after a CR tended to involve new sites. Repeat IL-2-based therapy was rarely effective in the recurrent setting [41].

IL-2 Therapy: Current Indications and Future Directions

Bolus intravenous HD IL-2 therapy is a reasonable option in selected patients with good performance status and clear cell histology on the basis of sustained CRs in approximately 5–10% of patients treated, despite the significant cost and toxicity entailed with treatment. Ongoing research efforts are aimed at exploring combinations of high-dose IL-2 with other agents and at identifying predictive factors that portend for a greater

benefit with IL-2 therapy to limit therapy to those most likely to benefit.

Interferon

Isaacs and Lindenmann discovered interferons after noticing that heat-inactivated influenza virus appeared to inhibit the growth of live influenza virus in vitro in 1957. In the two decades that followed, multiple experiments suggested that interferons had antitumor effects in a broad range of laboratory models. Following the purification and subsequent cloning of interferon genes in the 1980s, it became clear that far from being a single molecule, interferons were a large family of structurally related molecules with diverse effects. Once the interferon gene was inserted into bacteria using recombinant DNA technology, it was a mere matter of time before the commercial applications of interferon were discovered.

IFNs are subclassified as types I and II according to their structural and functional properties. Type II IFNs (IFN-γ in humans) are released by Th1 cells. Signaling via the IFN-γ receptor (IFN-γR), IFN-γ recruits leucocytes to infected areas resulting in inflammation, stimulates macrophages to phagocytose engulfed bacteria and up-regulates the Th2 response. Type I IFNs comprise a number of structurally similar molecules that all signal via the IFN-α receptor (IFN-αR). Whilst several subtypes have been identified, IFN-α, IFN-β, and IFN-ω are the most important ones in humans. Type I IFNs are produced in large quantities chiefly by the plasmacytoid dendritic cell in response to infectious and other noxious stimuli. Connecting the adaptive and innate arms of the immune response, type 1 IFNs have potent immunoregulatory, antiproliferative, differentiation-inducing, apoptotic, and antiangiogenic properties.

Several reports in the early 1980s suggested that IFN-α therapy resulted in objective responses in RCC and led to a series of trials that examined the role of IFN-α in the metastatic setting against two major comparators—immunotherapeutic (low-dose IL-2) and non-immunotherapeutic agents (medroxyprogesterone and vinblastine).

IFN-α: Single Agent Therapy

Single-agent IFN-α dosed between 8 and 18 MU/dose given three times weekly by subcutaneous injection is associated with response rates of approximately 15–20%, the vast majority of which are partial and do not generally persist beyond 12 months. In a Cochrane meta-analysis of four studies involving a total of 644 patients, IFN-α therapy was superior to comparator treatments and demonstrated a survival benefit with an OR for death at 1 year of 0.56 (95% CI 0.40–0.77) and an overall HR for death of 0.74 (95% CI 0.63–0.88) [42]. The average median improvement in survival with IFN-α treatment was 3.8 months. This improvement in survival, albeit modest, coupled with the cost savings and reduced treatment-related toxicity compared to IL-2 administration resulted in IFN-α becoming a widely used treatment for metastatic RCC worldwide.

IFN-α Therapy: Combinations

Knowing that IL-2 mediates its effects by potentiating the cytotoxic effects of effector cells and that IFN-α appears to function by increasing expression of HLA class I and tumor-associated antigens, it was hypothesized that IL-2 and IFN-α would work synergistically in combination. IFN-α was combined with various schedules of IL-2 including low-dose SC injections [24, 43–49], intermediate-dose continuous infusions [22] and high-dose intravenous boluses [50–55]. Although several phase II showed improved response rates than would be expected with high-dose IL-2, phase III results did not show any increase in either PFS nor OS benefit over IFN-α alone [56].

Subsequently several phase II studies ought to further refine the regimen and compare high-dose bolus IV IL-2 to various comparators. Generally, it was found that 5–7% of patients on the high-dose intravenous IL-2 arms experienced durable CRs compared with 0–2% on control arms. Compared to control, the administration of HD IL-2 was associated with an increased remission (Peto Odds Ratio 1.82–2.70 [39, 42]). Mortality benefit was inconsistently observed—one study showed an improved OR of 0.95 (Peto OR 0.95, 95% CI 0.59–1.53) vs. low-dose IV IL-2 whilst another study reported an OR of 0.71 (Peto OR 0.71, 95% CI 0.40–1.26) vs. combination of IFN-α and low dose subcutaneous IL-2.

Multiple combinations of IFN-α and conventional chemotherapy have been evaluated—IFN-α/5-fluorouracil [57–59], IFN/vinblastine [60, 61], and IFN-α/cis-retinoic acid [62, 63]. Whilst initial reports from the phase II setting suggested an increase activity for combination therapy, this benefit was not consistently observed in the phase III setting. The IFN-α/5-fluorouracil combination appears to be the most active with a response rate that ranged from 13% to 33% in two studies. However, this has yet to be evaluated in the phase III setting.

With the advent of the targeted therapies, interest expanded in combining these agents with IFN-α. Several trials looked at the combination of IFN-α/sorafenib [64, 65], IFN-α/sunitinib [66] and IFN-α/bevacizumab [67–69].

The initial phase I trials involved the multi-kinase inhibitors sunitinib and sorafenib in combination with IFN-α dosed between 3 and 9 MU subcutaneously three times a week. The IFN-α/sunitinib combination was poorly tolerated with dose reduction required in 18/25 (72%) patients with an objective response rate (ORR) of 12%—comparable to what was commonly observed with IFN-α-alone but less than the 31% observed in phase II and phase III studies of single-agent sunitinib [70]. Additionally, the adverse events reported in the study suggested that the toxicities of the respective agents were apparently additive—with a higher incidence of neutropenia than previously reported for either agent singly. As a result, this combination is no longer being pursued.

Conversely, the combination of sorafenib plus IFN-α resulted in response rates of 19–33% in two phase II studies [64, 65]. A third phase II study from Italy compared two different IFN-α dosing options (9 MU three times a week vs. 3 MU five times a week) combined with sorafenib (dosed at 400 mg BID). Overall, in both arms, 26 responses (3 complete, 23 partial) were seen resulting in a CRR of 26% [71]. Toxicities resulting in dose reductions were common, exceeded the incidence for either drug alone and were dominated by adverse events common to IFN administration. This suggested that outcomes could be improved by minimizing sorafenib dose reductions whilst maintaining tolerability. However, randomized phase III trial data to demonstrate any benefit for the sorafenib/IFN-α combination over sorafenib alone is still lacking.

Two large international randomized trials—avastin and interferon in renal cancer (AVOREN) and cancer and leukemia group B (CALGB) 90206—examined the clinical efficacy of the IFN-α/bevacizumab combination vs. IFN-α alone. In both studies, IFN-α was dosed at 9×10^6 MU thrice weekly whilst bevacizumab was dosed at 10 mg/kg. The CALGB 90206 trial recruited 732 patients and reported an ORR of 25.5% for the combination vs. 13.1% for IFN-α alone [68]. Combination therapy was associated with a higher PFS (8.5 months vs. 5.2 months) and an improved HR for the treatment arm (0.67, 95% CI 0.57–0.79; $p < 0.0001$). In the AVOREN study, 649 patients were enrolled and randomized either to IFN-α/bevacizumab or IFN-α alone [67]. The median duration of PFS was significantly better in the combination treatment arm (10.2 months vs. 5.4 months; $p = 0.0001$) and was noted to be irrespective of the MSKCC risk category. In the AVOREN study investigators were able to report a survival benefit for the combination therapy arm (23 months vs. 21.3 months, $p = 0.1291$) that did not meet the criteria for statistical significance. The results of these two pivotal studies led to the approval of this combination for the first-line treatment of patients with metastatic RCC by the FDA in August 2009.

A trial combining IL-2/IFN-α with bevacizumab, 5-fluorouracil, and gemcitabine was recently published. In this study IL-2 (1 MIU/m² bid subcutaneously days 8, 9, 15, 16 and 1 MIU/m²/d subcutaneously from days 10 to 12 and from 17 to 19) and IFN-α (3 MIU subcutaneously on days 10, 12, 17, 19) were combined with bevacizumab (10 mg/kg days 1 and 15) and escalated

doses of 5-fluorouracil and gemcitabine delivered on days 1 and 8 in a 28-day cycle. Twenty-seven patients were enrolled. Fifty-nine percent had received prior systemic therapy. Thirty-three percent of the subjects had a partial tumor response [72]. Median time to progression was 6.4 months, with 8% of patients progression-free at 30 months. Median overall survival was 22.6 months.

In summary, when combined with cytotoxic agents or IL-2, combination chemotherapy with IFN-α has failed to provide significant improvement in response rates and/or OS (see Table 16.2). Notably the success of the IFN-α/bevacizumab combination in demonstrating an improvement in PFS has led to this regimen being approved by the FDA.

IFN-α Therapy: Prognostic Factors and Predictors of Response

Five pretreatment clinical variables (low Karnofsky performance status, high lactate dehydrogenase, low serum hemoglobin, high corrected serum calcium, and time from initial RCC diagnosis to start of IFN-α therapy of less than 1 year) were identified as prognostic factors by MSKCC investigators when they analyzed 463 patients with advanced RCC who received IFN-α as first-line systemic therapy in six prospective clinical trials [81]. They were able to subclassify patients into three risk stratifications: zero risk factors (favorable risk), one or two (intermediate risk), and three or more (poor risk). Favorable risk patients had improved *median survival* (30 months vs. 14 months and 5 months for intermediate and poor risk patients), *survival at 1 year* (83% vs. 58% and 20%), *2 years* (55% vs. 31% and 6%), and *3 years* (45% vs. 17% and 2%).

As yet, we have not yet identified clinical or pathological variables that are able to predict response to IFN-α therapy. In the Italian RAPSODY study of sorafenib plus IFN-α, investigators analyzed biomarkers including serum thrombospondin-1 (TSP-1), VEGF, VEGF receptor-2 (VEGFR-2), and basic-fibroblast growth factor (b-FGF) to see whether levels would be correlated with response to therapy. Of the four,

Table 16.2 Selected studies of cytokine/targeted therapy combinations in advanced renal cell cancer

Author (year published)	Design	Participants	Interventions	Results
SWOG-S0412 [73] (2007)	Multicenter, nonrandomized, phase II	$N=62$; PS (ECOG 1) 40%; median age 61; clear cell unknown; prior nephrectomy 87%	Sorafenib 400 mg BID+SC IFN-α2b 10×10^6 IU/ m^2 thrice weekly	OR (CR+PR + unconfirmed PR) (19/62): 30% SD (24/62): 39%
Gollob [64] (2007)	Multicenter, nonrandomized, phase II	$N=40$; PS (ECOG-1) 15%; median age 57; clear cell 88%; prior nephrectomy 88%	Sorafenib 400 mg BID+SC IFN-α2b 10×10^6 IU/ m^2 thrice weekly	OR (CR+PR) (13/40): 33% SD (18/40): 45%
AVOREN [67, 74] (2007)	Multicenter, phase III, placebo-controlled RCT	$N=649$; median age 61; PS (KPS>80) 94%; MSKCC risk—intermediate (56%) and poor (9%); predominantly clear cell; post-nephrectomy 99%	1. SC IFN-α2b 9×10^6 IU/m^2 thrice weekly+Bevacizumab10 mg/kg every 2 weeks 2. SC IFN-α2b 9×10^6 IU/m^2 thrice weekly+placebo	OR (CR+PR) (2007): Bev+IFN-α 31% vs. IFN-α alone 13% OS (months) (updated 2010): Median (ITT) Bev+IFN-α 23.3 vs. IFN-α alone 21.3 By MSKCC risk category: *Favorable:* Bev+IFN-α 35.1 vs. IFN-α alone 37.2 *Intermediate:* Bev+IFN-α 22.6 vs. IFN-α alone 19.3 *Poor:* Bev+IFN-α 6.0 vs. IFN-α alone 5.1
CALGB 90-206 [68, 75] (2008)	Multicenter, phase III, open label RCT	$N=732$; PS (ECOG—0) 62%; median age 61 years; MSKCC risk—intermediate (64%) and poor (10%); predominantly clear cell; prior nephrectomy 85%	1. SC IFN-α2b 9×10^6 IU/m^2 thrice weekly+Bevacizumab 10 mg/kg every 2 weeks 2. SC IFN-α2b 9×10^6 IU/m^2 thrice weekly alone	OR (CR+PR) (2008): Bev+IFN-α 25.5% vs. IFN-α alone 13.1% OS (months) (updated 2010): Median Bev+IFN-α 18.3 vs. IFN-α alone 17.4 By MSKCC risk category: *Favorable:* Bev+IFN-α 32.5 vs. IFN-α alone 33.5 *Intermediate:* Bev+IFN-α 17.7 vs. IFN-α alone 16.1 *Poor:* Bev+IFN-α 6.6 vs. IFN-α alone 5.7
CWGS [30] (2010)	Multicenter, phase II, open label trial	$N=49$; PS—KPS≥80%; median age 55; predominantly clear cell; prior nephrectomy unknown	1. HD IL-2 18×10^6 MU/m^2/day (6×10^5 MU/m^2/ dose q8) during two 5-day courses starting on day 15 and 29 of each 84 day cycle 2. + Bevacizumab 10 mg/kg every 2 weeks	Responses: CR (4/49): 8%; PR (10/49): 20%; SD (21/49): 42% PFS (months): Median—9.0 2 year—15%

Study	Design	Patient characteristics	Treatment	Results
MRC RE04/ EORTC GU 30012 [56] (2010)	Multicenter, randomized, phase III	$N = 1,006$; PS (WHO PS 0) 54%; MSKCC risk group (58–60% medium, 17–19% high); prior nephrectomy 89–90%	1. SC IFN-α 10×10^6 IU/m^2 3 days/week 2. Combination therapy with IFN-α, IL-2 and 5-FU	Best overall response (BORR) at 3 years: 16% (1) vs. 23% (2) Survival: At 1 year: 67% (IFN-α) vs. 67% (combination) At 3 years: PFS—5.5 months (IFN-α) vs. 5.3 months (combination) OS—30% (IFN-α) vs. 26% (combination)
Niwakawa [76] (2011)	Phase I, open-label, nonrandomized dose-escalation study	$N = 18$; PS (KPS > 70%); predominantly clear cell histo; prior nephrectomy unknown	1. Sorafenib 200 mg BID + IM IFN-α 6×10^6 IU/m^2 thrice weekly 2. Sorafenib 400 mg BID + IM IFN-α 6×10^6 IU/m^2 thrice weekly 3. Sorafenib 400 mg BID + IM IFN-α 9×10^6 IU/m^2 thrice weekly	OR (CR + PR): 28% SD (11/18): 61%
TORAVA [77] (2011)	Multi-center, phase II, open label trial	$N = 171$; PS (ECOG 0–1) 88%; median age 62; MSKCC risk group—intermediate (44–53%) and poor (10–17%); predominantly clear cell; prior nephrectomy 83–98%	1. Temsirolimus 25 mg weekly + Bevacizumab 10 mg/kg q2weeks 2. Sunitinib 50 mg/day for 4 weeks followed by 2 weeks off 3. IFN-α 9×10^6 IU/m^2 thrice weekly + Bevacizumab 10 mg/kg q2weeks	*Responses:* BORR: 27% (A) vs. 29% (B) vs. 43% (C) CR: 2% (A) vs. 0% (B) vs. 0% (C) PR: 25% (A) vs. 29% (B) vs. 43% (C) SD: 52% (A) vs. 48% (B) vs. 33% (C) Duration (months): 7.7 (A) vs. 13.3 (B) vs. 13.9 (C) *Survival:* 12 months: 77% (A) vs. 74% (B) vs. 90% (C) *Long term data—pending*
RECORD-2 [78]	Multicenter, phase II RCT	First-line, metastatic RCC Trial in progress: $N = 360$; PS—KPS $\geq$ 70%; predominantly clear cell; partial or complete nephrectomy allowed	1. Everolimus 10 mg PO daily + Bevacizumab 10 mg/kg q2weeks 2. IFN-α 9×10^6 IU/m^2 thrice weekly + Bevacizumab 10 mg/kg q2weeks	Awaiting data
INTORACT [79]	Multicenter, phase III, open label trial	1st line, metastatic RCC	1. Temsirolimus 25 mg weekly + Bevacizumab 10 mg/kg q2weeks 2. IFN-α 9×10^6 IU/m^2 thrice weekly + Bevacizumab 10 mg/kg q2weeks	Awaiting data

only low baseline serum VEGFR-2 was associated with a significantly improved median PFS in patients treated with sorafenib plus IFN [71].

IFN-α Therapy: Current Indications and Future Directions

IFN-α has an overall response rate as high as 15–20% in metastatic RCC. Responses tend to be partial and typically are not sustained. Treatment-related toxicity, especially a "flu-like" illness, is common and frequently requires dose reductions though symptoms appear to lessen with successive cycles of therapy. IFN-α therapy tends to be safe with no reported treatment-related deaths (compared to the near 4% mortality associated with IL-2 administration). Formal quality-of-life (QOL) assessments reported by Negrier et al. showed that IFN-α therapy was associated with QOL impacts in up to 16% of patients at 3 months compared to 11% in medroxyprogesterone controls [25].

However, IFN-α monotherapy has been upstaged by the advent of targeted therapies. In this new paradigm, there still appears to be a role for the use of IFN-α as part of a combination with various targeted therapies—most successfully IFN-α/bevacizumab. As the mechanisms of IFN-α activity in RCC are better understood, rationale for additional combinations of IFN-α with other therapies may emerge.

Vaccines

Vaccines: Heat Shock Protein Vaccines

A novel tumor vaccination approach using heat shock proteins (HSPs) has been developed based upon the preclinical work of Dr. P. Srivastava [82]. One function of HSPs is to chaperone antigenic peptides for loading onto MHC molecules in the endoplasmic reticulum for presentation to T lymphocytes. HSPs participate in the process of immunological cross-priming, in which exogenous protein antigens are internalized and processed by APC, then loaded onto MHC class I

molecules for presentation to APC [83]. HSP–peptide complexes enriched from cellular lysates are able to prime CD8+ T cells in a number of protein, viral and tumor models, and can confer tumor-specific protective immunity [84]. Jonasch et al. performed a study of autologous HSP gp96–peptide complexes in patients with metastatic RCC [85]. Eligible subjects had metastatic RCC with primary tumor in place. Cytoreductive nephrectomy was performed, and HSP gp96–peptide complexes were enriched from homogenates prepared from the fresh-frozen tumor tissue. The resulting autologous HSP gp96–protein complexes (vitespen, HSPPC-96, Oncophage) were injected into subjects starting approximately 4 weeks after surgery (six subcutaneous injections over 6 weeks). There were 60 evaluable patients, of whom two had a partial tumor response and two achieved a complete response. The latter two were reported to have had some degree of tumor shrinkage prior to starting the vaccine series. Patients who had stable disease were able to continue the vaccine in combination with low-dose subcutaneous IL-2. A randomized phase III study was performed in patients with localized RCC to study whether vitespen would prolong the recurrence-free survival after nephrectomy. Subjects were randomized to receive vitespen injected intradermally weekly for 4 weeks then every 2 weeks until vaccine depletion or observation. There were 818 patients enrolled and 728 who were evaluable in total. Fourteen subjects (2%) had AJCC stage I disease (6th edition), 253 subjects (35%) had stage II disease, 420 (58%) had stage III disease, and 41 (6%) had stage IV disease at nephrectomy. After a median follow-up of 1.9 years, there was no difference in recurrence-free or OS between the two study groups. An exploratory analysis found a trend toward improved recurrence-free survival in subjects with AJCC stage I or stage II disease.

Vaccines: Oncofetal Antigen 5T4 Vaccines

The oncofetal antigen, 5T4, has been studied as a tumor antigen in vaccines in RCC and other cancers. 5T4 is normally expressed on trophoblasts in the placenta, and at low levels in the postnatal esophagus. High levels of expression are seen in RCC and other carcinomas [86, 87]. MVA-5T4 is an attenuated vaccinia virus that has been engineered to express the 5T4 antigen for the purpose of eliciting a cellular immune response. Phase II studies have been performed evaluating MVA-5T4 as a tumor vaccine in RCC. Studies have examined the agent in combination with IL-2 and with interferon alpha. One study randomized patients to receive MVA-5T4 with or without subcutaneous IFN-α. Fifteen subjects received the MVA-5T4 vaccine alone and 28 subjects received MVA-5T4 plus subcutaneous IFN-alpha [88]. Both antibody and cellular immune responses (by interferon ELISPOT) were detected against the 5T4 antigen following vaccination. Twenty-one out of 25 subjects mounted a humoral immune response, and 14 out of 23 analyzed subjects mounted cellular immune responses against 5T4 based on ELISPOT. A partial response was documented in one subject. The median PFS was 3.8 months and 14 patients had stable disease for some period of time.

Another phase II study treated 25 subjects with MVA-5T4 plus subcutaneous IL-2 [89]. Most had received prior treatments including sunitinib, sorafenib, bevacizumab, everolimus, IL-2, and IFN. There was one patient who had a partial tumor response and two patients who had complete tumor responses. Six additional patients had stable disease for >6 months. Median PFS was 3.37 months and median OS was 12.87+ months. A subsequent phase III study randomized patients to MVA-5T4 vs. placebo in combination with a "standard of care" regimen. The standard regimen could be subcutaneous IL-2, subcutaneous interferon-alpha or sunitinib, at the discretion of the investigator. Seven hundred and thirty-two were evaluable for the intent-to-treat analysis: 32.8% were given IL-2 as the standard treatment, 22.6 interferon-alpha, and 51.2% sunitinib [90]. OS was equivalent between the two arms of the study: 20.1 months for the vaccine-treated patients and 19.2 months for the placebo group. There was also no difference in PFS at 26 weeks or in response rates. Antibody responses against the

5 T4 antigen were detected post-treatment in 56% of MVA-5T4-treated patients, and antibody.

Carbonic-Anhydrase IX Monoclnal Antibody Treatment

G250 is a murine monoclonal antibody that recognizes CAIX, a cell surface antigen on RCC cells [91]. Normal renal epithelium and most normal tissues do not express the G250 antigen, with the exception of gastric mucosa and bile duct epithelial cells [92]. cG250 is a human-murine chimeric mAb that was engineered from G250 for clinical investigation. A phase II study of cG250 was conducted in patients with metastatic RCC [93]. Weekly intravenous doses of cG250 were administered for up to 12 weeks. Extended treatment was offered to patients with stable disease or tumor responses. Thirty-six patients were enrolled, and all generally tolerated treatment well. Ten subjects showed stable disease after 12 weeks of study treatment, and eight of these still had stable disease after 24 weeks. One complete tumor response and one minor response were observed. A study of radio-immunotherapy using ^{131}I-congugated cG250 was performed to assess dosimetry and pharmacokinetics [94]. Surprisingly, eight out of 27 subjects developed human antichimeric antibodies. A study of cG250 monoclonal antibody conjugated to Yttryum-90 is ongoing. (Clinincal trials.gov identifier NCT00199875).

Non-myeloablative Allo-Transplantation

Conventional allogeneic stem cell transplantation for hematopoietic malignancies involves a myeloablative conditioning regimen of high-dose cytotoxic chemotherapy and/or total body irradiation. Myeloablative conditioning is followed by reconstitution with allogeneic hematopoietic stem cells derived from the bone marrow or peripheral blood. In addition to the direct cytotoxic effect of the conditioning regimen on the malignancy, a graft-vs. leukemia (GVL) effect has been well documented in hematologic malignancies such as leukemias, lymphomas, and multiple myeloma. The increased rates of relapse in patients whose donor stem cells undergo ex vivo T cell depletion [to reduce graft vs. host disease (GVH)] supports this hypothesis, as does the decreased rate of recurrence in patients who develop GVH [95]. In addition, the rate of relapse was higher in patients who received stem cells from an identical twin (syngeneic) than those who received a nonidentical graft. The clinical impact of GVL and results of non-myeloablative transplantation in hematopoietic malignancies led to the hypothesis that non-myeloablative allogeneic transplantation might generate graft. vs. tumor responses in metastatic RCC. Richard Childs and colleagues from the National Institutes of Health reported a series of patients with metastatic RCC who underwent non-myeloablative peripheral stem cell transplantation [96]. Seventeen of the 19 patients had received prior cytokine therapy (IL-2 or interferon). Seventeen of the 19 patients received HLA-matched sibling transplants, and two received sibling transplants with a single HLA locus mismatch. The conditioning regimen consisted of cyclophosphamide (60 mg/kg IV on day 5 and day 6) plus fludarabine 25 mg/m^2 I.V. on day 5 through 1 prior to transplantation. Antithymocyte globulin was also given to the two patients who had an HLA mismatch. All patients received cyclosporine prophylaxis against GVHD starting on day 4. Three patients out of 19 had a complete radiographic response and seven had a partial response by W.H.O. criteria. Interestingly, six of the patients had initial tumor growth after transplantation, followed by tumor response after cyclosporine was withdrawn. Engraftment of myeloid and T cell populations was successful in all patients. Tumor responses correlated with the development of GVH.

After the publication of this promising pilot study, there were several studies of non-myeloablative transplantation in RCC conducted in Europe and the USA. These data are summarized in a recent review by Tykodi et al. [97]. Their review covered 389 patients reported in 17 separate case series. Overall, the clinical efficacy seen in the original series by Childs et al. was not replicated in the subsequent studies. The aggregate tumor response rate was only 22% (vs. 53% in the NIH series). There were fewer complete responses and less durability of response.

Therapeutic Manipulation of Co-stimulatory Signals

Stimulation of the T cell receptor (TCR) by major histocompatibility protein (MHC)-peptide complexes expressed on antigen-presenting cells (APCs) triggers antigen-specific T lymphocyte activation. However, a "second signal" delivered through the interaction between additional proteins on T lymphocytes and APC is essential to the outcome of these antigen-specific interactions. The second signal determines whether TCR ligation by peptide antigen leads to proliferation, cytokine secretion, differentiation, apoptosis, or tolerance/anergy. Co-stimulatory interactions are critical for mounting effective immune responses and for the maintenance of peripheral tolerance.

The primary positive co-stimulatory signal for naïve and resting T cells is ligation of CD28, a type I transmembrane protein expressed by T lymphocytes. CD28 is activated by binding to the counter-receptors B7-1(CD80) and B7-2 (CD86), which are type I transmembrane proteins expressed by professional APC. After activation, T cells upregulate CTLA-4, which binds to B7 with higher affinity than CD28, thereby inhibiting TCR signaling, interleukin (IL)-2 transcription, and T-cell proliferation. In addition, CTLA-4:B7 interaction results in the induction of indolamine 2, 3 dioxygenase in a subset of dendritic cells, which switch to potent and dominant T cell suppressive properties [98].

Co-stimulation: Cytotoxic T lymphocyte Antigen-4

Cytotoxic T lymphocyte antigen-4 (CTLA-4) (CD152) is a transmembrane protein that functions as a key negative regulator in CD4$^+$ and CD8$^+$ T cells [99, 100] as well as CD4$^+$CD25$^+$Foxp3$^+$

naturally occurring regulatory T cells (Tregs) [101]. The role of CTLA-4 in the maintenance of peripheral tolerance as a negative regulator of adaptive immune response is illustrated by the phenotype of CTLA-4 knockout mice, which have massive polyclonal expansion of T cells, and die at early age with multiorgan lymphocytic infiltration resulting in severe myocarditis and pancreatitis in the absence of CTLA-4 [102, 103].

It was hypothesized that blockade of the inhibitory signal delivered by CTLA-4 might allow development of antitumor T-cell immune responses in patients with cancer. Antibody blockade of CTLA-4, alone [104, 105] or in combination with a GM-CSF-containing tumor vaccine was able to eradicate established tumors in murine models including B16 melanoma [106] and mammary tumors [107]. Two monoclonal antibodies against CTLA-4 have entered clinical development. Ipilimumab (MDX-010) and tremelimumab (CP-675206) are fully human monoclonal antibodies that recognize CTLA-4 and block its interaction with B7 proteins. Tremelimumab (CP-675,206) was first studied in a phase I trial in 2002–2003, where 39 patients were accrued, of which 34 patients had melanoma, four patients had stage IV RCC, and one patient had stage IV colon cancer [108]. Although the trial was not designed to detect tumor response, 13 patients with melanoma had clinical benefit from tremelimumab, and durable objective tumor responses were observed 25+ to 36+ months (two patients with complete response and two patients with partial response). Not surprisingly, some patients developed autoimmune thyroiditis, colitis, vitiligo, and hypophysitis, indicative of breaking peripheral tolerance to "self" tissues.

Association between anti-CTLA-4 antibody-induced tumor response and autoimmune colitis was studied using ipilimumab in 189 patients with metastatic melanoma or RCC [109]. The overall response rate was 14%, and the ORR was 36% for melanoma patients with enterocolitis and 35% RCC patients with enterocolitis, compared with 11% and 2% in patients without enterocolitis, respectively ($p = 0.0065$ and 0.0016, respectively). The authors showed the pathology

of the colitis was due to neutrophil and lymphocyte infiltration and could be managed with high-dose corticosteroids or TNF alpha inhibitor, infliximab, in steroid-refractory cases without affecting tumor response.

Ipilimumab was approved by the FDA for treatment of metastatic melanoma based upon the results of a phase III study in which ipilimumab was shown to improve median OS compared to a peptide antigen derived from the melanosomal protein, glycoprotein 100 (gp100) [110]. This peptide has been shown to be presented by the HLA-A*0201 MHC, and so protocol eligibility was restricted to HLA-A*0201-positive individuals. Subjects were randomized in a 3:1:1 ratio to ipilimumab 3 mg/kg plus gp100 peptide vaccine, ipilimumab plus gp100 placebo or gp100 plus ipilimumab placebo. Each subject received assigned study treatment every 3 weeks × 4 doses. The median survival for the ipilimumab alone and ipilimumab plus gp100 groups were 10.1 and 10.0 months, respectively. A statistically significant difference between each of these ipilimumab-containing groups and the gp100 group (median survival 6.4 months) was demonstrated. PFS was also superior in the ipilimumab-containing groups. The overall response rate in the ipilimumab-alone group was 10.9 months. Interestingly, nine of 15 objective responses to ipilimumab were durable beyond 2 years.

The activity of ipilimumab in metastatic clear cell RCC was studied in a phase II trial reported by Yang et al. from the National Cancer Institute [111]. Ipilimumab was administered every 3 weeks intravenously. One cohort of 21 patients received a loading dose of 3 mg/kg followed by 1.5 mg/kg per dose. A second cohort of 40 patients received 3 mg/kg at each dosing. All of the subjects in the lower dose cohort and 26 of the patients in the higher dose cohort had received prior high dose IL-2. Eight subjects had received prior chemotherapy. Autoimmune toxicities were observed including enteritis and colonic perforation, rash, aseptic meningitis, hypophysitis, and hypopituitarism. The rate of grade III toxicity was 14% in the lower dose cohort and 35% in the higher dose cohort. Five of 40 patients (12.5%) in the cohort who received 3 mg/kg q3week dosing responded—the durations of these responses were 7, 8, 12, 17, and 21 months [111]. All of these responding subjects developed autoimmune toxicity, whereas none of the subjects who did not develop autoimmunity had an objective tumor response. The association of autoimmune toxicity from ipilimumab and tumor response was highly significant ($p = 0.0009$).

Rini and colleagues reported the results of a phase I dose escalation study in which tremelimumab was combined with the multitargeted kinase inhibitor, sunitinib in patients with metastatic RCC [112]. Tremelimumab was administered intravenously once every 12 weeks, and sunitinib as administered daily at 37.5 mg or at 50 mg on a 28-day on/14 day off schedule. The most common dose-limiting toxicity (DLT) was acute renal failure, which was seen in four patients. One of these underwent renal biopsy, which revealed interstitial nephritis with eosinophilic infiltration, consistent with hypersensitivity reaction. One subject developed a DLT of colitis, and another experienced a sudden death at home. The maximum tolerated dose (MTD) was determined to be 10 mg/kg of tremelimumab every 12 weeks in combination with sunitinib 37.5 mg daily. However, there was unacceptable toxicity in patients treated in the expansion cohort at the MTD, and the authors did not recommend pursuing these doses of the combination in phase II studies.

Co-stimulation: Programmed Death-1 (PD-1) and PD-1 Ligand (B7-H1)

The programmed death-1 (PD-1, CD279) protein is a member of the CD28 family that is expressed on activated, but not resting T cells, B cells, and myeloid cells [113, 114]. PD-1 binds to the B7 homolog, programmed cell death 1 ligand 1 (PD-L1), also known as B7 homolog (B7-H1) and as CD274. A second B7 homolog that binds PD-1 has been identified and is known as PD-L2 [115] and as B7-DC. Interaction of PD-1 with PD-L1 inhibits T cell proliferation, survival, and function, whereas blockade of PD-1 increases autoantibody production and generates auto-

reactive T cells [116]. Like CTLA-4, PD-1 also functions as a negative regulator of immune responses, as supported by the development of autoimmune glomerulonephritis, arthritis, and cardiomyopathy in PD-1 knockout mice [117, 118]. PD-L1 (B7-H1) is expressed abundantly on certain tumors and by cells of the tumor microenvironment [119, 120]. In RCC tumors, expression of B7-H1 is prognostic for aggressive tumor behavior and poor survival [119]. Furthermore, PD-1 expression on tumor infiltrating mononuclear cells was greater in patients with high-risk, larger, and/or symptomatic RCC tumors, higher nuclear grade, more advanced tumor-node-metastasis stage, coagulative necrosis, and sarcomatoid differentiation [121]. There was a correlation between expression of B7H-1 on RCC tumor cells and expression of PD-1 on tumor infiltrating mononuclear cells among the RCC specimens studied.

Analogous to CTLA-4 blockade by ipilimumab and temelimumab, monoclonal antibodies that block the interaction between PD-1 and B7-H1 are being developed to test the clinical impact of abrogating the negative signal delivered to T cells by PD ligand-expressing cancer cells. A phase I study of a fully humanized, anti-PD-1 IgG4 monoclonal antibody, MDX-1106 (BMS-936558/ONO-4538), was conducted in patients with refractory solid tumors [122]. Subjects received MDX-1106 intravenously and had restaging scans at 8 and 12 weeks. Repeat dosing could be administered at 12 and 16 weeks to patients who did not have intolerable toxicity, disease progression or development of antibodies against MDX-1106. Doses of 0.3, 1, 3, and 10 mg/kg were evaluated. There were no dose-limiting toxicities as defined by the study during the 28-day evaluation phase following the first dose of MDX-1106. There was one case of grade 3 inflammatory colitis in a patient who received five doses of study treatment, as well as a case of grade 2 hypothyroidism and two cases of polyarticular arthropathies. MDX-1106 was deemed tolerable at the doses evaluated. One subject with colorectal cancer achieved a complete response and one subject with melanoma achieved partial response. A patient who had multiorgan metastatic RCC, who had failed sunitinib, sorafenib and an experimental histone deacetylase inhibitor previously, had a partial response that lasted 16+ months [122].

A second phase I study of this monoclonal antibody included 18 patients with RCC—16 of whom were treated at a dose of 10 mg/kg. The toxicity profile of MDX-1106 (BMS936558) was similar to that observed in the previous study. Common adverse events included fatigue, diarrhea, rash, endocrinopathies. There was one case of drug-related pneumonitis. Five of these patients (31.3%) achieved confirmed partial responses, and another three (18.8%) achieved stable disease lasting more than 6 months [123].

Recently, the final phase I trial results of the anti-PD-1 (BMS-936558) and anti-PD-L1 (BMS-936559) antibodies were published [123, 124]. The phase I study of anti-PD-1 (BMS-936558) enrolled 296 patients with a variety of advanced solid tumors to receive PD-L1 antibody as an infusion every 2 weeks of an 8-week cycle in 3 dose-escalations (1, 3 and 10 mg/kg) with response assessments after each cycle. Authors reported objective evidence of response in a variety of tumor types including non-small cell lung cancer (NSCLC). Of the 33 patients enrolled with RCC, 9 responses were noted for an objective response rate of 27% compared to 24.1% for the trial overall. Notably responses were durable – greater than 12 months in 20 of 31 treated patients with greater than 1 year follow-up – and consistent with prior patterns of immune-related response previously described in patients treated with ipilimumab [125]. Tumor PD-L1 expression was not required and expression status was only available on 61 tumor specimens from 42 patients – 5 of whom had RCC. Interestingly, when responses were dichotomized according to PD-L1 expression, objective responses were noted in 9/25 PD-L1 positive patients but none in the 17 PD-L1 negative patients. Of the 5 patients with RCC on whom expression status was available (4 positive, 1 negative), responses were noted in 2 (both PD-L1 positive).

The study assessing PD-L1 blocking antibody (BMS-936559) which inhibits binding of PD-L1 to both PD-1 and CD80 was concurrently published. This phase I trial enrolled 207 patients (17 with renal cell cancer) with a variety of advanced solid tumors to receive BMS-936559 (dose range 0.3-10 mg/kg) in a standard 3+3 dose escalation design. As with the BMS-936558 trial, responses were noted in multiple tumor types including ovarian cancer and NSCLC with an overall response rate of 12.6% in the 135 patients in whom response was evaluable with a RCC-specific response rate of 12%.

These studies suggest that checkpoint inhibition is a viable option in advanced malignancies with relatively minimal toxicity (overall incidence of Grade 3/4 toxicity was 14% and 9% in the anti-PD-1 and anti-PD-L1 trials respectively) and durable responses even in traditionally non-immunogenic cancers malignancies such as ovarian cancer and NSCLC. PD-1 blockade appears to be associated with greater responses than PD-L1 blockade suggesting that these drugs are not identical in their downstream effects. Further trials planned include phase I biomarker study (NCT01358721), phase II dose-finding study in metastatic RCC (NCT01354431) and phase III trials in renal cell cancer, melanoma and NSCLC. Emerging evidence implicates PD-L1 mediated immune-downregulation in tumors evasion of immune surveillance suggesting that combinations of checkpoint inhibitors such as PD-1/PD-L1 antagonists and agents directly stimulating anti-tumor immunity may need to be combined for effective immunotherapy [126].

Effect of the Kinase Inhibitor, Sunitinib, on Immune Responses

Since the introduction of sunitinib, the effect of this multitargeted kinase inhibitor on immune function has been studied in efforts to better understand its mechanism and possible integration into immunotherapeutic options. It has been recognized that in RCC patients, there is a shift from a type-1-mediated CD4+ T cell response producing IFN-gamma, which is critical for antitumor effect, to a type-2 cytokine response (IL-4, IL-5, IL-10) that mediates humoral immunity [127, 128]. The type-2 bias of CD4+ T cells from patients with mRCC can be reversed with sunitinib, as it promotes type-1 cytokine response (IFN-gamma) and simultaneously decrease the type-2 response (IL-4) [129]. Furthermore, sunitinib suppresses the activity of CD3+CD4+CD25hiFoxp3+ Tregs without inhibiting the expansion of CD3+CD4+CD25− T effector cells. It is widely recognized that there is an increased frequency of CD4+CD25hi Tregs in tumor sites or the peripheral blood of patients with advanced, and depletion of Tregs in murine models with anti-CD25 antibody enhances antitumor activity [130].

The reduction in Tregs in mRCC patients treated with sunitinib is also associated with the reduction in CD15+CD14− and CD33+HLA-DR− myeloid-derived suppressor cells (MDSCs) [131]. MDSC represent a heterogeneous population of cells that impair T effector function [132] and stimulate Treg formation [133]. MDSC have been detected in peripheral blood of patients with tumors [134]. Elevated levels of MDSC were measured in mRCC patients compared to age-matched normal donors, which was decreased to normal levels with sunitinib. Furthermore, sunitinib-mediated reduction in MDSC was correlated with reversal of type-1 T cell suppression, as well as reversal of CD3+CD4+CD25hiFoxp3+ Treg elevation [131]. Neither the reversal of type-1 T cell suppression nor the reversal of Treg and MDSC elevation in mRCC patients correlated with tumor response or PFS in sunitinib-treated patients. To evaluate potential synergistic immune-stimulatory antitumor effects, a phase I trial of tremelimumab plus sunitinib was conducted in 28 patients with mRCC [112]. Rapid onset of renal toxicity was the most common DLT, one patient died of perforated colon and another patient suffered sudden death. Although the study was too small to fully assess tumor response, the observed partial response was 43%, somewhat higher than the historical phase 3 trial of sunitinib alone (31%) [70]. The clinical use of sunitinib as an adjunct in immuno-stimulatory therapeutic option remains to be described.

Conclusion

The inherent immunogenicity of RCC has seen led to many immunologically mediated antineoplastic approaches being tested in both the adjuvant and metastatic settings. Of the nonspecific cytokines, IL-2 and IFN-α have been the most extensively tested with only modest results in unselected patients populations. Once a mainstay of treatment, IFN-α, has been supplanted by targeted agents which have demonstrated PFS benefits in randomized clinical trials. High-dose IL-2 produces durable complete responses in a minority of patients with metastatic disease—however given the associated morbidity, use should be restricted to highly selected patients in appropriately experienced centers. Putative biomarkers of IL-2 efficacy have been suggested but lack validation in prospective studies.

Targeted therapies have redefined options for treatment of advanced RCC. The burgeoning of molecularly targeted agents in recent years does not negate a role for immunotherapy in RCC—rather it behooves us to consider identify predictive biomarkers for response to immunotherapy and pursue rational combinations of immunotherapeutic and targeted agents based on tumor and patient characteristics.

References

1. Rohdenburg GL. Fluctuations in the growth energy of malignant tumours in man, with special reference to spontaneous regression. J Cancer Res. 1918;3:193.
2. Vogelzang NJ, Priest ER, Borden L. Spontaneous regression of histologically proved pulmonary metastases from renal cell carcinoma: a case with 5-year followup. J Urol. 1992;148(4):1247–8.
3. Oliver RT, Nethersell AB, Bottomley JM. Unexplained spontaneous regression and alpha-interferon as treatment for metastatic renal carcinoma. Br J Urol. 1989; 63(2):128–31.
4. Middleton RG. Surgery for metastatic renal cell carcinoma. J Urol. 1967;97(6):973–7.
5. Bloom HJ. Hormone-induced and spontaneous regression of metastatic renal cancer. Cancer. 1973; 32(5):1066–71.
6. Elhilali MM, Gleave M, Fradet Y, et al. Placebo-associated remissions in a multicentre, randomized, double-blind trial of interferon gamma-1b for the treatment of metastatic renal cell carcinoma. The Canadian Urologic Oncology Group. BJU Int. 2000;86(6):613–8.
7. Gleave ME, Elhilali M, Fradet Y, et al. Interferon gamma-1b compared with placebo in metastatic renal-cell carcinoma. Canadian Urologic Oncology Group. N Engl J Med. 1998;338(18):1265–71.

8. Parada SA, Franklin JM, Uribe PS, Manoso MW. Renal cell carcinoma metastases to bone after a 33-year remission. Orthopedics. 2009;32(6):446.

9. Young RC. Metastatic renal-cell carcinoma: what causes occasional dramatic regressions? N Engl J Med. 1998;338(18):1305–6.

10. Morgan DA, Ruscetti FW, Gallo R. Selective in vitro growth of T lymphocytes from normal human bone marrows. Science. 1976;193(4257):1007–8.

11. Lotze MT, Robb RJ, Sharrow SO, Frana LW, Rosenberg SA. Systemic administration of interleukin-2 in humans. J Biol Response Mod. 1984;3(5):475–82.

12. Rosenberg SA, Grimm EA, McGrogan M, et al. Biological activity of recombinant human interleukin-2 produced in *Escherichia coli*. Science. 1984;223(4643):1412–4.

13. Taniguchi T, Matsui H, Fujita T, et al. Structure and expression of a cloned cDNA for human interleukin-2. Nature. 1983;302(5906):305–10.

14. Rosenberg SA, Mule JJ, Spiess PJ, Reichert CM, Schwarz SL. Regression of established pulmonary metastases and subcutaneous tumor mediated by the systemic administration of high-dose recombinant interleukin 2. J Exp Med. 1985;161(5):1169–88.

15. Lafreniere R, Rosenberg SA. Successful immunotherapy of murine experimental hepatic metastases with lymphokine-activated killer cells and recombinant interleukin 2. Cancer Res. 1985;45(8):3735–41.

16. Lotze MT, Chang AE, Seipp CA, Simpson C, Vetto JT, Rosenberg SA. High-dose recombinant interleukin 2 in the treatment of patients with disseminated cancer. Responses, treatment-related morbidity, and histologic findings. JAMA. 1986;256(22):3117–24.

17. Rosenberg SA, Lotze MT, Muul LM, et al. Observations on the systemic administration of autologous lymphokine-activated killer cells and recombinant interleukin-2 to patients with metastatic cancer. N Engl J Med. 1985;313(23):1485–92.

18. Fyfe G, Fisher RI, Rosenberg SA, Sznol M, Parkinson DR, Louie AC. Results of treatment of 255 patients with metastatic renal cell carcinoma who received high-dose recombinant interleukin-2 therapy. J Clin Oncol. 1995;13(3):688–96.

19. Rosenberg SA, Lotze MT, Yang JC, et al. Prospective randomized trial of high dose interleukin-2 alone or in conjunction with lymphokine-activated killer cells for the treatment of patients with advanced cancer. J Natl Cancer Inst. 1993;85(8):622–32.

20. Yang JC, Topalian SL, Parkinson D, et al. Randomized comparison of high-dose and low-dose intravenous interleukin-2 for the therapy of metastatic renal cell carcinoma: an interim report. J Clin Oncol. 1994;12(8):1572–6.

21. Yang JC, Topalian SL, Schwartzentruber DJ, et al. The use of polyethylene glycolmodified interleukin-2 (PEG-IL-2) in the treatment of patients with metastatic renal cell carcinoma and melanoma. A phase I study and a randomized prospective study comparing IL-2 alone versus IL-2 combined with PEG-IL-2. Cancer. 1995;76(4):687–94.

22. Negrier S, Escudier B, Lasset C, et al. Recombinant human interleukin-2, recombinant human interferon alfa-2a, or both in metastatic renal-cell carcinoma. Groupe Francais d'Immunotherapie. N Engl J Med. 1998;338(18):1272–8.

23. Yang JC, Sherry RM, Steinberg SM, et al. Randomized study of high-dose and low-dose interleukin-2 in patients with metastatic renal cancer. J Clin Oncol. 2003;21(16):3127–32.

24. McDermott DF, Regan MM, Clark JI, et al. Randomized phase III trial of high-dose interleukin-2 versus subcutaneous interleukin-2 and interferon in patients with metastatic renal cell carcinoma. J Clin Oncol. 2005;23(1):133–41.

25. Negrier S, Perol D, Ravaud A, et al. Medroxyprogesterone, interferon alfa-2a, interleukin 2, or combination of both cytokines in patients with metastatic renal carcinoma of intermediate prognosis: results of a randomized controlled trial. Cancer. 2007;110(11):2468–77.

26. McDermott DF, Ghebremichael MS, Signoretti S, et al. The high-dose aldesleukin (HD IL-2) "SELECT" trial in patients with metastatic renal cell carcinoma (mRCC). J Clin Oncol. 2010;28(Suppl):15s [Abstr 4514].

27. Lotze MT, Matory YL, Rayner AA, et al. Clinical effects and toxicity of interleukin-2 in patients with cancer. Cancer. 1986;58(12):2764–72.

28. Majhail NS, Wood L, Elson P, Finke J, Olencki T, Bukowski RM. Adjuvant subcutaneous interleukin-2 in patients with resected renal cell carcinoma: a pilot study. Clin Genitourin Cancer. 2006;5(1):50–6.

29. Clark JI, Atkins MB, Urba WJ, et al. Adjuvant high-dose bolus interleukin-2 for patients with high-risk renal cell carcinoma: a cytokine working group randomized trial. J Clin Oncol. 2003;21(16):3133–40.

30. Dandamudi UB, Ghebremichael MS, Sosman JA, et al. A phase II study of bevacizumab (B) and high-dose aldesleukin (IL-2) in patients (p) with metastatic renal cell carcinoma (mRCC): a Cytokine Working Group Study (CWGS). J Clin Oncol. 2010;28(Suppl 15S) [Abstr 4530].

31. Procopio G, Verzoni E, Bracarda S, et al. Sorafenib with interleukin-2 vs sorafenib alone in metastatic renal cell carcinoma: the ROSORC trial. Br J Cancer. 2011;104(8):1256–61.

32. Leibovich BC, Han K-R, Bui MHT, et al. Scoring algorithm to predict survival after nephrectomy and immunotherapy in patients with metastatic renal cell carcinoma. Cancer. 2003;98(12):2566–75.

33. Motzer RJ, Bacik J, Mariani T, Russo P, Mazumdar M, Reuter V. Treatment outcome and survival associated with metastatic renal cell carcinoma of non-clear-cell histology. J Clin Oncol. 2002;20(9):2376–81.

34. Upton MP, Parker RA, Youmans A, McDermott DF, Atkins MB. Histologic predictors of renal cell carcinoma response to interleukin-2-based therapy. J Immunother. 2005;28(5):488–95.

35. Pantuck AJ, Fang Z, Liu X, et al. Gene expression and tissue microarray analysis of interleukin-2 complete

responders in patients with metastatic renal cell carcinoma. J Clin Oncol. 2005;23(16S) [Abstr 4535].

36. Bui MH, Seligson D, Han KR, et al. Carbonic anhydrase IX is an independent predictor of survival in advanced renal clear cell carcinoma: implications for prognosis and therapy. Clin Cancer Res. 2003;9(2):802–11.

37. Atkins M, Regan M, McDermott D, et al. Carbonic anhydrase IX expression predicts outcome of interleukin 2 therapy for renal cancer. Clin Cancer Res. 2005;11(10):3714–21.

38. Jaeger E, Waldman F, Roydasgupta R, et al. Array-based comparative genomic hybridization (CGH) identifies chromosomal imbalances between Interleukin-2 complete and non-responders. J Clin Oncol. 2008;26(Suppl) [Aabstr 5043].

39. McDermott DF, Ghebremichael MS, Signoretti S, et al. The high-dose aldesleukin (HD IL-2) "SELECT" trial in patients with metastatic renal cell carcinoma (mRCC). J Clin Oncol. 2010;28(15S) [Abstr 4514].

40. Clement JM, McDermott DF. The high-dose aldesleukin (IL-2) "select" trial: a trial designed to prospectively validate predictive models of response to high-dose IL-2 treatment in patients with metastatic renal cell carcinoma. Clin Genitourin Cancer. 2009;7(2):E7–9.

41. Lee DS, White DE, Hurst R, Rosenberg SA, Yang JC. Patterns of relapse and response to retreatment in patients with metastatic melanoma or renal cell carcinoma who responded to interleukin-2-based immunotherapy. Cancer J Sci Am. 1998;4(2):86–93.

42. Coppin C, Porzsolt F, Awa A, Kumpf J, Coldman A, Wilt T. Immunotherapy for advanced renal cell cancer. Cochrane Database Syst Rev. 2005;1:CD001425.

43. Atzpodien J, Kirchner H, Jonas U, et al. Interleukin-2- and interferon alfa-2a-based immunochemotherapy in advanced renal cell carcinoma: a Prospectively Randomized Trial of the German Cooperative Renal Carcinoma Chemoimmunotherapy Group (DGCIN). J Clin Oncol. 2004;22(7):1188–94.

44. Atzpodien J, Lopez Hanninen E, Kirchner H, et al. Multiinstitutional home-therapy trial of recombinant human interleukin-2 and interferon alfa-2 in progressive metastatic renal cell carcinoma. J Clin Oncol. 1995;13(2):497–501.

45. Dutcher JP, Fisher RI, Weiss G, et al. Outpatient subcutaneous interleukin-2 and interferon-alpha for metastatic renal cell cancer: five-year follow-up of the Cytokine Working Group Study. Cancer J Sci Am. 1997;3(3):157–62.

46. Vogelzang NJ, Lipton A, Figlin RA. Subcutaneous interleukin-2 plus interferon alfa-2a in metastatic renal cancer: an outpatient multicenter trial. J Clin Oncol. 1993;11(9):1809–16.

47. van Herpen CM, Jansen RL, Kruit WH, et al. Immunochemotherapy with interleukin-2, interferon-alpha and 5-fluorouracil for progressive metastatic renal cell carcinoma: a multicenter phase II study. Dutch Immunotherapy Working Party. Br J Cancer. 2000;82(4):772–6.

48. Atkins MB, Dutcher J, Weiss G, et al. Kidney cancer: the Cytokine Working Group experience (1986–2001): part I. IL-2-based clinical trials. Med Oncol. 2001;18(3):197–207.

49. Rathmell WK, Malkowicz SB, Holroyde C, Luginbuhl W, Vaughn DJ. Phase II trial of 5-fluorouracil and leucovorin in combination with interferon-alpha and interleukin-2 for advanced renal cell cancer. Am J Clin Oncol. 2004;27(2):109–12.

50. Rosenberg SA, Lotze MT, Yang JC, et al. Combination therapy with interleukin-2 and alpha-interferon for the treatment of patients with advanced cancer. J Clin Oncol. 1989;7(12):1863–74.

51. Atkins MB, Sparano J, Fisher RI, et al. Randomized phase II trial of high-dose interleukin-2 either alone or in combination with interferon alfa-2b in advanced renal cell carcinoma. J Clin Oncol. 1993;11(4):661–70.

52. Sznol M, Mier JW, Sparano J, et al. A phase I study of high-dose interleukin-2 in combination with interferon-alpha 2b. J Biol Response Mod. 1990;9(6):529–37.

53. Bergmann L, Fenchel K, Weidmann E, et al. Daily alternating administration of high-dose alpha-2b-interferon and interleukin-2 bolus infusion in metastatic renal cell cancer. A phase II study. Cancer. 1993;72(5):1733–42.

54. Spencer WF, Linehan WM, Walther MM, et al. Immunotherapy with interleukin-2 and alpha-interferon in patients with metastatic renal cell cancer with in situ primary cancers: a pilot study. J Urol. 1992;147(1):24–30.

55. Budd GT, Murthy S, Finke J, et al. Phase I trial of high-dose bolus interleukin-2 and interferon alfa-2a in patients with metastatic malignancy. J Clin Oncol. 1992;10(5):804–9.

56. Gore ME, Griffin CL, Hancock B, et al. Interferon alfa-2a versus combination therapy with interferon alfa-2a, interleukin-2, and fluorouracil in patients with untreated metastatic renal cell carcinoma (MRC RE04/EORTC GU 30012): an open-label randomised trial. Lancet. 2010;375(9715):641–8.

57. Falcone A, Cianci C, Ricci S, Brunetti I, Bertuccelli M, Conte PF. Alpha-2B-interferon plus floxuridine in metastatic renal cell carcinoma. A phase I-II study. Cancer. 1993;72(2):564–8.

58. Igarashi T, Marumo K, Onishi T, et al. Interferon-alpha and 5-fluorouracil therapy in patients with metastatic renal cell cancer: an open multicenter trial. The Japanese Study Group Against Renal Cancer. Urology. 1999;53(1):53–9.

59. Elias L, Blumenstein BA, Kish J, et al. A phase II trial of interferon-alpha and 5-fluorouracil in patients with advanced renal cell carcinoma. A Southwest Oncology Group study. Cancer. 1996;78(5):1085–8.

60. Neidhart JA, Anderson SA, Harris JE, et al. Vinblastine fails to improve response of renal cancer to interferon alfa-n1: high response rate in patients with pulmonary metastases. J Clin Oncol. 1991;9(5):832–6.

61. Fossa SD, Martinelli G, Otto U, et al. Recombinant interferon alfa-2a with or without vinblastine in metastatic renal cell carcinoma: results of a European multicenter phase III study. Ann Oncol. 1992;3(4):301–5.

62. Motzer RJ, Murphy BA, Bacik J, et al. Phase III trial of interferon alfa-2a with or without 13-cis-retinoic acid for patients with advanced renal cell carcinoma. J Clin Oncol. 2000;18(16):2972–80.

63. Aass N, De Mulder PH, Mickisch GH, et al. Randomized phase II/III trial of interferon Alfa-2a with and without 13-cis-retinoic acid in patients with progressive metastatic renal cell Carcinoma: the European Organisation for Research and Treatment of Cancer Genito-Urinary Tract Cancer Group (EORTC 30951). J Clin Oncol. 2005;23(18):4172–8.

64. Gollob JA, Rathmell WK, Richmond TM, et al. Phase II trial of sorafenib plus interferon alfa-2b as first- or second-line therapy in patients with metastatic renal cell cancer. J Clin Oncol. 2007;25(22):3288–95.

65. Ryan CW, Goldman BH, Lara Jr PN, et al. Sorafenib with interferon alfa-2b as first-line treatment of advanced renal carcinoma: a phase II study of the Southwest Oncology Group. J Clin Oncol. 2007;25(22):3296–301.

66. Motzer RJ, Hudes G, Wilding G, et al. Phase I trial of sunitinib malate plus interferon-alpha for patients with metastatic renal cell carcinoma. Clin Genitourin Cancer. 2009;7(1):28–33.

67. Escudier B, Pluzanska A, Koralewski P, et al. Bevacizumab plus interferon alfa-2a for treatment of metastatic renal cell carcinoma: a randomised, double-blind phase III trial. Lancet. 2007;370(9605):2103–11.

68. Rini BI, Halabi S, Rosenberg JE, et al. Phase III trial of bevacizumab plus interferon alfa versus interferon alfa monotherapy in patients with metastatic renal cell carcinoma: final results of CALGB 90206. J Clin Oncol. 2010;28(13):2137–43.

69. Melichar B, Koralewski P, Ravaud A, et al. First-line bevacizumab combined with reduced dose interferon-alpha2a is active in patients with metastatic renal cell carcinoma. Ann Oncol. 2008;19(8):1470–6.

70. Motzer RJ, Hutson TE, Tomczak P, et al. Sunitinib versus interferon alfa in metastatic renal-cell carcinoma. N Engl J Med. 2007;356(2):115–24.

71. Bracarda S, Ludovini V, Porta C, et al. Serum thrombospondin-1 (TSP-1), vascular endothelial growth factor (VEGF), VEGF receptor-2 (VEGFR-2), and basic-fibroblast growth factor (b-FGF) as predictive factors for sorafenib plus interferon-alfa-2a (IFN) in metastatic renal cell carcinoma (MRCC): Biologic results from the randomized phase II RAPSODY trial. J Clin Oncol. 2010;28(15s) [Abstr 4628].

72. Buti S, Lazzarelli S, Chiesa MD, et al. Dose-finding trial of a combined regimen with bevacizumab, immunotherapy, and chemotherapy in patients with metastatic renal cell cancer: An Italian Oncology Group for Clinical Research (GOIRC) study. J Immunother. 2010;33(7):735–41.

73. Ryan CW, Goldman BH, Lara Jr PN, Mack PC, Beer TM, Tangen CM, Lemmon D, Pan CX, Drabkin HA, Crawford ED. Sorafenib with interferon alfa-2b as first-line treatment of advanced renal carcinoma: a phase II study of the Southwest Oncology Group. J Clin Oncol. 2007;25(22):3296–301.

74. Escudier B, Bellmunt J, Négrier S, et al. Phase III trial of bevacizumab plus interferon alfa-2a in patients with metastatic renal cell carcinoma (AVOREN): final analysis of overall survival. J Clin Oncol. 2010;28(13):2144–50.

75. Rini BI, Halabi S, Rosenberg JE, et al. Bevacizumab plus interferon alfa compared with interferon alfa monotherapy in patients with metastatic renal cell carcinoma: CALGB 90206. J Clin Oncol. 2008;26(33):5422–8.

76. Niwakawa M, Hashine K, Yamaguchi R, Fujii H, Hamamoto Y, Fukino K, Tanigawa T, Sumiyoshi Y. Phase I trial of sorafenib in combination with interferon-alpha in Japanese patients with unresectable or metastatic renal cell carcinoma. Invest New Drugs. 2011;30:1046–54.

77. Négrier S, Gravis G, Pérol D, et al. Temsirolimus and bevacizumab, or sunitinib, or interferon alfa and bevacizumab for patients with advanced renal cell carcinoma (TORAVA): a randomised phase 2 trial. Lancet Oncol. 2011;12(7):673–80.

78. Ravaud A, Bajetta E, Kay AC, et al. Everolimus with bevacizumab versus interferon alfa-2a plus bevacizumab as first-line therapy in patients with metastatic clear cell renal cell carcinoma. J Clin Oncol. 2010;28(Suppl):15s [Abstr TPS238].

79. NCT00631371. http://clinicaltrials.gov/ct2/show/NCT00631371.

80. NCT00378703. http://clinicaltrials.gov/ct2/show/NCT00378703.

81. Motzer RJ, Bacik J, Murphy BA, Russo P, Mazumdar M. Interferon-alfa as a comparative treatment for clinical trials of new therapies against advanced renal cell carcinoma. J Clin Oncol. 2002;20(1):289–96.

82. Srivastava P. Interaction of heat shock proteins with peptides and antigen presenting cells: chaperoning of the innate and adaptive immune responses. Annu Rev Immunol. 2002;20:395–425.

83. Binder RJ, Srivastava PK. Peptides chaperoned by heat-shock proteins are a necessary and sufficient source of antigen in the cross-priming of CD8+ T cells. Nat Immunol. 2005;6(6):593–9.

84. Tamura Y, Peng P, Liu K, Daou M, Srivastava PK. Immunotherapy of tumors with autologous tumor-derived heat shock protein preparations. Science. 1997;278(5335):117–20.

85. Jonasch E, Wood C, Tamboli P, et al. Vaccination of metastatic renal cell carcinoma patients with autologous tumour-derived vitespen vaccine: clinical findings. Br J Cancer. 2008;98(8):1336–41.

86. Southall PJ, Boxer GM, Bagshawe KD, Hole N, Bromley M, Stern PL. Immunohistological distribution of 5 T4 antigen in normal and malignant tissues. Br J Cancer. 1990;61(1):89–95.

87. Griffiths RW, Gilham DE, Dangoor A, et al. Expression of the 5 T4 oncofoetal antigen in renal cell carcinoma: a potential target for T-cell-based immunotherapy. Br J Cancer. 2005;93(6):670–7.

88. Amato RJ, Shingler W, Goonewardena M, et al. Vaccination of renal cell cancer patients with modified vaccinia Ankara delivering the tumor antigen 5 T4 (TroVax) alone or administered in combination with interferon-alpha (IFN-alpha): a phase 2 trial. J Immunother. 2009;32(7):765–72.

89. Amato RJ, Shingler W, Naylor S, et al. Vaccination of renal cell cancer patients with modified vaccinia ankara delivering tumor antigen 5 T4 (TroVax) administered with interleukin 2: a phase II trial. Clin Cancer Res. 2008;14(22):7504–10.

90. Amato RJ, Hawkins RE, Kaufman HL, et al. Vaccination of metastatic renal cancer patients with MVA-5 T4: a randomized, double-blind, placebo-controlled phase III study. Clin Cancer Res. 2010;16(22):5539–47.

91. Oosterwijk E, Ruiter DJ, Hoedemaeker PJ, et al. Monoclonal antibody G 250 recognizes a determinant present in renal-cell carcinoma and absent from normal kidney. Int J Cancer. 1986;38(4):489–94.

92. Oosterwijk E, Bander NH, Divgi CR, et al. Antibody localization in human renal cell carcinoma: a phase I study of monoclonal antibody G250. J Clin Oncol. 1993;11(4):738–50.

93. Bleumer I, Knuth A, Oosterwijk E, et al. A phase II trial of chimeric monoclonal antibody G250 for advanced renal cell carcinoma patients. Br J Cancer. 2004;90(5):985–90.

94. Brouwers AH, Buijs WC, Mulders PF, et al. Radioimmunotherapy with [131I]cG250 in patients with metastasized renal cell cancer: dosimetric analysis and immunologic response. Clin Cancer Res. 2005;11(19 Pt 2):7178s–86.

95. Childs RW, Clave E, Tisdale J, Plante M, Hensel N, Barrett J. Successful treatment of metastatic renal cell carcinoma with a nonmyeloablative allogeneic peripheral-blood progenitor-cell transplant: evidence for a graft-versus-tumor effect. J Clin Oncol. 1999;17(7):2044–9.

96. Childs R, Chernoff A, Contentin N, et al. Regression of metastatic renal-cell carcinoma after nonmyeloablative allogeneic peripheral-blood stem-cell transplantation. N Engl J Med. 2000;343(11):750–8.

97. Tykodi SS, Sandmaier BM, Warren EH, Thompson JA. Allogeneic hematopoietic cell transplantation for renal cell carcinoma: ten years after. Expert Opin Biol Ther. 2011;11(6):763–73.

98. Mellor AL, Chandler P, Baban B, et al. Specific subsets of murine dendritic cells acquire potent T cell regulatory functions following CTLA4-mediated induction of indoleamine 2,3 dioxygenase. Int Immunol. 2004;16(10):1391–401.

99. Chambers CA, Sullivan TJ, Truong T, Allison JP. Secondary but not primary T cell responses are enhanced in CTLA-4-deficient CD8+ T cells. Eur J Immunol. 1998;28(10):3137–43.

100. Chambers CA, Kuhns MS, Allison JP. Cytotoxic T lymphocyte antigen-4 (CTLA-4) regulates primary and secondary peptide-specific CD4(+) T cell responses. Proc Natl Acad Sci USA. 1999;96(15):8603–8.

101. Sutmuller RP, van Duivenvoorde LM, van Elsas A, et al. Synergism of cytotoxic T lymphocyte-associated antigen 4 blockade and depletion of CD25(+) regulatory T cells in antitumor therapy reveals alternative pathways for suppression of autoreactive cytotoxic T lymphocyte responses. J Exp Med. 2001;194(6):823–32.

102. Tivol EA, Borriello F, Schweitzer AN, Lynch WP, Bluestone JA, Sharpe AH. Loss of CTLA-4 leads to massive lymphoproliferation and fatal multiorgan tissue destruction, revealing a critical negative regulatory role of CTLA-4. Immunity. 1995;3(5):541–7.

103. Waterhouse P, Penninger JM, Timms E, et al. Lymphoproliferative disorders with early lethality in mice deficient in Ctla-4. Science. 1995;270(5238):985–8.

104. Leach DR, Krummel MF, Allison JP. Enhancement of antitumor immunity by CTLA-4 blockade. Science. 1996;271(5256):1734–6.

105. Yang YF, Zou JP, Mu J, et al. Enhanced induction of antitumor T-cell responses by cytotoxic T lymphocyte-associated molecule-4 blockade: the effect is manifested only at the restricted tumor-bearing stages. Cancer Res. 1997;57(18):4036–41.

106. van Elsas A, Hurwitz AA, Allison JP. Combination immunotherapy of B16 melanoma using anti-cytotoxic T lymphocyte-associated antigen 4 (CTLA-4) and granulocyte/macrophage colony-stimulating factor (GM-CSF)-producing vaccines induces rejection of subcutaneous and metastatic tumors accompanied by autoimmune depigmentation. J Exp Med. 1999;190(3):355–66.

107. Hurwitz AA, Yu TF, Leach DR, Allison JP. CTLA-4 blockade synergizes with tumor-derived granulocyte-macrophage colony-stimulating factor for treatment of an experimental mammary carcinoma. Proc Natl Acad Sci USA. 1998;95(17):10067–71.

108. Ribas A, Camacho LH, Lopez-Berestein G, et al. Antitumor activity in melanoma and anti-self responses in a phase I trial with the anti-cytotoxic T lymphocyte-associated antigen 4 monoclonal antibody CP-675,206. J Clin Oncol. 2005;23(35):8968–77.

109. Beck KE, Blansfield JA, Tran KQ, et al. Enterocolitis in patients with cancer after antibody blockade of cytotoxic T-lymphocyte-associated antigen 4. J Clin Oncol. 2006;24(15):2283–9.

110. Hodi FS, O'Day SJ, McDermott DF, et al. Improved survival with ipilimumab in patients with metastatic melanoma. N Engl J Med. 2010;363(8):711–23.

111. Yang JC, Hughes M, Kammula U, et al. Ipilimumab (anti-CTLA4 antibody) causes regression of metastatic renal cell cancer associated with enteritis and hypophysitis. J Immunother. 2007;30(8):825–30.

112. Rini BI, Stein M, Shannon P, et al. Phase 1 dose-escalation trial of tremelimumab plus sunitinib in patients with metastatic renal cell carcinoma. Cancer. 2011;117(4):758–67.

113. Agata Y, Kawasaki A, Nishimura H, et al. Expression of the PD-1 antigen on the surface of stimulated mouse T and B lymphocytes. Int Immunol. 1996;8(5):765–72.

114. Ishida Y, Agata Y, Shibahara K, Honjo T. Induced expression of PD-1, a novel member of the immunoglobulin gene superfamily, upon programmed cell death. EMBO J. 1992;11(11):3887–95.

115. Latchman Y, Wood CR, Chernova T, et al. PD-L2 is a second ligand for PD-1 and inhibits T cell activation. Nat Immunol. 2001;2(3):261–8.

116. Zha Y, Blank C, Gajewski TF. Negative regulation of T-cell function by PD-1. Crit Rev Immunol. 2004;24(4):229–37.

117. Nishimura H, Nose M, Hiai H, Minato N, Honjo T. Development of lupus-like autoimmune diseases by disruption of the PD-1 gene encoding an ITIM motif-carrying immunoreceptor. Immunity. 1999;11(2):141–51.

118. Nishimura H, Okazaki T, Tanaka Y, et al. Autoimmune dilated cardiomyopathy in PD-1 receptor-deficient mice. Science. 2001;291(5502):319–22.

119. Thompson RH, Gillett MD, Cheville JC, et al. Costimulatory B7-H1 in renal cell carcinoma patients: Indicator of tumor aggressiveness and potential therapeutic target. Proc Natl Acad Sci USA. 2004;101(49):17174–9.

120. Thompson RH, Gillett MD, Cheville JC, et al. Costimulatory molecule B7-H1 in primary and metastatic clear cell renal cell carcinoma. Cancer. 2005;104(10):2084–91.

121. Thompson RH, Dong H, Lohse CM, et al. PD-1 is expressed by tumor-infiltrating immune cells and is associated with poor outcome for patients with renal cell carcinoma. Clin Cancer Res. 2007;13(6):1757–61.

122. Brahmer JR, Drake CG, Wollner I, et al. Phase I study of single-agent anti–programmed death-1 (MDX-1106) in refractory solid tumors: safety, clinical activity, pharmacodynamics, and immunologic correlates. J Clin Oncol. 2010;28(19):3167–75.

123. Topalian SL, Hodi FS, Brahmer JR, et al. Safety, activity, and immune correlates of anti-PD-1 antibody in cancer. N Engl J Med. 2012;366(26):2443–54.

124. Brahmer JR, Tykodi SS, Chow LQ, et al. Safety and activity of anti-PD-L1 antibody in patients with advanced cancer. N Engl J Med. 2012;366(26):2455–65.

125. Wolchok JD, Hoos A, O'Day S, et al. Guidelines for the evaluation of immune therapy activity in solid tumors: immune-related response criteria. Clin Cancer Res. 2009;15(23):7412–20.

126. Taube JM, Anders RA, Young GD, et al. Colocalization of inflammatory response with B7-h1 expression in human melanocytic lesions supports an adaptive resistance mechanism of immune escape. Sci Transl Med. 2012;4(127):127–37.

127. Pardoll DM, Topalian SL. The role of CD4+ T cell responses in antitumor immunity. Curr Opin Immunol. 1998;10(5):588–94.

128. Onishi T, Ohishi Y, Imagawa K, Ohmoto Y, Murata K. An assessment of the immunological environment based on intratumoral cytokine production in renal cell carcinoma. BJU Int. 1999;83(4):488–92.

129. Finke JH, Rini B, Ireland J, et al. Sunitinib reverses type-1 immune suppression and decreases T-regulatory cells in renal cell carcinoma patients. Clin Cancer Res. 2008;14(20):6674–82.

130. Onizuka S, Tawara I, Shimizu J, Sakaguchi S, Fujita T, Nakayama E. Tumor rejection by in vivo administration of anti-CD25 (interleukin-2 receptor alpha) monoclonal antibody. Cancer Res. 1999;59(13):3128–33.

131. Ko JS, Zea AH, Rini BI, et al. Sunitinib mediates reversal of myeloid-derived suppressor cell accumulation in renal cell carcinoma patients. Clin Cancer Res. 2009;15(6):2148–57.

132. Kusmartsev S, Gabrilovich DI. Role of immature myeloid cells in mechanisms of immune evasion in cancer. Cancer Immunol Immunother. 2006;55(3):237–45.

133. Hoechst B, Ormandy LA, Ballmaier M, et al. A new population of myeloid-derived suppressor cells in hepatocellular carcinoma patients induces CD4(+)CD25(+)Foxp3(+) T cells. Gastroenterology. 2008;135(1):234–43.

134. Almand B, Clark JI, Nikitina E, et al. Increased production of immature myeloid cells in cancer patients: a mechanism of immunosuppression in cancer. J Immunol. 2001;166(1):678–89.

135. Wood et al. Lancet 2008, 372: 145.

Targeted Therapy: Vascular Endothelial Growth Factor

17

Linda Cerbone and Cora N. Sternberg

In the past few years better understanding of the main pathogenic mechanisms of development and progression of clear cell renal cell carcinoma (RCC) has led to novel therapeutic approaches with improvement in the prognosis of patients with metastatic disease (mRCC) (Table 17.1).

Inactivation of the Van Hippel–Lindau (VHL) gene and consequent vascular endothelial growth factor (VEGF) overexpression has been identified as the first step of tumor growth in the majority of patients with RCC. The importance of VEGF protein and its ligands vascular endothelial growth factor receptors (VEGFRs 1,2,3) has been thoroughly investigated and due to its crucial role in angiogenesis they have been considered the most relevant therapeutic targets to consider in patients with RCC [1]. There are numerous ways in which to inhibit VEGF, however, at present drug development has primarily focused upon the anti-VEGF antibody (Bevacizumab) and VEGF receptor tyrosine kinase inhibitors (TKIs): sunitinib, pazopanib, sorafenib, axitinib, and tivozanib (Fig. 17.1; Table 17.2).

Bevacizumab

Bevacizumab (Avastin®) is a recombinant human monoclonal antibody that binds and neutralizes all active isoforms of VEGF. After promising data in phase II trials, two randomized (1:1) phase III trials demonstrated that the addition of bevacizumab 10 mg/kg i.v. every 2 weeks to IFN-α (9 MIU × 3 s.c., weekly) leads to a statisically significant advantage in progression-free survival (PFS) in patients with previously untreated mRCC.

In both the European study (AVOREN, 649 patients [2] and the U.S. study (CALGB 90206, 732 patients) [3], the majority of patients were of good or intermediate risk according to MSKCC criteria [4] and less than 10% belonged to the poor prognosis category. In both studies, the addition of bevacizumab resulted in higher objective response rates (RR) compared with IFN-α alone (25.5% vs. 13.1% in the AVOREN trial; 31% vs. 13% in the CALGB trial). PFS in the AVOREN trial was 10.2 months vs. 5.4 months (HR=0.6; $p=0.0001$) and 8.5 months vs. 5.2 months in the CALGB trial (HR=0.71; $p<0.0001$). Neither of the studies demonstrated a statistically significant difference in overall survival (OS) between the two treatment arms. Survival in the CALGB trial was 18.3 months vs. 17.4 months ($p=0.097$) and 23.3 months vs. 21.3 months ($p=0.33$) in the AVOREN study. However, it should be noted that the majority of patients in both studies received further treatments

L. Cerbone • C.N. Sternberg (✉)
Department of Medical Oncology, San Camillo-Forlanini Hospital, Circonvallazione Gianicolense 87, Rome 00152, Italy
e-mail: cerbone.linda@gmail.com; cstern@mclink.it

S.C. Campbell and B.I. Rini (eds.), *Renal Cell Carcinoma: Clinical Management*, Current Clinical Urology, 303
DOI 10.1007/978-1-62703-062-5_17, © Springer Science+Business Media New York 2013

Table 17.1 mRCC treatment algorithm

Regimen	Setting	Therapy	Options
Treatment-naïve patient	MSKCC risk: good or intermediate	Sunitinib Bevacizumab+IFNα Pazopanib	High-dose IL-2 Sorafenib Clinical trials Observation
	MSKCC risk: poor	Temsirolimus	Sunitinib Clinical trials
Treatment-refractory patient (≥second line)	Cytokine refractory	Sorafenib (axitinib) Pazopanib	Bevacizumab Sunitinib Pazopanib
	TKI refractory	Everolimus (axitinib)	Clinical trials

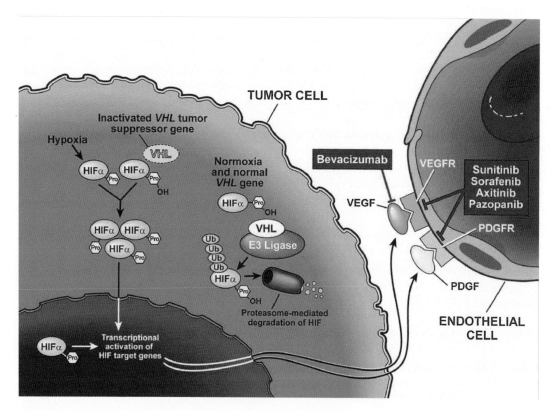

Fig. 17.1 Anti-VEGF mechanism of action (reprinted with permission from B Rini. Vascular endothelial growth factor-targeted therapy in metastatic renal cell carcinoma. Cancer (2009);2306–2312. John Wiley and Sons)

at the time of progression which impacted on survival. Based on these two phase III trials, the combination of Bevacizumab and IFN-α is considered a first-line therapeutic option for patients with mRCC with favorable and intermediate prognosis.

Sunitinib

Sunitinib (Sutent®) is an oral small molecule TKI that inhibits tyrosine kinases VEGFR-1,2,3, platelet-derived growth factor receptor (PGFR-α,β), c-kit, and FTL-3. It is considered a standard

Table 17.2 TKIs in mRCC: summary of survival and response

Treatment	No of patients	Objective response (%)	Median PFS (months)	Median OS (months)
Bevacizumab+INFα vs. INFα (AVOREN trial; Escudier 2007) (CALGB 90206 trial; Rini 2010)	649 732	25.5 31	10.2 vs. 5.4 TTP: 8.5 vs. 5.2	23.3 vs. 21.3 ($p=0.33$) 18.3 vs. 17.4 ($p=0.097$)
Sunitinib vs. IFNα (Motzer 2007)	750	31 vs. 6 ($p<0.001$)	11 vs. 5 ($p<0.000001$)	26.4 vs. 21.8 ($p=0.051$)
Pazopanib vs. placebo (Sternberg 2010)	435	30 vs. 3	9.2 vs. 4.2 ($p<0.0001$)	22.9 vs. 20.5 ($p=0.224$)
Sorafenib vs. placebo (Escudier 2007)	903	10	5.5 vs. 2.8 ($p<0.001$)	19.3 vs. 15.9 ($p=0.02$)
Axitinib vs. Sorafenib (Rini 2011)	732	19.4 vs. 9.4 ($p=0.0001$)	6.7 vs. 4.7 ($p<0.0001$)	

of care for first-line treatment in patients with mRCC. The use of this multikinase TKI is supported by the results of two phase II trials in cytokine pretreated patients [5] and a randomized phase III trial whose primary objective was to determine PFS in patients with previously untreated mRCC. Seven hundred and fifty patients were randomized (1:1) to receive sunitinib (50 mg orally daily, 4 weeks on and 2 weeks off) vs. IFN-α (9 MIU × 3 s.c., weekly). Sunitinib led to an advantage in terms of objective RR (31% vs. 6%, $p<0.001$) and PFS (11 months vs. 5 months, $p<0.000001$). The median OS was 26.4 months for patients treated with sunitinib vs. 21.8 months in the IFN-α arm ($p=0.051$). In this study, patients in the IFN arm also had access to subsequent treatment with sunitinib which may have impacted upon the OS results [6].

Pazopanib

Pazopanib (Votrient®) is an oral TKI of VEGFR 1,2,3, PDGFR-α,β, and c-kit. In a phase III study, 435 patients with mRCC who had no prior therapy or who had prior cytokine therapy were randomized in a 2:1 ratio to receive pazopanib (800 mg orally daily) or placebo [7]. Pazopanib resulted in a 54% reduction in the risk of progression or death (improvement in PFS), the primary endpoint of the study. The median PFS of pazopanib

compared to placebo was 9.2 months vs. 4.2 months, ($p<0.0001$). For patients who had no prior therapy, PFS was 11.1 months vs. 2.8 months ($p<0.001$) and for those who had prior cytokines PFS was 7.4 months vs. 4.2 months ($p<0.001$). Overall objective responses were reported in 30% of patients and the median duration of response was 58.7 weeks. No difference in OS was observed between the two arms (22.9 months vs. 20.5 months; $p=0.224$) [8]. This was most likely due to the fact that 54% of patients in the placebo arm crossed over to receive pazopanib and the fact that patients crossed over very early and remained on treatment for long periods of time.

Enrollment in the COMPARZ study (NCT00720941), a head-to-head trial comparing sunitinib and pazopanib in the first-line setting, was completed in August 2008 with 876 patients enrolled. The primary endpoint of the study is PFS and non-inferiority. Secondary endpoints include: OS, objective RR, duration of response, safety, and quality of life.

The PISCES trial (NCT01064310) has included approximately 160 patients in a randomized double-blind, crossover study of pazopanib vs. sunitinib in patients with locally advanced or mRCC who have received no prior systemic therapy. The trial's primary endpoint is patient preference (which will be assessed primarily by questionnaires) and secondary endpoints will include quality of life, safety, pharmacokinetics, and biomarkers. These two trials will help to inform the relative risks and benefits of each of these two common front-line agents in metastatic RCC.

Sorafenib

Sorafenib (Nexavar®) is an oral small molecule that inhibits VEGFR 2,3, PDGFR-β, raf kinase and FTL-3. A phase III trial, the TARGET trial, randomized 903 mRCC, patients who had received prior therapy, primarily cytokines, and who had a favorable or intermediate prognosis to receive Sorafenib (400 mg BID orally daily) vs. placebo [9]. The primary objective of the trial was overall survival, but patients who experienced progression on the placebo arm were allowed to cross over to sorafenib, most likely contributing to the lack of an overall survival difference (19.3 vs. 15.9 ($p = 0.02$)). In the sorafenib arm a benefit in PFS (5.5 months vs. 2.8 months, $p < 0.001$) was observed. Objective responses and stable disease were observed in 10% and 74% of cases. Sorafenib was the first TKI to be approved in many countries and reference treatment for second-line and later therapy. Its efficacy in the first-line setting has not been established. In a phase II trial, 189 untreated patients were randomized to receive Sorafenib (400 mg BID) or IFN (9 million units TIW). Dose escalation to Sorafenib 600 mg BID or crossover to Sorafenib 400 mg BID after disease progression were allowed. Disease control rate was 79% vs. 64% but the primary endpoint, PFS, was not reached (5.7 months vs. 5.6 months) [10].

Future Perspectives

Axitinib (AG 013736) is an oral potent inhibitor of VEGFR 1,2,3, PDGFR-α,β and c-kit that has shown promising activity in phase 2 trials both in patients pretreated with cytokines (44.2% RR and median time to progression of 15.7 months) and in patients refractory to sorafenib (PFS 7.4 months) [11]. A phase 3 trial (AXIS,

NCT00678392) randomized (1:1) 723 patients to evaluate the impact of axitinib (5 mg BID orally daily) vs. sorafenib as second-line treatment after any approved first-line therapy for mRCC. In both arms 94% of pts were of good-intermediate risk according to MSKCC criteria. This trial met its primary endpoint of improvement of PFS (6.7 months vs. 4.7 months, $p < 0.0001$); 19.4% of patients in the axitinib arm had a partial response vs. 9.4% in the sorafenib arm. Axitinib showed a similar safety profile compared to sorafenib with the exception of a greater incidence of hypertension (40% vs. 29%) and hypothyroidism (19% vs. 8%) and lower incidence of hand–foot syndrome (27% vs. 51%) [12].

There appears to be an association of diastolic blood pressure (dBP) > 90 mmHg with OS in patients treated with axitinib [13]. A prospective randomized phase II trial (NCT00835978) of axitinib dose escalation based upon achieving hypertension has completed accrual. Two-hundred treatment-naïve mRCC patients received an initial 4-week cycle of axitinib (5 mg BID). Patients who do not experience dBP ≥ 90 mmHg will be randomized 1:1 to receive axitinib + axitinib dose escalation or axitinib + placebo dose titration. The primary endpoint is overall RR; secondary endpoints are PFS, OS, response duration, safety, pharmacokinetics, BP, and biomarker correlations [14].

Tivozanib (AV951) is another potent VEGFR 1,2,3 and PDGFR inhibitor that has demonstrated promising activity in mRCC. In a phase II randomized discontinuation trial (NCT00502307) of 272 patients, PFS was 11.7 months and higher (14.8 months), in patients with clear cell carcinoma who had undergone a nephrectomy [15]. A phase III trial, the TIVO-1 trial (NCT01030783), has randomized (1:1) 500 patients with recurrent or mRCC, ECOG PS 0-1, treatment naïve or one prior non-VEGF targeted therapy to Tivozanib (1.5 mg orally daily 3 weeks on/1 week off) vs. Sorafenib (400 mg BID continuously). Crossover to tivozanib at the time of progression on sorafenib was permitted. The primary endpoint is PFS [16].

Dovitinib (TKI258) is a VEGFR 1,2,3 and FGFR inhibitor that has been evaluated in heavily pretreated patients (with sunitinib and/or sorafenib and/or mTOR inhibitor) in a phase I/II trial (NCT00715182). Promising results with PFS of 6.1 months and OS of 16 months were observed [17]. The FGFR pathway seems to be involved in tumor escape from VEGF and possibly mTOR inhibitor therapy [18]. A phase III randomized trial (NCT01223027) is comparing Dovitinib (500 mg orally daily 5 days on/2 days off scheduled in 28-day cycles) vs. Sorafenib (400 mg BID) in the third-line setting following VEGFR and mTOR inhibition. The primary endpoint is PFS. Secondary endpoints include OS, RR, safety, patient-reported outcomes, and pharmacokinetics.

Cediranib (AZD2171) is an oral inhibitor of VEGFR 1,2,3, PDGFR β (beta), c-kit and Flt-4 that has been studied in phase I–II trials. In combination or alone cediranib has demonstrated antitumor activity in mRCC in two phase I trials. It has been investigated in an open-label phase II trial (NCT00227760) in 43 untreated patients showing an 84% disease control rate (PR + SD) and a median PFS of 8.7 months. In a randomized, double-blind, phase II trial (NCT00423332) cediranib (45 mg daily) has been evaluated as first-line therapy in 71 patients with mRCC. Patients were treated with drug or placebo (3:1) for 12 weeks and then unblinded [19, 20]. The active treatment arm revealed a disease control rate of 81%. The median PFS was 12.1 months vs. 2.7 months. More trials are needed to confirm these data.

Toxicities and Management

The mechanism of action of novel targeted therapies is responsible for off target side effects. Many of these differ from those that oncologists are accustomed to manage, related to chemotherapy. To understand, recognize, and manage the side effects of VEGFR TKIs is critical for the long-term treatment of patients. Several studies have been published to update information on toxicity rates, and severity and to create common guidelines for their management. All concomitant therapies used to counteract side effects must take into account the risk of interaction with anti-VEGF drugs.

The major problems that have been described are constitutional (fatigue, anorexia, weight loss, and depression), cardiovascular (hypertension, decreased left ventricular ejection fraction, congestive failure), gastrointestinal (stomatitis, nausea, diarrhea, gastrointestinal perforation), metabolic (hypothyroidism), dermatological (hand-foot syndrome, rash, xerosis, skin and hair depigmentation, yellowing of the skin) renal (proteinuria, increased creatinine, decreased renal function), and hematologic and laboratory (neutropenia, lymphopenia, thrombocytopenia, anemia, increased transaminases and lipase) [21, 22] (Table 17.3).

Constitutional Toxicity

The main constitutional symptom described is fatigue. Across studies, fatigue has been reported with: Sunitinib 51% (high grade 7%), Sorafenib 37% (high grade 5%), bevacizumab plus INF-α 33% (high grade 12%) and pazopanib 19% (high grade 2%). Likewise, with Axitinib patients experience fatigue in 39% of cases and 11% are grades 3 and 4. To manage this side effect the first step is to understand whether there are other contributing factors such as anemia, hypothyroidism, or underlying depression. Recognition and treatment of these factors could decrease fatigue during therapy with TKIs. If depression is suspected, a psychiatric consultation is mandatory and drugs such as selective serotonin reuptake inhibitors (SSRIs) should be considered. Anorexia has been reported in 36% on bevacizumab plus IFN-α (3% grades 3 and 4), 34% on sunitinib (2% grades 3 and 4), 22% on pazopanib (2% grades 3 and 4), 14% on sorafenib (<1% grades 3 and 4), and in 39% with axitinib. These data can also partially explain the percentage of asthenia reported: 32% with bevacizumab plus IFN-α, 20% with sunitinib and 14% with pazopanib. No data are readily available for sorafenib and axinitinib [23–25].

Table 17.3 Anti-VEGF therapy: toxicities

	Sunitinib All grade % High grade %	Sorafenib All grade % High grade %	Bevacizumab+IFNα All grade % High grade %	Pazopanib All grade % High grade %	Axitinib All grade % High grade %
Fatigue	51 / 7	37 / 5	33 / 12	19 / 2	39
Anorexia	34 / 2	14 / <1	36 / 3	22 / 2	39
Hypertension	24 / 8	17 / 4	26 / 3	40 / 3	40 / 15
Arterial thrombotic events		2.9	2.4	3	
Hemorrhage	30 / 10	15 / 2	33 / 3	16 / 2	
Stomatitis	30 / 3	5			
Diarrhea	44–76 / 4	6.2–36.5 / 2	7 / 9	52 / 3	43–46
Hypothyroidism	18–85 / 2	5–23		<10	19
Hand–foot skin reaction	14.4 / 4.7	42 / 8.9		<10	14
Proteinuria	60		18 / 7	<10	18–36

Cardiovascular Toxicity

Arterial hypertension is the most common class side effect. Hypertension is secondary to inhibition of the VEGF/VEGFR pathway, leading to an increase in systemic vascular resistance by reducing microvessel density. Endothelial dysfunction reduces the production of nitric oxide and increased oxidative stress, perhaps altering neurohormonal factors involved in blood pressure regulation. These mechanisms are directly and indirectly mediated by activation of VEGFR-2, the main target of the anti-VEGFR therapies. As mentioned earlier, hypertension may be correlated with outcome [21]. Studies of sunitinib, sorafenib, bevacizumab plus IFN-α, pazopanib, axitinib, and cediranib report hypertension in 24%, 17%, 26%, 40%, 40%, and 35% respectively. Grade 3/4 hypertension has been observed with axitinib (16%), sunitinib (8%), sorafenib (4%), pazopanib (4%), and bevacizumab plus IFN-α (3%). Cediranib was studied in a phase II trial (NCT00264004) were 126 patients were randomized to receive two different dosages of drug (30 and 45 mg daily) with or without antihypertensive prophylaxis. Hypertension was most common grade 3 adverse event, but prophylaxis increased the number of patients who completed treatment at both dosages [30]. The different incidences are probably related to the degree of inhibition and selectivity among the different agents.

Bevacizumab inhibits VEGF-A allowing VEGFR-2 to be activated by VEGF-C, unlike other TKIs that selectively inhibit VEGFR-2. The "second generation" TKIs (axitinib and cediranib) have greater affinity for this receptor. Another factor that may affect severity of hypertension is the schedule of drug administration. A large meta-analysis showed a significant difference between continuous and intermittent schedules of Sunitinib in favor of intermittent dosing. Although this data requires validation, one can hypothesize that during the rest period vascular injuries could be partially resolved [31]. To improve management, many variables must be considered. It is important to know whether the patient has known risk factors for hypertension. Before starting therapy, in addition to a cardiovascular evaluation, renal function and the presence of proteinuria or microscopic hematuria must be investigated. This may be an expression of silent kidney disease that could predispose a patient to hypertension. Effective antihypertensive therapy must be instituted prior to anti-VEGFR agents. Although no randomized studies favor one particular antihypertensive drug, some considerations and an increasing literature provide suggestions. Nondihydropyridine calcium channel blockers such as Verapamil and Diltiazem should be avoided during therapy due to CYP3A4 inhibition that can interact with metabolism of TKIs. Antihypertensive drugs most often used are angiotensin-converting enzyme (ACE) inhibitors, beta blockers, dihydropyridine calcium channel blockers (dCCB), angiotensin 2 receptor antagonists (ARA), and diuretics. Blood pressure monitoring must be continued in all patients and in the case of hypertension, pharmacologic intervention is essential before stopping or reducing drug dosages [25, 32].

Cardiac toxicity is most likely related to hypertensive injury rather than to inhibition of intracellular pathways involved in cardiac repair. Decreased left ventricular ejection fraction (LVEF) has been described in 21% of patients treated with sunitinib; 4% experienced grades 3 and 4 toxicity. Left ventricular dysfunction and congestive heart failure has been observed in less than 1% of patients. Baseline evaluation of LVEF is suggested and control during treatment for patients with risk factors or in those developing symptoms such as chest pain or dyspnea is fundamental. Drug should be stopped if symptoms appear or reduced if LVEF decreases to <50% or decrease by >20% below baseline. In a single-center study evaluating cardiotoxicity with TKI therapy, the introduction of a beta blocker such as carvedilol in case of cardiologic damage was suggested based on the antioxidant properties of this drug and its protection against cardiomyopathy.

ECG modifications during therapy must be evaluated. QT prolongation occurred in <2% in the pazopanib trial. Torsade de pointes was observed in <1% and <0.1% in the pazopanib and sunitinib trials. Serum electrolyte levels should also be monitored [33–36].

Increased risk of thrombosis and bleeding may be related to the important role of VEGF in maintaining hemostasis. Arterial thrombotic events such as cardiac ischemia or infarction have been reported in 2.9% during sorafenib therapy, 2.4% with bevacizumab, and 3% with pazopanib. Hemorrhage occurred in 30% on sunitinib, 16% on pazopanib, 33% on bevacizumab and IFN-α, 15% on sorafenib, and was high grade in 10%, 2%, 3%, and 2% respectively [2, 3, 7–9]. It is important to investigate a history of coagulation disorders, avoid starting therapy if surgical scars are not completely healed, monitor patients on warfarin and if possible switch to low-molecular-weight heparin therapy.

Gastrointestinal Toxicity

The major intestinal toxicities are diarrhea, stomatitis, nausea, and anorexia. Most are a consequence of VEGF inhibition commonly expressed by normal intestinal mucosa. Diarrhea, often accompanied by abdominal pain, is observed in 20% of patients and has been reported as frequently as 50% with bevacizumab, sunitinib, and pazopanib. Sorafenib and axitinib are also associated with diarrhea in 43–46%. Management of diarrhea is essential to prevent dehydration, electrolyte imbalances, and fatigue. Drugs such as loperamide are useful, as are dietary modifications. Stomatitis has been reported with sunitinib (30%) and sorafenib (5%). Nausea is observed with all of the TKIs with an incidence ranging between 23% and 44%, though not with bevacizumab. All of the common antiemetics not metabolized by CYP3A4 can be used. Gastrointestinal perforation has been reported in 2.4% of patients treated with bevacizumab, in <1% treated with sorafenib and 0.9% with pazopanib [23–25].

Metabolic Toxicity

Hypothyroidism is the most common metabolic side effect of anti-VEGFR targeted therapies.

The mechanism of thyroid dysfunction is not clearly understood.

Hypothyroidism has also been described with Bevacizumab. This suggests that the pathogenesis could be related to inhibition of VEGFR 1 and 2 which are expressed on endothelial thyroid cells. Endothelial cells are involved in regulation, synthesis, and function of thyroid hormones. The true incidence of hypothyroidism has not yet been defined. In patients treated with sunitinib incidence ranges from 18% to 85%. For sorafenib, hypothyroidism has been reported in 18% and hyperthyroidism in 3%. Of note, less than 10% has been reported during therapy with pazopanib. Some of the variability can be explained by the fact that early studies on TKIs did not include prospective study of thyroid function and did not investigate baseline values. The real incidence should be prospectively evaluated in ongoing studies. Experience in recent years has shown that baseline screening of thyroid function is necessary and further testing on days 1 and 28 during the first four cycles is recommended. After that period, if thyroid function is normal, evaluation is encouraged every two cycles. When abnormal levels of TSH with or without mild symptoms of hypothyroidism are noted, monitoring is mandatory. When hypothyroidism occurs, levothyroxine should be initiated. There is an emerging body of data which correlate kidney and thyroid gland function in physiological and pathological non-cancer-related conditions and perhaps future studies may clarify the true causes of thyroid dysfunction during treatment for kidney tumors [26–29].

Dermatological Toxicity

Skin toxicity has often been reported with TKIs and includes rash, xerosis, cheilitis, pruritus, subungual splinter hemorrhages, modification of skin and hair pigmentation, yellowing skin and hand–foot skin reaction (HFSR). HFSR is defined as a localized cutaneous reaction characterized by erythema, numbness, dysesthesia, or paresthesia of the palms and/or soles. A recent meta-analysis of sunitinib revealed an incidence

of all grade HFSR of 14.4 with 4.7% high grade. For sorafenib, the all-grade incidence is 42% and high grade 8.9%. In phase I, cediranib produced HFSR in 10.8% of patients. Pazopanib and axitinib reported <10% and 14% of HFSR cases, respectively. The pathogenesis of this side effect is still unknown but there are two main hypotheses. TKIs seem to be secreted into eccrine glands and excreted in sweat causing direct skin toxicity, which is increased in the palms and soles where a major concentration of these glands exist. Another mechanism could be related to inhibition of VEGFR and PDGFR that affect normal vascular repair and cause damage in pressure sites. Although HFSR is not a life-threatening toxicity, it can heavily affect quality of life and determine a suspension or reduction of therapy. To prevent HFSR, pedicures should be recommended in patients with skin hyperkeratosis or calluses. Patients should avoid very hot water and not wear constrictive footwear. Pharmacological interventions have been suggested from such as keratolytic creams for grade 1 toxicity, topical clobetasol and analgesics for grade 2 toxicity and temporary interruption for grade 3 toxicity [37–39].

Renal Toxicity

Impact on renal function is characterized by proteinuria, an increase in creatinine and a decrease in clearance. Proteinuria is a consequence of VEGF inhibition that may affect glomerular endothelial function and cause damage to the glomerular filtration barrier. In this scenario, VEGF-A seems to play an important role, explaining the high incidence of proteinuria with bevacizumab (18% all grade and 7% grades 3 and 4). The mechanism behind proteinuria is not perfectly clear and proteinuria has also been reported with sunitinib (6%), pazopanib (<10%), and axitinib (18–36%). Proteinuria is dose dependent, may be related to hypertension, and in many cases decreases after drug suspension. Proteinuria is a cardiovascular risk factor and is also involved in long-term loss of renal function. Correct monitoring with urinalysis dipstick and a 24-h urine collection are helpful in detecting and managing this side effect before progression to renal damage. Although specific guidelines are not unavailable, drugs that block the renin–angiotensin system (ACE inhibitors and ARA) have shown antiproteinuric and renoprotective properties [21, 40].

Hematologic and Laboratory Toxicities

Common hematological toxicities correlated with VEGF/VEGFR therapy are leukopenia, ranging from 37% to 78%, neutropenia, ranging from 7% to 72%, lymphopenia, ranging from 23% to 60%, anemia, ranging from 10% to 71%, and thrombocytopenia ranging from 6% to 65%. Sunitinib has a higher incidence of hematologic toxicities than pazopanib due to its low affinity for FLT-3 expressed on hematopoietic cells. All grade increases in bilirubin, ALT and AST have been seen with pazopanib in 36%, 53%, and 53% respectively. This is, however, a class effect that is also seen with the other TKIs such as sunitinib with 46%, 52%, and 19% increases in AST, ALT and bilirubin, respectively. Liver function has to be monitored diligently during all TKI therapy. Reduction or suspension of drug has to be considered based on the grade and the duration of side effects. Other laboratory abnormalities such as hypophosphatemia, increased amylase and lipase have been observed during sunitinib therapy with an incidence of 31%, 35% and 56% [2–25].

Open Questions

Predictive Factors

The use of these novel agents permits a wide choice of therapy while raising many unanswered questions. We still lack fundamental knowledge which can help us to identify which patient would benefit from one drug rather than another. What is the best sequence of therapy to maximize survival? How can we overcome resistance which inevitably arises during treatment?

The emerging need to identify the best treatment for individual patients has focused research on biomarkers predictive of response to anti-VEGF therapies. Inactivation of the VHL gene has been extensively studied to understand its prognostic and/or predictive value, but in both cases its role remains unclear. Patients with VHL gene methylation or mutation do not appear to have a better clinical outcome to VEGF-targeting therapy than patients with VHL wild type [41]. A small study conducted on tumor specimens in 43 patients treated with sunitinib showed a predictive role for response with high HIF-2α expression.

Germline variants in angiogenesis- and exposure-related genes may predict treatment response to pazopanib. Genetic markers have been investigated in a retrospective analyses to evaluate correlation with pazopanib efficacy. Genetic variations in genes may be predictive of tumor angiogenesis (expression of variants of IL8, HIF1α, and sVEGFA that increase angiogenic activity) or of differences in metabolism [42]. It is interesting to note that data are emerging about the potential role as predictive markers of response to certain side effects such as the development of hypertension in patients treated with sunitinib and axitinib and the development of hypothyroidism in patients treated with sunitinib and sorafenib.

Optimal Duration of Treatment

Treatment with TKIs is continued until disease progression, and recently the debate of therapeutic management in patients with complete response (CR) has been raised. Discontinuation of therapy could have an important impact on quality of life. However, there are no data to support suspension of therapy. The only information is from small retrospective single-center studies in which patients with CR after treatment or surgery obtained with TKIs and unacceptable toxicities have been forced to suspend sunitinib or sorafenib. In patients with recurrent disease, the median TTP was 6 months and reintroduction of the drug was effective in all cases. There is, therefore, significant risk of relapse after CR. Validation of this therapeutic approach requires further study. The phenomenon underlying relapse, the so-called rebound or flare-up phenomenon, is recognized and its biological background has been described [43]. However, intermittent therapy related to unacceptable toxicity requires further investigation.

Resistance, Sequential and Combination Therapy

Patients develop either primary or acquired resistance to anti-VEGF therapy, the reason why anti-VEGF therapies are curative in only rare cases. Overcoming resistance is a serious topic of study. Among the mechanisms responsible for resistance, the first identified is activation or up-regulation of signals and alternative pathways of angiogenesis. To prevent this phenomenon, attempts have been made to block multiple pathways at the same time in a horizontal blockade or to block the same pathway in more than one site in a vertical blockade using combination therapies [44]. Two examples of vertical combinations with anti-VEGF agents have been evaluated. The first is a phase I/II trial (NCT00126503) investigating the association benefit of Sorafenib and Bevacizumab. In phase I an important increase of sorafenib-related toxicity (hypertension, proteinuria, hand–foot syndrome) was observed, with Sorafenib dose reduction in 74% of patients. The phase II is still ongoing. Another phase I trial (NCT00421512) was conducted to study the combination of Sunitinib and Bevacizumab. Even though the response rate was 52%, grades 3 and 4 hypertension, hematologic and vascular toxicities were prohibitive and the authors did not proceed to phase II [45]. A phase I trial (NCT00992121) studying the combination of pazopanib with bevacizumab is ongoing. The combination of TKIs can be expected to have drug interactions due to the common CYP3A4 hepatic metabolism [46, 47].

Sequential therapy is most likely more effective and safer. Available data on anti-VEGF sequential therapies are derived from retrospective studies which show that after progression during VEGF targeted therapy, patients may respond to another anti-VEGF treatment.

Sunitinib and sorafenib represent the most common sequence due to their earliest approval. For sunitinib after sorafenib progression a retrospective analysis showed a median PFS of 6.5 months, 15% PR and 51% SD, obtaining a total of 12.5 months of PFS for the complete treatment. Another small retrospective analysis evaluating the same sequence experienced an average TTP of 18.1 months with 21% PR and 38% SD during sunitinib therapy. Both studies investigated the inverse sequence. In the first analysis patients treated with sorafenib after sunitinib progression achieved a median PFS of 3.9 months, obtaining an overall PFS during all the treatment of 9 months. During sorafenib therapy 9% of PR and 54% of SD were observed. A very similar overall TTP was achieved in the other analysis (8.5 months) with lowest disease control during sorafenib therapy (5% PR; 30% SD). Another study achieved PFS of 10.3 months with sunitinib after sorafenib failure with an average PFS of 19 months [48, 49]. Considerable bias affects evaluation of such results. A retrospective analysis of the AVOREN trial evaluated the effect of TKI therapy after first-line bevacizumab plus IFN-α. Patients receiving second-line sunitinib achieved an OS of 43.6 months, patients receiving sorafenib an OS of 38.6 months. These results suggest but do not validate sequential therapy after bevacizumab plus cytokines [50]. Other interesting data concerning sequential therapy come from the previously described axitinib trial [12].

The idea of rechallenge has also been investigated in a retrospective analysis of 23 patients with mRCC retreated with Sunitinib. A partial response was demonstrated in 22% and a PFS of 7.2 months was achieved. Patients who experienced an interval between the two Sunitinib treatments greater than 6 months had better PFS (16.5 months vs. 6 months). A 6-month cutoff for rechallenge could be evaluated in clinical practice.

Conclusions

In recent years the therapeutic approach to mRCC has been revolutionized by the introduction of new and effective VEGF-targeted therapies. The current guidelines suggest Sunitinib, Bevacizumab plus IFNa or Pazopanib as first-line treatments for favorable and intermediate-risk patients with mRCC. Sorafenib, Sunitinib, Pazopanib and soon Axitinib can be recommended as second-line treatments for cytokine refractory mRCC. Research is now focused on identifying prognostic and predictive factors; clinical, biological, and genetic algorithms to create a treatment that would allow patients the best and personalized therapeutic approach, taking comorbidities into account.

The correct management of side effects is a crucial point to permit more efficacious treatment [51–53]. Current trials are investigating the best way to overcome drug resistance via sequential or combination approaches. All of the pivotal trials have shown a benefit in PFS that was not reflected in a strong benefit in OS due to cross-over and further treatments. A retrospective study of 1,158 patients treated with current targeted therapies has demonstrated a positive statistically significant correlation between 3 and 6 months PFS and OS [54].

References

1. Rini BI, Small EJ. Biology and clinical development of vascular endothelial growth factor-targeted therapy in renal cell carcinoma. J Clin Oncol. 2005;23:1028–43.
2. Escudier B, Pluzanska A, Koralewski P, et al. Bevacizumab plus interferon alfa-2a for treatment of metastatic renal cell carcinoma: a randomised, double-blind phase III trial. Lancet. 2007;370:2103–11.
3. Rini BI, Halabi S, Rosenberg JE, et al. Phase III trial of bevacizumab plus interferon-alpha versus interferon-alpha monotherapy in patients with metastatic renal carcinoma: final results of CALGB 90206. J Clin Oncol. 2010;28(13):2137–43.
4. Motzer RJ, Bacik J, Murphy BA, et al. Interferon-alfa as a comparative treatment for clinical trials of new therapies against advanced renal cell carcinoma. J Clin Oncol. 2002;20:289–96.
5. Motzer RJ, Redman BG, Rini BI, et al. Activity of SU11248, a multitargeted inhibitor of vascular endothelial growth factor receptor and platelet-derived growth factor receptor, in patients with metastatic renal cell carcinoma. J Clin Oncol. 2006;24(1):16–24.
6. Motzer RJ, Hutson TE, Tomczak P, et al. Sunitinib versus interferon alfa in metastatic renal-cell carcinoma. N Engl J Med. 2007;356:115–24.
7. Sternberg CN, Davis ID, Mardiak J, et al. Pazopanib in locally advanced or metastatic renal cell carcinoma: results of a randomized phase III trial. J Clin Oncol. 2010;28:1061–8.
8. Sternberg CN. Randomized, double-blind Phase III Study of Pazopanib in patients with advanced/metastatic renal cell carcinoma (mRCC): final overall survival (OS) results. 35th European Society for Medical Oncology ESMO Congress, October 2010 Milan Italy. Abstract LBA22.
9. Escudier B, Eisen T, Stadler WM, et al. Sorafenib in advanced clear-cell renal-cell carcinoma. N Engl J Med. 2007;356:125–34.
10. Szczylik C, Bukowski RM, Escudier B, et al. Randomized phase II trial of first line treatment with sorafenib versus interferon in patients with advanced renal cell carcinoma: final results. J Clin Oncol 2007;25 [Abstr 5025].
11. Rixe O, Bukowski RM, Michaelson MD, et al. Axitinib treatment in patients with cytokine-refractory metastatic renal-cell cancer: a phase II study. Lancet Oncol. 2007;8:975–84.
12. Rini BI, Escudier B, Tomczak P, et al. Axitinib versus sorafenib as second-line therapy for metastatic renal cell carcinoma (mRCC): results of phase III AXIS trial. J Clin Oncol. 2011; 29 [Abstr 4504].
13. Rini BI, Schiller JH, Fruehauf JP, et al. Diastolic blood pressure as a biomarkert of axitinib efficacy in solid tumors. Clin Cancer Res. 2011;17(11): 3841–9.
14. Jonasch E, Bair A, Rini BI, et al. Axitinib with or without dose titration as first-line therapy for metastatic renal cell carcinoma (mRCC). J Clin Oncol. 2010;28 [Abstr TPS235].
15. Nosov D, Bhargava P, Esteves WB, et al. Final analysis of the phase II randomized discontinuation trial (RDT) of tivozanib (AV-951) versus placebo in patients with renal cell carcinoma (RCC). J Clin Oncol. 2011; 29 [Abstr 4550].
16. Motzer RJ, Sternberg CN, Hutson TE, et al. A phase III, randomized, controlled study to compare tivozanib with sorafenib in patients (pts) with advanced renal cell carcinoma (RCC). J Clin Oncol. 2011; 29 [Abstr 310].
17. Angevin E, Grünwald V, Ravaud A, et al. A phase II study of dovitinib (TKI258), an FGFR- and VEGFR-inhibitor, in patients with advanced or metastatic renal cell cancer (mRCC). J Clin Oncol. 2011; 29 [Abst 4551].
18. Casanovas O, Hicklin D, Bergers G, et al. Drug resistance by evasion of antiangiogenic targeting of VEGF signaling in late-stage pancreatic islet tumors. Cancer Cell. 2005;8:299–309.
19. Sridhar SS, Mackenzie MJ, Hotte SJ, et al. Activity of cediranib (AZD2171) in patients (pts) with previously untreated metastatic renal cell cancer (RCC). A phase II trial of the PMH Consortium. J Clin Oncol. 2008; 26 [Abstr 5047].
20. Mulders P, Hawkins R, Nathan P, et al. Final results of a phase II randomised study of cediranib (RECENTIN™) in patients with advanced renal cell carcinoma (RCC). EJC Suppl. 2009;7:21.

21. Roodjart JM, Langeberg MH, Witteveen E, et al. The molecular basis of class side effects due to treatment with inhibitors of the VEGF/VEGFR pathway. Curr Clin Pharm. 2008;3:132–43.

22. Schmidinger M, Bellmunt J. Plethora of agents, plethora of targets, plethora of side effects in metastatic renal cell carcinoma. Cancer Treat Rev. 2010;36: 416–24.

23. Di Lorenzo G, Porta C, Sternberg C, et al. Toxicities of targeted therapy and their management in kidney cancer. Eur Urol. 2011;59:526–40.

24. Hutson TE, Figlin RA, Kuhn JG, et al. Targeted therapies for metastatic renal cell carcinoma: an overview of toxicity and dosing strategies. Oncologist. 2008;13:1084–96.

25. Bhojani N, Jeldres C, Patard J-J, et al. Toxicities associated with the administration of sorafenib, sunitinib, and temsirolimus and their management in patients with metastatic renal cell carcinoma. Eur Urol. 2008;53:917–30.

26. Rini BI, Tamaskar I, Shaheen P, et al. Hypothyroidism in patients with metastatic renal cell carcinoma treated with sunitinib. J Natl Cancer Inst. 2007;99:81–3.

27. Wolter P, Dumez H, Schöffski P. Sunitinib and hypothyroidism. N Engl J Med. 2007;356:1580–1.

28. Wolter P, Stefan C, Decallonne B, et al. The clinical implications of sunitinib-induced hypothyroidism: a prospective evaluation. Br J Cancer. 2008;99: 448–54.

29. Iglesias P, Diez JJ. Thyroid function and kidney disease. Eur J Endocrinol. 2009;160:503–15.

30. Langenberg MHG, Van Herpen CML, De Bono J, et al. Effective strategies for management of hypertension after vascular endothelial growth factor signaling inhibition therapy: results from a phase II randomized, factorial, double-blind study of cediranib in patients with advanced solid tumors. J Clin Oncol. 2009;27:6152–9.

31. Zhu X, Stergiopoulos K, Wu S. Risk of hypertension and renal dysfunction with an angiogenesis inhibitor sunitinib: systematic review and meta-analysis. Acta Oncol. 2009;48:9–17.

32. Izzedine H, Ederhy S, Goldwasser F, et al. Management of hypertension in angiogenesis inhibitor-treated patients. Ann Oncol. 2009;20:807–15.

33. Vaklavas C, Lenihan D, Kurzrock R, et al. Anti-vascular endothelial growth factor therapies and cardiovascular toxicity: what are the important clinical marker to target? Oncologist. 2010;15:130–41.

34. Schmidinger M, Zielinski CC, Vogl UM, et al. Cardiac toxicity of sunitinib and sorafenib in patients with metastatic renal cell carcinoma. J Clin Oncol. 2008;26:5204–12.

35. Lenihan DJ. Tyrosine kinase inhibitors: can promising new therapy associated with cardiac toxicity strengthen the concept of teamwork? J Clin Oncol. 2008;26:5154–5.

36. Bamias A, Lainakis G, Manios E, et al. Could rigorous diagnosis and management of hypertension reduce cardiac events in patients with renal cell carcinoma

treated with tyrosine kinase inhibitors? J Clin Oncol. 2009;27:2567–9.

37. Chu D, Lacouture ME, Weiner E, et al. Risk of hand–foot skin reaction with the multitargeted kinase inhibitor sunitinib in patients with renal cell and non-renal cell carcinoma: a meta-analysis. Clin Genitourin Cancer. 2009;7(1):11–9.

38. Lacouture ME, Wu S, Robert C, et al. Evolving strategies for the management of hand–foot skin reaction associated with the multitargeted kinase inhibitors sorafenib and sunitinib. Oncologist. 2008;13: 1001–11.

39. Dasanu CA, Dutcher J, Alexandrescu DT. Yellow skin discoloration associated with sorafenib use for treatment of metastatic renal cell carcinoma. South Med J. 2007;100(3):328–30.

40. Izzedine H, Massard C, Spano JP, et al. VEGF signaling inhibition-induced proteinuria: mechanism, significance and management. Eur J Cancer. 2010;46: 439–48.

41. Rini BI, Jaegert E, Weinberg V, et al. Clinical response to therapy targeted at vascular endothelial growth factor in metatstatic renal cell carcinoma: impact of patient characteristics and Von Hippel–Lindau gene status. BJU. 2007;98:756–62.

42. Xu CF, Bing NX, Sternberg CN, et al. Pazopanib efficacy in renal cell carcinoma: evidence for predictive genetic markers in angiogenesis-related and exposure-related genes. J Clin Oncol. 2011;29(18): 2557–64.

43. Johannsen M, Flörcken A, Bex A, et al. Can tyrosine kinase inhibitors be discontinued in patients with metastatic renal cell carcinoma and a complete response to treatment? A multicentre, retrospective analysis. Eur Urol. 2009;55:1430–9.

44. Grépin R, Pagès G. Molecular mechanism of resistance to tumour anti-angiogenic strategies. J Oncol. 2010;1–8.

45. Feldman DR, Baum MS, Ginsberg MS, et al. Phase I trial of bevacizumab plus escalated doses of sunitinib in patients with metastatic renal cell carcinoma. J Clin Oncol. 2009;27:1432–9.

46. Kwak EL, Clark JW, Chabner B. Targeted agents: the rules of combination. Clin Cancer Res. 2007;13: 5232–7.

47. Sosman JA, Puzanov I, Atkins MB. Opportunities and obstacles to combination targeted therapy in renal cell cancer. Clin Cancer Res. 2007;13:764s–9.

48. Hutson TE, Bukowski RM, Sternberg CN, et al. Sequential use of targeted agents in the treatment of renal cell carcinoma. Crit Rev Oncol Hematol. 2011;77:48–62.

49. Eichelberg C, Heuer R, Chun FK, et al. Sequential use of tyrosine kinase inhibitors sorafenib and sunitinib in metastatic renal cell carcinoma: a retrospective outcome analysis. Eur Urol. 2008;54:1373–8.

50. Bracarda S, Bellmunt J, Ravaud A, et al. Overall serviva in patients with metastatic renal cell carcinoma initially treated with bevacizumab plus interferon-α2a and subsequent therapy with tyrosine

kinase inhibitors: a retrospective analysis of the phase III AVOREN trial. BJU Int. 2010;107:214–9.

51. Rini BI. Metastatic renal cell carcinoma: many treatment options, one patient. J Clin Oncol. 2009;27:3225–34.

52. Escudier B, Albiges L, Blesius A, et al. How to select targeted therapy in renal cell cancer. Ann Oncol. 2010;21:vii59–62.

53. Bellmunt J, Flodgren P, Roigas J, et al. Optimal management of metastatic renal cell carcinoma: an algorithm for treatment. BJU Int. 2009;104:10–8.

54. Heng DYC, Xie W, Bjarnason GA, et al. Progression free survival as a predictor of overall survival in metastatic renal cell carcinoma treated with contemporary targeted therapy. Cancer. 2010;117(12):2637–42.

Mammalian Target of Rapamycin in Renal Cell Carcinoma

18

Eric Jonasch and Michel Choueiri

Introduction

Mammalian target of rapamycin (mTOR), the eukaryotic homolog of the yeast TOR, is involved in cell growth, metabolism, and response to stress. Located downstream of Akt in the PI3K/Akt/mTOR pathway, it is a plausible target for antineoplastic agents when this pathway is aberrantly activated in tumors including renal cell carcinoma (RCC). Rapamycin and its analogs inhibit the mTOR complex function and prevent progression from the G1 to the S phase. Two rapamycin analogs are currently approved for the management of patients with RCC; temsirolimus and everolimus. Temsirolimus has shown prolonged overall survival as a first-line agent in patients with poor prognostic features. Everolimus has resulted in improved progression-free survival vs. placebo in a phase III trial in patients who failed initial treatment with sunitinib or sorafenib. Based on these results, many clinical trials have been designed and many questions remain about the most suitable modalities to use these agents in conjunction with other available therapeutic options.

Signaling Pathways

mTOR/PI3K/Akt Pathway

Two yeast *Saccharomyces cerevisiae* TOR alleles, TOR1 and TOR2 were originally identified by Heitman in 1991, through mutations that conferred resistance to the growth inhibition effect by rapamycin [1]. In this study, Heitman showed that rapamycin requires an intracellular cofactor, FK506 binding protein 12 (FKBP12) to form a complex that subsequently binds and inhibits TOR function. The structure of the FKBP12-rapamycin complex was later described by Clardy et al. in 1996 [2]. This inhibition prevents the progression from the G phase into S phase.

The TOR gene is highly preserved and has thus far been identified in every eukaryote genome [3]. The eukaryote gene, mTOR, was first described as FRAP/RAFT-1 by Brown et al. in 1994 [4] and mTOR by Sabers et al. in 1995 [5]. It is a 289 kDa intracellular serine/threonine kinase and along with ataxia telangiectasia mutated (ATM), ATM and rad3 (ATR), and DNA protein kinases belongs to the phosphatidylinositol-3-kinase (PI3K) related kinases (PIKK) family [6, 7]. It shares a similar serine/threonine protein kinase domain at the carboxy-terminal with this family.

In the amino-terminal half, mTOR has tandem HEAT repeats and a FRAP-ATM-TTRAP (FAT) domain of unclear function. An FKBP12-rapamycin binding (FRB) domain links FAT to

E. Jonasch (✉) • M. Choueiri
Genitourinary Medical Oncology, UT MD Anderson Cancer Center, Unit 1374, PO Box 301439, Houston, TX 77230, USA
e-mail: ejonasch@mdanderson.org

S.C. Campbell and B.I. Rini (eds.), *Renal Cell Carcinoma: Clinical Management*, Current Clinical Urology,
DOI 10.1007/978-1-62703-062-5_18, © Springer Science+Business Media New York 2013

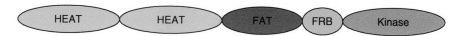

Fig. 18.1 Structure of mTOR. The amino-terminal contains tandem HEAT repeats and a FAT domain of unclear function. The kinase domain lies on the carboxy-terminal of mTOR and is linked to FAT by FKBP12-rapamycin binding domain (FRB)

the kinase site. Carboxy-terminal to the kinase domain is the FATC domain (Fig. 18.1).

In the cell, mTOR binds to different proteins to form two distinct complexes: mTOR complex 1 (mTORC1) and complex 2 (mTORC2) [8]. mTORC1 consists of mTOR, mammalian LST8 (mLST8), proline-rich Akt substrate 40 (PRAS40), and raptor [9–11]. Only mTORC1 is sensitive to rapamycin analogs [10] and has been more studied than mTORC2, on which our knowledge remains limited.

mTORC1 responds to stresses like nutrient availability, energy, stress, and growth factors [3, 12–17] to regulate cap-dependent translation, transcription cell progression, and survival. Downstream, mTORC1 activates ribosomal S6 kinase-1 (S6K1) and inactivates 4E-BP1 through phosphorylation. S6K1 is involved in translation whereas 4E-BP1 is the suppressor of the mRNA cap-binding protein eIF4E. Upon phosphorylation, 4E-BP1 dissociates from eIF4E, which becomes free to bind to a scaffolding protein, eIF4G. eIF4E, an mRNA cap-binding protein, selectively enables the translation of key proteins involved in cellular growth, angiogenesis, survival, and malignancy such as cyclin D1, Bcl-2, MMP-9, and vascular endothelial growth factor (VEGF) [18–20] (Fig. 18.2).

mTORC1 is activated through two pathways. The first pathway involves the binding of extracellular ligands such as insulin growth factor-1 (IGF-1), epidermal growth factor (EGF), transforming growth factor (TGF-α) to transmembrane tyrosine kinases triggering their autophosphorylation. These kinases activate PI3K, which then activates Akt. Akt inhibits two downstream complexes, the tuberous sclerosis complex 1 (TSC1) and complex 2 (TSC2) [21], which then release their inhibition on the downstream mTOR complex. Akt activation can be inhibited by the tumor suppressor phosphatase and tensin homolog

(PTEN) gene located on chromosome 10 [22]. The loss of PTEN function [23], or the presence of genetic mutations in the PI3K gene lead to constitutive phosphorylation of Akt and anomalous activation, and hence to mTOR activation.

Another parallel pathway, activated under nutrient or energy depletion conditions, involves the adenosine monophosphate (AMP) kinase activation of TSC1/TSC2, and suppression of mTOR kinase activity.

mTOR in RCC

In RCC, neoplasia is driven by the inactivation of the Von Hippel Lindau (VHL) gene, a tumor suppressor gene [24, 25]. The VHL protein is responsible for the proteasome-mediated degradation of the hypoxia-induced factor (HIF)-1α and is defective in the most common histologic subtype of RCC, clear cell carcinoma [26]. In the presence of an altered VHL protein, HIF accumulates and results in the nuclear transcription of genes that play a role in tumorigenesis such as VEGF-A, endothelial growth factor receptor (EGFR), platelet-derived growth factor (PDGF)-β, and transforming growth factor-α (TGF-α) [27–32].

In addition to the effects of a defective VHL protein, PTEN is also inactive in 20–30% of RCC tumors [33] and induce activation of mTOR through Akt, and consequently leads to HIF accumulation [27, 34]. mTOR increases the expression of HIF-1α through the downstream effects of S6K1 and eIF-4E which enhance the translation of ribosomal proteins and mRNA translation, respectively [35]. The inhibition of mTOR therefore is likely to decrease proliferation, angiogenesis in addition to a direct antitumor effect.

In an immunohistochemical study, phospho-mTOR staining showed moderate to strong signal

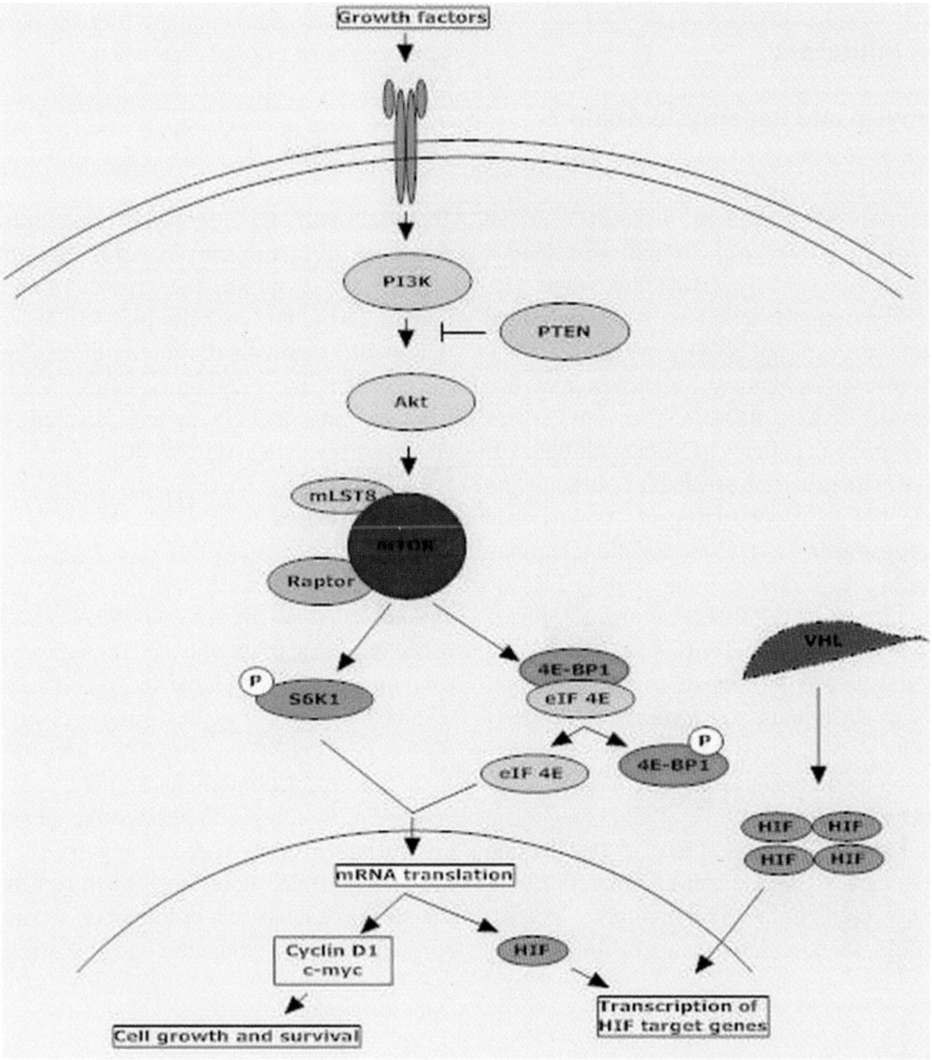

Fig. 18.2 Akt/PI3K/mTOR signaling pathway. mTOR binds to raptor and mLST8 to form mTORC1. MTORC1 is activated by Akt, which is activated by PI3K. PTEN inhibits the activation of Akt by PI3K. Downstream, mTOR phosphorylates p70S6K1 (S6K1) and 4E-BP1 leading to activation of pathways involved in cell growth and survival as well as translation of HIF. In RCC, inactivated VHL is unable to facilitate HIF-α proteolysis leading to HIF accumulation. HIF production is also induced by the activation of the mTOR pathway. The active intranuclear HIF-α induces transcription of HIF target genes such as VEGF and PDGF. Adapted from Rini et al. Lancet Oncol 2009;10:992–1000

in 17 out of 25 tissue microarrays from clear cell carcinomas, suggesting that mTOR is activated in a substantial percentage of patients with RCC [36]. In another immunohistochemical study [37] using antibodies against pAkt, PTEN, p27, and pS6 on a tissue microarray constructed from specimens from 375 patients with RCC, the mTOR pathway was more active in clear cell carcinoma, high-grade tumors, and tumors with poor prognostic features, indicating that these patients might be better candidates to treatment with mTOR inhibitors (mTORi). The mTOR-related proteins could also be helpful as predictors of response. In one study, Cho et al. found that p-S6K1 and pAkt might be predictive biomarkers for response to temsirolimus treatment and hence needed to be investigated further for possible application in patient selection models for mTORi [38].

mTOR Inhibitors

Rapamycin and Rapamycin Analogs

Rapamycin (sirolimus) is a macrolide secreted by *Streptomyces hygroscopicus*, isolated from an Easter Island ("Rapa Nui" island) soil sample and reported in 1975 by Vezina and Sehgal [39, 40]. It was initially found to have antifungal properties with special activity against Candida. Soon however, additional immunosuppressive [41] properties were found and rapamycin was used in transplant patients [42]. In addition, antitumor properties were described [43, 44], making it a potential antineoplastic agent. As described above, rapamycin exerts these functions through the binding to the intracellular protein FK-506 binding protein-12 (FKBP12) to form a complex that binds and inhibits mTORC1.

Rapamycin and three rapamycin analogs, temsirolimus, everolimus, ridaforolimus (formerly deforolimus), have therefore been investigated as possible antitumorigenic agents. The three rapamycin derivatives differ from the original rapamycin molecule at the C43 position through the addition of an ester, ether, or phosphonate group for temsirolimus, everolimus, and ridaforolimus, respectively (Fig. 18.3). Ridaforolimus is still at early stages of investigation and the former two agents have been more extensively studied.

Temsirolimus

Temsirolimus (CCI-779) is a water-soluble ester derivative of rapamycin. In vitro, temsirolimus was shown to inhibit the growth of multiple normal and tumorous cells [45–48]. In vivo, it inhibited the growth of various tumors including prostate cancer and breast cancer xenografts from cell lines lacking the expression of PTEN and overexpressing Akt [49, 50].

Phase I Studies
Dosing
The maximum tolerated dose, the dosing parameters, and safety profile of temsirolimus were established in clinical trials with patients with advanced solid tumors [51–54] (Table 18.1). The maximum tolerated dose with a cyclic dosing regimen (daily for 5 days every 2 weeks) was 15–19 mg/m^2 [55]. In a dose-escalation phase I study, a weekly, 30-min infusion regimen allowed the administration of higher doses (7.5–220 mg/m^2) [52]. The maximal tolerated dose was not truly achieved, despite the development of thrombocytopenia and reversible rash and stomatitis, and objective partial

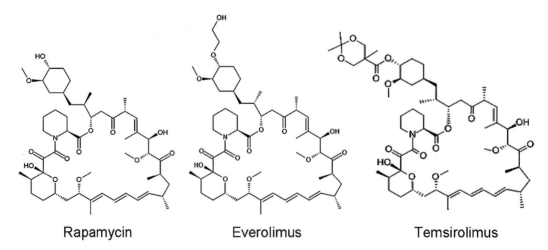

Fig. 18.3 Structure of rapamycin, everolimus, and temsirolimus. Everolimus and temsirolimus substitute the hydroxyl group on carbon 43 in rapamycin by an ether and ester group, respectively

Table 18.1 Dose escalation studies of temsirolimus in patients with advanced cancer including RCC

Reference	n	Dose	DLT (n)	Results
Hidalgo [51]	63 with advanced cancer (16 RCC)	0.75–24 mg/m²/day	Vomiting, diarrhea, asthenia, elevated transaminases (2) (19 mg/m²/day)	Half-life of 13–25 h
			Stomatitis (1) (24 mg/m²/day)	Unconfirmed PR in 2 pts with RCC on (3.7 and 19 mg/m²/day)
Raymond [52]	24 with advanced cancer (6 RCC)	7.5–220 mg/m²	Neutropenia, thrombocytopenia, hypophosphatemia (34 mg/ m²)	Maximal concentration and AUC increase sub-proportionally with dose
			Thrombocytopenia, asthenia, diarrhea (45 mg/m²)	6.5-month PR in 1 pt with RCC
			Manic-depressive syndrome, stomatitis (1), ALT elevation, asthenia stomatitis (1) (220 mg/m²)	

and minor responses were noted at doses below the maximal dose used. In addition, the variability predicted with flat doses was comparable with body surface area-normalized treatment, and flat doses were hence used [52].

Subsequent clinical trials on different advanced cancers hence used weekly IV doses of 25, 75, or 250 mg [56–58].

The temsirolimus dose needed for biologic activity, i.e., inhibition of mTOR activity was studied in peripheral blood mononuclear cells (PBMCs) [59]. In those cells, the activity was determined by a decrease in the activity of S6K1, and 25 mg was shown to be sufficient to induce inhibition.

Pharmacokinetics
Absorption
Temsirolimus administered intravenously at a dose of 25 mg weekly, results in a mean temsirolimus maximal concentration of 585 ng/mL in whole blood and a mean AUC in blood of 1,627 ng h/mL [60]. Its active metabolite, sirolimus, is approximately 40% bound to lipoproteins in the blood and hence elevated plasma lipoprotein levels may increase sirolimus plasma concentrations. In 18 patients with mild to moderate hepatic impairment who received a single dose of sirolimus, the clearance of sirolimus was decreased by more than 30% [61], and hence the dose of

temsirolimus should be decreased to 15 mg weekly in patients with hepatic impairment.

Metabolism
Temsirolimus is metabolized via oxidative hydrolysis to form sirolimus, its active metabolite [62]. Both temsirolimus and sirolimus are metabolized by the cytochrome P450 (CYP)3A4 pathway to form various demethylated and hydroxylated isomeric products [63, 64]. Sirolimus appears 15 min after temsirolimus infusion and reaches a peak at 0.5–2.0 h, followed by a monoexponential decrease [52]. The concentration of sirolimus is higher than temsirolimus with a mean AUC ratio (sirolimus/temsirolimus) of ~2.5–3.5. When temsirolimus was administered at doses higher than 34 mg/m², residual concentrations of sirolimus were noted before the scheduled treatment but did not result in rising concentrations of sirolimus after repeated cycles [52].

Elimination
Temsirolimus is excreted predominantly via the feces. When a single 25 mg dose of radiolabeled temsirolimus was administered, 78% of the radioactivity was recovered from the feces and 5% was recovered in the urine suggesting a minimal role for renal clearance of temsirolimus. Its mean half-life at a standard dose of 25 mg is approximately 13 h with a total plasma clearance (CL) of

16 L/h. Its active metabolite has a longer half-life with a mean between 61 and 69 h [65], and hence results in higher concentrations than temsirolimus. The clearance is moderate and increases substantially with higher doses and has a minimal patient intervariability. This is thought to be a result of saturable specific binding of CCI-779 to FKBP in the red blood cell [53].

Tumor Response and Toxicity

In addition to establishing the pharmacokinetics outlined above, the phase I studies yielded preliminary clinical results. In a study on 24 patients with advanced cancers, temsirolimus resulted in two confirmed partial responses (PR) in patients with breast cancer and RCC. The patient with RCC had documented tumor progression of lung and pleural metastasis on interferon-α (IFN) and interleukin 2 and received 15 mg/m^2 of temsirolimus [52]. The partial response lasted 6.5 months and was observed after 8 weeks of treatment. Two additional patients with RCC experienced minor responses after treatment with 15 and 45 mg/m^2, and had 34% and 39% tumor reductions respectively, with the partial responses lasting for 3 and 4.9 months.

In another dose-escalation study on 63 patients with advanced cancers, including 16 patients with RCC, six patients had evidence of clinical benefit, and two patients with RCC had unconfirmed PR. The first received 3.7 mg/m^2/day of temsirolimus, and the second received 19 mg/m^2/day temsirolimus for five cycles and then 15 mg/m^2/day [51]. Three patients had dose-limiting toxicities (stomatitis, vomiting/diarrhea, asthenia, and elevated liver transaminases). Five patients required dose reduction.

Additional phase I studies examined the role of temsirolimus in combination with agents targeting VEGF. In the first cohort of a study on three patients with mRCC, IV temsirolimus 15 mg weekly was administered concomitantly with oral sunitinib 25 mg daily (4 weeks on, 2 weeks off) but resulted in two DLTs (rash, thrombocytopenia, cellulitis, and gout) and the study was not pursued [66].

Another combination, bevacizumab/temsirolimus appears to have a better toxicity profile.

In two separate abstracts presented at ASCO in 2007 [67] and 2009 [68], Merchan et al. evaluated the safety and efficacy of this combination. In the phase I part involving 12 evaluable patients with stage IV clear cell RCC and who had progressed on up to two previous regimens, seven patients experienced a PR and two patients suffered DLTs (mucositis and hypertriglyceridemia). Following this phase I, a regimen of 10 mg/kg of bevacizumab IV every 2 weeks with temsirolimus 25 mg IV weekly was established. In the phase II component [68], 35 patients were evaluated. Four patients had PR and 18 patients had stable disease (SD), suggesting that 88% of the patients had experienced clinical benefits.

Phase II Studies

In phase II settings, temsirolimus role has been investigated in multiple advanced cancers including heavily pretreated breast cancer [58], melanoma [69], small cell lung cancer [57], glioblastoma multiforme [70], neuroendocrine tumors [71], and mantle cell lymphoma [72], with mixed results.

In RCC, phase II studies have determined the efficacy of temsirolimus monotherapy (Table 18.2) and combination regimens. Atkins et al. first investigated single-agent temsirolimus on 111 patients with cytokine-resistant RCC [65]. The patients were randomly assigned to weekly treatment with temsirolimus at a dose of 25, 75, or 250 mg. Tumor response, time to tumor progression, survival, and adverse events were recorded. An objective response rate of 7% (one complete response and seven partial responses) was observed and 26% of the patients experienced minor responses; 51% of patients overall experienced a PR or complete response, or SD lasting more than 24 weeks. The median PFS was 5.8 months and the median OS was 15 months. The most common grade 3 or 4 side effects were hyperglycemia (17%), hypophosphatemia (13%), anemia (9%), and hypertriglyceridemia (6%). Other grade 1 or 2 side effects included maculopapular rash, mucositis, asthenia, and nausea and occurred in more than two thirds of the patients. When these patients were stratified along good-, intermediate-, or poor-risk

Table 18.2 Phase 2 studies on temsirolimus in patients with advanced RCC

Reference	Treatment dose	n (total)	CR (total)	PR (total)	MR (total)	SD (total)	PD (total)	TTP (mo) (all pts)	OS (mo) (all pts)
Atkins [65]	25 mg weekly	36	0	2	5	20	6	6.3	13.8
	50 mg weekly	38	0	3	13	11	9	6.7	11.0
	250 mg weekly	37	1	2	11	11	7	5.2	17.5
		(111, 10 unknown)	(1)	(7)	(29)	(42)	(22)	(5.8)	(15.0)
Motzer [73]	IFN 6 MU + temsirolimus 5–25 mg weekly	71		8		25		9.1	18.8

CR complete response, *PR* partial response, *MR* minor response, *SD* stable disease, *PD* progressive disease, *TTP* time to progression, *OS* overall survival, *pts* patients

groups according to the MKCC criteria, OS were 23.8, 22.5, and 8.2 months, respectively. The OS in the poor risk group was longer than the traditional reported OS of 4.9 months in patients having received IFN [74] and justified further studying in this patient subset.

Another multicenter dose escalation phase I/II study examined the effect of temsirolimus/IFN combination [73]. An ascending dose (5, 10, 15, 20, or 25 mg) of temsirolimus was administered weekly in combination with IFN (6 or 9 million units) administered three times per week. Based on the dose-limiting toxicities, a dose of 15 mg/6 MU was recommended. Among the 39 patients who received the recommended dose, three patients achieved partial response and 14 had stable disease for at least 24 weeks, with a median PFS for all patients in the study of 9.1 months. The most common reported grade 3 or 4 side effects included leukopenia, hypophosphatemia, asthenia, anemia, and hypertriglyceridemia.

Phase III Trial

Because of the prolongation in OS noted in patients with poor risk features, a phase III trial was initiated. In 2007, Hudes et al. published the results of the multicenter global advanced renal cell carcinoma (Global ARCC) [75]. This trial compared temsirolimus to IFN and to the temsirolimus/IFN combination as a first-line treatment in patients with poor prognosis who were treatment naïve. The patients had three or more of six features: five MSKCC prognostic model criteria [76] and metastases in multiple organs [77]. The

eligibility criteria differed from other phase III trials on other targeted therapies by including all histologic subtypes of RCC. The trial also allowed for enrollment of patients with CNS metastases and patients were not required to have undergone a nephrectomy prior to enrollment. Six hundred and twenty-six patients were recruited and randomized to three treatment arms: (1) weekly 25 mg dose of IV temsirolimus weekly ($n=209$), (2) 3 MU IFN (with an escalation to 18 MU or maximum tolerated dose) subcutaneously three times weekly ($n=207$), and (3) a combination of temsirolimus (15 mg weekly) plus IFN (3 MU with an escalation to 6 MU three times weekly) ($n=210$). Twenty percent of the patients had non-clear cell histology and 67% had undergone previous nephrectomy.

The primary endpoint was OS and the secondary efficacy endpoints were PFS, the ORR, and the clinical benefit rate, defined as the proportion of patients with an objective response or stable disease for at least 24 weeks. No statistical difference was observed when the combination group and the IFN group were compared with OS of 8.4 and 7.3 months, respectively (HR 0.96, $p=0.70$). However, a prolonged OS of 10.9 months was observed in the temsirolimus monotherapy arm vs. 7.3 months in the IFN arm (HR 0.73, $p=0.008$). The objective response rates were not statistically different between the three groups, but more patients in the temsirolimus monotherapy (32.1%) experienced a clinical benefit compared to the combination group (28.1%) and IFN monotherapy (15.5%). An improvement in PFS was also

Table 18.3 Side effects occurring in >10% of patients receiving temsirolimus in the global ARCC trial [75]

Side effect	Grade 3 or 4 (%)	All grades
Asthenia	11	51
Rash	4	47
Nausea	2	37
Anorexia	3	32
Pain	5	28
Dyspnea	9	28
Infection	5	27
Diarrhea	1	27
Peripheral edema	2	27
Cough	1	26
Fever	1	24
Abdominal pain	4	21
Stomatitis	1	20
Constipation	0	20
Back pain	3	20
Vomiting	2	19
Weight loss	1	19
Headache	1	15
Laboratory abnormalities	20	45
Anemia	3	27
Hyperlipidemia	11	26
Hyperglycemia	1	24
Hypercholesterolemia	3	14
Elevated creatinine	1	14
Thrombocytopenia		

observed ($p<0.001$) in the temsirolimus arm compared to the IFN alone arm, and the reported PFS were 3.8, 1.9, and 3.7 months in the temsirolimus, IFN and combination arms, respectively.

Subsequent subset analyses were performed and the improvements in OS and PFS were independent of the histological type or the nephrectomy status [78, 79].

Patients receiving temsirolimus experienced a higher incidence of hyperglycemia, hyperlipidemia, and hypercholesterolemia compared to patients receiving IFN. They also experienced more rash, stomatitis, and peripheral edema but had a lower incidence of grade 3 and 4 side effects (Table 18.3).

Ongoing Trials

The availability of agents against the VEGF molecule and the VEGF receptor (VEGFR) raised the question about the possible role of combination therapies with the mTORi in RCC. A successful combination therapy should target different pathways simultaneously, improve clinical outcome, and have an acceptable safety profile. As described earlier, the combination of temsirolimus/bevacizumab yielded encouraging preliminary results, but the final results are still pending.

In contrast, the combination of temsirolimus with VEGFR TKIs appears to be less tolerated. For example, a study on three patients receiving temsirolimus (15 mg weekly) in conjunction with sunitinib (25 mg daily for 4 week-on therapy, 2 week-off therapy cycles) was terminated because of DLTs occurring in two patients (rash and cellulitis/thrombocytopenia) [80]. This combination is therefore not recommended.

The combination of temsirolimus and sorafenib, a VEGFR and Raf kinase inhibitor, is less conclusive [81]. DLT consisting of mucocutaneous side effects occurred at the full dose of 400 mg of sorafenib twice daily in conjunction with temsirolimus. But there was no evidence of pharmacokinetic drug–drug interaction. The DLTs necessitated a reduction in half of the sorafenib dose.

Many clinical trials have therefore been designed to study the efficacy of combination therapy in addition to clinical trials focused on sequential therapy options.

Combination Treatment
Investigation of TORISEL and Avastin Combination Therapy
Because of the clinical benefits observed in the phase II trials for the combination of bevacizumab/temsirolimus, trials were launched to further evaluate this regimen. The Investigation of TORISEL and Avastin Combination Therapy (INTORACT) trial is a phase 3b [82], randomized, open-label study comparing bevacizumab + temsirolimus to bevacizumab + IFN as a first-line treatment option in patients with advanced RCC (NCT00631371). The trial has completed accrual of 791 patients and the final results are pending. The primary outcome is independently assessed PFS and the secondary endpoints are safety, OS and investigator assessed PFS.

BeST
Another trial sponsored by ECOG, bevacizumab, sorafenib, and temsirolimus in advanced RCC (BeST), is a randomized phase II study comparing bevacizumab to the combinations of temsirolimus/bevacizumab, sorafenib/bevacizumab, and temsirolimus/sorafenib (NCT00378703) [83]. This study has also completed accrual and data should be forthcoming.

Sequential Treatment
Torisel 404
In addition to combination therapy, sequential treatment is being investigated in patients who have failed initial TKI treatment. The Torisel 404 phase III trial, sponsored by Wyeth [84], will compare temsirolimus to sorafenib as a second-line treatment in patients who have failed treat-

ment with sunitinib (NCT00474786). The trial is currently enrolling patients with an accrual goal of 480 patients. The primary endpoints are safety and tolerability of both temsirolimus and sorafenib in the second-line setting, and an independently assessed PFS. The secondary endpoints are OS, duration of response, and response rates.

Everolimus

Everolimus (RAD-001) differs from rapamycin through the addition of an ether group. It was first developed as an oral immunosuppressive agent to prevent allograft dysfunction following organ transplantation. It is well tolerated and is widely used for prophylaxis of rejection in patients who have undergone cardiac, liver, and renal transplants [85, 86]. The dose is 1.5 mg twice daily up to a dose of 6 mg/daily [87, 88].

Everolimus binds to a cytoplasmic protein, of FK-506 binding protein-12, to form a complex that interacts with mTOR. This interaction prevents the phosphorylation of S6K1 and 4E-BP1 and activation, and therefore affecting the tumor cell metabolism and growth.

In Vitro and Animal Studies
In addition to its immunosuppressant effects, everolimus displays antiproliferative properties against endothelial cells following injury and against tumor cells. In a rat model of renal microvascular injury, everolimus inhibited glomerular endothelial cell proliferation by up to 60%, an effect that was associated with a reduced phosphorylation of the p70S6 kinase and reduced VEGF levels in the glomeruli. It also inhibits the growth of human derived cell lines in culture and in xenograft models [89]. In a syngeneic rat pancreatic tumor model, everolimus showed dose-dependent antitumor activity with both daily and weekly administration schedules, and statistically significant decrease in the tumor size among the treated subjects of 70–95% depending on the dose. In this preclinical study, everolimus was well tolerated and had an antitumor potency similar to that of the cytotoxic agent 5-fluorouracil. Because everolimus also displays immunosuppressive

effects, it was important to find an adequate therapeutic window to balance the benefits of adequate tumor control with minimal immunosuppression. For that purpose, Boulay et al. biochemically profiled the mTOR signaling pathway in tumors, skin, and PBMCs, and found a decrease in the phosphorylation of 4E-BP1 and inactivation of S6K1 after a single administration of everolimus. This finding suggested that S6K1 from the PBMC could possibly be used as a marker for mTOR inhibition and as a means to assess everolimus treatment schedules in cancer patients.

Phase I Studies
Dosing Schedule
Based on these preliminary findings, a phase I study was conducted by Tanaka et al. [90] to predict optimal clinical regimens of everolimus. S6K1 from PBMC was used as a marker of mTOR inhibition. A pharmacokinetics/pharmacodynamics model was used to plot the association between everolimus concentrations and level of S6K1 inhibition in PBMCs in both human subjects and rats. A time- and dose-dependent S6K1 inhibition with everolimus was shown. In the rat model, a relationship was shown between S6K1 inhibition and antitumor effect. This model allowed the prediction of PBMC S6K1 inhibition-time profiles in patients receiving everolimus, and a daily administration was found to yield a greater effect than weekly administration at higher doses.

Pharmacokinetics
The pharmacokinetics evaluation of everolimus was done in conjunction with the pharmacodynamics evaluation described earlier.

Absorption
Everolimus is administered orally, has a low bioavailability in rats of 10% [91], but has a fast absorption. The peak everolimus concentration $(44.2 \pm 13.3 \, \mu g/L)$ is reached within 30 min to 1 h after administration with an area under the curve of $219.69 \pm \mu g \, h/L$ [92], with an approximate half-life of 30 h [93]. The steady state is reached within 7 days. High-fat meals decrease the absorption of everolimus by half [94], and hence the drug should be taken consistently either with food or without. The absorption is possibly also affected by the activity of P-glycoprotein, which reduces the oral bioavailability of drugs that are CYP3A substrates [95].

The protein binding of everolimus is not influenced by moderate hepatic impairment [96].

Metabolism
Unlike temsirolimus, everolimus is not degraded to sirolimus, but is metabolized essentially in the gut and liver by cytochrome P450 3A4, −3A5, and −2C8 and PgP enzymes into hydroxylated and demethylated metabolites [64, 97]. Hydroxy-everolimus is the most important metabolite, accounting for half of the dose-normalized AUC of the first 24 h (AUC24) of everolimus AUC24. The different metabolites appear within 1.2–2.0 h after administration, vs. 1.5 h for everolimus [98, 99].

To identify the optimal regimen and dosage of everolimus, O'Donnell et al. (Table 18.4) performed a dose-escalation study on 92 patients with advanced cancer with an everolimus dose range of 5–30 mg/week initially based on transplantation data. However, in view of the preclinical data favoring daily dosing, two regimens of 50 and 70 mg weekly and daily doses of 5 and 10 mg were investigated. S6 kinase 1 activity in PBMC was inhibited for at least 7 days at doses ≥ 20 mg/week. Evaluation of the stable predose serum trough concentration levels from 26 of the 31 patients treated with the weekly regimen indicated minimal accumulation at all weekly dose levels, with steady-state achieved by the second week of treatment. The area under the curve increased proportionally with the dose, but the maximal serum concentration increased less than proportionally at doses ≥ 20 mg/week. Evaluation of profiles from ten patients on the daily regimen patients showed that a steady-state level was reached within a week. Both maximal serum concentration and AUC increased in a dose proportional manner.

Excretion
No definite excretion study has been undertaken, but in patients receiving concurrent cyclosporine

Table 18.4 Dose escalation studies of everolimus in patients with advanced cancer including RCC

Reference	n	Dose	DLT (n)	Results
O'Donnell [93]	92 with advanced cancer (10 RCC)	Group 1: weekly dose 5 mg vs. 10 mg vs. 30 mg (n = 18)	No toxicity	S6K1 activity was inhibited for >7 days at doses higher than 20 mg/week
		Group 2: weekly dose 50 mg vs. 70 mg (n = 37)	Stomatitis and fatigue (1) (50 mg)	Everolimus was tolerated at dosages up to 70 mg/week and 10 mg/day
		Group 3: daily dose 5 mg vs. 10 mg (n = 37)	Hyperglycemia (1) (10 mg)	Five of ten patients with RCC had PFS ≥6 months
Tabernero [100]	55 with advanced cancer (2 RCC)	Group 1: weekly dose 20 mg vs. 50 mg vs. 70 mg (n = 31)	70 mg: stomatitis (2) neutropenia (1), hyperglycemia (1)	Complete inhibition of S6K1 and peIF-4G at 10 mg/day and ≥50 mg/week
		Group 2: daily dose 5 mg vs. 10 mg (n = 24)	Stomatitis (1) (10 mg)	One of two patients with RCC had stable disease for 14.6+ months at 50 mg weekly

radiolabeled everolimus, 80% of the radioactivity was recovered from the feces, and 5% was excreted in the urine, after the administration of a 3 mg single dose of everolimus (Everolimus-Summary of Product Characteristics. Novartis Pharma AG, Basel, Switzerland).

Tumor Response and Toxicity

Fifty-five patients were studied by Tabernero in a dose escalation phase I setting at doses of 20, 50, and 70 mg weekly or 5 and 10 mg daily [100]. A dose and schedule-dependent inhibition of the mTOR pathway was observed with complete inhibition of pS6K1 and p-eIF-4G at a daily dose of 10 mg or weekly dose of 50 mg or greater. Only two patients had RCC. Clinical benefit was noted in four patients including one patient with RCC who experienced stable disease of 14.6 months on 50 mg/week dose. One patient developed grade 3 stomatitis on the daily dose of 10 mg. On the weekly dose at 70 mg, two patients had grade 3 stomatitis, one had grade 3 neutropenia, and the last developed grade 3 hyperglycemia.

Among the 92 patients evaluated in the phase I trial by O'Donnell, four patients experienced partial responses, and 12 patients had a PFS of 6 months or more, including five of the ten patients with RCC. In the two previously described phase I studies, dose-limiting toxicity was seen in one out of six patients [93] receiving everolimus at a weekly dose of 50 mg (stomatitis and fatigue), and in four patients receiving 70 mg weekly. Among the patients treated with a daily regimen, one of the six patients receiving 10 mg developed hyperglycemia, and another patient also receiving 10 mg developed stomatitis [100].

Phase II Trials

Two phase II studies have recently investigated the safety and efficacy role of everolimus monotherapy [101] and the combination of everolimus and bevacizumab [102] in the treatment of patients with mRCC (Table 18.5).

Amato et al. conducted a 2-stage, single-arm, phase 2 trial to determine the PFS of patients with metastatic clear cell RCC receiving everolimus at a daily dose of 10 mg. Forty one patients were recruited, and 37 patients were evaluable for response. Eligibility criteria included ECOG PS ≤2, satisfactory hematologic, hepatic, renal, and cardiac function. Patients with brain metastases were excluded. The majority of the patients (83%) had received prior systemic treatment, mostly cytokine therapy with IL-2 and/or IFN-α (61%). 59, 37 and 5% had intermediate, good and poor risk per MSKCC criteria, respectively.

The results showed a median PFS of 11.2 months and a median OS of 22.1 months.

Table 18.5 Phase 2 studies on everolimus in patients with advanced RCC

Reference	Treatment dose	n	CR	SD	PR	PD	PFS (mo)	OS (mo)
Amato [101]	10 mg daily	41 (37 evaluated)		>6 months: 21 (57%)	5 (14%)		11	
Hainsworth [102]	10 mg daily + Bevacizumab (10 mg/kg every 2 weeks)	Group A: 50 (previously untreated)	1 (2%)	25 (50%)	14 (28%)	3 (6%)	9.1 (6.3–11.7)	21.3 (16.7—NR)
		Group B: 30 (Previous TKI treatment)	1 (3%)	19 (64%)	6 (20%)	3 (10%)	7.1 (3.7–10.9	14.5 (10.8—NR)

Five patients (14%) experienced a partial response, and 27 had a stable disease duration longer than 3 months, with 21 (57%) having a stable disease lasting more than 6 months. More than 70% of the patients therefore had partial response or SD>6 months. The most common grade ½ side effects were nausea (38%), anorexia (38%), diarrhea (31%), stomatitis (31%), pneumonitis (31%), and rash (26%). The grade 3/4 side effects included pneumonitis (18%), transaminase level elevations (10%), thrombocytopenia, hyperglycemia, and alkaline phosphatase elevations (8%), and hyperlipidemia (5%).

In the phase II study by Hainsworth et al., the efficacy and toxicity of the combination of bevacizumab and everolimus in mRCC or unresectable locally recurrent clear cell RCC with good performance status was evaluated [102]. Eighty patients were enrolled in the study and divided into two groups depending on whether they were targeted therapy-naïve ($n=50$) or had received previous treatment with either sorafenib and/or sunitinib ($n=30$). The patients received everolimus 10 mg orally daily and bevacizumab 10 mg/kg intravenously every 2 weeks, and were evaluated after 8 weeks of treatment. Patients who demonstrated either an objective response or stable disease were continued on treatment and reevaluated every 8 weeks until disease progression or development of severe toxicity.

The preliminary results from 59 patients were first partly presented at the 44th Annual Meeting of the American Society of Clinical Oncology in Chicago, IL in 2008 [103], and suggested a PFS of 12 and 11 months in the untreated group and treated groups, respectively. The final analysis, however, showed a median PFS of 9.1 and 7.1 months in the untreated and treated patients, respectively, with similar overall response rates were similar in both groups (30% and 23%). The discrepancy between the preliminary and the final report have put into question the role of using preliminary results from small phase II trials, and as a basis for designing phase III studies [104]. The most commonly reported nonhematologic grade 1/2 side effects were fatigue (76%), mucositis (60%), skin rash (47%), diarrhea (45%), hypertension (43%), nausea/vomiting (43%), proteinuria (41%), hyperlipidemia (40%), anorexia (33%), epistaxis (30%), constipation (24%), and the most common hematologic grade 1/2 side effects consisted of anemia (63%), thrombocytopenia (40%), and neutropenia (17%). The most common grade 3/4 side effects included proteinuria (26%) which was reversible after bevacizumab discontinuation, mucositis/stomatitis (15%), fatigue (12%), and diarrhea (9%). Eleven patients (14%) stopped treatment due to toxicity and 25 patients (31%) underwent dose adjustments but were able to tolerate treatments at lower doses.

Phase III Trials

In view of the phase II results using everolimus as a second-line agent in mRCC, a phase III study was designed to examine the role of everolimus in patients who had progressed on TKIs. The renal cell carcinoma treatment with oral RAD001 given orally (RECORD-1), launched in 2005, was a randomized double-blind phase III trial to investigate the role of everolimus in patients who had progressed within 6 months of stopping treatment with sunitinib or sorafenib or both. Four hundred and sixteen patients were therefore randomized in a 2:1 ratio to either everolimus at a daily dose of 10 mg/day ($n=277$) or placebo ($n=139$) with best supportive care. The primary endpoint was PFS by central review, and the secondary endpoints included safety, objective response rate, OS, and quality of life.

29, 56%, and 15% had favorable, intermediate, and poor MSKCC risk respectively, and 97% of the patients had undergone prior nephrectomy. 44, 30%, and 26% had received prior sunitinib, sorafenib or both drugs, respectively, and more than 85% had received immunotherapy, hormonal therapy, or other treatments.

At the second interim analysis, a significant difference in efficacy between the two study arms was observed and the trial was stopped after 191 progression events had been observed [105]. A median PFS of 4.0 months was observed in the everolimus group vs. 1.9 months in the placebo group (Fig. 18.4). These results prompted the approval of everolimus by the FDA for the treatment of patients with advanced RCC after failure of treatment with sunitinib or sorafenib, and a level 1 recommendation by the National

Comprehensive Cancer Network for treatment of patients with advanced RCC after failure of TKIs [106].

The preliminary results were confirmed in the final report [107], the median PFS was 4.9 months in the everolimus group vs. 1.9 months in the placebo group [hazard ratio (HR), 0.33; $p<0.001$] by independent central review. No difference was observed in OS with a median duration of 14.8 months in the everolimus group vs. 14.4 months in the placebo group ($p=0.126$). These values, however, were likely confounded by a crossover effect from the placebo group into the everolimus group. When the confounding factors were accounted for, the corrected OS for crossover was 1.9-fold longer with everolimus compared with placebo only.

The most common side effects (Table 18.6) were stomatitis (44%), infections (37%), asthenia (33%), fatigue (31%), diarrhea (30%), cough (30%), rash (29%), nausea (26%), anorexia (25%), and peripheral edema (25%). The common grade ¾ side effects (≥5%) included infections (10%), dyspnea (7%), and fatigue (5%). Four percent of the patients developed pneumonitis, necessitating interruption and/or reduction and corticosteroid use in selected patients.

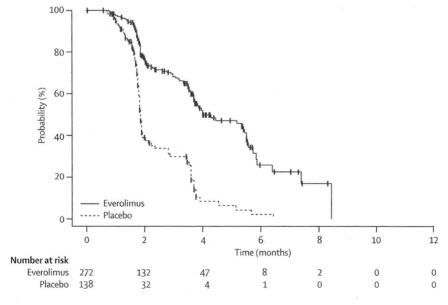

Fig. 18.4 Kaplan–Meier estimates of progression-free survival by the independent central radiology review in patients receiving everolimus in the RECORD-1 study. Reproduced from [105]

Table 18.6 Side effects occurring in >10% of patients receiving everolimus [105]

Side effect	Grade 3 or 4 (%)	All grades
Stomatitis	3	40
Rash	1	25
Fatigue	3	20
Asthenia	1	18
Diarrhea	1	17
Anorexia	1	16
Nausea	0	15
Mucosal inflammation	1	14
Vomiting	0	12
Coughing	0	12
Dry skin	1	12
Infections	2	10
Laboratory abnormalities	10	91
Anemia	3	76
Hypercholesterolemia	1	71
Hypertriglyceridemia	12	50
Hyperglycemia	1	46
Elevated creatinine	14	42
Lymphopenia	1	37
Elevated alkaline phosphatase	4	32
Hypophosphatemia	0	26
Leukopenia	1	21
Elevated AST	1	20
Thrombocytopenia	1	18
Elevated ALT	0	17
Hypocalcemia	0	11
Neutropenia		

Ongoing Trials

Based on the preliminary results suggesting a benefit for the everolimus/bevacizumab combination, and on the results showing a benefit for everolimus as a second-line treatment after TKIs, phase II and phase III studies were designed.

Phase II

The Renal Cell Cancer Treatment With Oral RAD 001 Given Daily-2 (RECORD-2) is a randomized, open-label, multi-center phase II study that aims at comparing the everolimus-bevacizumab to the established bevacizumab/IFN combination [108–111] as a first-line treatment (NCT00719264) [112]. This study, sponsored by Novartis Pharmaceuticals, has completed accrual with an estimated accrual of 360 patients but the final results are pending. The primary outcome is PFS with the secondary endpoints being OS, ORR, and safety profile of the combination regimen in addition to patient reported quality of life outcomes.

Another phase II study currently underway is the renal cell cancer treatment with oral RAD 001 given daily-3 (RECORD-3) which is a randomized, open-label, multi-center, phase 2 study investigating the role of sequential treatment with first-line everolimus followed by sunitinib vs. sunitinib followed by everolimus in patients with mRCC (NCT00903175). The study is sponsored by Novartis Pharmaceuticals and is currently recruiting patients with an estimated enrollment of 390 patients. The primary endpoint is non-inferiority of PFS after first-line of treatment with everolimus compared to PFS of patients who receive first-line sunitinib. The secondary endpoints include PFS after treatment with everolimus as second-line following sunitinib vs. PFS in patients receiving sunitinib as second-line after everolimus, safety profile of everolimus vs. sunitinib as first-line and overall for both the first-line and second-line. Other second endpoints are the patient reported outcomes in disease-related symptoms and overall quality of life during each line of treatment, ORR and duration of response differences during each line of treatment and OS rates during each line of treatment

A further study evaluating the sequencing of mTORi vs. antiangiogenic therapy is the sequential two-agent assessment in renal cell carcinoma therapy (START) trial, which randomizes previously untreated patients with mRCC between upfront everolimus, pazopanib, and bevacizumab (NCT01217931). This 240-patient study then rerandomizes individuals to one of the two remaining agents. The statistical design allows for prediction of the best sequence with a high degree of probability. Extensive biomarker analysis is being performed as part of this clinical trial, with the hope of developing predictive biomarkers to select individuals most likely to benefit from a particular sequence or class of agent.

Phase III
Based on the interim phase II results investigating the safety of the everolimus/bevacizumab combination, the Cancer and Leukemia Group B designed and sponsored a phase III, randomized, placebo-controlled, double-blind clinical trial to compare the efficacy of this combination to everolimus plus placebo in patients with mRCC who progressed after treatment with TKIs (NCT01198158). This study is currently recruiting patients and has an estimated enrollment of 700 patients. The primary endpoint will be OS and the secondary endpoints will include PFS, ORR, and toxicity. The patients should not have active brain metastases, and no renal, cardiac, or hepatic dysfunction to enroll. Samples might be collected from the blood, urine, and tumor tissue periodically for pharmacogenomic and correlative studies, and the patients will be followed up every 8 weeks after completion of the study treatment until disease progression and every 6 months afterwards.

Histologically, the tumor samples must have some component of clear cell elements.

Adjuvant Phase III
To better understand the role of mTORi in the adjuvant setting, the Southwest Oncology Group has launched the everolimus in treating patients with kidney cancer who have undergone surgery (EVEREST) study (NCT01120249). This trial is recruiting individuals with clear or non-clear cell RCC immediately post-nephrectomy whose tumors show intermediate high-risk to high risk features. Patients are randomized between 12 months of everolimus and placebo. The primary endpoint is recurrence free survival, and both tissue and blood samples are being collected for future biomarker studies.

Ridaforolimus

Another rapamycin analog, ridaforolimus (AP23573), contains phosphorus and is also being studied as an antineoplastic agent. Ridaforolimus was initially tested in sarcomas [113] with encouraging results. Its combination with capecitabine was recently evaluated in a phase Ib study on 32 patients with multiple advanced solid tumors, including seven patients with RCC [114]. Two recommend doses of 50 or 75 mg weekly were used with capecitabine and were tolerated. One patient with ovarian cancer had a partial response and ten patients experienced stable disease. Unlike temsirolimus and everolimus, the dose used is close to the maximal tolerated dose. Another phase II study has evaluated the ridaforolimus/paclitaxel combination on 29 patients with different cancers, including one patient with clear cell carcinoma. The patient with RCC did not respond but two partial responses were observed in pharyngeal squamous cell and pancreatic carcinoma and eight patients achieved stable disease ≥4 months [115]. The most common DLT is mucositis while other mild to moderate side effects include fatigue, nausea, rash, anemia, neutropenia, diarrhea, hyperlipidemia, and thrombocytopenia.

Mechanisms of Resistance

Unlike high-dose interleukin-2, no durable complete response has been observed with the mTORi, and although a clinical benefit has been noted with these agents, RCC invariably recurs. These agents appear to be cytostatic, and hence the mechanisms through which the RCC cells overcome mTOR inhibition are critical to understand to be able to formulate adequate treatment combinations.

The currently available agents inhibit mTOR in the mTORC1 complex. However, mTORC 2 phosphorylates Akt [116] in a positive biofeedback mechanism, and hence can limit the effectiveness of mTORi. Therefore, agents capable of inhibiting the kinase activity of both mTOR complexes could result in better antitumorigenic effect. Mutations affecting mTOR or FKBP12 can lead to an improper attachment to rapamycin and hence are associated with resistance to rapamycin [117–119]. In addition, defects or mutations in downstream effectors such as S6K1 [120, 121], and 4E-BP1 can result in rapamycin resistance [120]. In contrast, activation of the upstream Akt protein appears to induce sensitivity to the mTORi. Another mechanism of resistance involves the IGF receptor (IGFR)/PI3K/Akt pathway disruption. Insulin receptor substrates (IRS) 1 and 2 are activated by IGF-1 and insulin and induce PI3K and mTOR activation. As a downstream protein, S6K1 phosphorylates the IRSs in a negative feedback mechanism and hence decreases the insulin/IGF-1 activation of the PI3K/Akt pathway [122]. Under mTOR inhibition [123–125], this feedback mechanism is lost leading to unopposed IGFR/PI3K/Akt activation. This in turn could possibly decrease the effect of mTORi. Using IGFR inhibitors or inhibitors of PI3K and Akt could help overcome this resistance.

Conclusion

mTORi are a new class of antineoplastic agents against RCC. Because of the different available targeted agents in RCC, the exact place of the TORi in the treatment algorithms remains to be determined. Temsirolimus is currently beneficial as a first-line agent in patients with metastatic RCC and with poor risk features. Everolimus improves PFS as a second-line agent and can be used in patients who have progressed on sunitinib, sorafenib or both. Multiple clinical trials are currently underway and hence the use of the mTORi will probably change to parallel the results obtained in the phase III trials.

Despite the encouraging results with monotherapy, the improvements remain modest and hence sequential and combination treatments are being investigated as a means to improve clinical benefit. Combination therapies offer the benefit of inhibiting two different molecular pathways simultaneously. However, despite the theoretical benefit of combining mTORi with VEGF TKI, early data evaluating the temsirolimus/sunitinib combination suggest this treatment option might have unacceptable side effects. As an additional cautionary lesson that more therapy is not always better, the combination of temsirolimus with IFN was inferior to temsirolimus monotherapy in the global ARCC trial. In contrast, bevacizumab appears to be better tolerated when administered along with an mTORi, but single-arm trials published so far have not provided reassurance that the combination of bevacizumab and an mTORi is superior to monotherapy. Nevertheless, studies evaluating the role of mTORi in combination with bevacizumab have been performed, and include the mentioned INTORACT and RECORD-2 trials looking at combining bevacizumab with temsirolimus and everolimus, respectively. We look forward to the mature data from these trials to provide definitive evidence of the utility of combination anti-VEGF and mTORi therapy.

In addition to combination treatment, the recent approval of many antineoplastic agents against RCC has raised the question of how to best maximize the efficacy of those agents when used in sequence. The exact sequence of treatment will change when the many studies currently investigating different sequential options are concluded. For example, important studies include the RECORD-3 and START trials which will evaluate sequencing of mTORi and antiangiogenic agents. The results of these studies will shed light as to whether everolimus can be used as a first-line agent interchangeably with anti-VEGF therapy.

The role of mTORi in the adjuvant setting has not been defined. The SWOG EVEREST trial will provide valuable information on the role of this class of agents in the prevention or delay of metastatic disease development in the intermediate-high to high-risk patient population.

These new agents certainly offer hope for improved outcomes in patients with RCC. As more data become available, our predictive biomarkers improve, and newer generations of agents blocking mTOR and related pathways are developed the role of mTORi in the treatment of RCC will become increasingly clear.

References

1. Heitman J, Movva NR, Hall MN. Targets for cell cycle arrest by the immunosuppressant rapamycin in yeast. Science. 1991;253:905–9.
2. Choi J, Chen J, Schreiber SL, Clardy J. Structure of the FKBP12-rapamycin complex interacting with the binding domain of human FRAP. Science. 1996;273:239–42.
3. Wullschleger S, Loewith R, Hall MN. TOR signaling in growth and metabolism. Cell. 2006;124:471–84.
4. Brown EJ, Albers MW, Shin TB, et al. A mammalian protein targeted by G1-arresting rapamycin–receptor complex. Nature. 1994;369:756–8.
5. Sabers CJ, Martin MM, Brunn GJ, et al. Isolation of a protein target of the FKBP12-rapamycin complex in mammalian cells. J Biol Chem. 1995;270:815–22.
6. Helliwell SB, Wagner P, Kunz J, et al. TOR1 and TOR2 are structurally and functionally similar but not identical phosphatidylinositol kinase homologues in yeast. Mol Biol Cell. 1994;5:105–18.
7. Shiloh Y. ATM and related protein kinases: safeguarding genome integrity. Nat Rev Cancer. 2003;3:155–68.
8. Guertin DA, Sabatini DM. Defining the role of mTOR in cancer. Cancer Cell. 2007;12:9–22.
9. Hara K, Maruki Y, Long X, et al. Raptor, a binding partner of target of rapamycin (TOR), mediates TOR action. Cell. 2002;110:177–89.
10. Loewith R, Jacinto E, Wullschleger S, et al. Two TOR complexes, only one of which is rapamycin sensitive, have distinct roles in cell growth control. Mol Cell. 2002;10:457–68.
11. Kim DH, Sarbassov DD, Ali SM, et al. mTOR interacts with raptor to form a nutrient-sensitive complex that signals to the cell growth machinery. Cell. 2002;110:163–75.
12. Dudek H, Datta SR, Franke TF, et al. Regulation of neuronal survival by the serine-threonine protein kinase Akt. Science. 1997;275:661–5.
13. Hay N, Sonenberg N. Upstream and downstream of mTOR. Genes Dev. 2004;18:1926–45.
14. Inoki K, Zhu T, Guan KL. TSC2 mediates cellular energy response to control cell growth and survival. Cell. 2003;115:577–90.
15. Brugarolas J, Lei K, Hurley RL, et al. Regulation of mTOR function in response to hypoxia by REDD1 and the TSC1/TSC2 tumor suppressor complex. Genes Dev. 2004;18:2893–904.
16. Feng Z, Zhang H, Levine AJ, Jin S. The coordinate regulation of the p53 and mTOR pathways in cells. Proc Natl Acad Sci USA. 2005;102:8204–9.
17. Arsham AM, Howell JJ, Simon MC. A novel hypoxia-inducible factor-independent hypoxic response regulating mammalian target of rapamycin and its targets. J Biol Chem. 2003;278:29655–60.
18. De Benedetti A, Graff JR. eIF-4E expression and its role in malignancies and metastases. Oncogene. 2004;23:3189–99.
19. Soni A, Akcakanat A, Singh G, et al. eIF4E knockdown decreases breast cancer cell growth without activating Akt signaling. Mol Cancer Ther. 2008;7:1782–8.
20. Richter JD, Sonenberg N. Regulation of cap-dependent translation by eIF4E inhibitory proteins. Nature. 2005;433:477–80.
21. Potter CJ, Pedraza LG, Xu T. Akt regulates growth by directly phosphorylating Tsc2. Nat Cell Biol. 2002;4:658–65.
22. Tang JM, He QY, Guo RX, Chang XJ. Phosphorylated Akt overexpression and loss of PTEN expression in non-small cell lung cancer confers poor prognosis. Lung Cancer. 2006;51:181–91.
23. Neshat MS, Mellinghoff IK, Tran C, et al. Enhanced sensitivity of PTEN-deficient tumors to inhibition of FRAP/mTOR. Proc Natl Acad Sci USA. 2001;98:10314–9.
24. Clifford SC, Prowse AH, Affara NA, Buys CH, Maher ER. Inactivation of the von Hippel–Lindau (VHL) tumour suppressor gene and allelic losses at chromosome arm 3p in primary renal cell carcinoma: evidence for a VHL-independent pathway in clear cell renal tumourigenesis. Genes Chromosomes Cancer. 1998;22:200–9.
25. Latif F, Tory K, Gnarra J, et al. Identification of the von Hippel–Lindau disease tumor suppressor gene. Science. 1993;260:1317–20.
26. Patel PH, Chadalavada RS, Chaganti RS, Motzer RJ. Targeting von Hippel–Lindau pathway in renal cell carcinoma. Clin Cancer Res. 2006;12:7215–20.
27. Brugarolas J. Renal-cell carcinoma–molecular pathways and therapies. N Engl J Med. 2007;356:185–7.
28. Kim WY, Kaelin WG. Role of VHL gene mutation in human cancer. J Clin Oncol. 2004;22:4991–5004.

29. Maranchie JK, Vasselli JR, Riss J, et al. The contribution of VHL substrate binding and HIF1-alpha to the phenotype of VHL loss in renal cell carcinoma. Cancer Cell. 2002;1:247–55.

30. Thomas GV, Tran C, Mellinghoff IK, et al. Hypoxia-inducible factor determines sensitivity to inhibitors of mTOR in kidney cancer. Nat Med. 2006;12:122–7.

31. Kourembanas S, Hannan RL, Faller DV. Oxygen tension regulates the expression of the platelet-derived growth factor-B chain gene in human endothelial cells. J Clin Invest. 1990;86:670–4.

32. de Paulsen N, Brychzy A, Fournier MC, et al. Role of transforming growth factor-alpha in von Hippel–Lindau (VHL)(–/–) clear cell renal carcinoma cell proliferation: a possible mechanism coupling VHL tumor suppressor inactivation and tumorigenesis. Proc Natl Acad Sci USA. 2001;98:1387–92.

33. Brenner W, Farber G, Herget T, et al. Loss of tumor suppressor protein PTEN during renal carcinogenesis. Int J Cancer. 2002;99:53–7.

34. Abraham RT, Gibbons JJ. The mammalian target of rapamycin signaling pathway: twists and turns in the road to cancer therapy. Clin Cancer Res. 2007;13: 3109–14.

35. Rini BI, Atkins MB. Resistance to targeted therapy in renal-cell carcinoma. Lancet Oncol. 2009;10: 992–1000.

36. Robb VA, Karbowniczek M, Klein-Szanto AJ, Henske EP. Activation of the mTOR signaling pathway in renal clear cell carcinoma. J Urol. 2007;177:346–52.

37. Pantuck AJ, Seligson DB, Klatte T, et al. Prognostic relevance of the mTOR pathway in renal cell carcinoma: implications for molecular patient selection for targeted therapy. Cancer. 2007;109:2257–67.

38. Cho D, Signoretti S, Dabora S, et al. Potential histologic and molecular predictors of response to temsirolimus in patients with advanced renal cell carcinoma. Clin Genitourin Cancer. 2007;5:379–85.

39. Sehgal SN, Baker H, Vezina C. Rapamycin (AY-22,989), a new antifungal antibiotic. II. Fermentation, isolation and characterization. J Antibiot (Tokyo). 1975;28:727–32.

40. Vezina C, Kudelski A, Sehgal SN. Rapamycin (AY-22,989), a new antifungal antibiotic. I. Taxonomy of the producing streptomycete and isolation of the active principle. J Antibiot (Tokyo). 1975;28:721–6.

41. Martel RR, Klicius J, Galet S. Inhibition of the immune response by rapamycin, a new antifungal antibiotic. Can J Physiol Pharmacol. 1977;55:48–51.

42. Calne RY, Collier DS, Lim S, et al. Rapamycin for immunosuppression in organ allografting. Lancet. 1989;2:227.

43. Houchens DP, Ovejera AA, Riblet SM, Slagel DE. Human brain tumor xenografts in nude mice as a chemotherapy model. Eur J Cancer Clin Oncol. 1983;19:799–805.

44. Eng CP, Sehgal SN, Vezina C. Activity of rapamycin (AY-22,989) against transplanted tumors. J Antibiot (Tokyo). 1984;37:1231–7.

45. Albers MW, Williams RT, Brown EJ, et al. FKBP-rapamycin inhibits a cyclin-dependent kinase activity and a cyclin D1-Cdk association in early G1 of an osteosarcoma cell line. J Biol Chem. 1993;268: 22825–9.

46. Dilling MB, Dias P, Shapiro DN, et al. Rapamycin selectively inhibits the growth of childhood rhabdomyosarcoma cells through inhibition of signaling via the type I insulin-like growth factor receptor. Cancer Res. 1994;54:903–7.

47. Seufferlein T, Rozengurt E. Rapamycin inhibits constitutive p70s6k phosphorylation, cell proliferation, and colony formation in small cell lung cancer cells. Cancer Res. 1996;56:3895–7.

48. Marx SO, Jayaraman T, Go LO, Marks AR. Rapamycin-FKBP inhibits cell cycle regulators of proliferation in vascular smooth muscle cells. Circ Res. 1995;76:412–7.

49. Grunwald V, DeGraffenried L, Russel D, et al. Inhibitors of mTOR reverse doxorubicin resistance conferred by PTEN status in prostate cancer cells. Cancer Res. 2002;62:6141–5.

50. Yu K, Toral-Barza L, Discafani C, et al. mTOR, a novel target in breast cancer: the effect of CCI-779, an mTOR inhibitor, in preclinical models of breast cancer. Endocr Relat Cancer. 2001;8:249–58.

51. Hidalgo M, Buckner JC, Erlichman C, et al. A phase I and pharmacokinetic study of temsirolimus (CCI-779) administered intravenously daily for 5 days every 2 weeks to patients with advanced cancer. Clin Cancer Res. 2006;12:5755–63.

52. Raymond E, Alexandre J, Faivre S, et al. Safety and pharmacokinetics of escalated doses of weekly intravenous infusion of CCI-779, a novel mTOR inhibitor, in patients with cancer. J Clin Oncol. 2004;22: 2336–47.

53. Punt CJ, Boni J, Bruntsch U, Peters M, Thielert C. Phase I and pharmacokinetic study of CCI-779, a novel cytostatic cell-cycle inhibitor, in combination with 5-fluorouracil and leucovorin in patients with advanced solid tumors. Ann Oncol. 2003;14:931–7.

54. Boni JP, Hug B, Leister C, Sonnichsen D. Intravenous temsirolimus in cancer patients: clinical pharmacology and dosing considerations. Semin Oncol. 2009;36 Suppl 3:S18–25.

55. Skotnicki JS, Leone CL, Smith AL. Design, synthesis and biological evaluation of C-42 hydroxyesters of rapamycin: the identification of CCI-779 [abstract 477]. Clin Cancer Res. 2001;7:3749S–50.

56. Galanis E, Buckner JC, Maurer MJ, et al. Phase II trial of temsirolimus (CCI-779) in recurrent glioblastoma multiforme: a North Central Cancer Treatment Group Study. J Clin Oncol. 2005;23:5294–304.

57. Pandya KJ, Dahlberg S, Hidalgo M, et al. A randomized, phase II trial of two dose levels of temsirolimus (CCI-779) in patients with extensive-stage small-cell lung cancer who have responding or stable disease after induction chemotherapy: a trial of the Eastern Cooperative Oncology Group (E1500). J Thorac Oncol. 2007;2:1036–41.

58. Chan S, Scheulen ME, Johnston S, et al. Phase II study of temsirolimus (CCI-779), a novel inhibitor of mTOR, in heavily pretreated patients with locally advanced or metastatic breast cancer. J Clin Oncol. 2005;23:5314–22.

59. Peralba JM, DeGraffenried L, Friedrichs W, et al. Pharmacodynamic evaluation of CCI-779, an inhibitor of mTOR, in cancer patients. Clin Cancer Res. 2003;9:2887–92.

60. FDA.http://www.accessdata.fda.gov/drugsatfda_docs/label/2010/022088s008lbl.pdf.

61. Zimmerman JJ, Lasseter KC, Lim HK, et al. Pharmacokinetics of sirolimus (rapamycin) in subjects with mild to moderate hepatic impairment. J Clin Pharmacol. 2005;45:1368–72.

62. Boni JP, Leister C, Bender G, et al. Population pharmacokinetics of CCI-779: correlations to safety and pharmacogenomic responses in patients with advanced renal cancer. Clin Pharmacol Ther. 2005;77:76–89.

63. Sattler M, Guengerich FP, Yun CH, Christians U, Sewing KF. Cytochrome P-450 3A enzymes are responsible for biotransformation of FK506 and rapamycin in man and rat. Drug Metab Dispos. 1992;20:753–61.

64. Jacobsen W, Serkova N, Hausen B, et al. Comparison of the in vitro metabolism of the macrolide immunosuppressants sirolimus and RAD. Transplant Proc. 2001;33:514–5.

65. Atkins MB, Hidalgo M, Stadler WM, et al. Randomized phase II study of multiple dose levels of CCI-779, a novel mammalian target of rapamycin kinase inhibitor, in patients with advanced refractory renal cell carcinoma. J Clin Oncol. 2004;22:909–18.

66. Fischer P, Patel P, Carducci MA, et al. Phase I study combining treatment with temsirolimus and sunitinib malate in patients with advanced renal cell carcinoma. J Clin Oncol. 2008;26.

67. Merchan JR, Liu G FT, Picus J, et al. Phase I/II trial of CCI-779 and bevacizumab in stage IV renal cell carcinoma: phase I safety and activity results. J Clin Oncol 2007; ASCO annual meeting proceedings part I. 25, No. 18S (June 20 Supplement) 5034.

68. Merchan JR, Pitot HC, Qin R, et al. Phase I/II trial of CCI 779 and bevacizumab in advanced renal cell carcinoma (RCC): safety and activity in RTKI refractory RCC patients. J Clin Oncol. 2009;27(Suppl):15s [Abstr 5039].

69. Margolin K, Longmate J, Baratta T, et al. CCI-779 in metastatic melanoma: a phase II trial of the California Cancer Consortium. Cancer. 2005;104:1045–8.

70. Chang SM, Wen P, Cloughesy T, et al. Phase II study of CCI-779 in patients with recurrent glioblastoma multiforme. Invest New Drugs. 2005;23:357–61.

71. Duran I, Kortmansky J, Singh D, et al. A phase II clinical and pharmacodynamic study of temsirolimus in advanced neuroendocrine carcinomas. Br J Cancer. 2006;95:1148–54.

72. Witzig TE, Geyer SM, Ghobrial I, et al. Phase II trial of single-agent temsirolimus (CCI-779) for relapsed mantle cell lymphoma. J Clin Oncol. 2005;23:5347–56.

73. Motzer RJ, Hudes GR, Curti BD, et al. Phase I/II trial of temsirolimus combined with interferon alfa for advanced renal cell carcinoma. J Clin Oncol. 2007;25:3958–64.

74. Motzer RJ, Bacik J, Murphy BA, Russo P, Mazumdar M. Interferon-alfa as a comparative treatment for clinical trials of new therapies against advanced renal cell carcinoma. J Clin Oncol. 2002;20:289–96.

75. Hudes G, Carducci M, Tomczak P, et al. Temsirolimus, interferon alfa, or both for advanced renal-cell carcinoma. N Engl J Med. 2007;356:2271–81.

76. Motzer RJ, Mazumdar M, Bacik J, et al. Survival and prognostic stratification of 670 patients with advanced renal cell carcinoma. J Clin Oncol. 1999;17:2530–40.

77. Mekhail TM, Abou-Jawde RM, Boumerhi G, et al. Validation and extension of the Memorial Sloan-Kettering prognostic factors model for survival in patients with previously untreated metastatic renal cell carcinoma. J Clin Oncol. 2005;23:832–41.

78. Logan T, McDermott D, Dutcher J, et al. J Clin Oncol. 2008;26(Suppl) [Abstr 5050].

79. Dutcher JP, de Souza P, McDermott D, et al. Effect of temsirolimus versus interferon-alpha on outcome of patients with advanced renal cell carcinoma of different tumor histologies. Med Oncol. 2009;26:202–9.

80. Patel PH, Senico PL, Curiel RE, Motzer RJ. Phase I study combining treatment with temsirolimus and sunitinib malate in patients with advanced renal cell carcinoma. Clin Genitourin Cancer. 2009;7:24–7.

81. Patnaik A, ricart A, Cooper J, Papadopoulos K. A phase I, pharmacokinetic and pharmacodynamic study of sorafenib (S), a multi-targeted kinase inhibitor in combination with temsirolimus (T), an mTOR inhibitor in patients with advanced solid malignancies. J Clin Oncol. 2007;25(Suppl 18S):3512 [2007 ASCO annual meeting proceedings part I].

82. Wyeth. Phase 3b, randomized, open-label study of bevacizumab+temsirolimus vs. bevacizumab+interferon-alfa as first-line treatment in subjects with advanced renal cell carcinoma. In: ClinicalTrialsgov [Internet] Bethesda (MD): National Library of Medicine (US) 2000 [cited 2011 Feb 08]. http://clinicaltrials.gov/show/NCT00631371. NLM Identifier: 00631371.

83. ECOG. The BeST Trial: a randomized phase II study of VEGF, RAF Kinase, and mTOR combination targeted therapy (CTT) with bevacizumab, sorafenib and temsirolimus in advanced renal cell carcinoma [BeST]. In: ClinicalTrialsgov [Internet] Bethesda (MD): National Library of Medicine (US) 2000 [cited 2011 Feb 08]. http://clinicaltrials.gov/show/NCT0378703. NLM Identifier: 00378703.

84. Wyeth. A randomized trial of temsirolimus versus sorafenib as second-line therapy in patients with advanced renal cell carcinoma who have failed first-line sunitinib therapy. In: ClinicalTrialsgov [Internet] Bethesda (MD): National Library of Medicine (US) 2000 [cited 2011 Feb 08]. Available from: http://clinicaltrials.gov/show/NCT00474786. NLM Identifier: NCT00474786.

85. Neumayer HH, Paradis K, Korn A, et al. Entry-into-human study with the novel immunosuppressant SDZ RAD in stable renal transplant recipients. Br J Clin Pharmacol. 1999;48:694–703.

86. Eisen HJ, Tuzcu EM, Dorent R, et al. Everolimus for the prevention of allograft rejection and vasculopathy in cardiac-transplant recipients. N Engl J Med. 2003;349:847–58.

87. Pascual J. Everolimus in clinical practice – renal transplantation. Nephrol Dial Transplant. 2006;21 Suppl 3:iii18–23.

88. Sanchez-Fructuoso AI. Everolimus: an update on the mechanism of action, pharmacokinetics and recent clinical trials. Expert Opin Drug Metab Toxicol. 2008;4:807–19.

89. Boulay A, Zumstein-Mecker S, Stephan C, et al. Antitumor efficacy of intermittent treatment schedules with the rapamycin derivative RAD001 correlates with prolonged inactivation of ribosomal protein S6 kinase 1 in peripheral blood mononuclear cells. Cancer Res. 2004;64:252–61.

90. Tanaka C, O'Reilly T, Kovarik JM, et al. Identifying optimal biologic doses of everolimus (RAD001) in patients with cancer based on the modeling of pre-clinical and clinical pharmacokinetic and pharmaco-dynamic data. J Clin Oncol. 2008;26:1596–602.

91. Crowe A, Bruelisauer A, Duerr L, Guntz P, Lemaire M. Absorption and intestinal metabolism of SDZ-RAD and rapamycin in rats. Drug Metab Dispos. 1999;27:627–32.

92. Kovarik JM, Hartmann S, Figueiredo J, et al. Effect of rifampin on apparent clearance of everolimus. Ann Pharmacother. 2002;36:981–5.

93. O'Donnell A, Faivre S, Burris 3rd HA, et al. Phase I pharmacokinetic and pharmacodynamic study of the oral mammalian target of rapamycin inhibitor everoli-mus in patients with advanced solid tumors. J Clin Oncol. 2008;26:1588–95.

94. Kovarik JM, Noe A, Berthier S, et al. Clinical devel-opment of an everolimus pediatric formulation: rela-tive bioavailability, food effect, and steady-state pharmacokinetics. J Clin Pharmacol. 2003;43:141–7.

95. Lampen A, Zhang Y, Hackbarth I, et al. Metabolism and transport of the macrolide immunosuppressant sirolimus in the small intestine. J Pharmacol Exp Ther. 1998;285:1104–12.

96. Kovarik JM, Sabia HD, Figueiredo J, et al. Influence of hepatic impairment on everolimus pharmacokinet-ics: implications for dose adjustment. Clin Pharmacol Ther. 2001;70:425–30.

97. Strom T, Haschke M, Zhang YL, et al. Identification of everolimus metabolite patterns in trough blood samples of kidney transplant patients. Ther Drug Monit. 2007;29:592–9.

98. Kirchner GI, Meier-Wiedenbach I, Manns MP. Clinical pharmacokinetics of everolimus. Clin Pharmacokinet. 2004;43:83–95.

99. Taylor PJ, Franklin ME, Graham KS, Pillans PI. A HPLC-mass spectrometric method suitable for the therapeutic drug monitoring of everolimus. J Chromatogr B Analyt Technol Biomed Life Sci. 2007;848:208–14.

100. Tabernero J, Rojo F, Calvo E, et al. Dose- and sched-ule-dependent inhibition with the mammalian target of rapamycin pathway with everolimus: a phase I tumor pharmacodynamic study in patients with advanced solid tumors. J Clin Oncol. 2008;26:1603–10.

101. Amato RJ, Jac J, Giessinger S, Saxena S, Willis JP. A phase 2 study with a daily regimen of the oral mTOR inhibitor RAD001 (everolimus) in patients with metastatic clear cell renal cell cancer. Cancer. 2009;115:2438–46.

102. Hainsworth JD, Spigel DR, Burris 3rd HA, et al. Phase II trial of bevacizumab and everolimus in patients with advanced renal cell carcinoma. J Clin Oncol. 2010;28:2131–6.

103. Whorf RC, Hainsworth JD, Spigel DR, Yardley DA, Burris HA III, Waterhouse DM, Vazquez ER, Greco FA. Phase II study of bevacizumab and everolimus (RAD001) in the treatment of advanced renal cell carcinoma (RCC). J Clin Oncol 2008;26(Suppl) [Abstr 5010].

104. Escudier B. How to interpret phase II data for everolimus plus bevacizumab in renal cell carci-noma. J Clin Oncol. 2010;28:2125–6.

105. Motzer RJ, Escudier B, Oudard S, et al. Efficacy of everolimus in advanced renal cell carcinoma: a dou-ble-blind, randomised, placebo-controlled phase III trial. Lancet. 2008;372(9637):449–56.

106. National Comprehensive Cancer Network. NCCN Clinical Practice Guidelines in Oncology: Kidney Cancer v. http://www.nccn.org/professionals/physi-cian_gls/PDF/kidney.pdf. Accessed 28 Feb 2011

107. Motzer RJ, Escudier B, Oudard S, et al. Phase 3 trial of everolimus for metastatic renal cell carcinoma: final results and analysis of prognostic factors. Cancer. 2010;116:4256–65.

108. Escudier B, Pluzanska A, Koralewski P, et al. Bevacizumab plus interferon alfa-2a for treatment of metastatic renal cell carcinoma: a randomised, dou-ble-blind phase III trial. Lancet. 2007;370:2103–11.

109. Escudier B, Bellmunt J, Negrier S, et al. Phase III trial of bevacizumab plus interferon alfa-2a in patients with metastatic renal cell carcinoma (AVOREN): final analysis of overall survival. J Clin Oncol. 2010;28:2144–50.

110. Rini BI, Halabi S, Rosenberg JE, et al. Phase III trial of bevacizumab plus interferon alfa versus interferon alfa monotherapy in patients with metastatic renal cell carcinoma: final results of CALGB 90206. J Clin Oncol. 2010;28:2137–43.

111. Rini BI, Halabi S, Rosenberg JE, et al. Bevacizumab plus interferon alfa compared with interferon alfa monotherapy in patients with metastatic renal cell carcinoma: CALGB 90206. J Clin Oncol. 2008;26:5422–8.

112. Roche-Pharma NPA. A Randomized, open-label, multi-center phase II study to compare bevacizumab

plus RAD001 versus interferon alfa-2a plus bevaci-zumab for the first-line treatment of patients with metastatic clear cell carcinoma of the kidney. In: ClinicalTrialsgov [Internet] Bethesda (MD): National Library of Medicine (US); 2000 [cited in March 2011]. http://www.clinicaltrials.gov/ct2/show/NCT00719264.

113. Chawla SP, Sankhala KK, Chua V, Menendez LR, Eilber FC, Eckardt JJ. A phase II study of AP23573 (an mTOR inhibitor) in patients (pts) with advanced sarcomas. ASCO Meet Abstr. 2005;23:9068

114. Perotti A, Locatelli A, Sessa C, et al. Phase IB study of the mTOR inhibitor ridaforolimus with capecit-abine. J Clin Oncol. 2010;28:4554–61.

115. Sessa C, Tosi D, Vigano L, et al. Phase Ib study of weekly mammalian target of rapamycin inhibitor ridaforolimus (AP23573; MK-8669) with weekly paclitaxel. Ann Oncol. 2010;21:1315–22.

116. Sarbassov DD, Guertin DA, Ali SM, Sabatini DM. Phosphorylation and regulation of Akt/PKB by the rictor-mTOR complex. Science. 2005;307:1098–101.

117. Dumont FJ, Staruch MJ, Grammer T, et al. Dominant mutations confer resistance to the immunosuppres-sant, rapamycin, in variants of a T cell lymphoma. Cell Immunol. 1995;163:70–9.

118. Chen J, Zheng XF, Brown EJ, Schreiber SL. Identification of an 11-kDa FKBP12-rapamycin-binding domain within the 289-kDa FKBP12-rapamycin-associated protein and characterization of a critical serine residue. Proc Natl Acad Sci USA. 1995;92:4947–51.

119. Fruman DA, Wood MA, Gjertson CK, et al. FK506 binding protein 12 mediates sensitivity to both FK506 and rapamycin in murine mast cells. Eur J Immunol. 1995;25:563–71.

120. Sugiyama H, Papst P, Gelfand EW, Terada N. p70 S6 kinase sensitivity to rapamycin is eliminated by amino acid substitution of Thr229. J Immunol. 1996;157:656–60.

121. Mahalingam M, Templeton DJ. Constitutive activa-tion of S6 kinase by deletion of amino-terminal auto-inhibitory and rapamycin sensitivity domains. Mol Cell Biol. 1996;16:405–13.

122. Shah OJ, Wang Z, Hunter T. Inappropriate activa-tion of the TSC/Rheb/mTOR/S6K cassette induces IRS1/2 depletion, insulin resistance, and cell sur-vival deficiencies. Curr Biol. 2004;14:1650–6.

123. Wan X, Harkavy B, Shen N, Grohar P, Helman LJ. Rapamycin induces feedback activation of Akt sig-naling through an IGF-1R-dependent mechanism. Oncogene. 2007;26:1932–40.

124. O'Reilly KE, Rojo F, She QB, et al. mTOR inhibi-tion induces upstream receptor tyrosine kinase sig-naling and activates Akt. Cancer Res. 2006;66:1500–8.

125. Shi Y, Yan H, Frost P, Gera J, Lichtenstein A. Mammalian target of rapamycin inhibitors activate the AKT kinase in multiple myeloma cells by up-regulating the insulin-like growth factor receptor/insulin receptor substrate-1/phosphatidylinositol 3-kinase cascade. Mol Cancer Ther. 2005;4:1533–40.

Palliative and Supportive Care for Renal Cancer

19

Armida Parala-Metz* and Mellar Davis*

Introduction

A national cross-sectional study [1] of adult renal cell cancer patients showed that more than 50% of patients with both localized and metastatic disease reported pain, weakness, fatigue, sleep disturbance, urinary frequency, worry, irritability, and depression as being moderate to highly relevant. This is similar to other studies [2, 3] that have also mentioned fatigue, weakness, pain, lack of appetite, nausea, irritability, and sleep disturbance as commonly reported symptoms among patients with renal cell carcinoma. These symptoms need to be managed to improve the quality of life of these patients.

Advancements in targeted therapies for renal cancer have made this condition a chronic illness [4]. Renal cancer patients now live with their disease longer and may experience a multitude of symptoms that come with both advanced disease and treatment-related side effects.

*A World Health Organization Demonstration Project in Palliative Medicine.

A. Parala-Metz, MD • M. Davis, MD (✉)
The Harry R. Horvitz Center for Palliative Medicine and Supportive Oncology, Taussig Cancer Institute, Cleveland Clinic Health Systems, 9500 Euclid Avenue, Cleveland, OH, USA
e-mail: davism6@ccf.org

Cancer Pain Management

Pain is one of the most common and dreaded symptom of patients with cancer. However, it is often suboptimally treated in cancer patients [5, 6]. Under-treated pain impairs patients' daily functions and adversely affects their emotional and psychological health and may lead to suicide and the desire of hastened death [7].

Pain management has been guided by the World Health Organization's three-step analgesic ladder (Fig. 19.1) [8]. Analgesic choice is based upon pain intensity. For mild pain, non-opioid and/or adjuvant analgesics (Table 19.1) are used, weak opioids (Table 19.2) are substituted for non-opioids for moderate pain and strong opioids (Table 19.2) are substituted for weak opioids for severe pain. In countries where strong opioids are readily available and where palliative care is established, Step 2 is bypassed and low doses of potent opioids are used instead [9] (Table 19.3). Morphine is generally accepted as the opioid of choice for moderate to severe cancer pain [10, 11].

Cancer pain has different temporal patterns (Fig. 19.2) which dictate the opioid dosing strategy. Continuous pain is managed with around-the-clock (ATC) opioids either as sustained release morphine (or oxycodone or hydromorphone) every 12 or 24 h or with oral immediate release morphine (or oxycodone or hydromorphone) every 4 h. A majority of patients with continuous cancer pain will also have transient

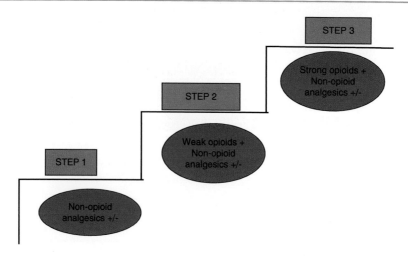

Fig. 19.1 WHO analgesic ladder

Table 19.1 Non-opioid analgesics and adjuvant analgesics

Non-opioid analgesics	Adjuvant analgesics
Acetaminophen	Systemic corticosteroids
NSAIDs	Antiepileptics (e.g., gabapentin, pregabalin, carbamazepine, lamotrigine, valproic acid)
Salicylates	Antidepressants (e.g., venlafaxine, duloxetine, amitriptyline)
	NMDA receptor blockers (e.g., ketamine, amantadine, magnesium sulfate, memantine)
	Alpha 2 adrenergic agonists (e.g., clonidine, dexmedetomidine)
	Skeletal muscle relaxants (e.g., diazepam, tizanidine, baclofen)
	Smooth muscle relaxants (e.g., glycopyrrolate, dicyclomine, atropine, scopolamine
	Bisphosphonates

Table 19.2 Weak opioids

Codeine
Hydrocodone (commercially available as Vicodin)
Tramadol
Tapentadol

Propoxyphene (Darvocet) was pulled out of the market in November 2010

flares of pain, known as breakthrough pain. Breakthrough or intermittent pain may be incident (i.e., related to movement or activity), non-incident (spontaneous), or end-of-dose-failure [12, 13]. Rescue (as needed) doses of short-acting opioids are given for breakthrough pain. Recommendations for rescue dosing are 25–50% of the 4 hourly dose, or the 4 hourly dose given hourly, or 10–20% of the daily dose [11, 12, 14]. End-of-dose failure is due to suboptimal doses of ATC opioids and is improved by titrating the

ATC opioid dose rather than shortening the dosing interval [12]. Successful cancer pain management requires ATC opioids plus rescue doses for intermittent pain, titrated against the patient's pain severity. Both non-opioid and/or adjuvant analgesics should be used to optimize analgesia at each step of the WHO analgesic ladder [15].

Effective pain management with opioids requires adequate analgesia without excessive adverse effects. Common initial side effects are mild nausea and vomiting, drowsiness, lightheadedness, and sedation [9]. These normally resolve several days after initiating the opioid. Nausea may require the use of antiemetics. Constipation is a common side effect that persists and does not improve with time. It should be treated proactively with stool softeners and laxatives. A minority of patients develop intolerable side effects

Table 19.3 Strong opioids and starting doses for opioid naïve patients

Opioid	Oral formulation		Parenteral formulation	
	Dose	Interval	Dose	Interval (prn dosing)
Morphine	5–10 mg	4 h	0.5–1 mg	1 h
Hydromorphone	2 mg	4 h	0.2 mg	1 h
Oxycodone	5–10 mg	4 h	N/A	N/A
Fentanyl	N/A	N/A	25 mcg	1 h
Methadone	5 mg (2.5 mg in the elderly)	12 h	0.2 mg	1 h

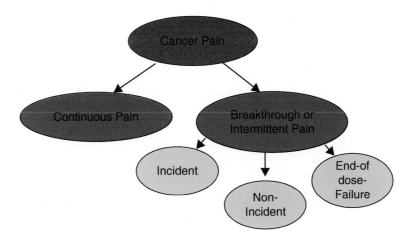

Fig. 19.2 Temporal pain patterns

prior to achieving pain relief. One strategy in this setting is opioid rotation, a planned switch from one opioid to another [16] to achieve a good balance of analgesia and side effects [17, 18]. A retrospective study [19] on terminal cancer patients showed that common reasons for opioid rotation were cognitive failure, hallucinations, myoclonus, nausea and vomiting, local toxicity, and refractory pain. Opioid rotation results in resolution of side effects and improved pain control in >50% of patients [19, 20]. In choosing a new opioid, it is important to consider relevant patient and disease-related factors, medical comorbidities, concomitant pharmacotherapy, patient's history of any drug sensitivities, the clinical care setting (outpatient, inpatient, long-term care, and hospice) and financial- or insurance-related issues [16, 21].

Switching to a different opioid is just one of the strategies that can be utilized when managing unacceptable outcomes associated with opioid administration. Other ways to manage opioid-related side effects include: (1) reducing the systemic opioid dose by 25–50% and simultaneously adding a non-opioid analgesic or adjuvant analgesic to maintain pain control [22]; (2) symptomatic management of opioid adverse effects (Table 19.4); and (3) changing the opioid route [23]. Around 10–30% [24–26] of cancer patients will not have acceptable pain control with systemic opioid therapy and will need other approaches to pain control such as radiation therapy and interventional treatments like neurolytic procedures, intrathecal drug therapy, kyphoplasty or vertebropalsty, or image-guided tumor ablation [27–32].

Hypercalcemia and Bisphosphonate Therapy

Hypercalcemia is a serious complication of malignant diseases. It most often occurs in renal cell carcinoma [33] and its incidence increases

Table 19.4 Common opioid adverse effects

Adverse effect	Intervention
Nausea and vomiting	May use metoclopramide, or neuroleptics (e.g., haloperidol, olanzapine) as needed. Common at the start of therapy and usually resolves in 7–10 days
Constipation	Stool softeners and laxatives. Prevention is key as no tolerance is developed to this side effect
Sedation	Reassurance. Need to review medication list to rule out other medications potentially causing sedation. Tolerance is developed days after starting opioid therapy. If persistent, consider reducing opioid dose and use a stimulant (e.g., methylphenidate)
Confusion	Reduce dose of opioid and start haloperidol as needed. Need Review medication list to remove other drugs that may cause delirium and rule out other potential causes (e.g., sepsis). Consider switching to a different opioid
Myoclonus	Reduce dose of opioid and prescribe clonazepam as needed. Consider adding an adjuvant analgesic to optimize pain control and lessen intolerable side effects

with the stage of the disease [34]. There are four proposed mechanisms of hypercalcemia associated with cancer [35]. Humoral hypercalcemia of malignancy (HHM) accounts for 80% of cases and is caused by secretion of parathyroid-related protein (PTHrP) by the tumor cells. PTHrP increases bone resorption and enhances reabsorption of calcium in the renal tubules. Other humoral factors which potentiate PTHrP activity and increase osteoclastic bone resorption have been implicated as well and include IL-1, IL-6, TNF-α, and tumor growth factors (TGF) α and β [36–38]. Another cause of hypercalcemia is osteolytic activity from sites of skeletal metastases which account for 20% of malignancy-related hypercalcemia. A less common cause is secretion of 1,25-dihydroxyvitamin D which increases osteoclastic bone resorption and intestinal calcium absorption. A rare cause of hypercalcemia is PTH secretion from ectopic hyperparathyroidism. Individuals with hypercalcemia associated with cancer should have low levels of PTH (with the rare exception of ectopic hyperparathyroidism). Individuals with elevated PTH levels should be assessed for primary hyperparathyroidism.

Common symptoms associated with hypercalcemia include nausea, vomiting, constipation, confusion, lethargy, and coma [39]. Symptom severity is dependent on the serum calcium level, the rate of increase of calcium, the presence of a comorbid neurologic or cognitive impairment, and concomitant use of sedatives and opioids which may have toxicity which mimics the neurologic symptoms of hypercalcemia [35].

When managing hypercalcemia, it is important to discontinue all calcium supplements and medications that can increase serum calcium level [35]. Intravenous hydration with normal saline corrects dehydration increases glomerular filtration rate (GFR) and inhibits calcium reabsorption [35, 39]. Loop diuretics (e.g., furosemide) should not be routinely given because if used prematurely, dehydration will get worse and GFR will be further reduced [35, 39]. They should be used only when managing clinical volume overload [4, 40].

Intravenous (IV) bisphosphonates (pamidronate and zoledronic acid) are the treatment of choice for hypercalcemia of malignancy [41]. Bisphosphonates have a very high affinity to bone mineral and achieve a high local concentration [42]. They work by inhibiting osteoclastic bone resorption [42, 43]. In most cases, serum calcium levels will normalize within 4–7 days and the response may last for 1–3 weeks [35]. Other agents like glucocorticoids, calcitonin, and gallium can be used if bisphosphonates are contraindicated or ineffective (Table 19.5). Denosumab, an anti-RANKL (receptor activator of nuclear factor-kappaB ligand) antibody, inhibits osteoclast-mediated bone resorption and reduces skeletal-related events (SREs) [44, 45]. Further research is needed to validate the use of denosumab in hypercalcemia.

Table 19.5 Management of malignant hypercalcemia

	Comment
(a) Initial intervention	
Intravenous saline hydration	200–300 mL/h. Consider a slower rate in patients with underlying cardiac or renal disease. Use loop diuretics (e.g., furosemide) if signs of fluid overload develops
Bisphosphonates	May use pamidronate (30–90 mg IV)or zolendronic acid (4 mg IV). Monitor serum creatinine level and ensure adequate hydration
(b) Second-line medications	
Calcitonin	4–8 units/kg subcutaneously every 4–6 h. Do not use for more than 48 h as tachyphylaxis develops. Use in symptomatic patients with serum calcium level of >14 mg/L. Use with saline hydration and bisphosphonates in the management of severe hypercalcemia
Glucocorticoids	For example, prednisone 20–40 mg/day
Gallium nitrate	200 mg/m^2/day for 5 days. Contraindicated in patients with severe renal impairment
Dialysis	Indicated for symptomatic patients with severe hypercalcemia and renal impairment or heart failure, in whom hydration cannot be safely administered

Bisphosphonates reduce pain [43] and prevent SREs associated with bone metastases (pathologic fractures, development of new osteolytic lesions, spinal cord compression, the need for radiation therapy or surgery caused by bone metastases) [43, 46]. In the absence of bone-targeted therapy, 30% patients with advanced renal cell carcinoma will experience symptomatic bone metastases [47]. The associated SREs adversely affect quality of life and decrease functional independence and may also increase mortality [48].

Parenteral pamidronate disodium and zolendronic acid are approved for use to prevent skeletal events in those with bone metastases. However, only zoledronic acid has been shown to prevent or delay SREs in a broad range of malignancies, including renal cell carcinoma [49]. A phase III, placebo-controlled, double blind, randomized controlled trial in patients with bone metastases from lung cancer and other solid tumors showed that zoledronic acid (4 or 8 mg) given every 3 weeks for 9 months, reduced SREs and increased the time to the first skeletal event by more than 2 months [50]. A follow-up study [51] on the same population which looked at long-term efficacy and safety revealed that fewer patients treated with zoledronic acid developed an SRE at 21 months compared with placebo.

There was also a significant delay in the median time to first SRE by more than 80 days. There was a significant reduction in the annual incidence of SREs with zoledronic acid (1.74 per year with the 4-mg dose vs. 2.71 per year with placebo; $p = 0.012$). Zoledronic acid was found to be well tolerated. A retrospective subset analysis [52] on 74 renal cell cancer patients from the original study showed a 50% reduction in the percentage of patients who developed SRE with zoledronic acid (37% vs. 74% placebo; $p = 0.015$). The risk for developing an SRE was also reduced by 61% and the time to first SRE was significantly delayed. Zoledronic acid should be considered in all patients with bone metastases from renal cell carcinoma [53].

Parenteral bisphosphonates cause systemic inflammatory reactions within 48 h after administration resulting in fever, arthralgia, myalgia, nausea and vomiting. These symptoms are usually mild and are treated with acetaminophen or NSAID and they generally resolve within 24–48 h [9]. Nephrotoxicity is a concern with intravenous bisphosphonates, particularly in patients who have had nephrectomy. It is recommended that serum creatinine levels be monitored, use the recommended dose and infusion rate, ensure adequate hydration, and avoid concurrent use of nephrotoxic drugs [9, 54].

Bisphosphonate-related osteonecrosis of the jaw (BRONJ) is a major but rare complication of parenteral bisphosphonate therapy. The American Academy of Oral and Maxillofacial Surgery (AAOMS) defined BRONJ by the presence of all of the following characteristics: (1) current or previous treatment with a bisphosphonate; (2) exposed bone in the maxillofacial region that has persisted for more than 8 weeks; and (3) no history of radiation therapy to the jaw bones [55]. The incidence in cancer patients is estimated to be between 0.6% and 15% and is most commonly seen in breast cancer (0.6–6.2%) and multiple myeloma (1.7–15%) patients [56]. A retrospective analysis of 4,000 patients treated with bisphosphonates reported BRONJ only in patients with multiple myeloma and breast cancer. There were no cases of BRONJ in other malignancies (lung, renal, or prostate cancer) or in benign diseases like osteoporosis and Paget's disease [57]. Risk factors for BRONJ include dental extractions, duration of bisphosphonate treatment, and type of bisphosphonate used. Management is aimed at decreasing pain, controlling oral infections, and minimizing the progression of bone necrosis [55]. Bisphosphonates should be stopped and patients should have close dental follow-up [9, 55]. Long-term outcomes for patients who develop BRONJ are generally poor with only a minority of patients reporting improvement or resolution of symptoms [58].

Anorexia and Cachexia

Most patients with advanced cancer suffer from lack of appetite and loss of weight [59], these predict poor outcomes and decreased survival in this setting [60, 61].

Cancer anorexia and cancer cachexia (presence of involuntary loss of lean body mass, weight, and appetite) occur by way of several overlapping mechanisms which include: (1) neurohormonal changes leading to loss of appetite, early satiety, chronic nausea, malabsorption, and autonomic failure; (2) metabolic alterations that lead to increased energy expenditure, increased glucose and protein turnover, and accelerated lipolysis leading to muscle wasting and loss of fat; and (3) induction of pro-inflammatory cytokines (i.e., tumor necrosis factor {TNF}, interleukin {IL} 1, IL-6, interferon (IFN) γ) and tumor-derived catabolic factors (proteolysis-inducing factor {PIF} and lipid-mobilizing factor) which are primarily responsible for reduction of muscle synthesis, increase in protein degradation, and lipolysis, causing muscle wasting in cancer patients [62–67].

It is important to identify reversible causes of anorexia and cachexia. Clinicians should make sure that their patients have a functional gastrointestinal tract (i.e., no obstruction or malabsorption), have optimal anti-emetic therapy, and that pain and depression have been addressed [62, 68]. It is also important that the patient has a desire to eat again and want their anorexia treated [68] before pharmacologic treatment is started. At best, appetite stimulants palliate anorexia but do not reverse cachexia [69]. It is important for clinicians to educate patients and families that anorexia is common symptom in cancer patients and is not due depression or "giving up" or to lack of willingness to eat on the patient's part or poor food choices on the family's part [69].

The most effective appetite stimulants are corticosteroids (e.g., dexamethasone, methylprednisolone, prednisone) and progestational agents (e.g., megesterol acetate, medroxyprogesterone acetate). The mechanism of action of corticosteroids is unclear but may be related to its euphorigenic effect, down-modulation of prostaglandin metabolism or cytokines release, or up-regulation of orexigenic hormones within the hypothalamus [62, 70]. Corticosteroids produce immediate improvement in appetite, however, their effects are short-lived and may only last a few weeks [71]. Corticosteroids are also associated with more side effects including, fluid retention, change in mental status, gastritis, cushingoid body habitus, and proximal myopathy with long-term use. Megesterol acetate (MA) is the best studied progestational agent in palliating anorexia in cancer patients. Its mechanism of action is not known but in animal models, MA appears to increase neuropeptide Y (a potent central appetite stimulant) synthesis, transport, and release

[72]. A meta-analysis [73] which included 30 studies, involving 4,123 patients showed a benefit of MA compared with placebo or other drugs, particularly with regard to appetite improvement and weight gain in cancer patients. MA is normally well tolerated. Side effects include hyperglycemia, fluid retention, hypertension, nausea, vomiting, impotence, reduced libido, and an increased risk of thromboembolism (5%) [62, 74]. The optimal dose of MA is between 400 and 800 mg/day. It is reasonable to use 160 mg/day in initial therapy of cancer anorexia [75]. A recent randomized study which compared MA alone with MA plus olanzapine (5 mg at night) found that the drug combination was significantly better than MA alone [76]. Promising agents in the management of cancer anorexia–cachexia include melatonin, thalidomide, oxandrolone, ghrelin, and antimyostatin therapies [68].

Fatigue

Cancer-related fatigue is a subjective sensation of tiredness which is disproportionate to the degree of activity and relatively unrelieved by rest. There is no consensus as to what cancer-related fatigue is [77]. Fatigue can be used for a sensation, a mental state, or a decrement in physical performance [77]. In general, among clinicians, it is regarded as a "subjective feeling of tiredness, weakness, or lack of energy" which interferes with normal activities [78].

Fatigue is a major symptom in 30% of cancer survivors, in most individuals undergoing chemotherapy or radiation and in more than 90% of advanced cancer patients [79]. Associated factors include pain, insomnia, dyspnea, depression, anxiety, and anorexia [79, 80]. Anemia during therapy worsens fatigue. The mechanism of cancer-related fatigue is poorly understood. Preliminary data suggests that it is at least due to failure to activate muscle (central fatigue) [81]. Assessment can be by way of numerical scale (0 no fatigue, 10 severe fatigue, with >4 being clinically significant). Multiple multidimensional questionnaires are available which also have been validated [82].

Initial management involves treating underlying associated symptoms such as pain, insomnia, and depression, correcting anemia, and screening for hypothyroidism. Psychostimulants such as methylphenidate have a small but significant benefit whereas antidepressants (paroxetine) and progestational steroids are ineffective [83,84]. Erythropoeitin to correct anemia during chemotherapy and exercise (resistance and aerobic) have modest benefits when used during chemotherapy [83, 84].

Summary

Renal carcinoma and its therapy are associated with a variety of symptoms that adversely affect patients' quality of life. Palliative and supportive therapies should be combined with oncologic treatment to optimize and improve patient care.

References

1. Harding G, Cella D, Robinson Jr D, Mahadevia PJ, Clark J, Revicki DA. Symptom burden among patients with renal cell carcinoma (RCC): content for a symptom index. Health Qual Life Outcomes. 2007;5:34.
2. Eton DT, Cella D, Bacik J, Motzer RJ. A brief symptom index for advanced renal cell carcinoma. Health Qual Life Outcomes. 2006;4:68.
3. Cella D, Li JZ, Cappelleri JC, Bushmakin A, Charbonneau C, Kim ST, Chen I, Motzer RJ. Quality of life in patients with metastatic renal cell carcinoma treated with sunitinib or interferon alfa: results from a phase III randomized trial. J Clin Oncol. 2008;26(22):3763–9.
4. Turner JS, Cheung EM, George J, Quinn DI. Pain management, supportive and palliative care in patients with renal cell carcinoma. BJU Int. 2007;99(5 Pt B):1305–12.
5. Cleeland CS, Gonin R, Hatfield AK, Edmonson JH, Blum RH, Stewart JA, Pandya KJ. Pain and its treatment in outpatients with metastatic cancer. N Engl J Med. 1994;330(9):592–6.
6. Breivik H, Cherny N, Collett B, de Conno F, Filbet M, Foubert AJ, Cohen R, Dow L. Cancer-related pain: a pan-European survey of prevalence, treatment, and patient attitudes. Ann Oncol. 2009;20(8): 1420–33.
7. Maessen M, Veldink JH, van den Berg LH, Schouten HJ, van der Wal G, Onwuteaka-Philipsen BD. Requests for euthanasia: origin of suffering in ALS, heart failure, and cancer patients. J Neurol. 2010;257(7):1192–8.
8. Ripamonti C, Bandieri E. Pain therapy. Crit Rev Oncol Hematol. 2009;70(2):145–59.

9. Twycross R, Wilcock A. Hospice and palliative care formulary USA. 2nd ed. UK: Palliativedugs.com Ltd; 2008. pp. 219, 363–72.

10. Quigley C. The role of opioids in cancer pain. BMJ. 2005;331(7520):825–9.

11. Hanks GW, Conno F, Cherny N, Hanna M, Kalso E, McQuay HJ, Mercadante S, Meynadier J, Poulain P, Ripamonti C, Radbruch L, Casas JR, Sawe J, Twycross RG, Ventafridda V. Morphine and alternative opioids in cancer pain: the EAPC recommendations. Expert Working Group of the Research Network of the European Association for Palliative Care. Br J Cancer. 2001;84(5):587–93.

12. Walsh D, Rivera NI, Davis MP, Lagman R, Legrand SB. Strategies for pain management: Cleveland Clinic Foundation guidelines for opioid dosing for cancer pain. Support Cancer Ther. 2004;1(3):157–64.

13. Payne R. Recognition and diagnosis of breakthrough pain. Pain Med. 2007;8 Suppl 1:S3–7.

14. Davis MP. Recent development in therapeutics for breakthrough pain. Expert Rev Neurother. 2010;10(5):757–73.

15. Zeppetella G. Impact and management of breakthrough pain in cancer. Curr Opin Support Palliat Care. 2009;3(1):1–6.

16. Fine PG, Portenoy RK. Ad hoc expert panel on evidence review and guidelines for opioid rotation. establishing "best practices" for opioid rotation: conclusions of an expert panel. J Pain Symptom Manage. 2009;38(3):418–25.

17. Vadalouca A, Moka E, Argyra E, Sikioti P, Siafaka I. Opioid rotation in patients with cancer: a review of the current literature. J Opioid Manag. 2008;4(4):213–50.

18. Vissers KC, Besse K, Hans G, Devulder J, Morlion B. Opioid rotation in the management of chronic pain: where is the evidence? Pain Pract. 2010;10(2):85–93.

19. de Stoutz ND, Bruera E, Suarez-Almazor M. Opioid rotation for toxicity reduction in terminal cancer patients. J Pain Symptom Manage. 1995;10(5): 378–84.

20. Mercadante S, Bruera E. Opioid switching: a systematic and critical review. Cancer Treat Rev. 2006;32(4):304–15.

21. Müller-Busch HC, Lindena G, Tietze K, Woskanjan S. Opioid switch in palliative care, opioid choice by clinical need and opioid availability. Eur J Pain. 2005;9(5):571–9.

22. Knotkova H, Pappagallo M. Adjuvant analgesics. Med Clin North Am. 2007;91(1):113–24.

23. Cherny N, Ripamonti C, Pereira J, Davis C, Fallon M, McQuay H, Mercadante S, Pasternak G, Ventafridda V. Strategies to manage the adverse effects of oral morphine: an evidence-based report. Expert Working Group of the European Association of Palliative Care Network. J Clin Oncol. 2001;19(9):2542–54.

24. Ventafridda V, Tamburini M, Caraceni A, De Conno F, Naldi F. A validation study of the WHO method for cancer pain relief. Cancer. 1987;59(4):850–6.

25. Schug SA, Zech D, Dörr U. Cancer pain management according to WHO analgesic guidelines. J Pain Symptom Manage. 1990;5(1):27–32.

26. Grond S, Zech D, Schug SA, Lynch J, Lehmann KA. Validation of World Health Organization guidelines for cancer pain relief during the last days and hours of life. J Pain Symptom Manage. 1991;6(7):411–22.

27. Watanabe A, Yamakage M. Intrathecal neurolytic block in a patient with refractory cancer pain. J Anesth. 2011;25:603–5.

28. Joshi M, Chambers WA. Pain relief in palliative care: a focus on interventional pain management. Expert Rev Neurother. 2010;10(5):747–56.

29. Chambers WA. Nerve blocks in palliative care. Br J Anaesth. 2008;101(1):95–100.

30. Dy SM. Evidence-based approaches to pain in advanced cancer. Cancer J. 2010;16(5):500–6.

31. Eleraky M, Papanastassiou I, Vrionis FD. Management of metastatic spine disease. Curr Opin Support Palliat Care. 2010;4(3):182–8.

32. Nazario J, Tam AL. Ablation of bone metastases. Surg Oncol Clin N Am. 2011;20(2):355–68. ix.

33. Vassilopoulou-Sellin R, Newman BM, Taylor SH, Guinee VF. Incidence of hypercalcemia in patients with malignancy referred to a comprehensive cancer center. Cancer. 1993;71(4):1309–12.

34. Fahn HJ, Lee YH, Chen MT, Huang JK, Chen KK, Chang LS. The incidence and prognostic significance of humoral hypercalcemia in renal cell carcinoma. J Urol. 1991;145(2):248–50.

35. Stewart AF. Clinical practice. Hypercalcemia associated with cancer. N Engl J Med. 2005;352(4):373–9.

36. Takahashi S, Hakuta M, Aiba K, Ito Y, Horikoshi N, Miura M, Hatake K, Ogata E. Elevation of circulating plasma cytokines in cancer patients with high plasma parathyroid hormone-related protein levels. Endocr Relat Cancer. 2003;10(3):403–7.

37. Palapattu GS, Kristo B, Rajfer J. Paraneoplastic syndromes in urologic malignancy: the many faces of renal cell carcinoma. Rev Urol. 2002;4(4):163–70.

38. Mundy GR, Guise TA. Hypercalcemia of malignancy. Am J Med. 1997;103(2):134–45.

39. Pelosof LC, Gerber DE. Paraneoplastic syndromes: an approach to diagnosis and treatment. Mayo Clin Proc. 2010;85(9):838–54.

40. LeGrand SB, Leskuski D, Zama I. Narrative review: furosemide for hypercalcemia: an unproven yet common practice. Ann Intern Med. 2008;149(4):259–63.

41. Lumachi F, Brunello A, Roma A, Basso U. Cancer-induced hypercalcemia. Anticancer Res. 2009;29(5): 1551–5.

42. Drake MT, Clarke BL, Khosla S. Bisphosphonates: mechanism of action and role in clinical practice. Mayo Clin Proc. 2008;83(9):1032–45.

43. Fleisch H. Bisphosphonates: mechanisms of action. Endocr Rev. 1998;19(1):80–100.

44. Miller PD. Denosumab: anti-RANKL antibody. Curr Osteoporos Rep. 2009;7(1):18–22.

45. Castellano D, Sepulveda JM, García-Escobar I, Rodriguez-Antolín A, Sundlöv A, Cortes-Funes H. The role of RANK-ligand inhibition in cancer: the story of denosumab. Oncologist. 2011;16(2):136–45.

46. Polascik TJ. Bisphosphonates in oncology: evidence for the prevention of skeletal events in patients

with bone metastases. Drug Des Devel Ther. 2009;3: 27–40.

47. Zekri J, Ahmed N, Coleman RE, Hancock BW. The skeletal metastatic complications of renal cell carcinoma. Int J Oncol. 2001;19(2):379–82.

48. Saad F, Lipton A, Cook R, Chen YM, Smith M, Coleman R. Pathologic fractures correlate with reduced survival in patients with malignant bone disease. Cancer. 2007;110(8):1860–7.

49. Saad F, Eastham JA. Zoledronic acid use in patients with bone metastases from renal cell carcinoma or bladder cancer. Semin Oncol. 2010;37 Suppl 1:S38–44.

50. Rosen LS, Gordon D, Tchekmedyian S, Yanagihara R, Hirsh V, Krzakowski M, Pawlicki M, de Souza P, Zheng M, Urbanowitz G, Reitsma D, Seaman JJ. Zoledronic acid versus placebo in the treatment of skeletal metastases in patients with lung cancer and other solid tumors: a phase III, double-blind, randomized trial—the Zoledronic Acid Lung Cancer and Other Solid Tumors Study Group. J Clin Oncol. 2003;21(16):3150–7.

51. Rosen LS, Gordon D, Tchekmedyian NS, Yanagihara R, Hirsh V, Krzakowski M, Pawlicki M, De Souza P, Zheng M, Urbanowitz G, Reitsma D, Seaman J. Long-term efficacy and safety of zoledronic acid in the treatment of skeletal metastases in patients with nonsmall cell lung carcinoma and other solid tumors: a randomized, Phase III, double-blind, placebo-controlled trial. Cancer. 2004;100(12):2613–21.

52. Lipton A, Zheng M, Seaman J. Zoledronic acid delays the onset of skeletal-related events and progression of skeletal disease in patients with advanced renal cell carcinoma. Cancer. 2003;98(5):962–9.

53. Aapro M, Abrahamsson PA, Body JJ, Coleman RE, Colomer R, Costa L, Crinò L, Dirix L, Gnant M, Gralow J, Hadji P, Hortobagyi GN, Jonat W, Lipton A, Monnier A, Paterson AH, Rizzoli R, Saad F, Thürlimann B. Guidance on the use of bisphosphonates in solid tumours: recommendations of an international expert panel. Ann Oncol. 2008;19(3): 420–32.

54. Conte P, Guarneri V. Safety of intravenous and oral bisphosphonates and compliance with dosing regimens. Oncologist. 2004;9 Suppl 4:28–37.

55. Ruggiero SL, Dodson TB, Assael LA, Landesberg R, Marx RE, Mehrotra B. Task force on bisphosphonate-related osteonecrosis of the jaws, American Association of Oral and Maxillofacial Surgeons. American Association of Oral and Maxillofacial Surgeons position paper on bisphosphonate-related osteonecrosis of the jaw – 2009 update. Aust Endod J. 2009;35(3):119–30.

56. Hoff AO, Toth B, Hu M, Hortobagyi GN, Gagel RF. Epidemiology and risk factors for osteonecrosis of the jaw in cancer patients. Ann N Y Acad Sci. 2011;1218(1):47–54.

57. Hoff AO, Toth BB, Altundag K, Johnson MM, Warneke CL, Hu M, Nooka A, Sayegh G, Guarneri V, Desrouleaux K, Cui J, Adamus A, Gagel RF, Hortobagyi GN. Frequency and risk factors associated with osteonecrosis of the jaw in cancer patients treated with intravenous bisphosphonates. J Bone Miner Res. 2008;23(6):826–36.

58. Tanvetyanon T, Stiff PJ. Management of the adverse effects associated with intravenous bisphosphonates. Ann Oncol. 2006;17(6):897–907.

59. Sarhill N, Mahmoud F, Walsh D, Nelson KA, Komurcu S, Davis M, LeGrand S, Abdullah O, Rybicki L. Evaluation of nutritional status in advanced metastatic cancer. Support Care Cancer. 2003;11(10):652–9.

60. Dewys WD, Begg C, Lavin PT, Band PR, Bennett JM, Bertino JR, Cohen MH, Douglass Jr HO, Engstrom PF, Ezdinli EZ, Horton J, Johnson GJ, Moertel CG, Oken MM, Perlia C, Rosenbaum C, Silverstein MN, Skeel RT, Sponzo RW, Tormey DC. Prognostic effect of weight loss prior to chemotherapy in cancer patients. Eastern Cooperative Oncology Group. Am J Med. 1980;69(4):491–7.

61. Loprinzi CL, Laurie JA, Wieand HS, Krook JE, Novotny PJ, Kugler JW, Bartel J, Law M, Bateman M, Klatt NE, et al. Prospective evaluation of prognostic variables from patient-completed questionnaires. North Central Cancer Treatment Group. J Clin Oncol. 1994;12(3):601–7.

62. Strasser F, Bruera ED. Update on anorexia and cachexia. Hematol Oncol Clin North Am. 2002;16(3): 589–617.

63. Nelson KA, Walsh D, Sheehan FA. The cancer anorexia–cachexia syndrome. J Clin Oncol. 1994;12(1): 213–25.

64. Tisdale MJ. Mechanisms of cancer cachexia. Physiol Rev. 2009;89(2):381–410.

65. Tisdale MJ. Cancer cachexia. Curr Opin Gastroenterol. 2010;26(2):146–51.

66. Braun TP, Marks DL. Pathophysiology and treatment of inflammatory anorexia in chronic disease. J Cachex Sarcopenia Muscle. 2010;1(2):135–45.

67. Blum D, Omlin A, Baracos VE, Solheim TS, Tan BH, Stone P, Kaasa S, Fearon K, Strasser F, European Palliative Care Research Collaborative. Cancer cachexia: a systematic literature review of items and domains associated with involuntary weight loss in cancer. Crit Rev Oncol Hematol. 2011;80:114–44.

68. Behl D, Jatoi A. Pharmacological options for advanced cancer patients with loss of appetite and weight. Expert Opin Pharmacother. 2007;8(8):1085–90.

69. Jatoi A. Pharmacologic therapy for the cancer anorexia/weight loss syndrome: a data-driven, practical approach. J Support Oncol. 2006;4(10):499–502.

70. Jatoi Jr. A, Loprinzi CL. Current management of cancer-associated anorexia and weight loss. Oncology (Williston Park). 2001;15(4):497–502.

71. Bruera E, Roca E, Cedaro L, Carraro S, Chacon R. Action of oral methylprednisolone in terminal cancer patients: a prospective randomized double-blind study. Cancer Treat Rep. 1985;69(7–8):751–4.

72. McCarthy HD, Crowder RE, Dryden S, Williams G. Megestrol acetate stimulates food and water intake in the rat: effects on regional hypothalamic neuropeptide Y concentrations. Eur J Pharmacol. 1994;265(1–2): 99–102.

73. Berenstein EG, Ortiz Z. Megestrol acetate for the treatment of anorexia-cachexia syndrome. Cochrane Database Syst Rev. 2005;18(2):CD004310.

74. Jatoi A, Windschitl HE, Loprinzi CL, Sloan JA, Dakhil SR, Mailliard JA, Pundaleeka S, Kardinal CG, Fitch TR, Krook JE, Novotny PJ, Christensen B. Dronabinol versus megestrol acetate versus combination therapy for cancer-associated anorexia: a North Central Cancer Treatment Group study. J Clin Oncol. 2002;20(2):567–73.

75. Loprinzi CL, Michalak JC, Schaid DJ, Mailliard JA, Athmann LM, Goldberg RM, Tschetter LK, Hatfield AK, Morton RF. Phase III evaluation of four doses of megestrol acetate as therapy for patients with cancer anorexia and/or cachexia. J Clin Oncol. 1993;11(4):762–7.

76. Navari RM, Brenner MC. Treatment of cancer-related anorexia with olanzapine and megestrol acetate: a randomized trial. Support Care Cancer. 2010;18(8):951–6.

77. Stone PC, Minton O. Cancer-related fatigue. Eur J Cancer. 2008;44(8):1097–104.

78. Radbruch L, Strasser F, Elsner F, Gonçalves JF, Løge J, Kaasa S, Nauck F, Stone P, Research Steering Committee of the European Association for Palliative Care (EAPC). Fatigue in palliative care patients – an EAPC approach. Palliat Med. 2008;22(1):13–32.

79. Davis MP, Khoshknabi D, Yue GH. Management of fatigue in cancer patients. Curr Pain Headache Rep. 2006;10(4):260–9.

80. Oh HS, Seo WS. Systematic review and meta-analysis of the correlates of cancer-related fatigue. Worldviews Evid Based Nurs. 2011;8(4):191–201.

81. Yavuzsen T, Davis MP, Ranganathan VK, Walsh D, Siemionow V, Kirkova J, Khoshknabi D, Lagman R, LeGrand S, Yue GH. Cancer-related fatigue: central or peripheral? J Pain Symptom Manage. 2009;38(4):587–96.

82. Seyidova-Khoshknabi D, Davis MP, Walsh D. Review article: a systematic review of cancer-related fatigue measurement questionnaires. Am J Hosp Palliat Care. 2011;28(2):119–29.

83. Minton O, Richardson A, Sharpe M, Hotopf M, Stone P. A systematic review and meta-analysis of the pharmacological treatment of cancer-related fatigue. J Natl Cancer Inst. 2008;100(16):1155–66.

84. Minton O, Richardson A, Sharpe M, Hotopf M, Stone P. Drug therapy for the management of cancer-related fatigue. Cochrane Database Syst Rev. 2010;7:CD006704.

Index

Printed by Printforce, the Netherlands